ANNALS OF
THE NEW YORK ACADEMY
OF SCIENCES

Volume 598

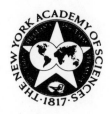

EDITORIAL STAFF

Executive Editor
BILL BOLAND

Managing Editor
JUSTINE CULLINAN

Associate Editor
COOK KIMBALL

The New York Academy of Sciences
2 East 63rd Street
New York, New York 10021

ATHEROSCLEROSIS II: RECENT PROGRESS IN ATHEROSCLEROSIS RESEARCH

The Second Saratoga International Conference on Atherosclerosis in Towada

ANNALS OF THE NEW YORK ACADEMY OF SCIENCES
Volume 598

ATHEROSCLEROSIS II: RECENT PROGRESS IN ATHEROSCLEROSIS RESEARCH
The Second Saratoga International Conference on Atherosclerosis in Towada

Edited by K. T. Lee, Kogo Onodera, and Kenzo Tanaka

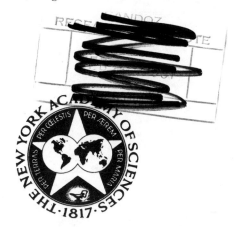

The New York Academy of Sciences
New York, New York
1990

Library of Congress Cataloging-in-Publication Data

Saratoga International Conference on Atherosclerosis (2nd : 1989 :
 Towada-shi, Japan)
    Atherosclerosis II : recent progress in atherosclerosis research:
 the Second Saratoga International Conference on Atherosclerosis in
 Towada / edited by K.T. Lee, Kogo Onodera, and Kenzo Tanaka.
       p.   cm—(Annals of the New York Academy of Sciences, ISSN
 0077-8923 ; v. 598)
    Conference held in Towada, Japan on October 11–13, 1989.
    Includes bibliographical references.
    Includes index.
    ISBN 0-89766-605-4 (cloth : alk. paper).—ISBN 0-89766-606-2
 (paper : alk. paper)
    1. Atherosclerosis—Congresses. I. Lee, K. T. II. Onodera,
 Kogo. III. Tanaka, Kenzō, 1922–   . IV. Title.   V. Title:
 Atherosclerosis two. VI. Title: Atherosclerosis 2. VII. Series.
    [DNLM: 1. Arteriosclerosis—congresses. W1 AN626YL v. 598 / WG
 550 S243a 1989]
 Q11.N5 vol. 598
 [RC692]
 500 s—dc20
 [616.1'36]
 DNLM/DLC
 for Library of Congress   90-6395
                                                                    CIP

B-B
Printed in the United States of America
ISBN 0-89766-605-4 (cloth)
ISBN 0-89766-606-2 (paper)
ISSN 0077-8923

ANNALS OF THE NEW YORK ACADEMY OF SCIENCES

Volume 598
August 31, 1990

ATHEROSCLEROSIS II: RECENT PROGRESS IN ATHEROSCLEROSIS RESEARCH

The Second Saratoga International Conference on Atherosclerosis in Towada[a]

Editors
K. T. Lee, Kogo Onodera, and Kenzo Tanaka

Conference Director
K. T. Lee

Conference Chairperson
Kogo Onodera

Organizing Committee
Kenzo Tanaka, K. T. Lee, Robert W. Wissler, Kogo Onodera, Chikayuki Naito, Fujio Numano, and Takemichi Kanazawa

CONTENTS

[a]The papers in this volume were presented at a conference entitled The Second Saratoga International Conference on Atherosclerosis in Towada, 1989, sponsored by the Second Department of Internal Medicine, Hirosaki University School of Medicine, Hirosaki, Japan, and held in Towada, Japan on October 11–13, 1989.

Part II. Major Responses of the Artery Wall to Atherogenic Stimuli
Chairpersons: Werner H. Hauss and Chikayuki Naito

Part III. Factors Leading to Accelerated and/or Progressive Atherosclerosis
Chairpersons: Russell Ross and Chuichi Kawai

Part IV. Evolving Approaches to Effective Intervention
Chairpersons: Paris Constantinides and Motoomi Nakamura

Part V. Areas for Future Research
Chairpersons: K. T. Lee and Kogo Onodera

Poster Papers

Late Paper

Introductory Remarks

K. T. LEE

Kosin Medical College Graduate School
Pusan 602-702, Korea
and
Department of Pathology
George Washington University
Washington, DC 20037

It may sound a bit strange to hold the Second "Saratoga" International Conference on Atherosclerosis in Japan. However, the name originates from the First International Conference on Atherosclerosis, held in Saratoga Springs, New York in 1984, of which I was chairperson (Ann. N.Y. Acad. Sci. Vol. 454). Many of my Japanese friends and colleagues participated in that conference and were impressed by its success and usefulness. Desiring to hold a similar conference in Japan for their many Japanese colleagues engaged in atherosclerosis research, they asked me if I would organize one. I was delighted to be asked and particularly to have the guidance and help of such distinguished colleagues as Professor Kogo Onodera as Conference Chairperson, and Professors Kenzo Tanaka, Robert W. Wissler, Chikayuki Naito, Fujio Numano, and Takemichi Kanazawa as members of the Organizing Committee.

We believe this type of conference is important for promoting the interchange of ideas and experimental data, particularly between leading scientists in the field of atherosclerosis from East and West. With the devoted efforts of all the members of the Organizing Committee we were able to assemble many internationally recognized scientists from Japan, the United States, the Soviet Union, West Germany, Romania, China, and Australia.

The meeting put into focus new developments and achievements in the field and encouraged the beneficial interaction of various disciplines in their ongoing attempts to achieve the goal of understanding atherosclerosis.

I wish to thank all the people who made this conference possible—our Conference Chairperson, who worked unselfishly for the past two years; the members of the Organizing Committee; and, needless to say, the invited speakers and designated discussants, who traveled so far in order to participate. My special thanks go to Dr. Kanazawa, who spent endless hours arranging and supervising all the details of the conference, to members of the Second Department of Internal Medicine at Hirosaki University School of Medicine, who assisted the conferees and organized the postconference tour, to the staff of the beautiful Blue Lake Hotel in Towada, whose devoted efforts made our stay so pleasant, to Ms. Reiko Komaki of Dodwell Travel Agency, who ably handled our travel needs, and to Ms. Won Kyung Lee of Kosin Medical Center, who managed most of the correspondence between my office and the participants. Finally, I would like to extend my sincere thanks to Mr. Bill Boland, Executive Editor of the New York Academy of Sciences, who graciously agreed to publish these proceedings, as he had those of the First Saratoga Conference several years ago.

Prelesional Modifications of the Vessel Wall in Hyperlipidemic Atherogenesis

Extracellular Accumulation of Modified and Reassembled Lipoproteins[a]

NICOLAE SIMIONESCU,[b] ROSALIA MORA, ELIZA VASILE,
FLOREA LUPU, DOINA A. FILIP, AND MAYA SIMIONESCU

*Institute of Cellular Biology and Pathology
Bucharest-79691, Romania*

INTRODUCTION

It is still uncertain whether atherosclerosis is generated by a single factor or by multiple factors; however, one of these, namely hypercholesterolemia is unanimously acknowledged to play a key role both as a risk and as an etiopathogenic factor. It has been well documented that both in humans and in experimental animals, elevated levels of plasma beta-lipoproteins are sufficient to induce lipid accumulation in the artery wall leading to the formation of fatty streak that can evolve into a fibrous plaque.[1-5]

Very little is known about the cellular and molecular mechanisms which link hypercholesterolemia to the formation of a restricted and preferentially located atherosclerotic lesion. So far, the earliest cellular change detected has been the focal adherence of mononuclear leukocytes, especially monocytes, to arterial[5,6] or valvular endothelium,[7] presumably in response to some chemoattractants and to some still not clearly identified adhesion molecules[5-10] Upon diapedesis and homing under endothelium, monocytes are activated as macrophages that are progressively loaded with cholesteryl ester-rich deposits to become foam cells, the hallmark of the fatty streaks. Surprisingly enough, the artery wall is constitutively poorly equipped with means of protection such as macrophages, polymorphonuclear neutrophilic leukocytes (PNMs), and lymphocytes. The defense against the massive influx of modified highly atherogenic lipoproteins is partially fulfilled by a continuous recruitment of monocytes converted to macrophages and a shift to a phagocytic phenotype of both the proliferated smooth muscle cells and endothelial cells. The hyperplasic reaction of the extracellular matrix components participates in localizing the pathologic process. Despite a successful restriction of the lesion, the progressive obstruction of the vessel lumen, usually supplemented by a thrombus, may vitally impede the tissue blood supply.

Although the pathogenesis of atherosclerosis has not been elucidated yet, in the last decade a continuously growing body of data has provided some promising clues to the

[a]This review article is based on work supported by the Ministry of Education, Romania and by National Institutes of Health Grant HL-26343.

[b]Address for correspondence: Professor Nicolae Simionescu, M.D., Institute of Cellular Biology and Pathology, 8 B.P. Hasdeu Street, Bucharest–79691, Romania.

understanding of some components underlying this complex process. There are several excellent reviews on various aspects of this issue such as an update of the response-to-injury hypothesis,[3] the clinical implications of the low-density lipoprotein (LDL) receptor concept,[11] concepts derived from studies of the metabolism of lipoproteins[12,13] or altered lipoproteins,[14–18] and the link between atherosclerosis and inflammation.[19,20]

In recent years, our laboratory has conducted studies aimed at identifying and characterizing the subtle biochemical and ultrastructural modifications which hypercholesterolemia induces in the lesion-prone regions of the artery wall *before monocyte migration,* during the *prelesional stage.*[21–28] Some of the findings which emerged from this inquiry are briefly reported herewith.

Experimental Design, Animal Models, and Tissue Sampling

The work was carried out on two animal models:

(i) Chinchilla male adult *rabbits* (499 experimental and 214 controls) in which the main cholesterol carrier is beta-VLDL; and (ii) Golden male adult *hamsters* (1,609 experimental and 770 controls) whose cholesterol is carried chiefly by LDL.

The experimental animals were fed a fat-rich diet (0.5–2.0% cholesterol and 5% butter) while controls received a standard chow only. The investigations were performed at 1–2 weeks (*prelesional stage*), up to 16 weeks (early lesional stage), or 1 year (*advanced lesions*) of diet.

In our experimental conditions, we observed that in more than 95% of cases, the lesions start in two locations: (a) the arterial aspect of the aortic valve, and (b) the inner lesser curvature of the aortic arch. These *lesion-prone areas* (previously determined by backwards screening of the lesional stages) were systematically examined, especially in the prelesional stage (at 1 week for the hamster aortic valve, and at 2 weeks for the rabbit aortic arch).

The inquiry, particularly focused on the state of lesion-prone areas in the prelesional stage, was aimed at the identification of the earliest subtle changes that can be detected in the following parameters:
- the charge, biochemistry, and functions of endothelial cells (EC) surface and plasma membrane;
- the transport of plasma lipoproteins and proteins;
- the EC biosynthetic activities; and
- the structure and chemistry of the extracellular matrix with the onset and progression of lipid accumulation.

We tried to understand how these *prelesional modifications* can be linked to the initiation of the atheromatous plaque.

INVESTIGATIONS

Several sets of investigations were performed, which, according to the nature of analysis, were carried out on either *in vivo, in situ,* or *in vitro* experiments (FIG. 1).

(1) *Hyperlipidemia* was assessed by measuring plasma total lipids, cholesterol, lipoproteins, triglycerides, and lipid peroxides as detailed in REFERENCE 24.

(2) *Endothelial Cell Surface Charge and Chemistry* was determined cytochemically by the detection of the following moieties with the appropriate markers:[25]

- cationic sites of high pK_a values, by using hemeundecapeptide or anionic heme-undecapeptide pI 4.8 and 4.3, respectively;
- anionic groups of strongly charged residues of low pK_a values, visualized with cationized ferritin pI 8.4;
- sialyl residues non-O-acetylated at C-8 or C-9 labeled with ferritin hydrazide on specimens previously oxidized by Na periodate;
- N-acetylneuraminic acid and N-acetylglucosamine with wheat germ agglutinin (WGA) followed by a mucin-gold conjugate;
- mannosyl and glucosyl residues visualized with Con A followed by HRP-gold conjugate;

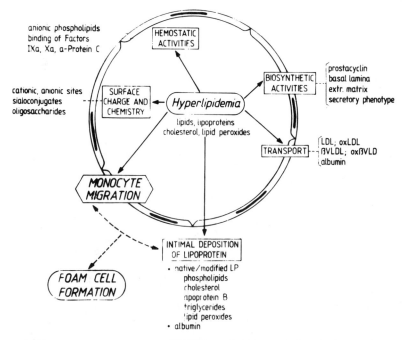

FIGURE 1. Diagrammatic representation of the investigations carried out in the experiments addressed to the early changes induced in the vessel wall during diet-induced hyperlipidemic atherogenesis.

- terminal galactosyl residues detected by peanut agglutinin (PA) in sequence with lactosaminated BSA-gold (Lac-N·BSA-Au);
- terminal galactose and N-acetylgalactosamine marked with the sequence galactose oxidase-ferritin hydrazide;
- subterminal galactosyl reacted with Ricinus communis agglutinin (RCA) followed by Lac-N·BSA-Au.

(3) *Biosynthetic Activities.* The EC production of prostacyclin and thromboxane A_2 (FIG. 2) was determined in collaboration with Dr. S. Tasca. Ultrastructurally we evaluated the extracellular matrix, especially the basal lamina, collagen fibers, and elastin bundles of the intima, as well as the EC switch to a secretory phenotype.

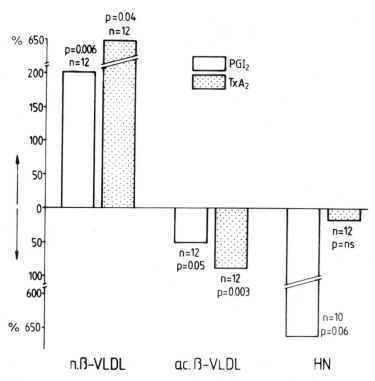

FIGURE 2. Production of prostacyclin and thromboxane A$_2$ by cultured bovine aortic endothelial cells incubated with native beta-VLDL, acetylated beta-VLDL, or 4-hydroxynonenal.

(4) *Transport.* A large number of experiments were devoted to endothelial interaction, endocytosis, and transcytosis of LDL, oxidized LDL, beta-VLDL, oxidized beta-VLDL, and albumin, employing *in vivo, in situ,* or *in vitro* systems.[26-28]

(5) *Transport of Lipoproteins and Albumin.* Two kinds of experiments were conducted (FIG. 3):

(a) *Experiments with exogenous probes* which were either added to the food (*i.e.,* [^{d}H]-cholesterol), or perfused *in vivo* or *in situ,* or put in the incubation medium of cultured endothelial cells (BAEC). As probes, we have chiefly used LDL and beta-VLDL in either native form or chemically modified (methylation, glycation, or oxidation). The probes were coupled with either the fluorescent probe DiI (1.1' = dioctadecyl-3,3,3',3'-tetramethylindocarbocyanine perchlorate) for examination by fluorescent microscopy, or radioiodinated for radioassay and autoradiography, or tagged with 5 nm gold particles for visualization in electron microscopy (EM) and morphometric analysis.[26-28]

(b) *Experiments with endogenous molecules* consisted in the *in situ* detection of apo B (beta-lipoproteins) and albumin by immunocytochemistry, or of the unesterified cholesterol upon specimen incubation with filipin or tomatine (known to bind specifically to 3-beta-hydroxysterols), followed by EM examination. Recently, we have been able to isolate and partially characterize the EL from rabbit aorta (Mora, R., *et al.,* submitted for publication) and hamster aortic valve (Filip, D. A., *et al.,* manuscript in preparation).

(6) *Intimal Deposition of Lipids.* Using various procedures, we have examined the fate

of the transcytosed native versus modified lipoproteins and their intact or modified—and reassembled—constituents.[4,7,21,22,24] We conducted two lines of investigations: (i) *In situ detection* of phospholipids, unesterified cholesterol, apoprotein B, albumin, and lipid peroxides, using fluorescent microscopy, electron microscopy, cytochemistry (filipin and tomatine as probes for unesterified cholesterol), freeze fracture, and immunocytochemistry (for apo B and albumin), and (ii) *Isolation, purification, and characterization* of the material accumulated in the intima, by using a four-step procedure that implied gel filtration, ultracentrifugation, and affinity chromatography. The material was examined by negative staining and assays for lipids, proteins, lipid peroxides, and chemotaxis (FIG. 4).

All these data were correlated with the appearance of monocyte recruitment and migration, and foam cell formation.[4]

RESULTS AND DISCUSSION

Plasma Lipids

Under relatively large individual variations, most animals developed rather rapidly hypercholesterolemia. In rabbits, plasma cholesterol level raised from 40 mg/ml to 250–

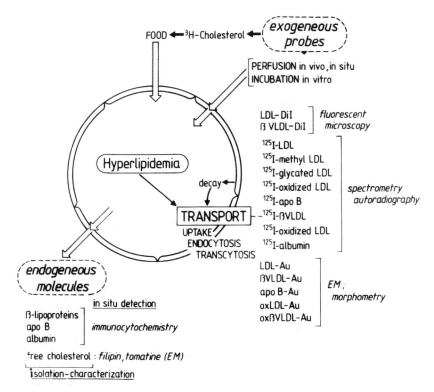

FIGURE 3. Schematic representation of the experimental design and probes used to assess the transport of lipoproteins and albumin by arterial endothelium in normal and hyperlipidemic animals.

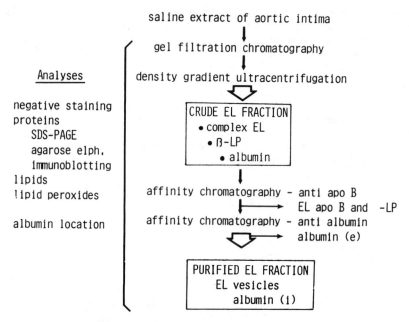

FIGURE 4. Flow diagram of the main steps of the protocol used for the isolation and purification of the extracellular liposome fraction obtained from aortic extracts of hyperlipidemic rabbits.

500 mg/ml (in the second week) to ~2,000 mg/ml (within 8 weeks of diet). In hamsters, serum cholesterol doubled in 3 weeks, increased 4-fold in the 4th week and progressively reached a 15-fold value after 10–12 months on diet.

Endothelial Cell Surface Charge and Chemistry

In the early stages of plaque formation, endothelium was morphologically intact and no platelet involvement could be detected. The findings revealed a remarkable resistance of the endothelial glycocalyx to very high levels of serum cholesterol. In lesion-prone areas and later, during the formation of fatty streaks, for an extended period of time, no significant alterations were visible in the distribution of the cationic, anionic, sialyl, and oligosaccharide moieties. A reduction in anionic sites and sialoconjugates could be detected in more advanced stages especially on EC loaded with lipid inclusions. Changes in EC surface content in sialyl residues were shown to increase the LDL uptake by EC.[29] In general, the circulating monocytes showed modulation in surface charge and chemistry which paralleled those of EC.[24,25] These findings showed that during hypercholesterolemic atherogenesis, the onset and progression of early intimal lesions are not preceeded by significant perturbations in the surface charge and general chemistry of arterial endothelium and monocytes. It is conceivable that more specific molecules are involved in monocyte recruitment and migration. However, under this intact endothelium displaying a grossly unaffected glycocalyx, the lesion-prone area became rapidly the site of the subendothelial accumulation of modified lipoproteins reassembled as vesicle-like structures which were named "extracellular liposomes" (EL).[24]

Biosynthetic Activities

The production of prostacyclin (Pc) and thromboxane A_2 (TxA_2) by cultured bovine endothelial cells (BAEC) was examined upon incubation with either native or acetylated beta-VLDL or with hydroxynonenal (HN) (S. Tasca). As shown in FIGURE 2, the Pc production was augmented by native beta-VLDL but was decreased by acetylated beta-VLDL and HN (presumably due to their lipid peroxides). The concomitant increase in TxA_2 secretion by the native beta-VLDL may be part of the procoagulant activation by hypercholesterolemia (Lupu, F., *et al.*, manuscript in preparation).

In the lesion-prone regions, while still devoid of monocyte-derived macrophages, there is a remarkable overproduction of successive layers of basal lamina material frequently interspersed with or alternating with rows of numerous EL.[4,22–24] Small, frequent bundles of elastin are difficult to define whether they result from hyperplasia or elastolysis of lamina elastica interna.

Endothelial cells overlying zones of EL accumulation frequently display a relatively thick cell body with elaborate smooth and rough endoplasmic reticulum, extensive perinuclear Golgi complex, sometimes intracytoplasmic membrane-bound vacuoles. This shift to a secretory phenotype is reminiscent of an activated EC described in inflammation and immune reactions.[30]

Transport of Lipoproteins and Albumin

(a) *Incorporation of Dietary [³H]-Cholesterol.* Rabbits fed for 10 or 25 days the fat-rich diet received in the last 46 h 1–5 mCi of [³H] = cholesterol added to 100 g food. After 40 h, plasma samples and aortic intima (separately the aortic arch) were collected. In animals on diet for 25 days, serum radioactivity was recovered mainly in the beta-VLDL fraction, and in the vessel wall, 60% of radioactivity was found in the intima at values double those in control animals. After ultracentrifugation, the material extracted from intima was recovered as a band in the range densities of VLDL and LDL.[4,24]

(b) *Experiments with ¹²⁵I] = Beta-VLDL Injected In Vivo.* Cholesterol-fed animals were weekly given i.v. 0.3–0.5 mCi radioiodinated beta-VLDL (obtained from rabbits at the same stage of diet). After 24 h, blood and aorta were collected and radioassayed. By comparison with the lipids accumulated in the vessel wall (TABLE 1) (chemically measured), the protein deposition was much lower, presumably due to the steep augmentation in the cholesterol content of VLDL particles (cholesterol/protein ratio increased from 1.5:1 in the first week to 3.8:1 in the 5th week and to 12.0:1 in the 8th week of diet).

(c) *Experiments with [¹²⁵I]-Beta-VLDL-DiI.* The probe was perfused *in situ* for 1–2 h and aortic segments were examined by radioassay and fluorescent microscopy: both revealed an augmented deposition of beta-VLDL in hypercholesterolemic vs control animals.[4,24]

(d) *Experiments with Beta-VLDL-Au Complex.* The probe was perfused *in situ* as in

TABLE 1. Uptake of ¹²⁵I-Beta-VLDL by the Rabbit Aortic Wall[a]

Experimental Condition	ng Beta-VLDL Protein /mg Wet Tissue
Normal	17.5 ± 2.3
Hyperlipidemia (2 w on H-diet)	25.1 ± 2.0

[a]24 h after tracer injection *in vivo*.

(c) for up to 15 min, and aortic segments examined by EM. Ligand was found predominantly in plasmalemmal vesicles and subendothelial space, but was absent from intercellular junctions. To a lesser extent, the probe decorated structures involved in endocytosis. Morphometric analysis indicated that transcytosis of beta-VLDL via plasmalemmal vesicles was the prevalent process and was markedly pronounced by hypercholesterolemia.[24] The beta-VLDL-Au particles were frequently found associated with EL. It has been shown that beta-VLDL by itself increases the permeability to LDL and albumin of rabbit aortic EC in culture.[31]

(e) *Experiments with Oxidized LDL and Beta-VLDL.* BAEC cultured in Millicell chambers in a bicompartmental system were incubated with native or copper-oxidized human LDL (o-LDL) or rabbit beta-VLDL (o-beta-VLDL). Similar probes were used to determine their *in situ* uptake and transport by aortic endothelium of normal and hypercholesterolemic rabbits. Aortas were examined by radioassay, autoradiography, or saline extracts were ultracentrifuged and assayed for lipid peroxides and lysophosphatidylcholine. It was found that *in vitro* transcytosis of oxidized LP occurred at values double those of native LP. Also, BAEC degraded twice as much o-beta-VLDL as its native counterpart. Similar differences were recorded *in situ.* The aortic intima of hypercholesterolemic animals, unlike controls, contained lipid peroxidation products (Vasile, E., *et al.,* manuscript in preparation).

From these data, it appears that both in normal and hypercholesterolemic conditions the transcytotic pathway for both LDL and beta-VLDL is via plasmalemmal vesicles.[4,24,26–28] Transcytosis is an important mechanism for monitoring the excessive LP accumulation in the plasma. In advanced lesions, opening of endothelial junctions may add a convective pathway while other cellular and extracellular alterations may impede the efflux of the LP-derived material, thus promoting plaque progression and complication.

Intimal Accumulation of Lipoprotein-Derived Components

In the lesion-prone areas of the aortic arch and aortic valve of animals fed for 1–2 weeks the cholesterol-rich diet, no grossly visible modifications of the vessel wall were observed. However, at the ultrastructural level, we noticed a progressive deposition of extracellular lipid material organized as small (100–300 nm) vesicles formed by phospholipid lamellae. These mostly unilamellar features termed ''extracellular liposomes'' (EL)[4,24] were rich in unesterified cholesterol (visualized with filipin),[24] and were surrounded by small deposits of apo B (identified by immunocytochemistry using an anti apo B antibody-HRP conjugate).[21,32] Combining the apo B immunocytochemical detection with reaction with tomatine (known to bind specifically to unesterified cholesterol (UC)) we have demonstrated that apo B and UC are colocalized in tight association with EL.[21,32] The intimal accumulation of EL was concurrent with the proliferation of successive layers of basal lamina-like material, microfibrils, and proteoglycans (visualized with safranin O). EL were detected in cell-free endothelium with no signs of cytolysis. In same areas, a certain number of apo B-reactive particles of the size of LDL or VLDL was also present. Vesicle-like structures in the early atherosclerotic lesions have been also described by other investigators in the WHH rabbits, identified by standard EM[33] or by ultrarapid freezing and freeze-etching,[34] in cholesterol-fed rabbits[33,35,36] as well as in the atherosclerotic lesions of human aortas.[36,38] The EL deposits may represent at ultrastructural level the equivalent of the filipin-positive particles seen in light microscopy by others.[24,37] In areas displaying solely a sero-fibrinous exudate, tomatine was also found to form spicules, suggesting that such extravasated material may contain unesterified cholesterol

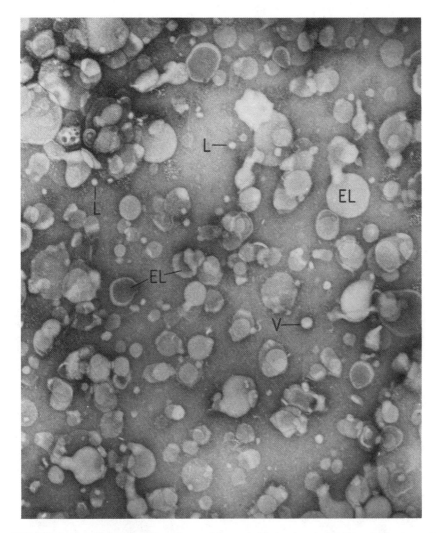

FIGURE 5. Negative staining of an aliquot of the crude EL fraction obtained by gel filtration and ultracentrifugation of an aortic extract from a hyperlipidemic rabbit. The material consists of particulate lipoproteins in the size range of LDL (L) and beta-VLDL (V) and a large population of extracellular liposomes. × 96,000.

carried by either lipoprotein particles or/and albumin. The latter was detected immuno-cytochemically in these locations (Mora, R., manuscript in preparation).

Isolation and partial characterization of lipid or lipo-proteic phases of advanced human or animal atherosclerotic plaques was reported by several laboratories.[39-44] The focus was chiefly on defining the modifications in the chemistry of the aortic beta-lipoproteins extracted from atherosclerotic lesions.

Reports on the extraction of material from aortic intima at the early stages of atherogenesis are extremely scarce.[36]

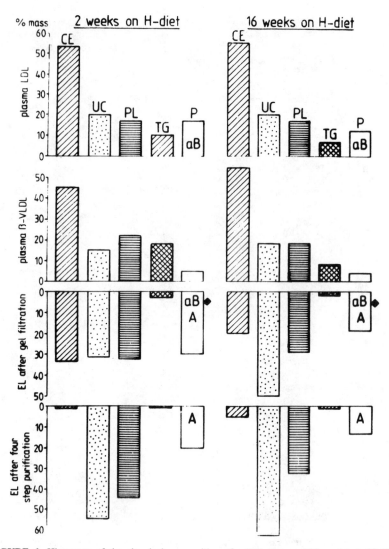

FIGURE 6. Histogram of the chemical composition of rabbit plasma LDL and beta-VLDL as compared with the crude and purified EL fractions. *CE,* cholesteryl esters; *UC,* unesterified cholesterol; *PL,* phospholipids; *TG,* triglycerides; *P,* proteins; *aB,* apoprotein B; *A,* albumin. ◆ = lipid peroxides. Values for lipids are mole % means ± SEM. P: protein % of total weight.

We developed a four-step isolation and purification procedure (FIG. 4) using aortas of Chinchilla rabbits fed a hyperlipidemic diet for 2 (prelesional stage) or 16 weeks (lesional stage) of diet. Isotonic saline extracts of aortic intima subjected to gel filtration chromatography yielded a crude EL fraction (EL$_c$) which, upon concentration of density gradient ultracentrifugation, floated in a broad density range (1.02–1.08 g/ml). EL$_c$ contained as proteins apo B and albumin which were further eliminated by affinity chromatography on anti apo B and anti-albumin-Sepharose columns, to obtain a purified EL fraction (EL_p). The EL fractions were examined by negative staining (FIG. 5), protein analysis (SDS-PAGE, immunoelectroblotting, autoradiography, uronic acid) and lipid analysis of total cholesterol (TC), unesterified cholesterol (UC), cholesteryl esters (CE), phospholipids (PL), triglycerides (TG), and lipid peroxides (LP) as malondialdehyde adducts (MDA).[16] As compared with serum LDL and beta-VLDL, the crude EL fraction was characterized by a higher relative percentage mass of PL, UC, and P (apo B and albumin), which became even more pronounced in lesional stages. The affinity-purified EL fraction was represented almost exclusively by PL, UC, and albumin (FIG. 6). Experiments with pronase digestion or delipidation followed by dot-blot immunolabeling and autoradiography showed that albumin was located in the core of EL. Control experiments with ^{125}I-albumin indicated that EL albumin was indeed trapped *in vivo*. EL crude fraction contained high amounts of lipid peroxides (determined as MDA equivalents), eluting mostly with the immunoadsorbed beta-lipoproteins (FIG. 6). The results showed that the aortic EL represent chemically modified lipoproteins reassembled extracellularly and trapping albumin (a natural antioxidant), probably upon its interaction with lysophosphatidylcholine generated by lipid peroxidation. Our observations revealed that monocyte recruitment and migration occur mostly in intimal regions containing extracellular liposomes (FIG. 7). Ultrastructural images suggest that EL are avidly taken up, presumably by phagocytosis, both by macrophages and smooth muscle cells, thus contributing to their conversion into foam cells.

TENTATIVE INTEGRATION OF FINDINGS—WORKING HYPOTHESIS

In our experimental conditions, despite very high levels of plasma cholesterol, arterial endothelium remains morphologically intact and no platelet involvement could be observed until advanced stages of fatty streak formation.

In the lesion-prone areas examined (aortic arch and aortic valve), during the prelesional stage (1–2 weeks of diet), one could notice *modulations* in endothelial functions

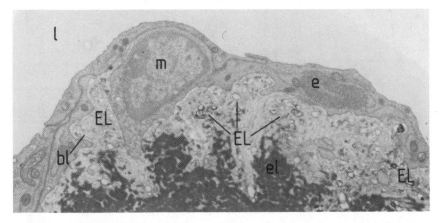

FIGURE 7. Segment of the aortic arch of a rabbit at two weeks of hypercholesterolemic diet. A monocyte (*m*) is migrated in the subendothelium of an intimal region containing extracellular liposomes (*EL*). *bl,* basal lamina; *e,* endothelium; *l,* vascular lumen. × 32,000.

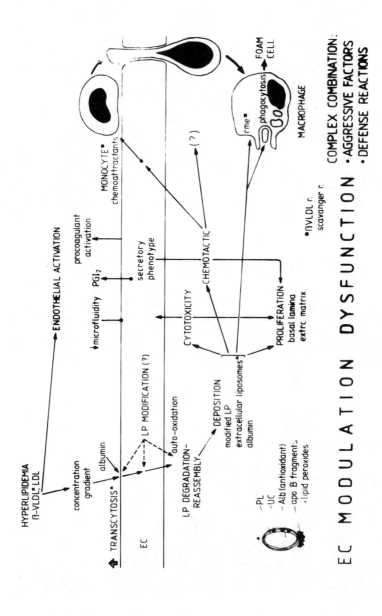

FIGURE 8. Diagrammatic illustration of a postulated sequence of events and mechanisms which may be involved in the prelesional modifications detected in the vessel wall during early stages of the hyperlipidemic atherogenesis (a working hypothesis).

such as an enhanced transcytosis of LDL (hamsters) or beta-VLDL (rabbits), presumably generated by a complex of factors among which the existence of a plasma-interstitial fluid concentration gradient that involves also albumin.

Upon interaction with endothelial cells, the lipoproteins (LP) undergo modifications, and it is unclear whether these occur at the cell surface, within plasmalemmal vesicles, or in the subendothelial extracellular compartment where LP can possibly suffer autoxidation[45] (FIG. 8).

Within the intima, the transcytosed LP occur as either particulate native LDL and beta-VLDL, or as degraded LP which upon interaction with components of the extracellular matrix are reassembled mostly as extracellular liposomes (EL). LP deposits also contain albumin and some other plasma proteins.

EL represent a key element in these prelesional modifications, being presumably formed from oxidatively-modified aggregated LP whose phospholipids are organized as uni- or multilamellar vesicles or drops. These lamellae entrap unesterified cholesterol that may represent a local defense reaction against the sclerogenc effect of cholesterol.[4] At a certain phase of their formation, the core of EL contains albumin, probably sequestrated there as natural antioxidant.[46,47] The EL contour is tightly associated with immunoreactive apo B or apo B fragments which also contain lipid peroxides.

There is a suggestive piece of evidence, although not yet fully proved, that altered LP, including the EL, have cytotoxic effects on EC and induce proliferation of basal lamina and extracellular matrix components especially proteoglycans.

At this early stage, EC seems to be affected from both sides: luminally by hyperlipidemia and abluminally by the subendothelial altered LP.[13-16] As a result, EC undergoes activation and *dysfunction* expressed by:

- a shift to secretory phenotype;
- increased production of basal lamina-like material and extracellular matrix;
- diminuation of plasma membrane microfluidity (Badea, M., manuscript in preparation);
- augmented secretion of prostacyclin and TxA_2;
- expression of chemoattractants (not completely characterized)[8-10,30] for monocytes which adhere, migrate, and within intima become activated as macrophages. So far it is unclear whether the LP or EL chemotactic effects are direct on monocytes or are mediated by EC activation.

The altered LP including EL are avidly taken up by macrophages presumably via the scavenger receptor, beta-VLDL receptor, and by phagocytosis, leading to the formation of foam cells that marks the initiation of the lesional stage.

During these prelesional events, EC goes progressively through *modulation, dysfunction,* and only in the advanced plaque may show *injury*. The prelesional modifications constitute a very dynamic, complex combination—sometimes difficult to discern—between *aggressive factors* and *defense reactions*. Therefore, much caution should be exercised in considering a biochemical or structural change as a *cause* of this disease, since it may just be a *consequence* of a defense mechanism.

REFERENCES

1. WISSLER, R. W. 1978. Progression and regression of atherosclerotic lesions. Adv. Exp. Med. Biol. **104:** 77–109.
2. FAGIOTTO, A. & R. ROSS. 1984. Studies on the hypercholesterolemia in the nonhuman primate. II. Fatty streak conversion to fibrous plaque. Arteriosclerosis **4:** 341–356.
3. ROSS, R. 1986. The pathogenesis of atherosclerosis. N. Engl. J. Med. **314:** 488–500.
4. SIMIONESCU, N. 1988. Prelesional changes of arterial endothelium in hyperlipoproteinemic

atherogenesis. *In* Endothelial Cell Biology in Health and Disease. N. Simionescu & M. Simionescu, Eds. 385–429. Plenum Press. New York, NY.

5. GERRITY, R. G., J. A. GOSS & L. SOBY. 1985. Control of monocyte recruitment by chemotactic factor(s) in lesion-prone areas of swine aorta. Arteriosclerosis **5:** 55–66.

6. JORIS, I., T. ZAND, J. L. NUNNARY, F. J. KROLIKOWSKI & G. MAJNO. 1983. Studies on the pathogenesis of atherosclerosis. I. Adhesion and emigration of mononuclear cells in the aorta of hypercholesterolemic rats. Am. J. Pathol. **113:** 341–358.

7. FILIP, D. A., A. NISTOR, A. BULLA, A. RADU, F. LUPU & M. SIMIONESCU. 1987. Cellular events in the development of valvular atherosclerotic lesions induced by experimental hyercholesterolemia. Atherosclerosis **67:** 199–214.

8. Mazzone, T., M. Jensen & A. CHAIT. 1983. Human arterial wall cells secrete factors that are chemotactic for monocytes. Proc. Natl. Acad. Sci. USA **80:** 5094–5097.

9. Bevilacqua, M. P., J. S. Pober, M. E. Wheeler, R. S. Cotran & M. A. GIMBRONE, JR. 1985. Interleukin I acts on cultured human endothelium to increase the adhesion of polymorphonuclear leukocytes, and related leukocyte cell lines. J. Clin. Invest. **76:** 2003–2011.

10. BERLINER, J. A., M. TERRITO, L. ALMADA, A. CARTER, E. SHAFONSKY & A. M. FOGELMAN. 1986. Monocyte chemotactic factor produced by large vessel endothelial cells *in vitro*. Arteriosclerosis **6:** 254–258.

11. BROWN, M. S. & J. L. GOLDSTEIN. 1983. Lipoprotein metabolism in the macrophage: implications for cholesterol deposition in atherosclerosis. Ann. Rev. Biochem. **52:**223–261.

12. MAHLEY, R. W. 1983. Development of accelerated atherosclerosis: concepts derived from cell biology and animal model studies. Arch. Pathol. Lab. Med. **107:** 393–399.

13. STEINBERG, D. 1988. Metabolism of lipoproteins and their role in the pathogenesis of atherosclerosis. *In* Atherosclerosis Reviews. A. M. Gotto, Jr. & R. Paoletti, Eds. Vol. 18. Hypercholesterolemia: Clinical and Therapeutic Implications. J. Stokes & M. Mancini, Eds. 1–23. Raven Press. New York, NY.

14. FOGELMAN, A. M., I. SCHECHTER, J. SEAGER, M. HOKOM, J. S. CHILD & P. A. EDWARDS. 1980. Malondialdehyde alteration of low density lipoprotein leads to cholesteryl ester accumulation in human monocyte-macrophages. Proc. Natl. Acad. Sci. USA **77:** 2214–2218.

15. STEINBERG, D., S. PARTHASARATHY, T. E. CAREW, J. C. KHOO & J. L. WITZTUM. 1989. Beyond cholesterol. Modifications of low density lipoprotein that increase its atherogenicity. N. Engl. J. Med. **320:** 915–924.

16. HABERLAND, M. E., D. FONG & L. CHENG. 1988. Malonaldehyde-altered protein occurs in atheroma of Watanabe heritable hyperlipidemic rabbits. Science **241:** 215–218.

17. HOFF, H. F. & J. W. GAUBATZ. 1982. Isolation, purification and characterization of a lipoprotein containing apo B from the human aorta. Atherosclerosis **42:** 273–291.

18. SHAIKH, M., S. MARTINI, J. R. QUINEY, P. BASKERVILLE, A. E. LA VILLE, N. L. BROWSE, R. DUFFIELD, P. R. TURNER & B. LEWIS. 1988. Modified plasma-derived lipoproteins in human atherosclerotic plaques. Atherosclerosis **69:** 165–172.

19. JORIS, I. & G. MAJNO. 1977. Atherosclerosis and inflammation. Adv. Exp. Med. Biol. **104:** 227–238.

20. MUNRO, J. M. & R. S. COTRAN. 1988. The pathogenesis of atherosclerosis: atherogenesis and inflammation. Lab. Invest. **58:** 249–261.

21. MORA, R., F. LUPU & M. SIMIONESCU. 1987. Prelesional events in atherogenesis: colocalization of apolipoprotein B, unesterified cholesterol and extracellular phospholipid liposomes in the aorta of hyperlipidemic rabbit. Atherosclerosis **67:** 143–154.

22. FILIP, D. A., A. NISTOR, A. BULLA, A. RADU, F. LUPU & M. SIMIONESCU. 1987. Cellular events in the development of valvular atherosclerotic lesions induced by experimental hypercholesterolemia. Atherosclerosis **67:** 199–214.

23. NISTOR, A., A. BULLA, D. A. FILIP & A. RADU. 1987. The hyperlipidemic hamster as a model of experimental atherosclerosis. Atherosclerosis **68:** 159–173.

24. SIMIONESCU, N., E. VASILE, F. LUPU, G. POPESCU & M. SIMIONESCU. 1986. Prelesional events in atherogenesis: accumulation of extracellular cholesterol-rich liposomes in the arterial intima and cardiac valves of the hyperlipidemic rabbit. Am. J. Pathol. **123:** 109–125.

25. LEABU, M., N. GHINEA, V. MURESAN, J. COLCEAG, M. HASU & N. SIMIONESCU. 1987. Cell surface chemistry of arterial endothelium and blood monocytes in the normolipidemic rabbit. J. Submicrosc. Cytol. **19:** 193–208.

26. VASILE, E., M. SIMIONESCU & N. SIMIONESCU. 1983. Visualization of the binding, endocytosis and transcytosis of low density lipoproteins in the arterial endothelium *in situ*. J. Cell Biol. **96:** 1677–1689.

27. VASILE, E. & N. SIMIONESCU. 1985. Transcytosis of low density lipoprotein through vascular endothelium. *In* Glomerular Dysfunction and Biopathology of the Vascular Wall. E. Seno, A. L. Copley, M. A. Venkatachalam, Y. Yamashida & T. Tsujii, Eds. 87–102. Academic Press. New York, NY.

28. VASILE, E., F. ANTOHE, M. SIMIONESCU & N. SIMIONESCU. 1989. Transport pathways of beta-VLDL by aortic endothelium of normal and hypercholesterolemic rabbits. Atherosclerosis **75:** 195–210.

29. GOROG, G. & G. V. R. BORN. 1982. Increased uptake of circulating low density lipoproteins and fibrinogen by arterial wall after removal of sialic acid from their endothelial surface. Br. J. Exp. Pathol. **63:** 447–451.

30. COTRAN, R. S. 1987. New role for the endothelium in inflammation and immunity. Am. J. Pathol. **129:** 407–413.

31. NAVAB, M., G. P. HOUGH, J. A. BERLINER, J. A. FRANK, A. M. FOGELMAN, M. E. HABERLAND & P. A. EDWARDS. 1986. Rabbit beta-migrating very low density lipoprotein increases endothelial macromolecular transport without altering electrical resistance. J. Clin. Invest. **78:** 389–397.

32. MORA, R., F. LUPU & N. SIMIONESCU. 1989. Cytochemical localization of beta-lipoproteins and their components in successive stages of hyperlipidemic atherogenesis of rabbit aorta. Atherosclerosis **79:** 183–195.

33. ROSENFELD, M. E., T. TSUKADA, A. M. GOWN & R. ROSS. 1987. Fatty streak initiation in Watanabe Heritable Hyperlipemic and comparably hypercholesterolemic fat-fed rabbits. Arteriosclerosis **1:** 9–23.

34. FRANK, J. S. & A. M. FOGELMAN. 1989. Ultrastructure of intima of WHHL and cholesterol-fed rabbit aorta prepared by ultrarapid freezing and freeze etching. J. Lipid Res. **30:** 967–978.

35. SEIFERT, P. S., F. HUGO, G. K. HANSSON & S. BHAKDI. 1989. Prelesional complement activation in experimental atherosclerosis. Terminal C5b-9 complement deposition coincides with cholesterol accumulation in the aortic intima of hypercholesterolemic rabbits. Lab. Invest. **60:** 747–754.

36. CHAO, F. F., L. M. AMENDE, E. J. BLANCHETTE-MACKIE, S. I. SKARLATOS, W. GAMBLE, J. H. RESAN, W. T. MERGUER & H. S. KRUTH. 1988. Unesterified cholesterol-rich lipid particles in atherosclerotic lesions of human and rabbit aortas. Am. J. Pathol. **131:** 73–86.

37. KRUTH, H. S. 1984. Filipin-positive, oil red O negative particles in atherosclerotic lesions induced by cholesterol feeding. Lab. Invest. **50:** 87–98.

38. GUYTON, J. R. & K. F. KLEMP. 1988. Ultrastructural discrimination of lipid droplets and vesicles in atherosclerosis: value of osmium-thiocarbohydrazide-osmium and tannic acid-paraphenylendiamine technique. J. Histochem. Cytochem. **36:** 1319–1328.

39. KATZ, S. S. & D. M. SMALL. 1980. Isolation and partial characterization of the lipid phases of human atherosclerotic plaques. J. Biol. Chem. **255:** 9753–9758.

40. SMITH, E. B. & E. M. STAPLES. 1980. Distribution of plasma proteins across the human aortic wall. Barrier functions of endothelium and internal elastic lamina. Atherosclerosis **37:** 579–592.

41. HOLLANDER, W., J. PADDOCK & M. COLOMBO. 1979. Lipoproteins in human atherosclerotic vessels. Part 1. Biochemical properties of arterial low density lipoproteins, very low density lipoproteins and high density lipoproteins. Exp. Mol. Pathol. **30:** 144–158.

42. HOFF, H. F. & J. W. GAUBATZ. 1982. Isolation, purification and characterization of a lipoprotein containing apo B from the human aorta. Atherosclerosis **42:** 273–282.

43. MORA, R., M. SIMIONESCU & N. SIMIONESCU. 1989. Purification and partial characterization of extracellular liposomes isolated from the hyperlipidemic rabbit aorta. J. Lipid Res. Submitted.

44. ROSENFELD, M. E., A. CHAIT, E. L. BIERMAN, W. KING, P. GOODWIN, C. E. WALDEN & R. ROSS. 1988. Lipid composition of aorta of Watanabe Heritable Hyperlipemic and comparably hypercholesterolemic fat-fed rabbits. Plasma lipid composition determines aortic lipid composition of hypercholesterolemic rabbits. Arteriosclerosis **8:** 338–347.

45. ESTERBAUER, H., G. JURGENS, O. QUCHENBERGER & E. KOLLER. 1987. Autoxidation of

human low density lipoprotein: loss of polyunsaturated fatty acids and vitamin E, and generation of aldehydes. J. Lipid Res. **28:** 495–509.

46. HALLIWELL, B. 1988. Albumin—an important extracellular antioxidant? Biochem. Pharmacol. **37:** 569–571.

47. PIRISINO, R., P. DiSIMPLICIO, G. IGNESTI, G. BIANCHI & P. BARBERA. 1988. Sulfhydryl groups and peroxidase-like activity of albumin as scavenger of organic peroxides. Pharmacol. Res. Commun. **20:** 545–552.

The Involvement of Lipoproteins in Atherogenesis

Evolving Concepts[a]

GODFREY S. GETZ

Department of Pathology
The University of Chicago
5841 South Maryland Avenue
Room BHS-329
Chicago, Illinois 60637

That hypercholesterolemia is a risk factor for atherosclerotic vascular disease, especially coronary heart disease, is beyond dispute.[1] Cholesterol is transported in the plasma in various lipoprotein complexes, and there is overwhelming evidence that the cholesterol that accumulates in the atherosclerotic plaque is derived from the plasma.[2] The cholesterol present in the diseased vessel wall may be esterified or free cholesterol. Cholesteryl ester has received the most attention, because it is the lipid component that exhibits the largest change in concentration during the early phases of atherogenesis. Most cholesteryl ester exists as lipid or nonpolar droplets. Though space-occupying, these droplets are probably not as hazardous to the cell as the free cholesterol which may be derived by the hydrolysis of the esters. Free cholesterol or its derivatives is probably more important as a hazard to the cells, since it is more likely to be incorporated into membranes where it may cause deviations in membrane fluidity and function. Perhaps more important, by being subject to peroxidation it may generate products toxic to cells. Other lipids may also be subject to oxidation, as has been clearly shown recently by Steinberg and colleagues.[3]

Lipoproteins and Atherogenesis

Lipoproteins that promote the deposition of plasma lipids in the artery wall and elicit the formation of a fatty streak and/or an atherosclerotic plaque may be referred to as atherogenic lipoproteins. It is likely that the atherogenicity of a lipoprotein is much more complex than has been hitherto appreciated. Three features about the relationship between lipoproteins and atherogenesis are noteworthy. First, there are new and provocative hypotheses about the early cellular pathogenesis of atherosclerosis.[2–5] Second, we now recognize that the cells and extracellular enivronment of the vessel wall may alter the properties of lipoproteins, making them more atherogenic.[2] Third, there is increasing appreciation of lipoprotein heterogeneity, and this has to be considered in relation to the evolution of the atherosclerotic plaque. Atherosclerotic plaques may be quite pleomorphic and each of the lipoprotein classes or subclasses that promote atherogenesis may result in variations in the life cycle of the resultant plaque(s).

Lipoproteins may contribute to the process of atherogenesis in at least three distinct ways. They are the obvious carriers of lesion lipids, especially cholesterol and perhaps

[a]Work of the author referred to in this paper was performed with the support of United States Public Health Service Grant HL 15062 (SCOR in Atherosclerosis).

17

slowly metabolized phospholipids like sphingomyelin. These lipids may be subject to modification in the vessel wall. Secondly, they may transport dietary fatty acid of various levels of saturation as raw materials for membrane synthesis affecting membrane fluidity and function, as well as providing the precursors for bioactive lipid "second" messengers. Thirdly, they may in other ways function as modulators or mediators of cell biological phenomena associated with atherogenesis.

Thinking about the atherogenicity of a lipoprotein has focused on two basic ideas. Lipid accumulation is a hallmark of atherosclerosis, so one idea about atherogenic lipoproteins relates to the extent to which such lipoproteins may account for the loading of cells in a vascular tissue with lipid, such as in the formation of the fatty streak. A second and equally prominent theme that defines a lipoprotein as atherogenic derives from the correlation of changes in the plasma concentration of a particular lipoprotein(s) with the risk of developing clinical atherosclerotic heart disease, namely, coronary atherosclerosis and ischemic heart disease. This correlation with the end point of atherosclerosis does not necessarily inform us about the role of the lipoprotein in early atherogenesis (FIG. 1). The vascular changes that underlie most ischemic heart disease are the end products of a very complex and multifaceted set of processes, probably beginning decades prior to the manifestation of clinical disease. These processes involve the initiation of atherosclerosis,

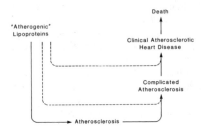

FIGURE 1. "Atherogenic" lipoproteins may act at various levels in the pathogenesis of clinical atherosclerotic heart disease: in primary atherogenesis; in promoting the evolution of an atherosclerotic plaque to a complicated lesion; or in provoking the progression of a complicated lesion beyond the clinical horizon, *e.g.,* via the promotion or stabilization of a thrombus.

probably by a fatty streak, followed by progression to a fibroatheromatous lesion, which in turn may be complicated by other processes such as thrombosis. While it is clear that lipoproteins carry lipid and cholesterol into the vessel wall, it is not established what other steps they influence in the cellular pathogenesis of atherosclerosis. Are they involved in the initiation of the processes only or are they equally involved in each of the stages of this pathogenetic chain? If they are involved at many stages of the genesis of the atherosclerotic plaque, it is likely that many mechanisms are at play. It is possible that the same lipoprotein class or subclass is not the responsible mediator at each step in the pathogenesis. We now recognize that the lipoproteins constitute a system of intimately interacting components and it is likely that no single lipoprotein subclass is uniquely responsible in the whole life history of an atherosclerotic plaque. As hypotheses relating to the cellular and molecular mechanisms of atherogenesis become more sophisticated, the opportunity for a refined analysis of the participation of individual subclasses of lipoproteins in each of these mechanisms becomes feasible and attractive.

LDL is the Prototype of Atherogenic Lipoproteins

LDL is the major lipoprotein in plasma and carries the bulk of the plasma cholesteryl ester, which is a source of lesion cholesterol. It is also readily filterable into the vessel wall. Its distinctive characteristics are its physical properties and the fact that it contains apoprotein B-100 as the only protein component. The evidence implicating LDL as the major atherogenic lipoprotein is based on five criteria. The most compelling evidence is the genetically determined elevation of LDL resulting from a single mutation in the LDL receptor gene.[6] The florid atheroslcerosis and notable premature cardiovascular disease that is the pathological hallmark of homozygous familial hypercholesterolemia points to LDL as the prototype of an atherogenic lipoprotein. A mutation in the pig, affecting the structure of apoprotein B and LDL and hence its clearance from the plasma is also associated with the spontaneous development of atherosclerosis.[7] Aside from this genetic caricature of human (and porcine) atherogenesis, in the larger human population there is a well established correlation between plasma concentrations of low density lipoprotein and the risk of atherosclerotic heart disease.[8] The induction of atherosclerosis in experimental animal models is also invariably associated with elevations of plasma LDL concentrations.[9] Examination of human and animal atherosclerotic plaques reveals the presence of reporters of LDL—apoprotein B, the protein of LDL and the associated cholesteryl ester. In some cases LDL-like lipoproteins have been extracted from the plaque.[10] Finally, LDL may influence the cells of the atherosclerotic plaque—endothelial cells, macrophages, smooth muscle cells, in appropriate ways to facilitate the evolution of the plaque. There will be much more about this issue later in this paper and elsewhere in this symposium.

On the face of it, the aggregate of evidence implicating LDL as the major if not the only atherogenic lipoprotein appears compelling. However, it is clear that much remains to be learned to account for issues surrounding each of the five points outlined above.

Genetic Elevations of LDL Are Frequently Not Isolated Lipoprotein Abnormalities

Even with markedly elevated LDL cholesterol in subjects with homozygous familial hypercholesterolemia there is considerable variation in the clinical manifestations in atherosclerosis, the extent of atherosclerosis itself not having been systematically measured. The artery wall is anything but an innocent bystander in the process of atherogenesis; it contains a variety of cell actors that significantly modify the response to attached or incoming lipoproteins. It is likely that a part of the phenotypic variation in atherosclerosis in homozygous familial hypercholesterolemia is attributable to the many genetic factors that influence the vessel wall response to elevated LDL. It is, nevertheless, possible that differences in the lipoprotein network may account for a portion of this variation. It is, for example, seen that receptor negative and receptor defective subjects have differing degrees of ischemic heart disease, even in the face of rather similar total serum cholesterol levels.[11] Lipoprotein(a) level also discriminates between familial hypercholesterolemic individuals with and without coronary artery disease.[12]

The plasma lipid transfer system represents a dynamic interacting network. Thus, when one discusses LDL as an atherogenic lipoprotein, this is within the context of the whole lipoprotein system. Even in homozygous familial hypercholesterolemia where the genetic defect of the LDL receptor focuses attention on the marked elevation of LDL, this is not an isolated lipoprotein change. There are concomitant but lesser elevations in VLDL and IDL, both in human and in rabbit homozygous familial hypercholesterolemia.[13] Also in genetic porcine atherosclerosis, LDL is elevated almost 10-fold along with a 4-fold increase of LDL cholesterol.[14] These changes in other apoprotein-B-containing lipoproteins cannot be discounted in explaining the atherogenicity of the lipoprotein profile in these genetic models. But it is not only apoprotein-B-containing lipoproteins that influence the clinical outcome in familial homozygous hypercholesterolemia. Plasma HDL levels are reduced by mechanisms yet unknown. Variation in HDL levels, even in the face of major elevations of plasma LDL may be correlated with the significant differences in the expression of ischemic heart disease in genetic hypercholesterolemic subjects.[11] In the Framingham human population aged 50–79, HDL cholesterol level is an inverse predictor of myocardial infarction, even at levels of total cholesterol below 200 mg/dl.[15] The protective or antiatherogenic properties of HDL are now well established, although the mechanisms by which these effects are promoted is not. These mechanisms merit a more extended consideration than can be developed here.

Experimental Atherosclerosis

The relationship of the atherosclerotic lesion induced in experimental animals to that observed in human subjects has been an issue. Atherosclerosis, as it occurs in man, is a tissue response which evolves over decades at modestly elevated serum cholesterol levels, and some have questioned whether the animal counterparts truly model the human disease. It has, however, been possible by manipulation of the dietary context in which experimental atherosclerosis has been induced to generate experimental lesions of varying morphology that resemble the fatty streak as well as the complicated fibroatheroma seen in the advanced disease of man.[16] In view of the protracted time scale over which advanced atherosclerosis develops, it is difficult in the life span of a single experimentalist to map out the natural history of atherosclerosis as it is encountered in man. McGill[17] discussed the relationship of the fatty streak, a subendothelial lesion rich in macrophage foam cells, so readily produced in experimental animals, to the clinically significant advanced atherosclerotic plaque. While we know relatively little about the factors that regulate the transformation of the fatty streak to the more advanced lesion, the evidence now seems compelling that the fatty streak is the precursor of the latter, though not all fatty streaks become advanced lesions. This evidence comes largely from three sources. The very careful temporal studies of experimental atherosclerosis in the pigtail monkeys[18] have focused on the evolution of the atherosclerotic plaque through the early raised macrophage foam cell lesion. Second is the careful study of coronary atherosclerosis in young humans without clinical manifestations of the disease by Stary,[19] who also shows the coincident localization of macrophage-rich fatty lesions with the more advanced fibroatheroma. Furthermore, he describes coronary artery lesions whose morphology is entirely consistent with the evolution of the fatty streak to the advanced lesion. Third, the study of homozygous familial hypercholesterolemia in the Watanabe rabbit permitted the demonstration that macrophage-rich foam cell lesions and advanced atherosclerotic plaques were both outcomes of a defect in LDL metabolism determined at a single gene locus.[20,21]

Are Lipoproteins or Lipoprotein Components in Atherosclerotic Lesions Derived Exclusively from LDL?

The detection of lipoprotein particles or their ghosts in the atherosclerotic plaques is circumstantial evidence for the role of these lipoproteins in initiation and progression of atherogenesis.[10,22] The lipoprotein components that are most readily detected in the artery wall are cholesterol and its ester and apoprotein B, neither of which is specific only to LDL. These two reporters of lipoproteins are major components of a significant spectrum of aproprotein-B-containing lipoproteins and most studies of the artery wall do not distinguish among these lipoproteins. They also have not always distinguished between those lipoproteins that contain apoprotein B-100 or apoprotein B-48. Lipoprotein particles have been isolated from vessel walls that closely resemble in composition that of plasma LDL.

Components most readily demonstrable in the lesion are not necessarily those most active as mediating agents, though this could well be the case in the atherosclerotic plaque. Less abundant mediators cannot be discounted just because they do not happen to be in the lesion when we look or in the way that we look. It is well known that activity may not correlate with mass. This might particularly apply to lipoprotein subfractions or derivative particles. This is a particularly significant caveat for the slowly evolving atherosclerotic lesion in a context of a variety of cells which have the capacity to respond to and modify the microenvironment and its associated lipid particles.

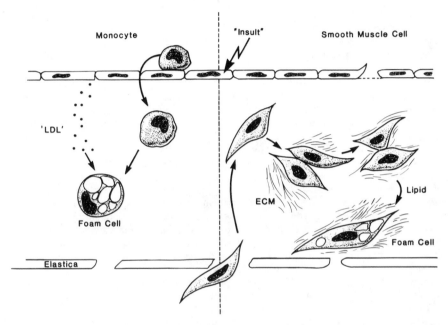

FIGURE 2. Early atherogenesis: monocyte and smooth muscle participation. Monocytes adhere to modified ('insult') endothelium, migrate into the subendothelial space, where they become loaded with lipid derived from modified 'LDL' to form foam cells. Subendothelial monocytes may liberate chemotactic factors and growth factors, which promote further influx of monocytes and also medial smooth muscle cells. The intimal smooth muscle cells are modulated, proliferating and synthesizing and secreting matrix macromolecules. These smooth muscle cells also become loaded with lipid, perhaps from dying monocyte-macrophages in the microenvironment. The liberation of lipases and proteases as well as cytotoxic lipids and activated oxygen species may damage the endothelium further.

The Cellular Pathogenesis of Atherosclerosis

The outlines of the cellular steps of the early phases of atherogenesis are becoming clearer. This is reflected in FIGURE 2, which was kindly provided by Dr. Peter Davies. The steps involve adherence of monocytes to the endothelial cell, a phenomenon that is favored by hyperlipidemia and is manifest shortly after its induction. Some of these monocytes are incorporated into the subendothelial space where they remain, become loaded with lipid from lipoproteins to form foam cells, and are activated to liberate chemotactic factors for monocytes and smooth muscle cells, drawing these latter into the intima. The influx of monocytes may also promote the migration of lipoprotein.[23] Modified endothelial cells, intimal macrophages, and intimal smooth muscle cells may liberate growth factors which promote the proliferation of intimal smooth muscle cells.[24] The migration of monocytes from the plasma through the endothelium may be the result of metabolic damage to the endothelium, which may promote increased permeability to macromolecules, such as lipoproteins. The influxing lipoprotein may be native or modified. There is no known mechanism by which native LDL can directly support foam cell formation. This is in contrast to modified LDL, most of which can promote foam cell formation. During passage into the intima, native lipoproteins may be modified by endothelial cells, macrophages, or smooth muscle cells, all of which are capable of promoting the oxidation of LDL to a form which is recognized by macrophage scavenger and other receptors and able to load these cells with lipid to form foam cells.[25] The role of oxidized LDL will be dealt with later in this volume by Dr. Steinberg. Other modified LDL molecules, e.g., glycosylated LDL in diabetic plasma, aggregated LDL, or proteoglycan LDL complexes, may all form in and around the cells and matrix of the evolving early atherogenic lesion. Also, leukocytes may promote the dimerization of LDL which can then load the macrophage with lipid via the LDL receptor.[26] Foam cells derived from smooth muscle cells tend to form later than those that derive from the intimal macrophages.

The transformation of the initial lesion "pre-atheroma" to a mature atheroma involves the synthetic capacity of the intimal smooth muscle cells whose relocation seems to modulate their behavior and result in the production of all of the components of the matrix of the fibroatheroma, namely, collagen, elastin, proteoglycan, etc. Development of the atheroma is probably the result of the death of foam cells and the liberation of stored sterol as extracellular lipid core, perhaps also trapping further plasma lipoprotein. The precise involvement of lipoproteins in each of the steps just described is not clear and needs to be studied further. Lipoprotein may function as an initiator of some steps and as a modulator of others. One of the most attractive features of the oxidized LDL hypothesis as proposed by Steinberg and collaborators,[25] whether it is correct in all of its details or not, is that it sets forth a framework within which to test pathogenetic hypotheses involving lipoproteins as mediators of chemotaxis, of macrophage retention, of foam cell formation, and of cytotoxicity.

Of the various steps in this pathogenetic chain, LDL has been shown to be a potential modulator or mediator of several. However, except for the case of lipoprotein uptake by the macrophage, the molecular details of each of these effects are essentially unknown. Hyperlipidemia can clearly promote the adhesion of monocytes to the endothelium. This is probably an effect both on the monocyte[27] and the endothelial cell[28] and is observable shortly after the induction of hyperlipidemia. LDL from postprandial human plasma has been shown to promote monocyte adhesion to endothelial cells in culture.[29] Native LDL does not, but modified LDL can promote the formation of foam cells from intimal macrophages using the scavenger receptor of these cells and other less well characterized receptors, including perhaps the F_c receptor, which may mediate the uptake of immune complexes involving modified LDL, which upon conjugation with lipid oxidation products, can serve as a neo-antigen.[25] The endocytic pathways leading to the formation of cytoplasmic droplets of cholesteryl ester, mainly cholesterol oleate, are reasonably well understood. Finally, lipoproteins from hyperlipemic serum can also promote cholesterol esterification in smooth muscle cells in culture.[30,31] Hyperlipidemic LDL is also capable of promoting smooth muscle cell proliferation in tissue culture.[32]

Improved understanding of the cellular and molecular mechanisms of atherogenesis emphasizes the role of the vascular wall and its cells. The vessel wall is not a bystander in the process of atherogenesis. Indeed, the cells and other components of the vessel wall may actually contribute to the atherogenic properties of resident lipoprotein particles by modification of lipoproteins as discussed above. Apoprotein E synthesized in cholesterol-loaded macrophages[44] resident in the lesion may be added to resident lipoproteins, also enhancing their receptor-mediated uptake by local cells, perhaps even via the recently described LDL receptor-like protein.[34]

Heterogeneity of LDL

The development of new techniques for the fine resolution of LDL subclasses has raised the question of whether some subspecies of LDL might be more actively atherogenic than others. The use of sophisticated density gradient ultracentrifugation, as well as nondenaturing gel electrophoresis, has allowed the separation of LDL subspecies by size.[35,36] Four major subspecies of LDL may be considered ranging in size from 220 to 275 angstroms in diameter.[37] The largest LDL species overlaps in size and even density and composition with a fraction of IDL. Two major patterns of LDL which may be genetically determined have been described.[38] Pattern A, present in the majority of the studied population, involves a predominance of buoyant lipoprotein, while pattern B has a predominance of smaller, denser LDL. Individuals with pattern B had increased levels of triglyceride, very low density lipoprotein and intermediate density lipoprotein and decreased levels of HDL_2. Pattern B is encountered in hyperapobetalipoproteinemia and in familial combined hyperlipidemia and is associated with a higher risk of coronary artery disease.[39] At a given cholesterol level, the number of LDL particles in a subject exhibiting pattern B would be higher than would be the case in a subject with larger, more buoyant LDL. On the other hand, more buoyant LDL and larger LDL enriched with cholesteryl ester may be found in hypercholesterolemia of humans and experimental animals. Buoyant LDL accumulates in pigs genetically prone to atherosclerosis.[7] The mutation designated Lpb5/5, affects apoprotein B, and is associated with changes in the clearance and production of the buoyant LDL.[14] The buoyant LDL appears to be cleared from the plasma by receptor-independent mechanisms. It is not clear whether the atherogenicity of these particles is attributable to their special characteristics or simply to the elevation in their particle number. Large and relatively buoyant LDL is also found in the nonhuman primate in diet-induced atherosclerosis.[40,41] In both the African green and Cynomolgus monkeys the extent of coronary artery atherosclerosis is correlated with the size (enlargement) and cholesteryl ester enrichment of these LDL particles.

The complex of apo(a) with LDL to form Lp(a) is a special example of heterogeneity that has received much attention in recent times. Apo(a) is related to plasminogen[42] which contains five disulfide linked "kringles." Apo(a) is made up of multiple repeats of one of these kringles, kringle 4. Apo(a) is highly polymorphic in relation to its structure as well as its plasma concentration.[12] The structural polymorphism is genetic in origin and is expressed in most populations that have been studied, including nonhuman primates like baboons[43] and Rhesus monkeys. Since the structural and mass polymorphism are thought not to be influenced by diet or to be related to lifestyle, it is unlikely that Lp(a) accounts for a significant part of the geographic variation in ischemic heart disease. However, the level of Lp(a) in the plasma is positively related to the incidence of myocardial infarction.[44] Lp(a) represents a major fraction of the apoprotein-B-containing lipoprotein extractable from aortic atherosclerotic lesions of individuals undergoing aorta coronary bypass.[45] Apo(a) also accumulates in atherosclerotic saphenous vein grafts.[46]

While much further work is required on the association of Lp(a) with atherosclerosis, the available evidence would seem to suggest that Lp(a) is not, on its own, capable of initiating atherosclerosis. It is much more likely that it operates in the context of a larger lipoprotein profile and may potentiate or complicate atherogenesis induced by other atherogenic lipoproteins. It has been suggested that thrombosis may collaborate in the process of atherogenesis, especially in the proliferation and modulation of smooth muscle cells that characterizes the formation of the fibrous cap. It may be at this point that Lp(a), a homologue of plasminogen, by attenuating the lysis of fibrin, collaborates in the formation of the complicated atherosclerotic plaque.[47]

The significance of LDL heterogeneity has not been systematically addressed in relation to the cell and molecular events that may accompany atherogenesis. LDL is formed as a late or end product from precursor lipoproteins such as VLDL and IDL. This transformation involves lipolysis of core triglyceride, exchange of core cholesteryl ester and triglyceride and modulation of the surface apoprotein composition and conformation. During this transformation cascade, there are changes in apoproteins B and E which are important in the interaction of lipoproteins with cells and in promoting the storage of cholesteryl ester in foam cells. Both the amount and conformation of apoprotein E may be important. The changes in apoprotein B epitope expression that accompany the dynamic transformations to form LDL could be important to the various steps of the atherogenic process, for example, the promotion of monocyte adhesion to endothelial cells, the oxidizability of LDL, the interaction with proteoglycans and retention within the intimal extracellular space, the interaction with one another to form dimers, the susceptibility to proteases which also promote aggregation, etc. Changes in surface and core components of LDL may also accompany postprandial lipid metabolism. The systematic study of these potential sites of involvement in the process of atherogenesis are worthy of further study with defined subspecies of LDL particles. The size of LDL particles could be important in facilitating influx into the intima. Though there are wide variations in the flux rates of lipoproteins into the artery wall that are probably the result of local arterial permeability differences, as well as rheological factors, there is a tendency for small lipoproteins to have a higher plasma clearance rate into the vessel wall than larger lipoproteins.[48] This could in part account for the atherogenicity of small LDL.

Atherogenic Lipoproteins Other Than LDL

Whatever other characteristics define the atherogenicity of lipoproteins, they all contain apoprotein B. This may relate to the interaction of apoprotein B with matrix components or its propensity to be modified as by oxidation. Lipoproteins that do not gain access to the subendothelial space are by themselves unlikely to be atherogenic. However, one cannot exclude the possibility that they contribute to the process of atherogenesis by interacting at the endothelial surface. It does seem clear that chylomicrons, as encountered in type I hyperlipoproteinemia,[49] and large VLDL, as encountered in hypercholesterolemic, alloxan diabetic rabbits (particles larger than 75 nm in diameter), do not appear to be atherogenic.[50]

VLDL

VLDL is at least an atherogenic lipoprotein precursor. β-VLDL, a VLDL with β rather than pre-β mobility that is enriched in both cholesteryl ester and apoprotein E, appears with atherosclerosis in experimental animals fed cholesterol-rich diets and in type III hyperlipoproteinemia in man.[60] For this and other reasons, this lipoprotein is thought to be atherogenic. It promotes cholesteryl ester storage in macrophages in culture and is a potential source of lipid for foam cell formation entering the macrophage by the LDL receptor using apoprotein E as a high affinity ligand.[51,52] Such VLDL may also promote monocyte adhesion to endothelial cells[27-29,53] as well as transendothelial transport of

LDL.[54] The β-electrophoretic mobility of this lipoprotein is not an essential prerequisite for its cholesteryl ester loading properties.[55] Like LDL, VLDL is structurally and functionally heterogeneous. It varies in size over the range of 300–500 angstroms, as well as in lipid composition and apoprotein composition. VLDL size will influence its potential rate of entry into the blood vessel wall with the largest VLDL being essentially excluded from the subendothelial area.[50] Each VLDL particle contains a single molecule of apoprotein B, but may contain from zero to many molecules of apoprotein E. The enrichment of apoprotein E relative to apoprotein B is an important determinant of lipoprotein uptake by macrophages.[55,56] The apoprotein E content and conformation in hypertriglyceridemic VLDL, especially the large VLDL subspecies, influences the interaction of these lipoproteins with the LDL receptor of cultured fibroblasts.[57]

VLDL that has gained entry into the blood vessel may be locally modified in several other important ways. Subendothelial monocyte/macrophages probably secrete lipoprotein lipase,[58] which could convert triglyceride-containing VLDL to remnants that may be subject to all of the fates of LDL as discussed above. Cholesterol ester loaded macrophages also produce and secrete apoprotein E,[33] which may enrich cholesteryl-ester-rich VLDL-like particles already in the environment, perhaps sufficiently to promote their uptake by the newly described LDL receptor related protein[34] present on many cells and perhaps on smooth muscle cells as well. This may be an alternate pathway for the cholesteryl ester enrichment of intimal smooth muscle cells.

IDL

Although few specific studies have been carried out on the cellular pathogenesis of atherosclerosis with IDL, mainly because of the technical problems of isolating large enough quantities of this lipoprotein, its potential atherogenicity was first noted by Gofman *et al.*[59] It is present in increased concentration in the Watanabe and the fat-fed rabbit, as well as in the mutant pigs who have apoprotein B mutations associated with atherosclerosis.[13,14,20] Increased intermediate density lipoprotein is also found in type III hyperlipoproteinemia[60] and is a component of the related changes associated with the atherogenic pattern B lipoprotein profile.[39] The concentration of intermediate density lipoprotein appears to be predictive of the progression of atherosclerosis in men with established atherosclerotic heart disease.[61]

Chylomicron Remnants

Chylomicrons are not atherogenic. On the other hand, the situation with chylomicron remnants is less clear. Such particles accumulate in the plasma of subjects with type III hyperlipoproteinemia[60] and also in many experimental animals fed high-cholesterol, high-fat diets, notably in the fat-fed rabbit.[62] Furthermore, in the normally feeding human, the arteries are subject to fairly steady though probably not high concentrations of chylomicron remnants through a major portion of the day. Remnants may also be generated in the artery or in its local environment by the lipoprotein lipase produced by endothelial cells[63] or monocyte macrophages.[58] Remnants are capable of promoting cholesterol esterification and cholesteryl-ester storage in macrophages.[64] Most of the lipoprotein profiles hitherto associated with atherosclerosis have been assayed in the postabsorptive state. This takes little account of chylomicron remnants which need to be evaluated in the postprandial state. Satisfactory methods for the physical isolation and measurement of chylomicron remnants distinctly from other lipoproteins are much needed as is the capacity to distinguish apoproteins B-100 and B-48 quantitatively in the atherosclerotic lesion. Such methods would facilitate the evaluation of the role of chylomicron remnants.

CONCLUSIONS

Although there can be no doubt about the central role of lipoproteins in atherogenesis, the precise mechanisms by which they influence this process requires very much further study. Their role in the formation of foam cells and in the carriage of plasma lipid into the vessel wall is well established. Their ability to influence monocyte adhesion to endothelial cells is becoming better supported, although the precise mechanism for this effect is quite uncertain. They are likely to be involved in many other steps in the cellular pathogenesis of atherosclerosis. As this process becomes better understood and more discrete steps in the process become better defined, the opportunity is open for the study of the potential role of individual lipoproteins, lipoprotein products and derivatives, and lipoprotein subclasses in these processes. Meanwhile, with the better delineation of the heterogeneity of lipoproteins and lipoprotein profiles comes the prospect of improved understanding of the relationships between plasma lipoproteins and atherogenesis. The renewed study of postprandial lipoproteins will further help to clarify their potential role in atherogenesis. Finally, the appreciation of the important role of the blood vessel wall itself as an active participant, not only in the cellular pathogenesis of atherosclerosis, but also in modifying the atherogenicity of lipoproteins that enter it, is a very significant advance.

ACKNOWLEDGMENTS

I am deeply grateful to Ms. Karen Sande for her help in the preparation of the manuscript and to my colleagues, particularly Peter Davies, for constructive criticism.

REFERENCES

1. Report of the National Cholesterol Education Program Expert Panel on Detection, Evaluation and Treatment of High Blood Cholesterol in Adults. 1988. Arch. Intern. Med. 148: 36–69.
2. NEWMAN, H. A. I. & D. B. ZILVERSMIT. 1962. J. Biol. Chem. 237: 2078–2084.
3. STEINBERG, D., S. PARTHASARATHY, T. E. CAREW, J. C. KHOO & J. L. WITZTUM. 1989. N. Engl. J. Med. 320: 915–924.
4. ROSS, R. 1986. N. Engl. J. Med. 314: 488–500.
5. BENDITT, E. P. & J. M. BENDITT. 1973. Proc. Natl. Acad. Sci. USA 70: 1753–1756.
6. GOLDSTEIN, J. L. & M. S. BROWN. 1977. Ann. Rev. Biochem. 46: 897–930.
7. RAPACZ, J., J. HASLER-RAPACZ, K. M. TAYLOR, W. J. CHECOVICH & A. D. ATTIE. 1986. Science 234: 1573–1577.
8. Lipid Research Clinics Program: The Lipid Research Clinics Coronary Primary Prevention Trial Results II. 1984. J. Am. Med. Assoc. 251: 365–374.
9. WISSLER, R. W. & D. VESSELINOVITCH. 1968. Ann. N.Y. Acad. Sci. 149: 907–922.
10. SMITH, E. B. & R. S. SLATER. 1973. In Atherogenesis: Initiating Factors (Ciba Foundation Symposium No. 12). 39. Elsevier Publishing Co. Amsterdam.
11. YAMAMOTO, A., T. KAMIYA, T. YAMAMURA, S. YOKOYAMA, Y. HORIGUCHI, T. FUNAHASHI, A. KAWAGUCHI, Y. MIYAKE, S. BEPPU, K. ISHIKAWA, Y. MATSUZAWA & S. TAKAICHI. 1989. Arteriosclerosis 9: 66–74.
12. UTERMANN, G. 1989. Science 246: 904–910.
13. HAVEL, R. J., N. YAMADA & D. M. SHAMES. 1989. Arteriosclerosis 9: 33–38.

14. CHECOVICH, W. J., W. L. FITCH, R. M. KRAUSS, M. P. SMITH, J. RAPACZ, C. L. SMITH & A. D. ATTIE. 1988. Biochemistry **27:** 1934–1941.
15. ABBOTT, R. D., P. W. F. WILSON, W. B. KANNEL & W. P. CASTELLI. 1988. Arteriosclerosis **8:** 207–211.
16. WISSLER, R. W. 1984. *In* Heart Disease: A Textbook of Cardiovascular Medicine, Second Edition. E. Braunwald, Ed. 1183–1204. W. B. Saunders Co. Philadelphia, PA.
17. MCGILL, H. C., JR. 1984. Arteriosclerosis **4:** 443–451.
18. FAGGIOTO, A., R. ROSS & L. HARKER. 1984. Arteriosclerosis **4:**323–340.
19. STARY, H. C. 1989. Arteriosclerosis **9:** 19–32.
20. ROSENFELD, M. E., T. TSUKADA, A. M. GOWN & R. ROSS. 1987. Arteriosclerosis **7:** 9–23.
21. BUJA, L. M., T. KITA, J. L. GOLDSTEIN, Y. WATANABE & M. S. BROWN. 1983. Arteriosclerosis **3:** 87–101.
22. HOFF, H. F. & J. W. GAUBATZ. 1982. Atherosclerosis **42:** 273–297.
23. TERRITO, M., J. A. BERLINER & A. M. FOGELMAN. 1984. J. Clin. Invest. **74:** 2279–2284.
24. ROSS, R. 1986. N. Engl. J. Med. **314:** 488–500.
25. STEINBERG, D., S. PARTHASARATHY, T. E. CAREW, J. C. KHOO & J. L. WITZTUM. 1989. N. Engl. J. Med. **320:** 915–924.
26. POLACEK, D., R. E. BRYNE & A. M. SCANU. 1988. J. Lipid Res. **29:** 797–808.
27. ROGERS, K. M., R. L. HOOVER, J. J. CASTELLOT, J. M. ROBINSON & M. J. KARNOVSKY. 1986. Am. J. Pathol. **125:** 284–291.
28. ALDERSON, L. M., G. ENDEMANN, S. LINDSEY, A. PRONCZUK, R. L. HOOVER & K. C. HAYES. 1986. Am. J. Pathol. **123:** 334–342.
29. ENDEMANN, G., A. PRONCZUK, G. FRIEDMAN, S. LINDSEY, L. ALDERSON & K. C. HAYES. 1987. Am. J. Pathol. **126:** 1–6.
30. ST. CLAIR, R. W., B. P. SMITH & L. L. WOOD. 1977. Circ. Res. **40:** 166–173.
31. BATES, S. R. & R. W. WISSLER. 1976. Biochim. Biophys. Acta **450:** 78–88.
32. MITSUMATA, M., K. FISCHER-DZOGA, G. S. GETZ & R. W. WISSLER. 1988. Exp. Mol. Pathol. **48:** 24–36.
33. MAZZONE, T., H. GUMP, P. DILLER & G. S. GETZ. 1987. J. Biol. Chem. **262:** 11657–11662.
34. KOWAL, R. C., J. HERZ, J. L. GOLDSTEIN, V. ESSER & M. S. BROWN. 1989. Proc. Natl. Acad. Sci. USA **86:**5810–5814.
35. NICHOLS, A. V., R. M. KRAUSS & T. A. MUSLINER. 1986. Meth. Enzymol. **128:** 417–431.
36. CHUNG, B. H., J. P. SEGREST, M. J. RAY, J. D. BRUNZELL, J. E. HOKANSON, R. M. KRAUSS, K. BEAUDRIE & J. T. CONE. 1986. Meth. Enzymol. **128:** 181–209.
37. MUSLINER, T. A. & R. M. KRAUSS. 1988. Clin. Chem. **34:** B78–B83.
38. AUSTIN, M. A., M.-C. KING, K. M. VRANIZAN, B. NEWMAN & R. M. KRAUSS. 1988. Am. J. Hum. Genet. **43:** 838–846.
39. AUSTIN, M. A., J. A. BRESLOW, C. H. HENNEKENS, J. E. BURING, W. C. WILLETT & R. M. KRAUSS. 1988. J. Am. Med. Assoc. **260:** 1917–1921.
40. RUDEL, L. L. & L. L. PITTS II. 1978. J. Lipid Res. **19:** 992–1003.
41. RUDEL, L. L., & B. C. BULLOCK. 1981. Fed. Proc. **40:** 345(A).
42. MCLEAN, J. W., J. E. TOMLINSON, W. J. KUANG, D. L. EATON, E. Y. CHEN, G. M. FLESS, A. M. SCANU & R. M. LAWN. 1987. Nature **330:** 132–137.
43. RAINWATER, D. L., G. S. MANIS & J. L. VANDEBERG. 1989. J. Lipid Res. **30:** 549–558.
44. HOEFLER, G., F. HARNONCOURT, E. PASCHKE, W. MIRTL, K. H. PFEIFFER & G. M. KOSTNER. 1988. Arteriosclerosis **8:** 398–401.
45. RATH, M., A. NIENDORF, T. REBLIN, M. DIETEL, H.-J. KREBBER & U. BEISIEGEL. 1989. Arteriosclerosis **9:** 579–592.
46. CUSHING, G. L., J. W. GAUBATZ, M. L. NAVA, B. J. BURDICK, T. M. A. BOCAN, J. R. GUYTON, D. WEILBAECHER, M. E. DEBAKEY, G. M. LAWRIE & J. D. MORRISETT. 1989. Arteriosclerosis **9:** 593–603.
47. BROWN, M. S. & J. L. GOLDSTEIN. 1987. Nature **330:** 113–114.
48. STENDER, S. & D. B. ZILVERSMIT. 1981. Arteriosclerosis **1:** 38–49.
49. BRUNZELL, J. D. 1989. *In* The Metabolic Basis of Inherited Disease, 6th edit. J. B. Stanbury, J. B. Wyngaarden & D. S. Fredrickson, Eds. Chap. **45:** 1165–1180. McGraw-Hill, Inc. New York, NY.
50. NORDESTGAARD, B. G., S. STENDER & K. KJELDSEN. 1988. Arteriosclerosis **8:** 421–428.

51. INNERARITY, T. L., K. S. ARNOLD, K. H. WEISGRABER & R. W. MAHLEY. 1986. Arteriosclerosis **6:** 114–122.
52. KOO, C., M. E. WERNETTE-HAMMOND & T. L. INNERARITY. 1986. J. Biol. Chem. **261:** 1194–1201.
53. TERRITO, M. C., J. A. BERLINER, L. ALMADA, R. RAMIREZ & A. M. FOGELMAN. 1989. Arteriosclerosis **9:** 824–838.
54. NAVAB, M., G. P. HOUGH, J. A. BERLINER, J. A. FRANK, A. M. FOGELMAN, M. E. HABERLAND & P. A. EDWARDS. 1986. J. Clin. Invest. **78:** 389–397.
55. SOLTYS, P. A., H. GUMP, L. HENNESSY, T. MAZZONE, K. D. CAREY, H. C. McGILL, G. S. GETZ & S. R. BATES. 1988. J. Lipid Res. **29:** 191–201.
56. GETZ, G. S., T. MAZZONE, P. SOLTYS & S. R. BATES. 1988. Arch. Pathol. Lab. Med. **112:** 1048–1055.
57. BRADLEY, W. A., S.-L. C. HWANG, J. B. KARLIN, A. A. Y. LIN, S. C. PRASAD, A. M. GOTTO, JR. & S. H. GIANTURCO. 1984. J. Biol. Chem. **259:** 14728–14735.
58. KHOO, J. C., E. M. MAHONEY & J. L. WITZTUM. 1981. J. Biol. Chem. **256:** 7105–7108.
59. GOFMAN, J. W., F. LINDGREN, H. ELLIOT, W. MANTZ, J. HEWITT, B. STRISOWER, V. HERRING & T. P. LYON. 1950. Science **111:** 166–171.
60. MAHLEY, R. W. 1982. Med. Clin. North Am. **66:** 375–402.
61. KRAUSS, R. M., P. T. WILLIAMS, J. BRENSIKE, K. M. DETRE, F. T. LINDGREN, S. F. KELSEY, K. VRANIZAN & R. I. LEVY. 1987. Lancet **2:** 62–66.
62. ROSS, A. C. & D. B. ZILVERSMIT. 1977. J. Lipid Res. **18:** 169–181.
63. ZILVERSMIT, D. B. 1973. Circ. Res. **33:** 633–638.
64. VAN LENTEN, B. J., A. M. FOGELMAN, R. L. JACKSON, S. SHAPIRO, M. E. HABERLAND & P. A. EDWARDS. 1985. J. Biol. Chem. **260:** 8783–8788.

Studies on Lipid Particles in Atherosclerotic Lesions

HIROSHI SEKIMOTO AND YOSHIKAZU GORIYA[a]

Department of Gerontology
Kanazawa Medical University
Ishikawa, Japan

INTRODUCTION

The role of macrophages in the regression of atherosclerosis has been confirmed by numerous experimental data and clinical observations.[1,2] In pursuit of its mechanism, much attention has been paid to those studies which dealt with the removal of lipids in arterial walls, particularly, intracellular clearing of lipids by foam cells, whereas little attention has been paid to another possible regression system which mobilizes lipids from the intracellular space to the extracellular space, *i.e.,* the blood stream. Therefore, in this present study we tried to demonstrate the presence of such a regression system morphologically in experimental animals and human autopsies in which macrophages derived from circulating monocytes served as a lipid-container by passing through the vascular endothelial junctions, engulfing lipid particles, and then re-entering into the blood stream. Moreover, effects of macrophages on the regression of atherosclerosis was investigated by the biochemical analysis of lipid particles engulfed by macrophages. Finally, phagocytic activity of macrophages was studied to see the effects of aging on the development and the regression of atherosclerosis.

MATERIALS AND METHODS

Morphological Study

The phagocytic action of mononuclear macrophages in atherosclerotic lesions of arterial walls was observed using an electron microscope in experimental animals including rats and rabbits fed a 5% lanolin containing diet for 10 weeks and also in human autopsy specimens.

Analysis of Lipid Particles

Lipid particles taken up by macrophages were obtained from atherosclerotic lesions of human aorta by way of enzymatic separations of cell membranes and protoplasm. Lipid particles thus obtained were then super-centrifuged to be divided into three classes according to their densities, namely, VLDL (<1.006 g/ml), LDL ($1.006-1.063$ g/ml), and

[a]Address for correspondence: Dr. Yoshikazu Goriya, Department of Gerontology, Kanazawa Medical University, 1-1, Daigaku, Uchinada, Kahoku, Ishikawa 920-02, Japan.

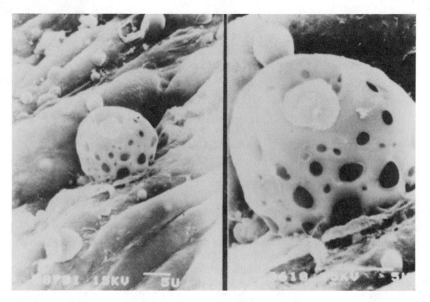

FIGURE 1. Scanning electron micrograph of macrophages with lipid particles re-entering the blood stream from the atheromatous lesions of a human coronary artery.

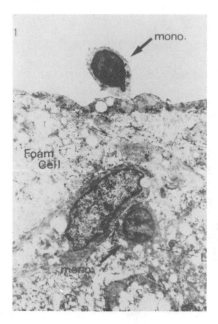

FIGURE 2. Transmission electron micrograph of monocytes entering the endothelial junctions of atheromatous lesions in rats.

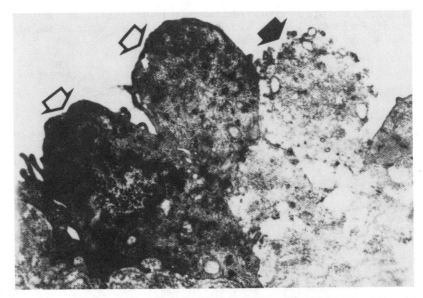

FIGURE 3. Monocytes entering the arterial wall (*white arrows*) and macrophage with lipid particles returning to the blood stream from atherosclerotic lesions of human coronary artery (*black arrow*).

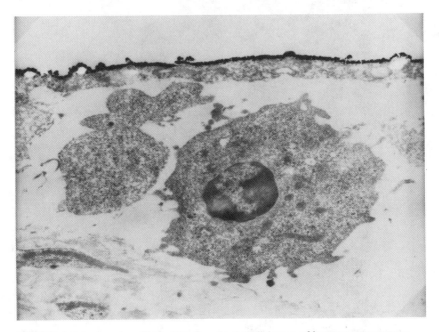

FIGURE 4. Monocyte patrolling within the subendothelial space of human coronary artery.

HDL (1.063–1.210 g/ml). Moreover, the diameters of lipid particles in each class were measured using a scanning electron microscope and the distance from the intimal surface of atherosclerotic lesions were also measured.

Phagocytic Activity of Macrophages

Monocytes were separated from peripheral venous blood taken from healthy young adults (20–40 years) and elderly persons (60–93 years). Phagocytic activity of mononuclear macrophages was assayed by counting the fluorescence per macrophage after the incubation of the monocytes with fluorescent latex beads, as described in the previous report.[3]

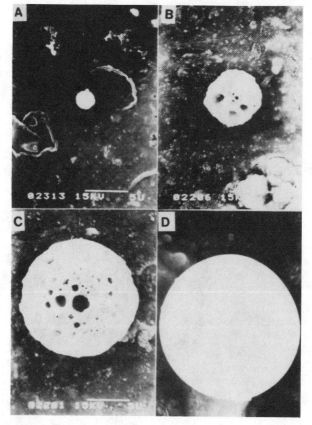

FIGURE 5. Lipid particles of various sizes separated from atherosclerotic lesions of human aorta.

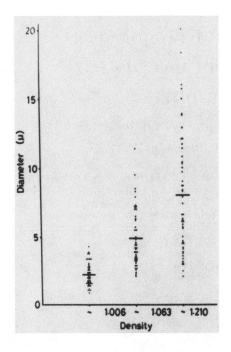

FIGURE 6. The relationship between the density and the diameter of lipid particles of macrophages in atherosclerotic lesions of human aorta.

RESULTS

Morphological Study

As shown in FIGURE 1, re-entering of macrophages, which engulfed lipid particles, into the blood stream from the atheromatous lesions of a human coronary artery could be observed. In cholesterol-loaded rats, the invasion of numerous monocytes into the endothelial junctions occurred from the beginning of a cholesterol loading (FIG. 2). In rabbits, on the contrary, neutrophils acted as professional phagocytes instead of monocytes. Their action on lipids removal, however, did not work well compared to monocytes, thus leading to the process of depository degeneration in atheromatous lesions. As in experimental animals, the similar action of macrophages could be seen in human autopsy specimens. Mononuclear macrophages acting at the endothelial junctions of atherosclerotic lesions in human coronary artery are shown in FIGURE 3. Monocytes patrolling within the subendothelial space of human coronary artery are shown in FIGURE 4. The phagocytic action of this monocyte was not yet sufficient to be called a macrophage.

Analysis of Lipid Particles

Lipid particles with four representative sizes which were obtained from atherosclerotic lesions of human aorta by enzymatic separations are shown in FIGURE 5. Diameters of these particles ranged from 2 to 10 microns. The smallest particle, A, could be found initially with the appearance of macrophages. Various sizes of craters could be found in lipid particles with moderate sizes, B and C, demonstrating the pre-existence of the protein portion. These remnant particles were such lipids as fused themselves together

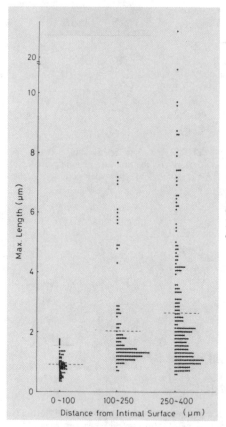

FIGURE 7. The relationship between the distance from the intimal surface of atherosclerotic lesions of human aorta and the maximum length of lipid particles.

later. The largest particle, D, which was obtained from the media of an arterial wall, occupied a greater part within the engulfed cell and was surrounded with thick membranous materials of high density.

The relationship of the density and the diameter of lipid particles of macrophages in atherosclerotic lesions of human aorta is presented in FIGURE 6. A positive correlation between the density and the diameter of lipid particles could be found. Similarly, the relationship of the diameter from the intimal surface of atherosclerotic lesions of human aorta and the maximum length of lipid particles is shown in FIGURE 7. It was found that the longer the distance from the intimal surface was, the larger the size of lipid particles became.

Phagocytic Activity of Macrophages

The relationship of phagocytic activity of macrophages and age is shown in FIGURE 8. The phagocytic activity of macrophages tended to decrease with age, in the 80s becoming half of what it was in the 20s.

DISCUSSION

Although it has been thought that macrophages would remove lipids deposited in atherosclerotic lesions by means of intracellular clearing of lipids, we could demonstrate another lipids clearing system in which macrophages from circulating monocytes penetrated under endothelial space and took up the deposited lipids and then returned to the blood stream, containing lipid-rich particles. Thus, the degree of activity of monocytic macrophages from the subendothelial space of arterial walls to the blood stream seemed to be a key factor in the development of atherosclerosis.[4] However, differences in the species in this "monocyte-macrophage system" were found to exist. Contrary to rats and humans, neutrophils occupied the greatest part of white blood cells in rabbits and acted as professional phagocytes instead of monocytes. The action of lipid removal of these neutrophils, however, did not work so well as monocytes, because they could hardly return to the blood stream, and they lost the mobility as white blood cells due to an over-intaking of lipids.[5,6]

From the study of lipid particles, we observed a difference in lipid constituents which was associated with their sizes. The smaller lipid particles contained more triglyceride and less cholesterol, whereas the larger ones contained more cholesterol and less triglyceride. Moreover, the relationship between the diameter from the intimal surface and the size of lipid particle could also be demonstrated. In other words, lipid particles which are close to the vascular subendothelial space tend to contain much triglyceride, and those which contain much cholesterol tend to increase in number toward the media. This may mean that lipid particles with triglyceride can be easily cleared within the subendothelial space and intimal media, while those with steroid structures which can hardly be cleared tend to remain in the deeper portion of arterial walls, suggesting the subendothelial space to be the main portion of atheroma formation in arteries.

From these observations, it can be concluded that with regard to macrophages and atherosclerosis, the clearing of blood vessels can be maintained by means of the mono-

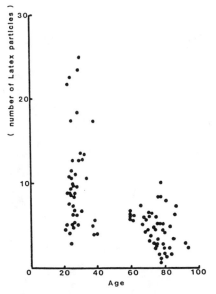

FIGURE 8. The relationship between phagocytic activity of macrophages and age.

cyte-macrophage system and that fibroblast and smooth muscle cells would start their phagocytic actions just when the invasion of lipids into the subendothelial space occurs in amounts which exceed the capacity of this system.

Furthermore, it can be said that for the understanding of vascular changes by aging it is important to consider that the observed deterioration of the monocyte-macrophage system with age would lead to the acceleration of atherosclerosis and to the decline of its regression activity.

REFERENCES

1. POOL, J. C. & H. W. FLOREY. 1958. Changes in the endothelium of the aorta and the behavior of macrophages in experimental atheroma of rabbits. J. Pathol. Bacteriol. **75:** 245–252.
2. GOLDSTEIN, J. L., Y. K. HO, S. K. BASU & M. S. BROWN, 1979. Binding site on macrophages that mediates uptake and degradation of acetylated low density lipoprotein, producing massive cholesterol deposition. Proc. Natl. Acad. Sci. USA **76:** 333–337.
3. SEKIMOTO, H., M. MATSUMOTO, E. MORIMOTO, T. NAKANO, Y. MIYAZAWA & M. OKUIZUMI. 1988. Studies on aging macrophage function of human. J. Jpn. Atheroscler. Soc. **15:** 1625–1630.
4. SEKIMOTO, H., M. NAKANISHI, O. SHIMADA, E. UEMURA & I. Nakada. 1982. Studies on regression of atherosclerosis: role of lipid containers. Jpn. Circ. J. **46:** 27–34.
5. BEESLEY, J. E., J. D. PEARSON, J. S. CARLETON, A. HUTCHINGS & J. L. GORDEN. 1978. Interaction of leukocytes with vascular cells in culture. J. Cell Sci. **33:** 85–101.
6. LUTAS, E. M. & D. ZUCKER-FRANKLIN. 1977. Formation of lipid inclusions in normal human leukocytes. Blood **49:** 309–320.

Atherogenic Lipoproteins Resulting from Genetic Defects of Apolipoproteins B and E

KARL H. WEISGRABER, THOMAS L. INNERARITY,
STANLEY C. RALL, JR., AND ROBERT W. MAHLEY

Gladstone Foundation Laboratories for Cardiovascular Disease
Cardiovascular Research Institute
Departments of Pathology and Medicine
University of California, San Francisco
San Francisco, California 94140-0608

INTRODUCTION

Since a positive association was established between elevated concentrations of plasma cholesterol and an increased risk of atherosclerosis,[1] much attention has been devoted to identifying specific lipoprotein classes that are potentially atherogenic. Studies of human genetic disorders of lipid metabolism and of diet-induced changes in lipoproteins in several animal models have implicated two classes of lipoproteins as playing a major role in the pathogenesis of atherosclerosis. These classes comprise the cholesterol-rich remnants of chylomicrons and very low density lipoproteins (VLDL), collectively referred to as β-VLDL, and low density lipoproteins (LDL) (for review, see REFS. 2–9). One of the key developments that led to our current understanding was an appreciation of the importance of the interaction of lipoprotein receptors with specific apolipoproteins in directing the metabolism of lipoproteins and controlling their plasma concentrations. The best-characterized receptor is the LDL receptor, originally described by Brown and Goldstein.[7] The two ligands for this receptor are apolipoproteins (apo) B[7] and E[3,10] (hence the LDL receptor is also referred to as the apo B,E(LDL) receptor). This review will focus on genetic disorders associated with mutations of apo E and B that result in defective interactions with lipoprotein receptors. These defective interactions lead to the accumulation of the atherogenic lipoproteins β-VLDL and LDL.

ROLE OF APOLIPOPROTEINS E AND B IN LIPOPROTEIN METABOLISM

Normal Metabolism

In the absence of an excessive intake of cholesterol and saturated fats or of mutations in key proteins involved in lipid metabolism, the metabolism and transport of lipid is an efficient process. A central regulatory component of this process is the interaction of apo E and B with lipoprotein receptors. Before discussing the origin and role of specific lipoproteins associated with atherogenesis, it is necessary to consider briefly several normally occurring major plasma lipoproteins and their metabolism.

Chylomicrons are synthesized by the intestine to transport dietary triglycerides and cholesterol. As they circulate in the plasma compartment, the triglycerides are hydrolyzed by the action of lipoprotein lipase, resulting in the production of cholesterol-enriched chylomicron remnants. The chylomicron remnants are rapidly cleared from the plasma by

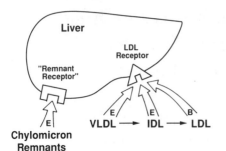

FIGURE 1. General scheme of lipoprotein metabolism showing the central role that hepatic cell-surface receptors play in the uptake and clearance of lipoprotein classes. Apolipoproteins E and B serve as ligands for these receptors.

the liver in a process mediated by apo E[3,10] (see FIG. 1). Although the pathway responsible for the uptake of the chylomicron remnants is incompletely characterized, it probably involves a chylomicron remnant (apo E) receptor.[10] The chylomicron remnant cholesterol is converted to bile acids and excreted or is used in synthesizing membranes and hepatic lipoproteins.

Very low density lipoproteins are triglyceride-rich particles synthesized by the liver. They contain both apo E and B. As the VLDL circulate, their triglycerides are also hydrolyzed by lipases, liberating fatty acids for use as an energy source in various tissues. In this lipolytic cascade, VLDL are converted to VLDL remnants, including intermediate density lipoproteins (IDL). Although apo B is present on these remnant particles, their clearance by hepatic LDL receptors is mediated by apo E. However, not all IDL are removed by the liver; in humans, the major fraction of IDL is converted to LDL by further action of lipases. The removal of triglycerides from the VLDL results in cholesterol-enriched IDL and LDL.

The LDL are the end product of VLDL catabolism and are the major cholesterol-transporting lipoproteins in the plasma. As a result of lipolytic processing, apo B remains as the predominant apolipoprotein component of LDL. The LDL are catabolized by both liver and extrahepatic tissues in a process that involves LDL receptors and is mediated by apo B.

As can be appreciated from FIG. 1, a dysfunction in either the apo E or apo B ligand or in hepatic receptors can result in abnormal lipid metabolism, resulting in the accumulation of specific lipoprotein classes. Thus, defective forms of apo E and B are associated with genetic diseases that lead to the formation and accumulation of lipoproteins that have atherogenic potential.

Apolipoprotein E

As indicated in FIG. 1, apo E is contained in several lipoprotein classes. The mature apo E protein consists of 299 amino acids ($M_r \sim 34,000$) and is polymorphic as a result of multiple alleles at a single gene locus.[5,10] Three common isoforms are present in the population and are designated by their isoelectric focusing position: apo E2, apo E3, and apo E4. This polymorphism results in six common phenotypes: three homozygous (E2/2, E3/3, and E4/4) and three heterozygous (E4/2, E4/3, and E3/2). The E3/3 phenotype is the most common one, occurring in approximately 60% of the population. Structurally, the three isoforms differ by cysteine-arginine interchanges at two positions in the protein, residues 112 and 158: apo E3 contains cysteine at 112 and arginine at 158, apo E2 contains cysteine at both positions, and apo E4 contains arginine at both positions.

Several other rare variants of apo E have been described. TABLE 1 summarizes the forms of apo E whose abilities to bind to the LDL receptor have been determined. As determined in an *in vitro* competitive binding assay in which the purified apo E is combined with phospholipid to produce an artificial particle, only apo E3 and apo E4(Cys$_{112}$ → Arg) bind normally; the other variants possess only 1 to 40% of normal binding activity. The significance of association of these dysfunctional proteins with the accumulation of β-VLDL will be discussed in a later section.

Determining the location and nature of the amino acid substitutions in the defective variants has helped to map the region of apo E that interacts with the LDL receptor. Complementary approaches, including examination of the binding of apo E fragments,[11] monoclonal antibody studies,[12] and site-directed mutagenesis,[13] have indicated that the region of apo E that interacts with the LDL receptor is located in the center of the protein, in the vicinity of residues 140–160.

The predicted secondary structure of this region is shown in FIG. 2. The key features are the presence of an α-helix, encompassing residues 130–150, that is enriched in basic amino acids. This putative helix is followed by a β-turn and then β-structure. It has been postulated that the basic amino acids within the helix bind directly to the acidic regions of ligand-binding domains of the LDL receptor via ionic interactions.[14] The cysteine-for-arginine substitution at residue 158 results in defective binding by perturbing the conformation of the receptor-binding region rather than by disrupting the interaction of apo E with the receptor.[15]

Apolipoprotein B

The mature apo B protein consists of 4536 amino acids ($M_r \sim 500,000$) and represents one of the largest mammalian proteins sequenced to date.[16–19] Two forms of apo B exist in the plasma: a truncated form, apo B48, which represents approximately 48% of the amino terminus of the protein and is a component of chylomicrons and their remnants; and a full-length form, apo B100, which is a component of VLDL, IDL, and LDL. Only the full-length form exhibits receptor-binding activity.

Although much effort has been focused on determining the receptor-binding domain of apo B, its location is not as clearly defined as that of apo E. Thrombin cleaves apo B100 into three fragments (FIG. 3), which serve as useful points of reference when discussing the structure and function of apo B. One of the more informative approaches to defining the receptor-binding domain of apo B has been monoclonal antibody studies. The epitopes of antibodies that completely inhibited LDL binding to the LDL receptor clustered near the thrombin cleavage site at residue 3249 (the T3/T2 junction) (FIG. 3).[18] Antibodies whose epitopes were located in other regions of the protein had little effect on receptor binding. It was also demonstrated that once LDL bound to the LDL receptors, antibodies with epitopes in the region of residues 3000–4000 bound poorly, if at all.[20]

TABLE 1. Summary of the Receptor-Binding Activity of Various Forms of Apolipoprotein E

Normal Binding	Defective Binding
Apo E3	Apo E2(Arg$_{158}$ → Cys)
Apo E4(Cys$_{112}$ → Arg)	Apo E2(Arg$_{145}$ → Cys)
	Apo E2(Lys$_{146}$ → Gln)
	Apo E1(Lys$_{146}$ → Glu)
	Apo E3$_{Leiden}$
	Apo E3(Cys$_{112}$ → Arg, Arg$_{142}$ → Cys)

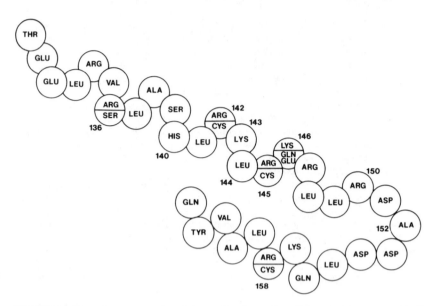

FIGURE 2. Schematic representation of the predicted secondary structure of the receptor binding region of apo E, indicating the location and the identity of the amino acid substitutions that occur in this region of the protein.

Thus, while the antibody studies have localized receptor binding to a region of apo B100, this region includes approximately 1000 amino acids.

ATHEROGENIC LIPOPROTEINS

Three genetic diseases of lipoprotein metabolism (type III hyperlipoproteinemia, familial hypercholesterolemia, and familial defective apo B100) provide key insights into the role of specific lipoproteins in atherogenesis. The importance of understanding these disorders lies in the close parallels between the lipoproteins seen in these genetic disorders and those induced by the consumption of diets high in saturated fat and cholesterol.

Chylomicron Remnants and Very Low Density Lipoprotein Remnants

Type III Hyperlipoproteinemia

Type III hyperlipoproteinemia is associated with hypertriglyceridemia and hypercholesterolemia and is characterized by the accumulation of β-VLDL (the cholesterol-rich

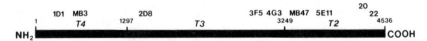

FIGURE 3. Linear representation of apo B100 indicating the two thrombin cleavage sites at residues 1297 and 3249 that generate the T4, T3, and T2 thrombolytic fragments. The location of the epitopes of several monoclonal antibodies raised against LDL or apo B100 are indicated *above the bar*. Antibodies 3F5, 4G3, MB47, and 5E11 completely inhibit the binding of LDL to the LDL receptor, whereas antibodies 1D1, MB3, 2D8, 20, and 22 have little or no effect on binding.

remnants of chylomicrons and VLDL or IDL) in the plasma. Patients with type III hyperlipoproteinemia develop accelerated atherosclerosis involving both coronary and peripheral arteries. In considering the potentially atherogenic lipoproteins seen in this disorder, it is important to note that affected patients usually have low levels of LDL and high density lipoproteins (HDL) and that the hyperlipidemia is associated exclusively with an elevated concentration of β-VLDL. The underlying genetic defect responsible for the lipoprotein abnormalities is the occurrence of abnormal forms of apo E. These variants do not bind normally to the LDL receptor or, presumably, the remnant (apo E) receptor (for a more complete discussion of type III hyperlipoproteinemia, see REFS. 6, 21, and 22). The disorder is most often associated with homozygosity for the apo $E2(Arg_{158} \rightarrow Cys)$ variant.

The defective forms of apo E disrupt the normal metabolism of chylomicron and VLDL remnants (FIG. 1), causing these remnant lipoproteins to accumulate in the plasma. These defective forms of apo E also interfere with the normal formation of LDL from VLDL and IDL in patients with the type III disorder (FIG. 1).[23] This could contribute to the low level of LDL seen in these patients and contribute further to the accumulation of β-VLDL in their plasma. These accumulated cholesterol-rich remnants have to be cleared from the plasma by an alternative pathway. The alternative route may well involve macrophages (scavenger cells), including macrophages of the arterial wall that participate in foam-cell production in atherosclerotic lesions.

Several lines of evidence implicate β-VLDL in atherogenesis and suggest that macrophages are involved in the process (for review, see REFS. 3, 4, 6, 8, and 21). Macrophages are capable of taking up β-VLDL via their LDL receptors. Both chylomicron and VLDL remnants cause massive cholesteryl ester accumulation in cultured macrophages, whereas LDL and other cholesterol-rich lipoproteins (HDL_c) do not.[24] In addition, it has been shown that foam cells in the arterial wall can take up β-VLDL.[25]

In further support of the postulate that β-VLDL may be atherogenic, animals fed diets high in saturated fat and cholesterol have markedly elevated levels of β-VLDL in their plasma and develop accelerated atherosclerosis.[6,21] These diet-induced β-VLDL also cause cholesteryl ester accumulation in macrophages. Furthermore, lipoproteins resembling β-VLDL are seen in human plasma after subjects have consumed a single high-fat, high-cholesterol meal, and it is reasonable to speculate that these transient lipoproteins may contribute to the increased risk of atherogenesis in populations consuming such diets.[6,21]

Unlike type III hyperlipoproteinemia, in which the accumulation of β-VLDL is due to the presence of defective-binding apo E, the β-VLDL accumulation observed after saturated fat and cholesterol feeding appears to be secondary to a reduction (down-regulation) in the number of LDL receptors.[3,7,9] While excessive fat/cholesterol feeding decreases the number of LDL receptors in the liver, it may not decrease the expression of remnant (apo E) receptors.[3,26] Presumably, lipoprotein overproduction induced by the dietary fat and cholesterol, in association with a decrease in LDL receptors, exceeds the ability of the lipoprotein receptors to clear the extra particles from the plasma, and both the chylomicron and VLDL remnants accumulate. Both conditions are associated with accelerated atherosclerosis.

Dominant and Recessive Expression of Type III Hyperlipoproteinemia

The question of dominant versus recessive expression of type III hyperlipoproteinemia has recently come into focus. The recessive mode of transmission is more frequent and can be illustrated with the common $E2(Arg_{158} \rightarrow Cys)$ variant. As noted, type III hyperlipoproteinemia is most often associated with the E2/2 phenotype. But while homozygosity is required for expression, not all E2/2 subjects express the hyperlipidemia. Its expression requires the presence of an additional genetic or environmental factor, such as diabetes, hypothyroidism, or obesity. Thus, the presence of the defective apo E does not by itself result in expression of the hyperlipidemia, *i.e.*, the allele has a low degree of penetrance. In dominant expression, in contrast, heterozygotes express the disorder and all subjects with the defective form of apo E express the hyperlipidemia, *i.e.*, the alleles appear to have a high degree of penetrance. Dominant expression is not associated with the E2(Arg$_{158}$ → Cys) variant; it has only been observed with the 142, 146, and apo E3$_{Leiden}$ variants (TABLE 1).[27–30]

A key feature appears to distinguish the two modes of transmission: in recessive expression, the binding activity of the E2(Arg$_{158}$ → Cys) variant appears to be modulated by its lipid environment or by chemical manipulation. Evidence for modulation by the lipid environment was obtained from a dietary intervention study in a type III hyperlipoproteinemic subject who was homozygous for the E2(Arg$_{158}$ → Cys) variant.[31] Before the diet, the subject's plasma cholesterol and triglyceride levels were elevated (725 and 670 mg/dl, respectively) and the subject weighed 270 lb. After dietary intervention, there was a dramatic reduction in plasma lipid levels (cholesterol, 92 mg/dl; triglyceride, 77 mg/dl) and the subject lost 33 lb. In the d <1.006 g/ml density fraction, which contains the β-VLDL, the cholesterol-to-triglyceride ratio showed a sixfold decrease after weight loss, demonstrating a change in the lipid composition of these particles.

That study demonstrated that the post-diet β-VLDL bound to fibroblast LDL receptors with a 30-fold higher affinity than the pre-diet β-VLDL. The binding of both the pre- and post-diet β-VLDL was mediated by apo E, as determined by inhibition with the monoclonal antibody 1D7. The binding activity of the pre-diet β-VLDL was also increased by cysteamine modification, which had little effect on post-diet β-VLDL. (Cysteamine is a sulfhydryl reagent that converts cysteine to a lysine analogue). The results from that study demonstrate that the binding activity of the apo E2(Arg → Cys) variant can be increased by a change in lipid composition of the β-VLDL or by chemical modification with cysteamine. Thus, under certain conditions this variant binds very well to receptors, perhaps almost to the normal level. This would account for the need for both homozygosity and an additional, exacerbating factor for expression of type III hyperlipoproteinemia in subjects with the E2/2 phenotype.

A similar dietary intervention study is not available for any of the apo E variants associated with dominant expression, but the effect of cysteamine modification has been studied on the E3(Cys$_{112}$ → Arg, Arg$_{142}$ → Cys) variant in parallel with the E2(Arg$_{158}$ → Cys) variant. Relative to apo E3, both variants are defective, but only the E2(Arg$_{158}$ → Cys) variant was activated by cysteamine treatment. Thus, in contrast to the latter variant, the binding activity of the E3(Cys$_{112}$ → Arg, Arg$_{142}$ → Cys) variant is not modulated by chemical modification. This implies that the E3(Cys$_{112}$ → Arg, Arg$_{142}$ → Cys) variant exhibits a binding defect under all conditions, which may account for the expression of type III hyperlipoproteinemia in the heterozygous state, even in the presence of one normal apo E allele.

Examining the location of the substitution sites in the dominantly expressed E3(Cys$_{112}$ → Arg, Arg$_{142}$ → Cys) variant and the recessively expressed E2(Arg$_{158}$ → Cys) variant reveals an interesting feature. As noted, the arginine-to-cysteine substitution at position 158 is located outside the basic helix that is thought to interact directly with the LDL receptor. Binding studies suggest that while the residue at position 158 may not form a direct contact with the receptor, it helps to maintain the conformation of the binding region and thereby allows binding to occur.[15] Either arginine or the lysine analogue generated by cysteamine at this position will stabilize the receptor-binding region. However, the lysine analogue cannot substitute for arginine within the helix (residues 130–150), presumably because its presence would prevent a proper fit between the ligand and receptor and thereby prevent their interaction. Therefore, arginine is specifically required at residue 142 in the helix to ensure this proper fit. Because one other mutation at residue 146 also appears to result in a dominant mode of expression of type III hyperlipo-proteinemia,[30] it appears that being located within the helix may be a critical factor in determining whether a mutation will be dominantly expressed. Other natural mutations also occur within the helix (at residues 136, 145, and 146)[32–34]; however, family studies have not been performed to determine whether they are also expressed in a dominant manner.

Low Density Lipoproteins

Familial Hypercholesterolemia

Much of the evidence implicating LDL in the development of accelerated atheroscle-rosis has resulted from studies of patients with familial hypercholesterolemia. As dem-onstrated by the classic studies of Goldstein and Brown (for review, see REFS. 2, 4, 7, and 9), patients with this disorder lack or have defective LDL receptors that prevent normal LDL uptake and catabolism. Although this disorder involves a receptor dysfunction and not a ligand dysfunction, it is discussed here because familial hypercholesterolemia pro-vided additional clues to the atherogenicity of LDL. Patients homozygous for this disorder often die in the second decade of life from coronary artery disease. It should be kept in mind that these subjects also have abnormally high levels of VLDL remnants and IDL, which could contribute to the atherogenic process through the mechanisms discussed above.

Low density lipoproteins accumulate not only in the plasma of individuals with familial hypercholesterolemia, but also in the plasma of animals fed diets high in saturated fat and cholesterol.[6,21] The increase in plasma LDL in the various animal models is very likely secondary to the down-regulation in expression of the LDL receptors. The decrease in the number of these receptors would be expected to decrease LDL catabolism and to result in an increased plasma concentration of LDL. This may well be the mechanism whereby the consumption of high-fat, high-cholesterol diets raises plasma cholesterol levels in humans and predisposes them to an increased risk of developing coronary artery heart disease.

The precise mechanism whereby LDL may be atherogenic is not known (for review, see REFS. 4, 6, and 8). High levels of LDL may lead to endothelial damage (including the possibility of a subtle derangement in endothelial cell metabolism) and thereby to an influx of LDL into the arterial wall. The LDL do accumulate in the arterial wall in association with atherosclerotic lesions, and these lesions are associated with cholesterol accumulation in smooth muscle cells and macrophages. However, it is difficult to explain how the smooth muscle cells could acquire excess cholesterol since, at least in tissue culture, the LDL receptors are efficiently down-regulated by delivery of cholesterol to these cells and the cells will not accumulate excess cholesterol. Furthermore, *in vitro* studies have shown that macrophages do not accumulate massive amounts of cholesteryl ester after incubation with even high concentrations of normal LDL.

An intriguing hypothesis has been advanced to explain how macrophages may become loaded with cholesterol in response to high levels of LDL. It has been shown that chemically modified LDL can be recognized by unique receptors on macrophages; these receptors are referred to as the acetyl LDL receptors or as the receptors for chemically modified LDL (for review, see REFS. 3, 4, and 6). Low density lipoproteins modified by acetylation, acetoacetylation, malondialdehyde modification, or oxidation can be recog-nized by this receptor and can cause massive cholesteryl ester accumulation within macrophages. Cell-mediated oxidation of LDL can occur by incubating this lipoprotein with endothelial cells, smooth muscle cells, or macrophages.[35-38] Such modifications of LDL could occur in the plasma as the lipoproteins circulate or in the arterial wall as they perfuse through the tissue.

Two recent observations support the hypothesis that chemical modification of LDL might be of physiological relevance. First, studies by Kita et al.[39] and Carew et al.[40] have demonstrated that probucol, a hypolipidemic agent with the property of an antioxidant, retards atherosclerosis in Watanabe heritable hyperlipidemic (WHHL) rabbits. These studies have been interpreted as suggesting that the drug, which is actually incorporated into the LDL, prevents LDL oxidation and thus retards atherosclerosis. A second observation suggests that modified LDL, specifically malondialdehyde-LDL presumably produced by lipid peroxidation, can be identified by antibodies within the lesions of WHHL rabbits.[41] There was an immunochemical co-localization of protein modified by malondialdehyde and the extracellular deposit of apo B100 in the rabbit atheroma. Despite the attractiveness of these postulated mechanisms, more data are required to establish the importance of chemical modification of LDL in the pathogenesis of atherosclerosis. Even the demonstration of modified lipoproteins in the arterial wall does not establish that they cause atherosclerosis.

Familial Defective Apolipoprotein B100

Familial defective apo B100 is a newly described genetic defect that arises from a mutation in the apo B gene and results in an abnormal form of LDL that binds defectively to LDL receptors.[42] The disorder has been observed in 11 unrelated families (with a total of 41 affected subjects) and is inherited as an autosomal codominant trait. All the subjects that have been identified are heterozygous for the defect. Because each LDL particle possesses a single molecule of apo B100, two populations of LDL are present in affected subjects, one with defective binding and one with normal binding.

Because the apo B100 monoclonal antibody MB47 could distinguish the LDL obtained from affected subjects,[43] the region of the protein in the vicinity of the MB47 epitope (residues 3490 to 3510) was regarded as the likely location of the mutation. Sequencing an affected subject's genomic DNA clones that code for the apo B protein sequence between residues 2488 and 3901 uncovered one unique mutation in the codon for residue 3500 in one allele.[44] The CGG codon was changed to CAG, causing a glutamine-for-arginine substitution in the expressed protein. A rapid screening method combining in vitro amplification of genomic DNA by the polymerase chain reaction with detection by allele-specific synthetic oligonucleotide probes has been developed.[44] Screening efforts to date have centered in four cities: San Francisco, Dallas, Montreal, and Salzburg, Austria. These efforts have led to the identification of the aforementioned 11 probands and 41 affected subjects. In all cases there is an absolute correlation between the mutation at residue 3500 and the functional defect in LDL receptor-binding activity. This provides strong evidence that this mutation is responsible for the defect, although definitive proof will require expressing a full-length apo B100 construct differing only in this mutation and testing its binding ability.

Because the populations in the four cities were nonrandomly selected, an exact determination of the overall frequency of the mutation is not possible. However, preliminary estimates place the frequency in the 1/500 range. If this estimate is supported by screening of randomly selected populations, an effort now under way, then this disorder is as prevalent as familial hypercholesterolemia. This would be noteworthy because familial hypercholesterolemia is an unusual clinical abnormality: it is one of the most common disorders to result from the mutation of a single gene.

Clinical features of familial defective apo B100 include a moderately elevated hyper-cholesterolemia (250 to 350 mg/dl) associated with elevated LDL cholesterol concentrations (~80 mg/dl higher than in age- and sex-matched controls). This disorder differs from familial hypercholesterolemia in an important aspect. Because only the binding activity of apo B is affected in familial defective apo B100, the LDL are the only lipoprotein fraction to be elevated. In familial hypercholesterolemia, where the receptor is defective, VLDL remnants and IDL also accumulate as a result of impaired uptake. This, in turn, results in more of these particles being converted to LDL. This difference in metabolism between the two disorders probably accounts for the more moderately elevated levels of LDL cholesterol (196 mg/dl) in familial defective apo B100 heterozy-gotes than in familial hypercholesterolemic heterozygotes (241 mg/dl). Thus, familial defective apo B100 offers the unique opportunity to examine the atherogenic potential of LDL directly, without the added complication of a parallel accumulation of VLDL remnants that occurs with familial hypercholesterolemia. With the moderate-size population that has been identified, further studies can be directed at assessing the risk of athero-sclerosis associated with this disorder.

SUMMARY

Accelerated atherosclerosis occurs in patients with type III hyperlipoproteinemia and familial hypercholesterolemia. These genetic disorders focus attention on specific types of lipoproteins as being responsible for the development of accelerated coronary artery heart disease. The accumulation of chylomicron remnants of intestinal origin and of VLDL remnants or IDL of hepatic origin observed in type III hyperlipoproteinemia appears to correlate with coronary disease. The presence of defective forms of apo E prevents normal receptor-mediated catabolism of these lipoproteins. Patients with familial hypercholester-olemia have an elevation of plasma LDL (and to a lesser extent an increase in VLDL remnants and IDL) secondary to defective LDL receptors that impair normal catabolism. Familial defective apo B100 is secondary to an abnormality of apo B100 that prevents the normal interaction of LDL with the LDL receptor and increases plasma LDL. However, it has not yet been established that familial defective apo B100 predisposes affected individuals to accelerated atherosclerosis. Animals fed diets high in saturated fat and cholesterol have an accumulation of β-VLDL, IDL, and LDL that resembles the changes in lipoproteins observed in patients with these genetic disorders.

Macrophages (which are presumably derived from circulating monocytes) have emerged as a likely key component in atherogenesis because they appear to be progenitors of foam cells in arterial lesions. Macrophages in the arterial wall express receptors that recognize chylomicron remnants and VLDL remnants (β-VLDL) and chemically modi-fied LDL. Thus, in the presence of these specific lipoproteins, macrophages are converted to cells that resemble foam cells. The precise stimulus that causes monocyte-derived macrophages to enter specific regions of the arterial wall remains to be determined.

ACKNOWLEDGMENTS

The authors thank Al Averbach and Sally Gullatt Seehafer for editorial assistance, Tom Rolain and Charles Benedict for graphics, and Kerry Humphrey for manuscript preparation.

REFERENCES

1. CONSENSUS CONFERENCE. 1985. Lowering blood cholesterol to prevent heart disease. J. Am. Med. Assoc. **253:** 2080–2086.

2. HAVEL, R. J., J. L. GOLDSTEIN & M. S. BROWN. 1980. Lipoproteins and lipid transport. *In* Metabolic Control of Disease. P. K. Bondy & L. E. Rosenberg, Eds.: 393–494. W. B. Saunders Company. Philadelphia, PA.
3. MAHLEY, R. W. & T. L. INNERARITY. 1983. Lipoprotein receptors and cholesterol homeostasis. Biochim. Biophys. Acta. **737:** 197–222.
4. BROWN, M. S. & J. L. GOLDSTEIN. 1983. Lipoprotein metabolism in the macrophage: implications for cholesterol deposition in atherosclerosis. Annu. Rev. Biochem. **52:** 223–261.
5. MAHLEY, R. W., T. L. INNERARITY, S. C. RALL, JR. & K. H. WEISGRABER. 1984. Plasma lipoproteins: apolipoprotein structure and function. J. Lipid Res. **25:** 1277–1294.
6. MAHLEY, R. W. 1985. Atherogenic lipoproteins and coronary artery disease: concepts derived from recent advances in cellular and molecular biology. Circulation **72:** 943–948.
7. BROWN, M. S. & J. L. GOLDSTEIN. 1986. A receptor-mediated pathway for cholesterol homeostasis. Science **232:** 34–47.
8. STEINBERG, D. 1983. Lipoproteins and atherosclerosis. A look back and a look ahead. Arteriosclerosis **3:** 283–301.
9. BROWN, M. S. & J. L. GOLDSTEIN. 1984. How LDL receptors influence cholesterol and atherosclerosis. Sci. Am. **251:** 58–66.
10. MAHLEY, R. W. 1988. Apolipoprotein E: cholesterol transport protein with expanding role in cell biology. Science **240:** 622–630.
11. INNERARITY, T. L., E. J. FRIEDLANDER, S. C. RALL, JR., K. H. WEISGRABER & R. W. MAHLEY. 1983. The receptor-binding domain of human apolipoprotein E. Binding of apolipoprotein E fragments. J. Biol. Chem. **258:** 12341–12347.
12. WEISGRABER, K. H., T. L. INNERARITY, K. J. HARDER, R. W. MAHLEY, R. W. MILNE, Y. L. MARCEL & J. T. SPARROW. 1983. The receptor-binding domain of human apolipoprotein E. Monoclonal antibody inhibition of binding. J. Biol. Chem. **258:** 12348–12354.
13. LALAZAR, A., K. H. WEISGRABER, S. C. RALL, JR., H. GILADI, T. L. INNERARITY, A. Z. LEVANON, J. K. BOYLES, B. AMIT, M. GORECKI, R. W. MAHLEY & T. VOGEL. 1988. Site-specific mutagenesis of human apolipoprotein E. Receptor binding activity of variants with single amino acid substitutions. J. Biol. Chem. **263:** 3542–3545.
14. MAHLEY, R. W., T. L. INNERARITY, K. H. WEISGRABER, S. C. RALL, JR., D. Y. HUI, A. LALAZAR, J. K. BOYLES, J. M. TAYLOR & B. LEVY-WILSON. 1986. Cellular and molecular biology of lipoprotein metabolism: characterization of lipoprotein receptor-ligand interactions. Cold Spring Harbor Symp. Quant. Biol. **51:** 821–828.
15. INNERARITY, T. L., K. H. WEISGRABER, K. S. ARNOLD, S. C. RALL, JR. & R. W. MAHLEY. 1984. Normalization of receptor binding of apolipoprotein E2. Evidence for modulation of the binding site conformation. J. Biol. Chem. **259:** 7261–7267.
16. CHEN, S.-H., C.-Y. YANG, P.-F. CHEN, D. SETZER, M. TANIMURA, W.-H. LI, A. M. GOTTO, JR. & L. CHAN. 1986. The complete cDNA and amino acid sequence of human apolipoprotein B-100. J. Biol. Chem. **261:** 12918–12921.
17. CLADARAS, C., M. HADZOPOULOU-CLADARAS, R. T. NOLTE, D. ATKINSON & V. I. ZANNIS. 1986. The complete sequence and structural analysis of human apolipoprotein B-100: relationship between apoB-100 and apoB-48 forms. EMBO J. **5:** 3495–3507.
18. KNOTT, T. J., R. J. PEASE, L. M. POWELL, S. C. WALLIS, S. C. RALL, JR., T. L. INNERARITY, B. BLACKHART, W. H. TAYLOR, Y. MARCEL, R. MILNE, D. JOHNSON, M. FULLER, A. J. LUSIS, B. J. MCCARTHY, R. W. MAHLEY, B. LEVY-WILSON & J. SCOTT. 1986. Complete protein sequence and identification of structural domains of human apolipoprotein B. Nature **323:** 734–738.
19. LAW, S. W., S. M. GRANT, K. HIGUCHI, A. HOSPATTANKAR, K. LACKNER, N. LEE & H. B. BREWER, JR. 1986. Human liver apolipoprotein B-100 cDNA: complete nucleic acid and derived amino acid sequence. Proc. Natl. Acad. Sci. USA **83:** 8142–8146.
20. MILNE, R., R. THEOLIS, JR., R. MAURICE, R. J. PEASE, P. K. WEECH, E. RASSART, J.-C. FRUCHART, J. SCOTT & Y. MARCEL. 1989. The use of monoclonal antibodies to localize the low density lipoprotein receptor-binding domain of apolipoprotein B. J. Biol. Chem. **264:** 19754–19760.
21. MAHLEY, R. W., T. L. INNERARITY, S. C. RALL, JR. & K. H. WEISGRABER. 1985. Lipoproteins of special significance in atherosclerosis: insights provided by studies of type III hyperlipoproteinemia. Ann. N.Y. Acad. Sci. **454:** 209–221.

22. MAHLEY, R. W. & S. C. RALL, JR. 1989. Type III hyperlipoproteinemia (dysbetalipoproteinemia): the role of apolipoprotein E in normal and abnormal lipoprotein metabolism. *In* The Metabolic Basis of Inherited Disease. 6th edit. C. R. Scriver, A. L. Beaudet, W. S. Sly & D. Valle, Eds.:1195–1213. McGraw-Hill. New York, NY.

23. EHNHOLM, C., R. W. MAHLEY, D. A. CHAPPELL, K. H. WEISGRABER, E. LUDWIG & J. L. WITZTUM. 1984. Role of apolipoprotein E in the lipolytic conversion of β-very low density lipoproteins to low density lipoproteins in type III hyperlipoproteinemia. Proc. Natl. Acad. Sci. USA **81:** 5566–5570.

24. KOO, C., M. E. WERNETTE-HAMMOND & T. L. INNERARITY. 1986. Uptake of canine β-very low density lipoproteins by mouse peritoneal macrophages is mediated by a low density lipoprotein receptor. J. Biol. Chem. **261:** 11194–11201.

25. PITAS, R. E., T. L. INNERARITY & R. W. MAHLEY. 1983. Foam cells in explants of atherosclerotic rabbit aortas have receptors for β-very low density lipoproteins and modified low density lipoproteins. Arteriosclerosis **3:** 2–12.

26. MAHLEY, R. W., D. Y. HUI, T. L. INNERARITY & U. BEISIEGEL. 1989. Chylomicron remnant metabolism. Role of hepatic lipoprotein receptors in mediating uptake. Arteriosclerosis **9 (Suppl. I):** I-14–I-18.

27. HAVEL, R. J., L. KOTITE, J. P. KANE, P. TUN & T. BERSOT. 1983. Atypical familial dysbetalipoproteinemia associated with apolipoprotein phenotype E3/3. J. Clin. Invest. **72:** 379–387.

28. RALL, S. C., JR., Y. M. NEWHOUSE, H. R. G. CLARKE, K. H. WEISGRABER, B. J. MCCARTHY, R. W. MAHLEY & T. P. BERSOT. 1989. Type III hyperlipoproteinemia associated with apolipoprotein E phenotype E3/3: structure and genetics of an apolipoprotein E3 variant. J. Clin. Invest. **83:** 1095–1101.

29. HAVEKES, L., E. DE WIT, J. GEVERS LEUVEN, E. KLASEN, G. UTERMANN, W. WEBER & U. BEISIEGEL. 1986. Apolipoprotein E3-Leiden. A new variant of human apolipoprotein E associated with familial type III hyperlipoproteinemia. Hum. Genet. **73:** 157–163.

30. MANN, A. W., R. E. GREGG, R. RONAN, T. FAIRWELL, J. M. HOEG & H. B. BREWER, JR. 1989. Apolipoprotein E-1$_{Harrisburg}$, a mutation in the receptor binding domain, that is dominant for dysbetalipoproteinemia results in defective ligand-receptor interactions. Clin. Res. **37:** 520A. Abstract.

31. INNERARITY, T. L., D. Y. HUI, T. P. BERSOT & R. W. MAHLEY. 1986. Type III hyperlipoproteinemia: a focus on lipoprotein receptor-apolipoprotein E2 interactions. *In* Lipoprotein Deficiency Syndromes. A. Angel & J. Frohlich, Eds.: 273–288. Plenum Publishing Company. New York, NY.

32. WARDELL, M. R., S. O. BRENNAN, E. D. JANUS, R. FRASER & R. W. CARRELL. 1987. Apolipoprotein E2-Christchurch (136 Arg → Ser). New variant of human apolipoprotein E in a patient with type III hyperlipoproteinemia. J. Clin. Invest. **80:** 483–490.

33. RALL, S. C., JR., K. H. WEISGRABER, T. L. INNERARITY & R. W. MAHLEY. 1982. Structural basis for receptor binding heterogeneity of apolipoprotein E from type III hyperlipoproteinemic subjects. Proc. Natl. Acad. Sci. USA **79:** 4696–4700.

34. RALL, S. C., JR., K. H. WEISGRABER, T. L. INNERARITY, T. P. BERSOT, R. W. MAHLEY & C. B. BLUM. 1983. Identification of a new structural variant of human apolipoprotein E, E2(Lys$_{146}$ → Gln), in a type III hyperlipoproteinemic subject with the E3/2 phenotype. J. Clin. Invest. **72:** 1288–1297.

35. HENRIKSEN, T., E. M. MAHONEY & D. STEINBERG. 1981. Enhanced macrophage degradation of low density lipoprotein previously incubated with cultured endothelial cells: recognition by receptors for acetylated low density lipoproteins. Proc. Natl. Acad. Sci. USA **78:** 6499–6503.

36. PARTHASARATHY, S., D. J. PRINTZ, D. BOYD, L. JOY & D. STEINBERG. 1986. Macrophage oxidation of low density lipoprotein generates a modified form recognized by the scavenger receptor. Arteriosclerosis **6:** 505–510.

37. HEINECKE, J. W., H. ROSEN & A. CHAIT. 1984. Iron and copper promote modification of low density lipoprotein by human arterial smooth muscle cells in culture. J. Clin. Invest. **74:** 1890–1894.

38. STEINBRECHER, U. P. 1988. Role of superoxide in endothelial-cell modification of low-density lipoproteins. Biochim. Biophys. Acta **959:** 20–30.

39. KITA, T., Y. NAGANO, M. YOKODE, K. ISHII, N. KUME, A. OOSHIMA, H. YOSHIDA & C. KAWAI. 1987. Probucol prevents the progression of atherosclerosis in Watanabe heritable hyperlipidemic rabbit, an animal model for familial hypercholesterolemia. Proc. Natl. Acad. Sci. USA **84:** 5928–5931.
40. CAREW, T. E., D. C. SCHWENKE & D. STEINBERG. 1987. Antiatherogenic effect of probucol unrelated to its hypocholesterolemic effect: evidence that antioxidants *in vivo* can selectively inhibit low density lipoprotein degradation in macrophage-rich fatty streaks and slow the progression of atherosclerosis in the Watanabe heritable hyperlipidemic rabbit. Proc. Natl. Acad. Sci. USA **84:** 7725–7729.
41. HABERLAND, M. E., D. FONG & L. CHENG. 1988. Malondialdehyde-altered protein occurs in atheroma of Watanabe heritable hyperlipidemic rabbits. Science **241:** 215–218.
42. INNERARITY, T. L., K. H. WEISGRABER, K. S. ARNOLD, R. W. MAHLEY, R. M. KRAUSS, G. L. VEGA & S. M. GRUNDY. 1987. Familial defective apolipoprotein B-100: low density lipoproteins with abnormal receptor binding. Proc. Natl. Acad. Sci. USA **84:** 6919–6923.
43. WEISGRABER, K. H., T. L. INNERARITY, Y. M. NEWHOUSE, S. G. YOUNG, K. S. ARNOLD, R. M. KRAUSS, G. L. VEGA, S. M. GRUNDY & R. W. MAHLEY. 1988. Familial defective apolipoprotein B-100: enhanced binding of monoclonal antibody MB47 to abnormal low density lipoproteins. Proc. Natl. Acad. Sci. USA **85:** 9758–9762.
44. SORIA, L. F., E. H. LUDWIG, H. R. G. CLARKE, G. L. VEGA, S. M. GRUNDY & B. J. MCCARTHY. 1989. Association between a specific apolipoprotein B mutation and familial defective apolipoprotein B-100. Proc. Natl. Acad. Sci. USA **86:** 587–591.

Disproportionally High Concentrations of Apolipoprotein E in the Interstitial Fluid of Normal Pulmonary Artery in Man

YOSHIYA HATA[a] AND KUMIKO NAKAJIMA[a]

Department of Medicine
Keio University School of Medicine
35 Shinano-machi, Shinjuku
Tokyo 160, Japan

INTRODUCTION

[1]Apoprotein E is one of the apolipoproteins present in blood plasma.[1,2] It is primarily synthesized in the liver and secreted into plasma as a peptide of 299 amino acids with a molecular weight of 34,200.[2,3] As it has become clear that apo E is synthesized not only in the liver, but also in other organs such as brain, lung, spleen, kidney, adrenal, ovary, testis, and muscle in several different species,[3] considerable attention has been drawn to the physiological functions of apo E in the body.

Recently, Mahley classified them into three categories,[4] i) Distribution of lipids through systemic circulation among cells of different organs. Plasma lipoproteins with E are the vehicles for this process. Chylomicron and the remnants convey dietary triglycerides to peripheral tissues and dietary cholesterol to the liver.[5] Very low density lipoprotein (VLDL) and intermediate density lipoprotein (IDL) deliver endogenously synthesized lipids to peripheral organs.[5] High density lipoprotein (HDL) with E transports excess cholesterol in reverse from peripheral tissues to the liver.[6] ii) Redistribution of lipids via interstitial fluid among cells within tissues.[4,7] Apo E appears to carry cholesterol from cells with excess cholesterol to those requiring it within the tissue. Recent studies have shown that the coordinated storage and redistribution of cholesterol are mediated by apo E, for instance, in injured and regenerating peripheral nerve cells.[4] iii) Regulation of cellular activities at cell site such as growth, repair, migration, hormone secretion, and immune responses.[2,4] In smooth muscle cells, for instance, apo E production goes parallel with growth arrest, cell differentiation, and migration in tissue.[8] In ovary cells, it exerts a permissive effect on hormone secretion,[9] and on T lymphocytes, it stimulates immune activation and proliferation into the tissue.[4]

These indicate that apo E has an expanding role not only in delivery of lipids among organs, but also in redistribution of them within tissues, and moreover they determine biological functions of various cells from several tissues.

In arterial tissues, the accumulation of cholesteryl ester leads to formation of foam cells in the intima,[10,11] whose cholesterol moiety originates from serum LDL.[12] There-

[a]Address for correspondence: Department of Medicine and Gerontology, Kyorin University School of Medicine, 6-20-2, Shinkawa, Mitaka, Tokyo 181, Japan.

fore, LDL cholesterol and the protein moiety of apo B have been studied on both normal and diseased tissues.[13,14] However, as far as apo E is concerned, no information is available for both normal intima and atherosclerotic lesions, in spite of the fact that foam cell formation may arise from a disturbance in redistribution of cholesterol among cells in the intimal tissue.

We have investigated localization, form, and concentration of apo E, together with apo C-III for comparison, in the interstitial fluid of normal intima of pulmonary arteries in man, and found that apo E occurs in a disproportionally high concentration in the interstitial fluid of normal arterial tissues.

SUBJECTS AND METHODS

We used grossly normal pulmonary arteries from a total of 19 autopsied subjects (10 males and 9 females). Their average age was 57 ± 15 (male 63 ± 17, female 50 ± 6). Blood pressure on admission averaged $134 \pm 21/82 \pm 11$ mmHg, and fasting blood glucose 119 ± 40 mg/dl. Total cholesterol determined before death was 168 ± 41 mg/dl and triglycerides 121 ± 30 mg/dl.

The grossly normal portions of pulmonary artery were dissected after washing carefully with 0.15 M saline solution. To demonstrate the presence and localization of serum apolipoproteins in the tissues, thin sections of 5 u in thickness were made for immunofluorescence study using antibodies for apo E and C-III labeled with 5-fluorescein isothiocyanate (FITC).[15] The remaining dissected tissues were used for conventional histology with hematoxylin eosin (HE) and oil red 0 staining to check whether there was any atherosclerotic lesion. The endothelial cell linings were examined by scanning electron microscopy (SEM) after fixation with 2.5% glutaraldehyde and 1% osmium tetroxide.

The intima of grossly normal tissues dissected was minced with ophthalmological scissors into fine pieces about 1 cubic mm, then homogenized gently with a homogenizer having a teflon pest in 0.13 M Tris HCl buffer (pH 7.4) for 3 minutes at 4°C. We employed Tris HCl buffer for the isolation medium, because the yield of lipids released from tissues was not different when compared among 0.15 M saline solution, 0.13 M Tris HCl buffer (pH 7.4), and 1/15 M phosphate buffer (pH 7.4). We employed gentle homogenization for recovery of tissue apoproteins, because they are known to be digested by lysosomal enzymes within 90 minutes once they are taken up into cytoplasm.[16] We homogenized the tissues for 3 minutes to release apoproteins, because a preliminary time course study showed that the release of apoproteins reached a plateau after 3 minutes and gave a sufficient yield of tissue apoproteins. The recovery of apo E and C-III from the tissue by this method was 94% and 95%, respectively.

The tissue fluid thus recovered was ultracentrifuged with a Beckman SW 50.1 rotor for 24 hours after adjustment of background density at 1.21. The upper phase was taken and dialyzed against 0.15 M saline solution.

To show biochemically the presence of serum apolipoproteins in recovered tissue fluids, sodium dodecyl sulfate (SDS) gradient (3–20%) polyacrylamide gel electrophoresis (PAGE) was performed.[17] The gel was stained with 0.0025% Comassie brilliant blue for 18–24 hours and destained with 10% acetic acid for 18–24 hours.

To demonstrate the complexity of tissue apoproteins with lipids, the specimens were prestained with Sudan black B, and a disc electrophoresis with 3.5% PAG was performed.[18]

To quantify the contents of apo E and C-III in the tissue fluids, the specimens were quantitatively condensed *in vaccuo,* then measured by the single radial immunodiffusion (SRID) method.[19] The apoprotein contents gained in a unit of mg/g wet tissue were converted into mg/dl of extracellular, interstitial fluid by using factors for water content of normal intima of pulmonary artery as $81 \pm 1\%$ and extracellular volume as $68 \pm 11\%$ of water content, which were determined by preliminary studies using lyophylization and ^{14}C-inulin space methods with an assumption that the inulin space of tissue water is the extracellular, interstitial fluid. The apoprotein concentrations were compared with normal serum apoprotein levels of Japanese population.[20]

RESULTS

Light microscopy of grossly normal tissue specimens stained with HE and oil red 0 staining revealed that they had neither an accumulation of lipids nor formation of lesions, though there was a slight thickening in the intima. SEM showed that the intimal surface

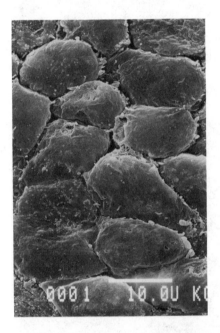

FIGURE 1. Scanning electron micrograph of a normal pulmonary artery in man stained with 2.5% glutaraldehyde and 1% osmium tetroxide.

was covered with spindle-shaped cells and that the intimal cell lining was maintained in an integrated form, as in FIGURE 1.

Presence and localization of apo E and C-III in the normal intima were demonstrated by an immunofluorescence study. Specific fluorescence of apo E and C-III were diffusely present both in the intima and media of pulmonary artery, as in FIGURE 2.

Presence of apo E and C-III was also demonstrated in the recovered tissue fluid by SDS gradient PAGE. Bands of molecular weights of 33 K and 8 K, equivalent to those of apo E and C-III, were detected, as in FIGURE 3.

The form of apoproteins in the tissue fluid was examined by disc PAGE. The tissue fluid prestained for lipid moiety with Sudan black B migrated according to electric charges of protein moiety in two bands with mobility equivalent to those of serum VLDL and LDL. These indicated that apo E and C-III occurred in the tissue fluid in a complex

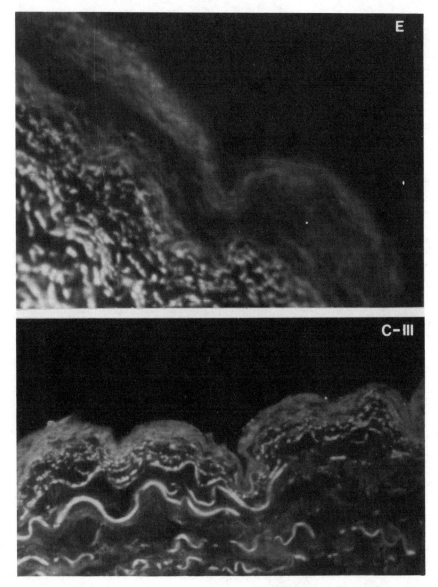

FIGURE 2. Immunofluorescence of apo E and C-III in the normal pulmonary artery in man.

with lipids, namely, as lipoproteins in FIGURE 4. The spherical form of apolipoprotein complex with lipids is shown in FIGURE 5. We can see spherical particles of homogeneous size in a diameter of approximately 200A, mixed occasionally with larger particles of about 800–900 A in diameter.

The extracted tissue fluids were quantitatively condensed *in vaccuo,* and determined for apo E and C-III by the SRID method. Apo E contents averaged as 0.004 ± 0.003 mg/g wet tissue and Apo C-III 0.002 ± 0.004 mg/g wet tissue. When they were converted to the unit of mg/dl by the conversion factors described above. Then apo E concentration was 0.6 ± 0.6 mg/dl and apo C-III 0.2 ± 0.3 mg/dl. For comparison, normal serum apolipoprotein levels are given in TABLE 1.

DISCUSSION

The localization, form, and concentrations of interstitial apolipoprotein E and C-III were determined for normal pulmonary arteries secured from autopsied subjects. The results have shown that i) in the normal pulmonary arteries, apo E and C-III are present in both the intima and media in the form of spherical lipoproteins, ii) the apo E and C-III concentrations in the interstitial fluid are distinctly different from the serum counterpart, and iii) the apo E concentration is disproportionally high in the interstitial fluids, when compared with other interstitial apoproteins like C-III.

We chose the pulmonary artery for demonstration and determinations of serum apoproteins in the interstitial fluid of arterial tissue, because comparative pathology on atherosclerosis has shown that the pulmonary arteries are rarely affected with atherosclerotic lesions even in the aged.[21] This is probably due to the fact that the vascular resistance is low in pulmonary circulation,[22] pulmonary blood pressure is therefore as low as 1/6 of systemic blood pressure,[22] pulmonary hypertension is a rare clinical condition,[22] and

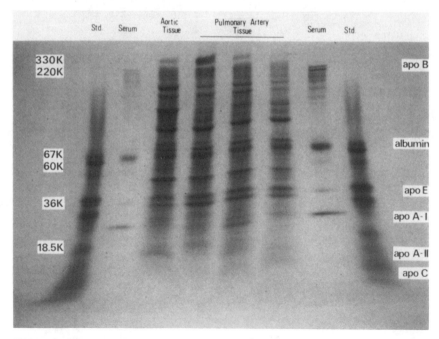

FIGURE 3. SDS gradient PAGE of the recovered tissue fluids from normal pulmonary artery in man.

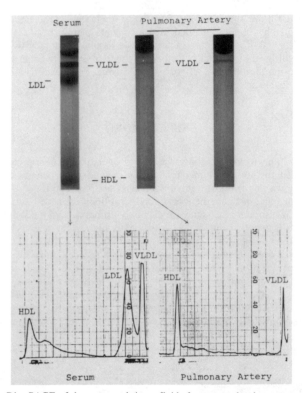

FIGURE 4. Disc PAGE of the recovered tissue fluids from normal pulmonary artery in man.

hypertension is one of the most common causes for endothelial damages.[8] Actually, the specimens we used revealed an intact endothelium without formation of any atherosclerotic lesion as examined by light microscopy and SEM (FIG. 1), though the age of subjects was 57 ± 15 years. This implies that the interstitial apoprotein concentrations measured in the intima of pulmonary artery are very close to the natural state of *milieu interior* of the arterial tissues.

Owing to the intact endothelium, there is a distinct difference in apo E and C-III concentrations between serum and pulmonary interstitial fluid, as they are 1/7 and 1/19 of normal serum counterparts, respectively (see TABLE 1). This indicates that intimal smooth muscle cells are incubated with the interstitial fluid containing lipoproteins different in the amount from serum apoproteins, This confirms that the endothelium in its integrated form serves as a barrier for maintenance of *milieu interior* in the arterial tissue.

TABLE 1. Concentrations of Interstitial Apo E and C-III in Normal Pulmonary Artery

	Interstitial Fluid		Serum	
	mg/gWet Tissue	mg/dl	mg/dl	ISF[a]/Serum
Apo E	0.004 ± 0.003	0.6 ± 0.6	4.1 ± 1.2	1:7
Apo C-III	0.002 ± 0.004	0.4 ± 0.7	7.5 ± 3.0	1:19

[a]ISF: interstitial fluid.

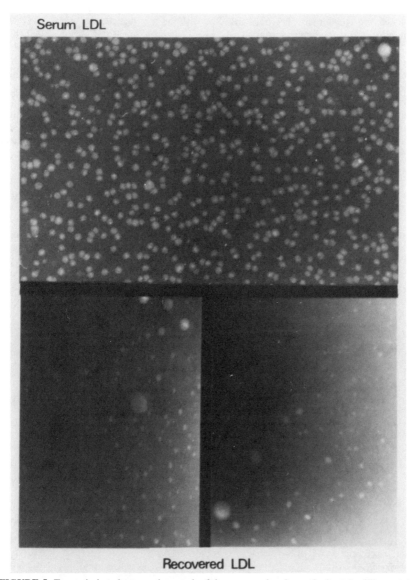

FIGURE 5. Transmission electron micrograph of the recovered and negatively stained lipoproteins from normal pulmonary artery in man.

When we look at the ratio of serum apolipoproteins in TABLE 1, the apo E/C-III ratio is 0.55 in normal serum, while it is 1.50 in the interstitial fluids. This difference in the ratio between serum and interstitial fluids can be interpreted as either apo E is disproportionally raised or apo C-III is extremely low in the intima.

We consider the former to be the case, since when it is assumed that interstitial apo C-III comes solely with serum VLDL, the interstitial VLDL must be at the level of 1/19 of the serum counterpart. This falls into line with the fact that the size of the peak with a mobility corresponding to serum VLDL is very small on disc PAGE of interstitial fluid, and that the particles with diameters of 800–900 A are sparse in TEM (FIG. 5).

As for interstitial apo E, it is carried into the tissue by both VLDL and HDL with E. When we assume that they permeate into the tissue, keeping the ratio of 0.55 in serum, then apo E contents in the interstitial fluid has to be 1/35 of serum apo E. However, the interstitial apo E measured is 1/7 of serum apo E, which is 5 times higher than that estimated. We think this elevation is not due to accumulation of HDL with E *in situ*, since neither the peak corresponding to serum HDL has been deeply stained on disc PAGE, nor have apo A-I and A-II bands been intensified on SDS gradient PAGE. It can be concluded therefore that apo E is elevated in the interstitial fluid of the normal arterial tissue, not due to accumulation of HDL with E or increased infiltration of serum VLDL.

It is known that both arterial smooth muscle cells and macrophages derived from circulating monocytes can produce apo E at tissue site.[3,4,23] The interstitial apo E could therefore originate not only from serum VLDL or HDL with E, but at least a part of it is locally synthesized by those cells. Apo E synthesized *in situ* may be contributing to the redistribution of cholesterol from cells with excess cholesterol either to cells requiring it or to the acceptors for cholesterol excretion, with which reverse cholesterol transport starts.[6] The interstitial apo E may thus be playing a salient role in restoration of cholesterol homeostasis in the intima to protect the genesis of atherosclerosis, though the precise mechanism remains to be elucidated.

REFERENCES

1. MAHLEY, R. W. & T. L. INNERARITY. 1983. Lipoprotein receptors and cholesterol homeostasis. Biochim. Biophys. Acta **737:** 197–222.
2. MAHLEY, R. W., T. L. INNERARITY, S. C. RALL, JR. & K. H. WEISGRABER. 1984. Plasma lipoproteins: Apolipoprotein structure and function. J. Lipid Res. **24:** 1277–1294.
3. DRISCOL, D. M. & G. S. GETZ. 1984. Extrahepatic synthesis of apolipoprotein E. J. Lipid Res. **25:** 1368–1379.
4. MAHLEY, R. W. 1988. Apolipoprotein E: Cholesterol transport protein with expanding role in cell biology. Science **240:** 622–630.
5. BROWN, M. S., P. T. KOVANEN & J. L. GOLDSTEIN. 1981. Regulation of plasma cholesterol by lipoprotein receptors. Science **212:** 628–635.
6. MILLER, N. E. 1978. Current concept of the role of HDL in reverse cholesterol transports. *In* Clinical and Metabolic Aspects of High-density Lipoproteins, N. E. Miller & G. J. Miller, Eds. 187–216. Elsevier. Amsterdam.
7. MAHLEY, R. W., J. K. BOYLES & R. E. PITAS. 1989. Role of apolipoprotein E and high density lipoproteins in lipid redistribution locally within tissues. *In* High Density Lipoproteins and Atherosclerosis II. N. E. Miller, Ed. 263–268. Excerpta Medica. Amsterdam.
8. ROSS, R. 1986. The pathogenesis of atherosclerosis—An update. N. Engl. J. Med. **314:** 488–500.
9. DYER, C. A. & L. K. CURTIS. 1988. Apoprotein E-rich high density lipoproteins inhibit ovarian androgen synthesis. J. Biol. Chem. **263:** 10965–10973.
10. HATA, Y., J. HOWER & W. INSULL, JR. 1974. Cholesteryl ester-rich inclusions from human fatty streak and fibrous plaque lesions of atherosclerosis. I. Crystalline properties, size and internal structure. Am. J. Pathol. **75:** 423–456.
11. GERRITY, R. G. 1981. The role of the monocytes in atherogenesis. I. Transition of blood borne monocytes into foam cells in fatty lesions. Am. J. Pathol. **103:** 181–190.
12. DAYTON, S. & S. HASHIMOTO. 1970. Recent advance in molecular pathology: A review. Cholesterol flux and metabolism in arterial tissue and in atheroma. Exp. Mol. Pathol. **13:** 253–268.
13. SMITH, E. B. 1974. The relationship between plasma and tissue lipids in human atherosclerosis. Adv. Lipid Res. **12:** 1–9.

14. LINDEN, T., O. WIKLUND & G. FAGER. 1986. A new microimmunoassay for apolipoprotein B in arterial tissue. Atherosclerosis **62:** 227–237.
15. STAUDER, W. T. & S. H. ONG. 1983. Apoprotein B localization in control and streptozocin-diabetic rat skeletal muscles. Histochem. J. **15:** 15–20.
16. GOLDSTEIN, J. L. & M. S. BROWN. 1976. The LDL pathway in human fibroblasts. A receptor-mediated mechanism for the regulation of cholesterol metabolism. Curr. Top. Cell. Regul. **11:** 147–181.
17. KING, J. & U. K. LAEMMLI. 1971. Polypeptide of tail fibers of bacteriophage T4. J. Mol. Biol. **62:** 465–473.
18. NARAYAN, K. A., S. NARAYAN & F. A. KUMMEROW. 1965. Disc electrophoresis of human serum lipoproteins. Nature **205:**246–248.
19. GOTO, Y., Y. AKANUMA, Y. HARANO, Y. HATA, H. ITAKURA et al. 1986. Determination by SRID method of normal values of serum apoproteins (A-I, A-II, B, C-II, C-III and E) in normolipidemic healthy Japanese subjects. J. Clin. Biochem. Nutr. **1:** 73–88.
20. NOMA, A., Y. HATA & Y. GOTO Quantitation of serum apolipoproteins A-I, A-II, B, C-II, C-III and E in normal healthy Japanese subjects by turbidimetric immunoassay: Reference values and age and sex differences. Atherosclerosis. In press.
21. ROBERTS, J. C., JR., C. MOSES & R. H. WILKINS. 1959. Autopsy studies in atherosclerosis. I. Distribution and severity of atherosclerosis in patients dying without morphologic evidence of atherosclerotic catastrophe. Circulation **20:** 511–519.
22. LEE, G. D. & B. BAJAGOPALLAN. 1981. Pulmonary blood flow. In Structure and Function of the Circulation, Vol. 2. C. J. Schwartz, N. T. Werthessn & S. Wolf, Eds. 363–403. Plenum Press. New York, NY.
23. BROWN, M. S. & J. L. GOLDSTEIN. 1983. Lipoprotein metabolism in the macrophage: Implications for cholesterol deposition in atherosclerosis. Annu. Rev. Biochem. **52:** 223–261.

Risk Factors for Atherosclerotic Vascular Diseases with Special Reference to the Relationship between Apolipoprotein E Mutations and Hyperlipidemia

AKIRA YAMAMOTO, TAKU YAMAMURA, AND SHOJI TAJIMA

Department of Etiology and Pathophysiology
National Cardiovascular Center Research Institute
5-7-1 Fujishiro-dai, Suita
Osaka 565, Japan

INTRODUCTION

Apolipoprotein E (apo E) is a determinant that mediates the metabolism of intermediate density lipoprotein (IDL), chylomicron remnants, and high density lipoprotein (HDL) through low density lipoprotein (LDL)-receptors and another kind of still uncharacterized lipoprotein receptors.[1,2] It is generally recognized that apo E plays an important role in the reverse cholesterol transport from peripheral tissues to the liver and also for the redistribution of cholesterol in some localized areas in peripheral tissues.[3]

There are three major isoforms and several mutants in apo E molecules.[4,5] Important findings have been obtained by Utermann and some others that those people with apo E-4 (ϵ4 allele) have higher LDL-cholesterol levels than those with apo E-3 (ϵ3 allele), while the latter still have higher LDL-cholesterol levels compared to those with apo E-2 (ϵ2 allele).[6]

During the course of our study on apo E isoform distribution among the Japanese population and patients with hyperlipidemia and ischemic heart diseases, two peculiar mutants were found; apo E-5[7] and E-7,[8] both of which are more alkaline than the common isoform, E-4. These two mutants were originally found in patients with myocardial infarction or angina pectoris and our further study demonstrated that the frequency of these mutants is not so small in the general population in Japan as that of the other ones, like apo E-1,[9] E-2',[10] and E-3',[11] which had been found in Europe or America.

In this study we compared the apo E phenotype distribution for patients with myocardial infarction and a control group of apparently healthy subjects.[12] We characterized the sites of mutation on the apo E gene in E-5[13] and E-7[14] and also studied the affinity of apo E-5 and E-7 on LDL-receptors to see how these two mutant apo Es interfere with LDL-receptors.[15]

MATERIALS AND METHODS

Subjects of the Study and Lipoprotein Analysis

One hundred and ninety-nine patients administered in the CCU and 56 patients in the SCU of the National Cardiovascular Center Hospital were the subjects of the present study. Most of the patients in the former group had been attacked by myocardial infarction and the latter group were a mixture of those who had been attacked by cerebral hemorrhage and those attacked by cerebral infarction. Two hundred and eleven apparently healthy subjects who visited a health care hospital in the Suita area for physical check-ups were used as the control group.

Blood was taken after overnight fast and the very low density lipoprotein (VLDL) fraction was obtained from serum by ultracentrifugation at a density = 1.006. Cholesterol and triglycerides in serum and in VLDL fraction were measured by enzymatic assays. HDL-cholesterol was determined in a supernatant after precipitation of LDL and VLDL by the addition of heparin and Ca^{++} to appropriately diluted serum samples. Analysis of apo E was done by isoelectric focussing of apolipoproteins extracted from the VLDL fraction.[7,8]

Analysis of Apo E-5 and E-7 Genes

Genomic DNA was isolated from patients' white blood cells. The 11 kb Hind III digestion fragments from the heterozygous genes of apo E (either E5/3 or E7/3) were ligated into the Hind III sites of a λ phage vector, (λ 2001) and cloned. A 5.6-kb Bam HI fragment was obtained from the clone and a fragment containing all four exons of apo E gene (15 base pairs downstream from the TATA box to 1 kbp downstream from the polyadenylation signal, FIG. 1) was subcloned into pGEM-3. The Bam HI fragment was then ligated into the Bam HI sites of a murine retrovirus shuttle vector pZIP-Neo SV (X) and transfected into mouse strain cells (ψ-2) to express apo E protein. For transfection, the calcium phosphate-DNA coprecipitation technique was used. Cells were incubated in a medium containing 10% fetal calf serum with 0.4 mg/ml of G418 (GIBCO). The density of the cultured medium of transfected ψ2 cells expressing apo E-3 or E-5 (or E-7) was subjected to isoelectric focussing to determine the type of apo E, and those colonies of pGEM-3 expressing E-5 or E-7 were subjected to DNA sequencing.[13,14]

For sequencing the exons of the apo E-5 and E-7 genes, the pGEM-3 was partially deleted with Exonuclease III and directly sequenced by the dideoxy method. The first exon was sequenced from the 5' end of the plasmid without deletion. For the second and third exons, the Bam HI/Eco RI fragment was recloned into pGEM-3. For the fourth exon and the second and third exons for the opposite directions, a X-baI/Bam HI fragment was recloned. The sequence of the fourth exon was also determined by subcloning the PstI fragment into M13mp18 or mp19.

The Activity of Binding of Apo E-5 to LDL-Receptors

Apo E-dimyristoylphosphatidylcholine (DMPC, Sigma) complexes were prepared according to the method of Rall *et al.*[16] Apo E and a sonicated preparation of DMPC were mixed and incubated for 1 hr at 25°C and the complexes were isolated by ultracentrifugation in a fraction of d = 1.006–1.21 at 49000 rpm for 20 hr at 15°C. The isolated complexes (apo E·DMPC) had average phospholipid/protein ratio of 3.7:1 (wt/wt).

Human skin fibroblasts were cultured and the competitive binding of apo E·DMPC with ^{125}I-LDL was assayed at 4°C on ice as described by Innerarity *et al.*[17]

RESULTS

Apo E Phenotype Distribution in Patients with Ischemic Heart Diseases: Comparison to Normal Subjects

The frequency of E4/4 was higher and E3/2 lower in CCU patients compared to the control group. The frequencies of E4/3 and E2/2 were almost the same for the patients and

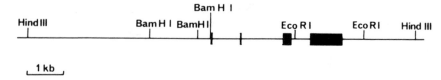

FIGURE 1. Restriction endonuclease map of the apo E gene. The relative positions of the exons are shown by *boxes*. Restriction sites for Bam HI, Hind III, Eco RI, XbaI, and PstI are indicated.

the control, and therefore, the total ε4 allele frequency in CCU patients was significantly higher than in the group of healthy subjects. Although the frequency of E4/4 was higher and E3/2 lower also in SCU patients, that of E4/3 was lower and E2/2 higher in these patients than in the control and, therefore, no significant difference in apo E gene allele frequency was found between SCU patients and the group of healthy subjects.

CCU patients were divided into men and women. About 80% of the patients were men. We further divided the male patients into a relatively young age group (below 60 years) and an older age group (at or above 60 years). Although the apo E phenotype distribution in the older age men's group was about the same as the distribution in healthy control group, the distribution in the younger men and also that in the women were significantly different; the frequency of E4/4 and E4/3 was higher and E3/2 lower compared to the healthy controls (TABLE 1). There was no E2/2 in the younger men and no E3/2 or E2/2 in the female patients. The frequencies of our new mutants E-5 and E-7, both of which were in heterozygous form combined with E-3 (E5/3 and E7/3), were 2 to 3 times higher in the younger men patients compared to healthy subjects.

When we divided the CCU patients into those who were suddenly attacked by acute myocardial infarction without being preceded by angina pectoris (Group A) and those who had experienced anginal pains before the attack of myocardial infarction (Group B), the deviation in apo E allele frequency was significant only in Group B patients.

LDL-Cholesterol and VLDL-Triglyceride Concentrations among Different Groups

There was a tendency for LDL-cholesterol to increase in the order of apo E phenotypes; E3/2 < E3/3 < E4/3 and E4/4 (FIG. 2). VLDL-triglycerides increased in the

TABLE 1. Apo E Phenotype Distribution in CCU Patients[a]

Apo E Phenotype	Control Total %	(n)	Male Total %	(n)	<60 y.o. %	(n)	60 y.o. %	(n)	Female Total %	(n)
E 4/4	1.0	(2)	4.4	(7)	5.3	(3)	3.9	(4)	7.7	(3)
E 4/3	17.5	(37)	15.0	(24)	19.3	(11)	12.6	(13)	25.6	(10)
E 4/2	1.0	(2)	0.6	(1)	1.8	(1)	—	(0)	2.6	(1)
E 3/3	67.2	(142)	68.7	(110)	64.8	(37)	70.9	(73)	61.5	(24)
E 3/2	11.3	(24)	8.1	(13)	3.5	(2)	10.7	(11)	—	(0)
E 2/2	0.5	(1)	1.3	(2)	—	(0)	1.9	(2)	—	(0)
E 7/3	1.0	(2)	1.3	(2)	3.5	(2)	—	(0)	2.6	(1)
E 5/3	0.5	(1)	0.6	(1)	1.8	(1)	—	(0)	—	(0)
Total	100.0	(211)	100.0	(160)	100.0	(57)	100.0	(103)	100.0	(39)

[a]Male patients were divided into two groups; 1) relatively young patients under 60 years, and 2) older patients aged 60 or above.

reverse direction; E4/3 and E4/4 < E3/3 < E3/2. The average LDL-cholesterol level in CCU patients was significantly higher than that in healthy subjects for each of the three apo E phenotype subgroups. VLDL-triglycerides also showed a tendency to be at a higher level on average compared to the normal subjects, although the difference was not very significant, as it was in LDL-cholesterol. A large number of the CCU patients had type IIa or IIb hyperlipoproteinemia. Distribution of Type IV hyperlipoproteinemia in CCU patients was not significantly different from that in normal subjects.

The LDL-cholesterol level in CCU patients according to the apo E phenotypes showed the same tendency as observed in normal subjects to elevate in the order of E3/2 < E3/3 < E4/3 and E4/4. The average LDL-cholesterol level in a group of CCU patients with the E3/2 phenotype (the lowest LDL-cholesterol among the three apo E phenotypes) was still higher than the LDL-cholesterol in a group of normal subjects with E4/3 and E4/4

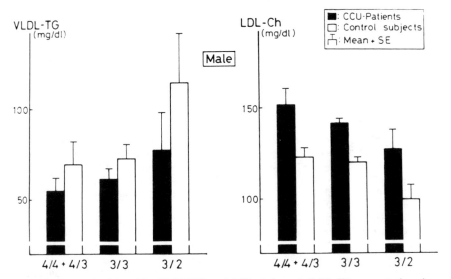

FIGURE 2. VLDL-triglyceride (VLDL-TG) and LDL-cholesterol (LDL-Ch) concentrations in plasma of CCU patients and control subjects according to apo E phenotypes. Data obtained from male patients and controls are shown.

phenotypes (the highest level among the three apo E phenotypes). VLDL-triglyceride levels were higher in E3/2 group than in E3/3 and E4/3 and a high level of VLDL-triglycerides in CCU patients with the E3/2 phenotype was prominent.

Analysis of Apo E-5 and E-7 Genes

The analysis of the nucleotide sequence of the exons and exon-intron boundary regions of apo E-5 gene showed G to A substitution in the 18th nucleotide from the 5' end of the third exon. This single base substitution changes the amino acid residue Glu to Lys at the third amino acid from amino-terminus of the mature protein and gives two additional units of positive charge to the molecule (FIG. 3). The apo E-5 showed a molecular

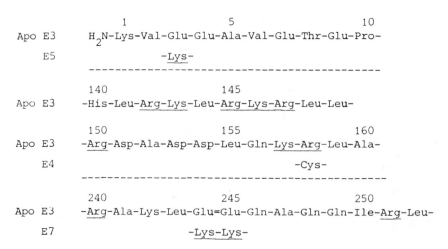

FIGURE 3. Mutation sites in peptide structure of the major apo E isoforms and apo E-5 and 7.

weight a little (about 2,000 daltons) smaller than apo E-3 and E-4 on SDS-PAGE. But we could not find any abnormality in the gene which would cause the apparent reduction of the molecular weight. It is unlikely that apo E-5 is posttranslationally proteolyzed at the amino-terminal region without changing the charge balance of the whole molecule. It is also unlikely that the one amino acid change in the amino-terminal region causes the proteolysis of the carboxy-terminal region. Apo E-2, which is one of the isoforms apo E caused by the substitution of Arg 158 to Lys, gives about 1,500 higher apparent molecular weight than that of apo E-3 on SDS-PAGE. The charged amino acids might effect the amount of SDS bound on the molecule.

The analysis of the nucleotide sequence of apo E-7 showed two G to A nucleotide substitutions at the 548 and 551 nucleotide position from the 5' end of the fourth exon. These two base substitutions change the amino acid residue -Glu-Glu- to -Lys-Lys- at the 244 and 245 positions from amino-terminus of the mature protein, and give four additional units of positive charge to the molecule. This mutation creates a highly basic stretch containing 4 basic amino acid residues within 6 residues between positions 240 and 245. The stretches of consecutive basic amino acids are -Arg-Lys-(142-143), -Arg-Lys-Arg-(145-147), and -Lys-Arg-(157-158) in apo E-3. The new basic stretch in apo E-7 (240-245) might give another receptor binding domain to the apo E molecule.

The Affinity of Apo E-5 and E-7 on LDL-Receptors of Human Skin Fibroblasts

APO E-5·DMPC competed with ^{125}I-LDL binding on human skin fibroblasts with a strength similar to apo E-3·DMPC at the concentration between 0.1–1.0 μg protein (apo E)/ml. When we tested the ability to compete with LDL at a lower concentration of apo E·DMPC, apo E-5 showed a higher binding activity than apo E-3. A logit-log plot of binding data was used to determine the 50% competition. The concentration of apo E·DMPC at which 50% of ^{125}I-LDL was displaced was 29–30 ng protein/ml for apo E-5 and 63–66 ng protein/ml for E-3 (Fig. 4). Apo E-5 is twice as active in its binding to LDL-receptors as apo E-3.

In contrast to apo E-5, apo E-7·DMPC competed with ^{125}I-LDL binding on LDL-receptors more weakly than apo E-3·DMPC. The logit-log plot of binding data showed the concentration of apo E-7·DMPC for 50% displacement 220 ng/ml; the affinity of apo E-7 to LDL-receptors was only 23% of apo E-3.

DISCUSSION

Apo E is one of the important factors that regulate lipoprotein metabolism through affinity binding with LDL-receptors and so-called remnant receptors.[1-3] There are three major isoforms of apo E; E-2, E-3, and E-4.[4,5] Among them E-2 lacks the ability to bind with the receptors and some individuals homozygous to apo E-2 (E2/2) develop a peculiar type of hyperlipoproteinemia (Type III) characterized by the retention of β-VLDL.[18] If we exclude such special cases, there is a tendency for LDL-cholesterol to increase as the positive charge of the apo E molecule increases in the order of E-2 < E-3 < E-4.[6,19,20] Although the difference was not so remarkable as in the European population, the results of our study[21] and another study carried out in other areas of Japan[22] also showed the same tendency.

Our data showed that the prevalence of apo E-4, 5, and 7 among relatively young men and among women with myocardial infarction was significantly higher and that of E-2 lower than in the normal population. A large number of patients in CCU in this study had type IIa or IIb hyperlipoproteinemia and it is reasonable to speculate that the development of coronary atherosclerosis was accelerated in those patients with an increase in the extent of hyperlipidemia. The distribution of apo E phenotypes among older male patients was almost equal to that in the normal population, probably because the influence of other risk factors, glucose intolerance, hypertension, etc., was much stronger in aged persons. It is generally accepted that the risk of coronary heart diseases among hyperlipidemics was

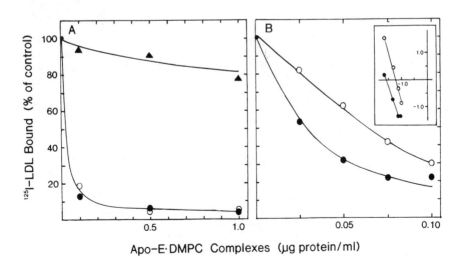

FIGURE 4. LDL-receptor-binding of ^{125}I-labelled LDL competed by apo E-3·DMPC complexes (○) and apo E-5·DMPC complexes (●). The 100% value corresponded to 50 ng of ^{125}I-LDL protein bound/mg of cellular protein. The *inset* shows a logit-log plot of binding data. The concentration of apo E at which 50% of ^{125}I-LDL was displaced was 29 ng/ml for apo E-5 (●) and 63 ng/ml for apo E-3 (○).

much stronger in younger generations. In Japan, smoking is still not so popular with women, especially in older generations and the participation of other risk factors is also not so strong in them as in men. This is probably the reason why more remarkable deviation from normal population in apo E phenotype distribution was observed in women with ischemic heart diseases than in men patients.

There was a tendency for LDL-cholesterol to increase in the order of E-2 < E-3 < E-4 in CCU patients as is also seen in the normal population. The LDL-cholesterol level in a group of CCU patients with the E3/2 phenotype was still higher than that in a group of healthy subjects with E4/3 and E4/4 phenotypes. This suggests that other factors, besides the apo E gene, influenced the development of coronary atherosclerosis. Probably, more common predispositions for hyperlipidemia presented risk factors independent of apo E phenotypes.

Apo E-5 and E-7 had originally been found among the patients with ischemic heart diseases. It is interesting that all three mutation sites involved the same base change G to A, which causes the change in amino acid from glutamic acid into lysin. The same change occurs in apo E-7 at two neighboring positions. At this time, no apo E-5 which has a single Glu→ Lys change at residue 244 or 245 has been detected. The E-5 and E-7 mutations found in other laboratories in Japan are the same as ours.[22,23]

It has been shown that apo E strongly competes with LDL for binding with LDL receptors. Recently Funahashi et al. reported that the affinity to LDL-receptors of lipid particles provided with apo E-3 is proportionate to the apo E concentration.[24] When there were 4 molecules of apo E on one lipid particle with the size of LDL, the affinity to LDL-receptors was almost comparable to the affinity of LDL. When the surface of the lipid particle was saturated with 7 molecules of apo E, the affinity was 7 times that of LDL. Our present study of the competitive binding of apo E-5 shows that it has a little higher affinity of LDL receptors than apo E-3. It is reasonable to suggest that our patients with apo E-5 mostly had combined hyperlipidemia instead of type III, which is caused by a defective binding of apo E-2[25] or some other rare mutants[9-11] to lipoprotein receptors. Although the difference is small, a higher affinity of apo E-5 on LDL-receptors may result in a stronger interference for the binding of LDL on the receptors.

As apo E-7 is much more alkaline than apo E-4 and the molecule is provided with a new stretch of consecutive basic amino acids, we anticipated that apo E-7 might provide stronger competition for the receptors than apo E-3. However, our experimental data showed that the affinity of apo E-7 to LDL-receptors was reduced to 23% of the affinity of apo E-3. The fragment rich in basic amino acid must produce a strong conformational change in the apo E molecule. Our patients were all heterozygous to apo E-7. We are continuing clinical and basal studies on why and how apo E-7 is associated with hyperlipidemia and atherosclerosis.

REFERENCES

1. MAHLEY, R. W. & T. L. INNERARITY. 1983. Lipoprotein receptors and cholesterol homeostasis. Biochim. Biophys. Acta **737:** 197–222.
2. INNERARITY, T. L., K. S. ARNOLD, K. H. WEISGRABER, & R. W. MAHLEY. 1986. Apolipoprotein E is the determinant that mediates the receptor uptake of β-very low density lipoproteins by mouse macrophages. Arteriosclerosis **6:** 114–122.
3. MAHLEY, R. W. 1988. Apolipoprotein E: cholesterol transport protein with expanding role in cell biology. Science **240:** 622–630.
4. UTERMANN, G., U. LANGENBECK, U. BEISIEGEL & W. WEBER. 1980. Genetics of the apolipoprotein E system in man. Am. J. Hum. Genet. **32:** 339–347.
5. BRESLOW, J. L., J. MCPHERSON, A. L. NUSSBAUM, H. W. WILLIAMS, F. LOFQUIST-KAHL, S. K. KARATHANASIS, & V. I. ZANNIS. 1982. Identification and DNA sequence of a human apolipoprotein E cDNA clone. J. Biol. Chem. **257:** 14639–14641.

6. DAVIGNON, J., R. E. GREGG & C. F. SING. 1988. Apolipoprotein polymorphism and athero-sclerosis. Arteriosclerosis **8**: 1–21.
7. YAMAMURA, T., A. YAMAMOTO, K. HIRAMORI & S. NAMBU. 1984. A new isoform of apoli-poprotein E—apo E5—associated with hyperlipidemia and atherosclerosis. Atherosclerosis **50**: 159–172.
8. YAMAMURA, T., A. YAMAMOTO, T. SUMIYOSHI, K. HIRAMORI, Y. NISHIOEDA & S. NAMBU. 1984. New mutants of apolipoprotein E associated with atherosclerotic disease but not to type III hyperlipoproteinemia. J. Clin. Invest. **74**: 1229–1237.
9. WEISGRABER, K. H., S. C. RALL, JR., T. L. INNERARITY, R. W. MAHLEY, T. KUUSI & C. EHNHOLM. 1984. A novel electrophoretic variant of human apolipoprotein E. Identifica-tion and characterization of apolipoprotein E1. J. Clin. Invest. **73**: 1024–1033.
10. RALL, S. C., Jr., K. H. WEISGRABER, T. L. INNERARITY, T. P. BERSOT, R. W. MAHLEY & C. B. BLUM. 1983. Identification of a new structural variant of human apolipoprotein E, E2 (Lys146→Gln), in a type III hyperlipoproteinemic subject with the E3/2 phenotype. J. Clin. Invest. **72**: 1288–1297.
11. HAVEKES, L. M., J. A. GEVERS-LEUVEN, E. VAN CORVEN, E. DE WIT & J. J. EMEIS. 1984. Functionally inactive apolipoprotein E3 in a type III hyperlipoproteinemic patient. Eur. J. Clin. Invest. **14**: 7–11.
12. YAMAMURA, T., S. TAJIMA & A. YAMAMOTO. 1989. Genetics of apolipoprotein E polymor-phism and atherosclerosis. J. Jpn. Atheroscler. Soc. **16**: 1047–1051 (in Japanese).
13. TAJIMA, S., T. YAMAMURA & A. YAMAMOTO. 1988. Analysis of apolipoprotein E5 gene from a patient with hyperlipoproteinemia. J. Biochem. **104**: 48–52.
14. TAJIMA, S., T. YAMAMURA, M. MENJU & A. YAMAMOTO. 1989. Analysis of apolipoprotein E7 (apolipoprotein E-Suita) gene from a patient with hyperlipoproteinemia. J. Biochem. **105**: 249–253.
15. DONG, L-M., T. YAMAMURA & A. YAMAMOTO. 1989. Analysis of the activity of binding of an apolipoprotein E mutant, Apo E5, to LDL receptors on human fibroblasts. Biochem. Biophys. Res. Commun. In press.
16. RALL, S. C., JR., K. H. WEISGRABER, T. L. INNERARITY & R. W. MAHLEY. 1982. Structural basis for receptor binding heterogeneity of apolipoprotein E from type III hyperlipoprotein-emic subjects. Proc. Natl. Acad. Sci. USA **79**: 4696–4700.
17. INNERARITY, T. L., R. E. PITAS & R. W. MAHLEY. 1979. Binding of arginine-rich (E) apoprotein after recombination with phospholipid vesicles to the low density lipoprotein receptors of fibroblasts. J. Biol. Chem. **254**: 4186–4190.
18. HAVEL, R. J. 1982. Familial dysbetalipoproteinemia. Med. Clin. Nor. Am. **66(2)**: 441–454.
19. EHNHOLM, C., M. LUKKA, T. KUUSI, E. NIKKILÄ & G. UTERMANN. 1986. Apolipoprotein E polymorphism in the Finnish population: gene frequencies and relation to lipoprotein con-centrations. J. Lipid Res. **27**: 227–235.
20. YAMAMURA, T. 1986. Lipoprotein and apolipoprotein abnormalities associated with ischemic heart diseases. J. Jpn. Atheroscler. Soc. **14**: 19–23 (in Japanese).
21. ETO, M., K. WATANABE & K. ISHII. 1986. Reciprocal effects of apolipoprotein E allele (ϵ2 and ϵ4) on plasma lipid levels in normolipidemic subjects. Clin. Genet. **29**: 477–484.
22. MAEDA, H., H. NAKAMURA, S. KOBORI, M. OKADA, H. NIKI, T. OGURA & S. HIRAGA. 1989. Molecular cloning of a human apolipoprotein E variant: E5 (Glu 3→ Lys 3). J. Biochem. **105**: 491–493.
23. MAEDA, H., H. NAKAMURA, S. KOBORI, M. OKADA, H. MORI, H. NIKI, T. OGURA & S. HIROGA. 1989. Identification of human apolipoprotein E variant gene: apolipoprotein E7 (Glu 244,245→Lys 244,245). J. Biochem. **105**: 51–54.
24. FUNAHASHI, T., S. YOKOYAMA & A. YAMAMOTO. 1989. Association of apolipoprotein E with the low density lipoprotein receptor: demonstration of its co-operativity on lipid microemul-sion particles. J. Biochem. **105**: 582–587.
25. WEISGRABER, K. H., T. L. INNERARITY, K. J. HARDER, R. W. MAHLEY, R. W. MILNE, Y. MARCEL & J. T. SPARROW. 1983. The receptor-binding domain of human apolipoprotein E. Monoclonal antibody inhibition of binding. J. Biol. Chem. **258**: 12348–12354.

Increased Triglyceride May Determine the Sites of Coronary Arterial Lesions

HARUO NAKAMURA,[a] KYOICHI MIZUNO, TOSHIO SHIBUYA,
AND KO ARAKAWA

First Department of Medicine
National Defense Medical College
Tokorozawa, Japan 359

There is much controversy on the significance of elevated triglyceride in the development of coronary atherosclerosis. Many epidemiological studies indicate that triglyceride is not an independent risk. However, clinical studies or *in vitro* studies suggest that triglyceride or certain triglyceride-rich lipoproteins might be atherogenic. In order to clarify the clinical significance of hypertriglyceridemia, we compared angiographic findings in the patients with various types of hyperlipidemia.

SUBJECTS AND METHODS

Patients with ischemic heart disease consecutively underwent coronary angiography, and then a coronary atherosclerotic index was calculated according to the sum of stenotic points as indicated in TABLE 1.

Atherosclerotic patterns were arbitrarily classified into three types. The proximal type (P type) was characterized by the presence of coronary sclerotic lesions in segments 1, 2, 5, 6, 7 and 11 (FIG. 1). The multiple type (M type) signified the presence of 7 or more stenotic sites. The long type (L type) implied the presence of stenosis longer than 2 cm (TABLE 2).

Hyperlipidemias were classified according to the criteria of the World Health Organization (WHO), based on the determination of plasma lipids in the fasting state. Apolipoproteins were also measured by the method of the single radial immunodiffusion.

RESULTS

Clinical profiles of each type of hyperlipidemia indicated that there were no significant differences in age, male and female ratio, height, weight, smoking habits, incidence of hypertension, and diabetes mellitus.

Total cholesterol level was mildly elevated in type IIa and IIb, while triglyceride was also mildly elevated in type IIb and type IV.

HDL-cholesterol was significantly decreased in type IV. However, fasting blood sugar and uric acid level were not significantly different (TABLE 3).

In type IIa, a significant increase in apolipoprotein B was present, while in type IV,

[a]Address for correspondence: Haruo Nakamura, M.D., 1st Department of Medicine, National Defense Medical College, 3-2 Namiki, Tokorozawa 359, Japan.

TABLE 1. Coronary Atherosclerotic Index[a]

Stenosis (%,AHA)	Point
0	0
25	1
50	2
75	3
90	4
99–100	5

[a]Sum of points (LAD max + LCX max + RCA max).

TABLE 2. Atherosclerotic Pattern

Proximal type (P):	segment 1, 2, 5, 6, 7, 11
Multiple type (M):	stenotic sites 7 or more
Long type (L):	stenosis longer than 2 cm

a significant increase in C-III and E was observed compared to those in type IIa. Apoprotein A-I levels were not significantly different in 3 types of hyperlipidemia (TABLE 4).

Atherosclerotic patterns in the coronary angiographic findings indicated that relatively increased incidence of M type and L type in type IIa was observed, while relatively increased incidence of P type in type IV was noticed.

In type IIb, P type as well as M type were frequently encountered.

It was interesting to note that coronary atherosclerotic indexes were not significantly different in the 3 hyperlipidemic types (TABLE 5).

In order to further investigate these relations, clinical profiles of the patients with 3 different atherosclerotic patterns were examined.

There were no significant differences in ages, male and female ratio, smoking habits, incidence of hypertension and diabetes mellitus.

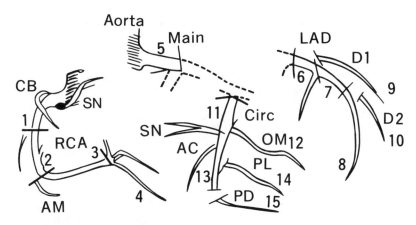

FIGURE 1. Segments of coronary artery. AC: atrial circumflex, AM: acute marginal, CB: conus branch, Circ: circumflex, D_1: first diagonal, D_2: second diagonal, LAD: left anterior descending, Main: left main, OM: obtuse marginal, PO: posterior descending, PL: posterolateral, RCA: right coronary artery, SN: sinus node.

TABLE 3. Characteristics of Subjects with Hyperlipidemias[a]

	IIa	IIb	IV
N	27	29	44
Age (y/o)	56.8 ± 10.2	52.4 ± 11.3	55.3 ± 8.0
Height (cm)	162.6 ± 7.1	164.6 ± 5.8	163.6 ± 4.9
Weight (kg)	61.4 ± 10.0	64.1 ± 8.0	61.5 ± 12.3
Smoking			
(pack, year)	36.8 ± 23.6	35.7 ± 24.5.	39.0 ± 26.8
Hypertension (+)	12	16	17
(−)	15	13	27
DM (+)	8	5	14
(IGT)	2	2	2
(−)	17	22	28
FBS (mg/dl)	106.5 ± 49.7	100.3 ± 31.4	109.7 ± 33.3
TC (mg/dl)	252.6 ± 29.5b**	262.0 ± 35.7 c**	189.4 ± 26.7b**,c**
TG (mg/dl)	113.6 ± 21.9a**,b**	198.1 ± 43.4 a**	212.1 ± 56.5b**
HDL-C (mg/dl)	40.1 ± 12.7b**	37.0 ± 9.2 c*	31.8 ± 9.6b**,c*
UA (mg/dl)	5.7 ± 1.6	6.3 ± 1.2	6.4 ± 1.3

[a]Mean ± SD. a*,b*,c* p <0.05; a**,b**,c** p <0.01.

TABLE 4. Type of Hyperlipidemia and Apoproteins[a]

	IIa	IIb	IV
Apo A-I	113.9 ± 22.1	117.4 ± 19.6	109.2 ± 24.9
A-II	26.6 ± 4.7 a*	29.6 ± 5.6 a*,c*	26.7 ± 5.7c*
B	132.1 ± 28.4b**	142.6 ± 25.5c**	108.1 ± 18.6b**,c**
C-II	4.5 ± 1.6 a*	5.6 ± 1.9 a*	5.2 ± 1.8
C-III	7.9 ± 2.2 a**,b**	11.0 ± 4.2 a**	10.8 ± 4.2b**
E	4.2 ± 1.0 a**,b*	5.3 ± 1.6 a**	4.9 ± 1.7b*

[a]Mean ± SD, mg/dl. a*,b*,c* p <0.05; a**,b**,c** p <0.01.

Significant increase in height and weight was observed in type IV. However, there were no significant differences in the body mass index.

Significant increase in apoprotein B was observed in both type IIa and IIb. There were no significant alterations in apo A-I, A-II, C-II, C-III, or E (TABLE 6).

Coronary atherosclerotic patterns were examined based on plasma lipids, other metabolic parameters, and the coronary atherosclerotic index.

The number of vessels affected and the coronary atherosclerotic index showed significant reductions in type IV compared to those in type IIa and IIb.

TABLE 5. Type of Hyperlipidemia and Coronary Atherosclerosis[a]

	IIa	IIb	IV
N	27	29	44
Vessel disease	1.5 ± 0.8	1.7 ± 0.8	1.7 ± 0.8
Type L	5 (18.5)	4 (13.8)	5 (11.4)
M	7 (25.9)	7 (24.1)	5 (11.4)
P	2 (7.4)	8 (27.6)	16 (36.4)
CAI	7.4 ± 2.9	7.4 ± 3.5	7.5 ± 3.2

[a]Mean ± SD (%).

TABLE 6. Type of Coronary Atherosclerosis and the Profile of Subjects[a]

	L	M	P
N	14	18	26
Age (y/o)	59.4 ± 8.8	57.7 ± 7.8	54.2 ± 10.6
Height (cm)	160.6 ± 4.2 b*	162.6 ± 6.0	164.1 ± 5.1b*
Weight (kg)	57.3 ± 7.5 b*	60.0 ± 7.7	63.4 ± 8.9b*
Smoking (pack-year)	41.2 ± 28.1	38.6 ± 19.6	36.0 ± 23.9
Hypertension (+)	3	10	13
(−)	1	0	1
DM (+)	4	5	6
(IGT)	1	0	1
(−)	9	13	19
Apo A-I (mg/dl)	115.7 ± 21.1	111.8 ± 23.6	115.6 ± 24.9
A-II (mg/dl)	27.1 ± 4.9	26.0 ± 5.6	27.6 ± 6.2
B (mg/dl)	129.4 ± 20.0b*	130.8 ± 30.7c*	114.0 ± 21.3b*,c*
C-II (mg/dl)	4.7 ± 2.1	4.5 ± 1.6	5.2 ± 2.1
C-III (mg/dl)	8.7 ± 3.7	9.3 ± 3.4	10.1 ± 4.3
E (mg/dl)	4.7 ± 1.1	4.4 ± 1.6	5.1 ± 1.9

[a]Mean ± SD. b*,c* $p < 0.05$.

Fasting blood sugar and uric acid levels were not significantly different in the 3 atherosclerotic patterns.

It was again interesting to note that the triglyceride level alone was increased significantly in P type without reducing HDL-cholesterol (TABLE 7).

DISCUSSION

The present study indicated the close relationship between hypertriglyceridemia and the sites of coronary arterial lesions.

As was pointed out previously, mildly or moderately elevated cholesterol increased coronary atherosclerotic lesions with multiple or long stenoses.[1]

Since there were no systematic observations on plasma lipid and atherosclerotic pattern, it was interesting to observe that proximal atherosclerosis was revealed mostly in hypertriglyceridemic subjects. And those patients showed no significant reduction in HDL-cholesterol in spite of having a reduced coronary atherosclerotic index compared to those in pure hypercholesterolemia and combined hyperlipidemia.

TABLE 7. Type of Coronary Atherosclerosis[a]

	L	M	P
FBS (mg/dl)	116.4 ± 58.3	110.4 ± 51.1	96.7 ± 18.3
TC (mg/dl)	235.1 ± 27.6b*	252.6 ± 55.5c*	212.2 ± 34.0b*,c*
TG (mg/dl)	165.1 ± 60.0b*	159.9 ± 51.5c*	206.5 ± 62.3b*,c*
HDL-C (mg/dl)	35.6 ± 9.5	37.7 ± 12.2	34.2 ± 9.2
UA (mg/dl)	5.7 ± 1.2	5.8 ± 1.9	6.4 ± 1.4
Vessel disease	1.9 ± 0.8 b**	2.2 ± 0.8 c**	1.1 ± 0.3b**,c**
CAI	8.9 ± 3.4 b**	10.1 ± 3.4 c**	4.5 ± 1.7b**,c**

[a]Mean ± SD. b*,c* $p < 0.05$; b**,c** $p < 0.01$.

CONCLUSION

Atherosclerotic lesions in the proximal portion of coronary artery were found frequently in the patients with hypertriglyceridemia based on the examination of angiographic findings and plasma lipids.

REFERENCE

1.   SHIBUYA, T.1988. Characteristics of coronary angiographic findings in diabetes mellitus and each type of hyperlipidemia. Jpn. J. Med. **77**(4): 472–480.

Diffuse Intimal Thickening and Other Mesenchymal Changes

YUTAKA NAGAI,[a] TETSU YAMANE,[b] HIDETO WATANABE,[a]
AND YOJI YOSHIDA[b]

[a]Department of Tissue Physiology
Medical Research Institute
Tokyo Medical and Dental University
2-3-10 Kandasurugadai, Chiyoda-ku
Tokyo 101, Japan
and
[b]Department of Pathology
Yamanashi Medical College
Yamanashi 409-38, Japan

INTRODUCTION

Atherosclerosis is a disease of the arteries that is known to be a focalized growth of the vessel wall into the vessel lumen. A characteristic feature of the atherosclerotic lesion is a massive deposition of lipid within the affected tissue, where inflammatory cells such as monocyte-macrophages are infiltrated forming foam cells. In addition, in the early stage of atherogenesis, proliferation of smooth muscle cells in the intima of the artery is known to be significant. Although intimal smooth muscle cells originate from the media, the cells show high levels of growth activity and production of interstitial collagens compared to those in the media.[1]

Our previous studies on the stromal reaction in inflammatory states such as articular tissue destruction in rheumatoid arthritis and skin diseases have shown that infiltrated polymorphonuclear leukocytes release factor(s) (PMN-factor), the major component of which is now known to be interleukin-1β (IL-1β)[2], stimulate productions of collagenase[3] and prostaglandin E_2 (PGE$_2$)[4] of connective tissue cells. These include synovial cells, fibroblasts, chondrocytes,[5] and even hepatocytes. Both PMN and monocytes from peripheral blood do not contain any stimulating factor of this sort, but can be activated with lipopolysaccharide or zymosan, indicating that inflammatory cells acquire the factor(s) during and/or after infiltration into tissues. In general, members of the IL-1 family affect connective tissue cells to stimulate cell proliferation and productions of collagenase and PGE$_2$, but suppress productions of both collagenous and noncollagenous proteins. In this article, we will discuss the effects of inflammatory factors on the cell growth rate and collagen production of smooth muscle cells in culture, and immunolocalization of IL-1, interstitial collagenase and tissue inhibitor of metalloproteinases (TIMP) in atherosclerotic lesions.

Effects of Inflammatory Factors on the Production of Collagen and Metalloproteinases by Smooth Muscle Cells in Culture

Smooth muscle cells isolated from the thoracic aorta of new born babies obtained at autopsy were cultured in Dulbecco's modified Eagle's medium containing 10% fetal bovine serum with or without recombinant IL-1α, β (10^{-9} g/ml each, Otsuka Pharma-

71

ceutical Co., Tokushima), human PMN-factor (50 μl/ml) or platelet-derived growth factor (PDGF) for 3 days and collagenase activity in the media was determined using FITC-labeled bovine type I collagen as a substrate. To determine DNA synthesis and collagen production, incorporations of ^{3}H-thymidine into DNA fraction (for 2 hr) and of ^{3}H-Pro into collagen (bacterial collagenase-sensitive) fraction (for 24 hr) were analyzed respectively.[6]

DNA synthesis of smooth muscle cells was markedly stimulated by the addition of PDGF (twofold) or IL-1α (1.5-fold), but not by the other two stimulants used. There were no significant differences in collagen synthesis/cell employed with or without any stimulants, except for IL-1α, which slightly enhanced total protein synthesis of the cells, and relative ratios of collagen/total protein synthesized remains constant (about 5%) in all the cases tested. The same was true with relative ratios of collagen types synthesized by the cells, that is, type I (84%), type III (15%), and type V (detectable).

We also tried to see the effect of inflammatory factors on smooth muscle cell collagenase production by determining apparent enzyme activity in conditioned media. However, no enzyme activity was detected in any case, which is quite a contrast to the case of skin fibroblasts employed as positive control that showed a marked increase in colla-

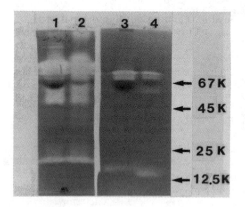

FIGURE 1. Typical patterns of the zymogram of proteinases in day-3 conditioned medium (HB102) of human aortic smooth muscle cells *(lanes 1 and 3)* and skin fibroblasts *(lanes 2 and 4)* after *(lanes 1 and 2)* or before *(lanes 3 and 4)* activation with trypsin.

genase activity under the same experimental conditions as reported. The reason for no detectable collagenase activity in conditioned media was ascribed to the presence of an excess amount of TIMP produced by smooth muscle cells, which was confirmed by an inhibition test for exogenously added enzyme. Smooth muscle cells produce metalloproteinases as much as fibroblasts do, as shown in FIGURE 1.

Immunolocalization of Collagenase, TIMP, and IL-1

Since we noticed that smooth muscle cells in culture, which are the synthetic type in contrast to cells in media (contractile), produced an unexpectedly large amount of TIMP regardless of the presence or absence of inflammatory factors, and that this may partly explain the progressing accumulation of interstitial collagens in the intima in atherosclerosis, we tried to see the distributions of collagenase, TIMP, and IL-1 in atherosclerotic lesions by using the peroxidase-antiperoxidase staining method.[7]

Tissue specimens of ten cases (2 years old–83 years old) were analyzed by using monoclonal antibodies to human skin collagenase, rTIMP (a gift from Toray Research

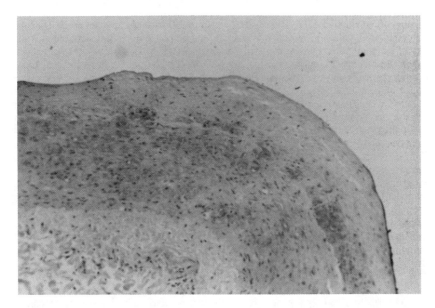

FIGURE 2. A light micrograph immunostained for interstitial collagenase. An aortic tissue specimen with atherosclerosis (39-year-old female) showing dense distribution of collagenase in the diffuse intimal thickening region and focal distributions around foam-cell-rich regions.

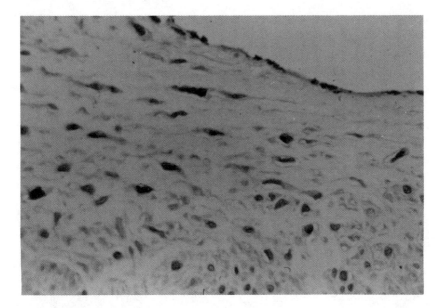

FIGURE 3. A light micrograph immunostained for interstitial collagenase. A high power view of artery tissue with severe thickening (2-year-old female) showing active production of collagenase by highly populated intimal smooth muscle cells. The cytoplasm of endothelial cells was also stained with anti-collagenase antibodies.

Institute, Kamakura) and PMN elastase and polyclonal antibodies to human rIL-1α and β. All antibodies were prepared in our laboratory, except for anti-rIL-1 antibodies, which were kindly supplied by Otsuka Pharmaceutical Co.

In atherosclerotic lesions, collagenase was densely distributed in the musculoelastic layer and focally in the surroundings of the atheroma, especially round cell- or macrophage-rich regions, although the enzyme is diffusely distributed in the medial smooth muscle layer (FIG. 2). In the case of infant tissue where highly populated cells were present, the cytoplasm of individual cells including endothelial cells was well stained with anti-collagenase antibody (FIG. 3). With advancing age, however, collagenase deposition became much less in the intima, except for the regions of the atheroma and musculoelastic layer where dense deposition of the enzyme was focally observed. This suggests that cells present in the surroundings of the atheroma and infiltrating cells in the intima are actively producing collagenase. In the lesion of diffuse intimal thickening, collagenase in the media decreased with age, but remained in the intima where some cells in the fibrous cap showed positive.

In contrast to collagenase, TIMP was densely distributed in the media and focally in the musculoelastic layer, showing that proliferating smooth muscle cells are actively producing TIMP (FIG. 4). Much less TIMP was detected in the upper layer of thickened intima.

To examine a possible involvement of inflammatory factor(s) in collagenase production by cells present in the atherosclerotic lesion, serial sections of tissue specimens were stained for IL-1α and β. Both IL-1α and β were similarly distributed in the thickened intima, mainly localizing in the area of foam-cell-rich regions and musculoelastic layer where dense staining for collagenase was observed (FIG. 5), strongly suggesting that cells

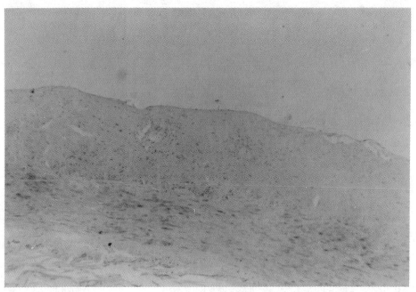

FIGURE 4. A light micrograph immunostained for TIMP. The same tissue specimen as in FIGURE 2 showing dense distributions in the media and musculoelastic layer where proliferating smooth muscle cells were migrating into the intima, but much less around foam-cell-rich regions.

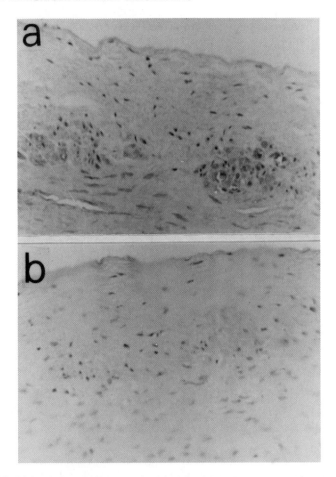

FIGURE 5. Light micrographs immunostained for interstitial collagenase and IL-1β. A high power view of aortic tissue with atherosclerosis (39-year-old female) showing focal distributions of collagenase around foam-cell-rich regions (a) where IL-1β was also detected selectively (b).

present in these regions are under the influence of IL-1-producing cells, probably macrophages.

Of particular interest in this study was that some cells in the deep layer of the thickened intima and in the inner side of the atheroma were stained with anti-PMN elastase antibody. This suggests that PMN may also be a candidate cell participating in the pathophysiology of atherosclerosis or that intimal smooth muscle cells in the lesion had acquired a capacity to produce an elastase-like enzyme immunoreactive with anti-PMN elastase antibody, which may also contribute to the progression of atherosclerosis. Further studies along this line are now in progress in our laboratory.

REFERENCES

1. YOSHIDA, Y., M. MITSUMATA, T. YAMANE, M. TOMIKAWA & K. NISHIDA. 1988. Arch. Pathol. Lab. Med. **112:** 987–996.

2. MORI, S., F. GOTO, K. GOTO, S. OHKAWARA, S. MAEDA, K. SHIMADA & M. YOSHINAGA.
    1988. Biochem. Biophys. Res. Commun. **150:** 1237–1243.
3. HASHIDA, R., K. TERATO, K. MIYAMOTO, T. MORIMOTO, H. HORI & Y. NAGAI. 1982. Biomed.
    Res. **3:** 506–516.
4. HASHIDA, R., S. KOBAYASHI, H. SHIROTA, K. YOSHIMATSU, S. OHSAWA, H. HORI, S. HATTORI
    & Y. NAGAI. 1984. Prostaglandins **27:** 697–709.
5. OHSAWA, S., H. HORI, R. HATA & Y. NAGAI. 1984. Biomed. Res. **5:** 177–186.
6. HATA, R., Y. NINOMIYA & Y. NAGAI. 1980. Biochemistry **19:** 169–176.
7. ARAI, K., K. UEHARA & Y. NAGAI. 1989. Jpn. J. Cancer Res. **80:** 840–847.

Endothelial-Dependent Mechanisms of Leukocyte Adhesion in Inflammation and Atherosclerosis[a]

MICHAEL A. GIMBRONE, JR.,[b] MICHAEL P. BEVILACQUA,
AND MYRON I. CYBULSKY

Vascular Research Division
Department of Pathology
Brigham and Women's Hospital
and
Harvard Medical School
Boston, Massachusetts 02115

INTRODUCTION

Adhesion of circulating leukocytes to the blood vessel wall is an essential component of acute and chronic inflammatory reactions, and various vascular disease processes, including vasculitis, allograft rejection, ischemia-reperfusion injury, and atherosclerosis. In particular, the focal adherence of blood monocytes at certain sites in the aortic tree, and their subsequent transmigration into the intima, appear to be consistent early events in the formation of foam cell-rich lesions during atherogenesis in humans and experimental animals.[1-16] There is increasing evidence that vascular endothelial cells play an active role in these processes. Our research group has been especially interested in defining endothelial-dependent mechanisms of leukocyte adhesion, and exploring their relevance for human vascular pathophysiology. In this paper, we shall summarize our recent progress in characterizing inducible endothelial cell surface structures involved in leukocyte adhesion—endothelial-leukocyte adhesion molecules ("ELAMs"). We will also provide a brief summary of the pathophysiologic implications of leukocyte-endothelial interactions for the atherosclerotic disease process, and indicate promising future directions for research in this area.

Endothelial-Dependent Leukocyte Adhesion: the ELAM Hypothesis

As an *in vitro* experimental model, our laboratory has used cultured human endothelial cells (HEC)[17] in standardized monolayer adhesion assays,[18-20] to study factors that can alter leukocyte-endothelial adhesion and to explore the molecular mechanisms involved. In particular, we have examined the hypothesis that certain inflammatory substances can

[a]This research was supported primarily by grants from the National Institutes of Health. Michael P. Bevilacqua, M.D., Ph.D. is a Pew Scholar and Myron I. Cybulsky, M.D. is a fellow of the Canadian Medical Research Council.

[b]Address for correspondence: Dr. Michael A. Gimbrone, Jr., Department of Pathology, Brigham and Women's Hospital, 75 Francis Street, Boston, MA 02115.

act directly on vascular endothelial cells to increase the adhesion of blood leukocytes.[19,21] We initially found that human monocyte-derived interleukin-1 (IL-1) could act on cultured HEC in a time- and protein synthesis-dependent fashion to increase the adhesion of human blood polymorphonuclear leukocytes (PMN), monocytes, and related cell lines (HL-60 and U937).[19,21] Subsequently, we studied the effects of other cytokines, including recombinant IL-1-α, IL-1-β, tumor necrosis factor (TNF), and lymphotoxin (LT) as well as bacterial endotoxin (lipopolysaccharide, LPS).[22] Other laboratories have made similar observations using various mediators and leukocyte types.[23-28] Together, these studies suggested that "activation" of vascular endothelium by certain inflammatory stimuli results in increased expression of cell surface adhesive molecules that can bind blood leukocytes. We have referred to these putative structures as "endothelial-leukocyte adhesion molecules" (ELAMs).[21] We reasoned that the inducible expression of ELAMs by the endothelial lining of blood vessels could contribute to the spatial and temporal patterns of leukocyte adhesion observed in various pathophysiological settings *in vivo*. Further, we envisioned that a recognition mechanism involving leukocyte-specific ELAMs, functioning as receptors for ligands on the surface of different leukocytes types (PMN, monocyte, lymphocyte) could add additional selectivity to this process. To test the "ELAM hypothesis" directly and to better define cytokine-induced alterations in endothelial cell surface properties, we developed monoclonal antibodies to cytokine-activated HEC.[29] This strategy has yielded useful reagents for the immunochemical and functional characterization of putative ELAMs *in vitro*, their molecular cloning, and investigation of their expression in human and animal tissues in pathophysiologic settings.

Identification of Endothelial-Leukocyte Adhesion Molecule 1 (ELAM-1)

Studies by Bevilacqua and co-workers[29-32] led to the characterization of two monoclonal antibodies, designated H4/18 and H18/7, which recognize an inducible endothelial cell surface protein. Its expression is upregulated from undetectable levels on unstimulated HEC by endotoxin and the same cytokine mediators (IL-1, TNF, LT) that act on HEC to increase leukocyte adhesion. Peak HEC expression of the epitopes recognized by H4/18 and H18/7 occurs after approximately four hours of stimulation and is correlated with peak expression of HEC adhesiveness for leukocytes. Other cytokines, including interferon-α, -β, or γ, and IL-2, do not stimulate leukocyte adhesion or monoclonal antibody binding to HEC. Various other cell types including blood cells (PMN, monocytes, lymphocytes, HL-60 cells), before and after stimulation with phorbol ester, as well as cultured human dermal fibroblasts, before and after incubation with IL-1, fail to bind these monoclonal antibodies.

Immunoprecipitation of total cell extracts from metabolically labeled IL-1 or TNF-stimulated HEC with monoclonal antibodies H18/7 and H4/18 yielded two polypeptides (Mr 115kD, 95kD on reduced SDS-PAGE) which were not detected in unstimulated HEC.[30] Exhaustive treatment of HEC lysates by H18/7 removed all H4/18 reactive polypeptides and vice-versa, thus indicating that these two monoclonal antibodies were recognizing the same molecule in cytokine-activated HEC.

When tested in leukocyte adhesion assays, Mab H4/18 partially blocked HL-60 cell adhesion to IL-1-activated HEC, but failed to inhibit PMN adhesion.[30] In contrast, H18/7 significantly and consistently blocked the adhesion of both HL-60 cells and PMN to IL-1-activated HEC.[30] In contrast, neither monoclonal antibody appeared to be effective in blocking peripheral blood monocyte or lymphocyte adhesion to HEC, under basal or cytokine activated conditions. Based on the ability of H18/7 to block the adhesion of PMN and HL-60 cells to cytokine-activated HEC, we have designated the molecule recognized by this antibody as "endothelial-leukocyte adhesion molecule 1" (ELAM-1).[30,32] Several characteristics distinguish ELAM-1 from previously identified cell surface adhesive struc-tures, such as platelet glycoprotein IIb/IIIa-like proteins, intercellular adhesion molecule 1 (ICAM-1), and HLA-DR, which also are expressed on endothelial cells.[33,34] These characteristics include: 1) the lack of basal (*i.e.*, unstimulated) endothelial expression of ELAM-1; 2) the mediator specificity and kinetics of its induction; and 3) its molecular weight characteristics.

In order to establish the primary structure of ELAM-1 and to clarify its potential relationship to other adhesion proteins, in collaboration with Dr. Brian Seed's laboratory, we undertook its molecular cloning. Using a monoclonal antibody-directed, expression-cloning strategy in COS cells,[35] a full-length complementary DNA (cDNA) for ELAM-1 was isolated.[31,32] Cells transiently transfected with the putative ELAM-1 clone expressed a cell surface structure recognized by both ELAM-1-specific monoclonal antibodies (H4/ 18 and H18/7) and supported the adhesion of isolated human blood PMN and HL-60 cells. Expression of ELAM-1 transcripts in cultured human endothelial cells was inducible by cytokines, reaching a maximum at 2–4 hours and decaying by 24 hours. Cell surface expression of ELAM-1 protein paralleled that of the mRNA. The primary sequence of ELAM-1, predicted from its cDNA, indicated a transmembrane protein whose extracel-lular portion consisted of a complex mosaic of three different domain types: an amino-terminal lectin-like domain, an EGF domain, and six tandem repetitive motifs (about 60 amino acids each) related to those found in complement regulatory proteins. These unique structural characteristics, interestingly, were found to be shared by the recently cloned mouse protein MEL-14,[36,37] a lymphocyte cell surface homing receptor, and a human platelet granule membrane protein GMP-140.[38] The latter protein also has been recently described in endothelial cells, and, in both cell types appears to be rapidly mobilized, upon activation by thrombin and other stimuli, from storage granules to the cell surface (hence, its alternative designation PADGEM, "platelet activation dependent granule-external membrane protein").[39] The identification of these three cell surface molecules of similar, complex domain structure thus appears to describe a new gene family, for which the name "Vascular Selectins" has been proposed.[40] Two of the members of this family, ELAM-1 and MEL-14 antigen, have a defined role in leukocyte-endothelial adhesion. ELAM-1, expressed on activated endothelium, mediates the adhesion of blood neutro-phils, while MEL-14 antigen, a molecule expressed by granulocytes, monocytes, and lymphocyte subsets, mediates lymphocyte adhesion to specialized lymph node endothelial cells. Recently, GMP-140 expression on the surface of thrombin-activated human plate-lets has been shown to support the adhesion of neutrophils and monocytes.[39] Its potential role in blood cell-endothelial adhesive interactions is now being investigated. Studies also are in progress to determine the adhesive function(s) of the various components of the complex mosaic structure of ELAM-1, to identify its interacting ligand(s) on leukocytes, and to identify homologous ELAMs in other species.

Using monoclonal antibodies to immunohistochemically stain human tissues, mi-crovascular endothelium has been shown to express ELAM-1 transiently in.certain patho-logical settings, in particular acute and chronic inflammatory processes in which cytokine generation is thought to occur.[41–43] Interestingly, ELAM-1 is not expressed in unin-flamed endothelial cells in various vessel types nor in other normal tissue components. To date, ELAM-1 has not been detected in the endothelium associated with human atherosclerotic plaques at various stages of progression (M. Munro, personal communi-cation). Studies with explants of human foreskin, which have been treated *ex vivo* with recombinant cytokines, indicate that the expression of ELAM-1 is topographically limited to the postcapillary venular region of the microcirculation.[44] An experimental animal model of ELAM-1 expression in the baboon has been established,[45] which should lend itself to further studies of the expression of ELAM-1 in various pathophysiological set-tings.

Expression of a Monocyte-Selective ELAM in Atherogenesis (ATHERO-ELAM)

To further explore the ELAM hypothesis and to facilitate its *in vivo* testing in well defined experimental models of inflammation and atherosclerosis, the existence of inducible, leukocyte-selective adhesion mechanisms in rabbit endothelium has been investigated both *in vitro* and *in vivo*. Cybulsky and Gimbrone[46,47] have reported the immunochemical identification of a putative "monocyte-directed ELAM" (ATHERO-ELAM) that is inducible by bacterial endotoxin in cultured large vessel endothelial cells from New Zealand White rabbits. Monoclonal antibody Rb1/9 recognizes this cell surface structure in living cell binding assays, and differentially blocks the attachment of monocyte-like U937 cells, but not promelocytic HL-60 cells, to the hyperadhesive "activated" endothelial monolayer.[46] Immunochemical studies with Rb1/9 have identified two polypeptide species (Mr118, 98; on reduced SDS-PAGE) in both metabolically labelled and surface-iodinated rabbit endothelial cells. Further structural characterization of this putative rabbit MONO-ELAM is in progress.

Recently, evidence has been obtained for the expression of this ATHERO-ELAM *in vivo* in rabbit aortic endothelium during atherogenesis.[47] The intact endothelial covering of early, foam cell-rich intimal lesions in New Zealand White rabbits, maintained on a hypercholesterolemic diet for 8 to 12 weeks, shows specific immunohistochemical staining with monoclonal antibody Rb1/9. In the same animals, adjacent uninvolved aortic endothelium fails to stain with Rb1/9, as does the aortic lining of normal, dietary control animals. A similar pattern of lesion-localized, endothelial-selective staining is also observed in developing atherosclerotic lesions in Watanabe heritable hyperlipidemic (WHHL) rabbits. Taken together, these observations indicate that this putative ATHERO-ELAM is inducibly expressed in rabbit aortic endothelium during early lesion formation in both dietary-induced and congenital hyperlipidemic models of atherosclerosis. The possible pathogenetic role of this or related ELAMs in monocyte-vessel wall interactions in atherogenesis, as well as their potential diagnostic and/or therapeutic usefulness as markers of endothelial dysfunction in early lesions are worthy of further investigation.

Other Endothelial-Dependent Mechanisms Involved in Leukocyte Adhesion

In addition to inducible cell surface adhesion molecules, endothelial cells also can synthesize a wide variety of soluble substances that potentially can influence leukocyte interactions with the blood vessel wall.[48] These include: growth factors (*e.g.*, PDGF), cytokines (*e.g.*, GM-CSF), arachidonate metabolites (*e.g.*, lipoxygenase products), and other lipid mediators (*e.g.*, PAF). The overall biological effect of these mediators tends to be *pro-adhesive*, usually through leukocyte-directed actions. Several laboratories have also reported on the isolation and partial characterization of both lipid and peptide chemoattractants from the vessel wall and cultured endothelial (and/or smooth muscle cells),[49-56] several of which show monocyte-selective effects *in vitro*.

Recent studies indicate that the endothelial cell also can be a source of *anti-adhesive* factors. In particular, Gimbrone and co-workers[57,58] have identified a soluble product of human enodthelial cells that can inhibit the adhesion of human blood leukocytes to hyperadhesive, cytokine-activated endothelial monolayers. Purification of this "leukocyte adhesion inhibitor" (LAI) has revealed that it is a novel homologue of interleukin-8 (IL-8),[58] an inflammatory cytokine that previously had been characterized solely as a neutrophil-activating factor and chemoattractant.[59] Thus, it is becoming apparent that a complex interplay of pro-adhesive and anti-adhesive factors potentially can influence leukocyte adhesion at the endothelial interface with circulating blood.

Pathophysiologic Implications and Future Directions

Interaction of blood leukocytes with the cellular components of the blood vessel wall (endothelium and smooth muscle) clearly plays a prominent role in the pathobiology of atherosclerosis and its complications. Various leukocyte types are associated with atherosclerotic lesions at different stages in their life history, and the pathophysiological implications of their presence appear to be multiple. The propensity for circulating blood monocytes to adhere to the endothelial lining in the region of "young lesions," their subsequent emigration into the subendothelial space and transformation into foam cells, constitute important morphologic correlates of the atherogenic process. Careful immunohistochemical, ultrastructural, and autoradiographic studies in various animal models and human tissues have helped to establish the relationship between adhering/migrating monocytes and the foam cells that progressively accumulate in atherosclerotic lesions. In addition, cell biological and molecular biological approaches have suggested multiple potential roles for this unusual macrophage population in lesion progression, including: the localized generation of growth factors, (*e.g.*, PDGF, FGF), cytokines (*e.g.*, IL-1, TNF), coagulation and fibrinolytic factors, arachidonate-derived mediators, and reactive oxygen products.[14,48] Recent immunohistochemical studies have also provided evidence for a second type of mononuclear leukocyte in the human atherosclerotic plaque, the T-lymphocyte.[60] The pathophysiological implications of this subpopulation of infiltrating leukocytes, which is virtually absent from normal human arteries, also are multiple. Cytokines, such as gamma-interferon, released by activated lymphocytes can modulate the functions of various cell types, including vascular endothelium and smooth muscles.[48] In particular the inducible expression of Class II MHC antigens on these cells may modify their immunological status.[34] The observation that smooth muscle cells in atherosclerotic plaques (but not in normal arteries) express HLA-DR strongly suggests that this humoral cell-cell interaction can occur.[60] Lymphocyte products similarly can influence the metabolism of lipoproteins by macrophages and other cells. All these interactions are potentially relevant to the progression/regression of more advanced lesions. The third leukocyte type involved in the atherosclerotic process is the neutrophil. Although there is little, if any, clearly defined role for neutrophils in lesion initiation (except perhaps transiently in certain mechanical injury models), they are a feature of the complicated plaque, in which cellular necrosis and neovascularization is occurring. Their route of influx may involve the newly formed microvessels at the base of the plaque, and their presence may simply signify ongoing acute inflammation. Neutrophil-endothelial interactions play a prominent role in the tissue injury that often accompanies the clinical problem of thrombosis/ischemia/reperfusion as a complication of occlusive atherosclerotic vascular disease.

Although the leukocyte types found in lesions and their potential functional implications are multiple and diverse, all of these interactions share a common initial event— adhesion of a circulating blood leukocyte to the endothelial surface. Recently, we have gained considerable insight into the cellular and molecular mechanisms responsible for enhanced neutrophil adhesion to cytokine-activated endothelium. In this case, the interplay of pro-adhesive and anti-adhesive endothelial mechanisms appears to contribute to local regulation of adhesion. Recent evidence also suggests that analogous endothelial-dependent mechanisms may be responsible for the localized adhesion of blood monocytes in early lesion formation. The inducible expression of a putative monocyte-directed ELAM in the aortic lining of hypercholesterolemic rabbits suggests a number of experimentally testable questions: 1) Does monocyte ELAM expression *precede* foam cell accumulation? 2) Is ELAM expression *necessary* for monocyte attachment, and can foam cell accumulation be blocked by antibodies directed to these endothelial surface receptors? 3) What are the stimuli for monocyte ELAM expression and what relationship do they bear to known atherosclerotic risk factors? 4) Can this monocyte ELAM provide a marker of early "endothelial dysfunction" that can be used for diagnostic purposes? 5) Are selective monocyte adhesion inhibitors produced by the normal blood vessel wall? 6) What influences the balance of adhesive surface changes, chemoattractants, and adhesion inhibitors at various stages of atherosclerotic lesion progression/regression? The answers to these and other questions related to the endothelial-dependent mechanisms of leukocyte adhesion should provide new pathogenetic insights, and hopefully, useful diagnostic and therapeutic tools for the treatment of atherosclerotic and inflammatory vascular diseases.

ACKNOWLEDGMENTS

We thank our colleagues and collaborators and the technical support staff of the Vascular Research Division, Department of Pathology, who have contributed in essential ways to these studies, and Randi White for her help in preparation of the manuscript.

REFERENCES

1. GERRITY, R. G., H. K. NAITO, M. RICHARDSON & C. J. SCHWARTZ. 1979. Dietary induced atherogenesis in swine: morphology of the intima in prelesion stages. Am. J. Pathol. **95:** 775–792.
2. GERRITY, R. G. 1981. The role of the monocyte in atherogenesis: I. Transition of blood-borne monocytes into foam cells in fatty lesions. Am. J. Pathol. **103:** 181–190.
3. GERRITY, R. G. 1981. The role of the monocyte in atherogenesis: II. Migration of foam cells from atherosclerotic lesions. Am. J. Pathol. **103:** 191–200.
4. JORIS, I., T. ZAND, J. J. NUNNARI, F. J. KROLIKOWSKI & G. MAJNO. 1983. Studies on the pathogenesis of atherosclerosis. I. Adhesion of mononuclear cells in the aorta of hypercholesterolemic rats. Am. J. Pathol. **113:** 341–358.
5. KLURFELD, D. M. 1985. Identification of foam cells in human atherosclerotic lesions as macrophages using monoclonal antibodies. Arch. Pathol. Lab. Med. **109:** 445–449.
6. SCHAFFNER, T., K. TAYLOR, E. J. BARTUCCI et al. 1980. Arterial foam cells with distinctive immunomorphologic and histochemical features of macrophages. Am. J. Pathol. **100:** 57–80.
7. GOWN, A. M., T. TSUKADA & R. ROSS. 1986. Human atherosclerosis. II. Immunocytochemical analysis of the cellular composition of human atherosclerotic lesions. Am. J. Pathol. **125:** 191–207.
8. FAGGIOTTO, A., R. ROSS & L. HARKER. 1984. Studies of hypercholesterolemia in the nonhuman primate I. Changes that lead to fatty streak formation. Arteriosclerosis **4:** 323–340.
9. FAGGIOTTO, A. & R. ROSS. 1984. Studies of hypercholesterolemia in the nonhuman primate. II. Fatty streak conversion into fibrous plaque. Arteriosclerosis **4:** 341–356.
10. FOWLER, S., H. SHIO & N. J. HALEY. 1979. Characterization of lipid-laden aortic cells from cholesterol-fed rabbits. IV. Investigation of macrophage-like properties of aortic cell populations. Lab. Invest. **41:** 372–378.
11. WATANABE, T., M. HIRATA, Y. YOSHIKAWA, Y. NAGAFUCHI, H. TOYOSHIMA & T. WATANABE. 1985. Role of macrophages in atherosclerosis: Sequential observations of cholesterol-induced rabbit aortic lesion by the immunoperoxidase technique using monoclonal antimacrophage antibody. Lab. Invest. **53:** 80–90.
12. SCHWARTZ, C. J., E. A. SPRAGUE, J. L. KELLEY, A. J. VALENTE & C. A. SUENRAM. 1985. Aortic intimal monocyte recruitment in the normal and hypercholesterolemic baboon (Papio cynocephalus): An ultrastructural study: Implications in atherogenesis. Virchows Arch. (Pathol. Anat.) **405:** 175–191.
13. LEWIS, C. J., R. G. TAYLOR & W. G. JEROME. 1985. Foam cell characteristics in coronary arteries and aortas of White Carneau pigeons with moderate hypercholesterolemia. Ann. N.Y. Acad. Sci. **454:** 91–100.

14. Ross, R. 1986. The pathogenesis of atherosclerosis—an update. N. Engl. J. Med. **314:** 488–500.

15. Davies, P. F. 1986. Vascular cell interactions with special reference to the pathogenesis of atherosclerosis. Lab. Invest. **55:** 5–24.

16. Munro, J. M. & R. S. Cotran. 1988. The pathogenesis of atherosclerosis: Atherogenesis and inflammation. Lab. Invest. **58(3):** 249–261.

17. Gimbrone, M. A. Jr. 1976. Culture of vascular endothelium. *In* Progress in Hemostasis and Thrombosis. T. Spaet, Ed. Vol. 3: 1–28. Grune and Stratton. New York, NY.

18. Gimbrone, M. A., Jr. & M. R. Buchanan. 1982. Interactions of platelets and leukocytes with vascular endothelium: *in vitro* studies. *In* Symposium on Endothelium. A. P. Fishman, Ed. Ann. N.Y. Acad. Sci. **401:** 171–183.

19. Bevilacqua, M. P., J. S. Pober, M. E. Wheeler, R. S. Cotran & M. A. Gimbrone, Jr. 1985. Interleukin 1 (IL-1) acts on cultured vascular endothelium to increase the adhesion of polymorphonuclear leukocytes, monocytes and related cell lines. J. Clin. Invest. **76(5):** 2003–2011.

20. Luscinskas, F. W., A. F. Brock, M. A. Arnaout & M. A. Gimbrone, Jr. 1989. Endothelial-leukocyte adhesion molecule-1 (ELAM-1)-dependent and leukocyte CD11/18-dependent mechanisms contribute to polymorphonuclear leukocyte adhesion to cytokine-activated human vascular endothelium. J. Immunol. **142:** 2257–2263.

21. Bevilacqua, M. P., M. E. Wheeler, J. S. Pober, W. Fiers, D. L. Mendrick, R. S. Cotran & M. A. Gimbrone, Jr. 1985. Interleukin 1 (IL-1) activation of vascular endothelium: Effects on procoagulant activity and leukocyte adhesion. Am. J. Pathol. **121:** 393–403.

22. Bevilacqua, M. P., M. E. Wheeler, J. S. Pober, W. Fiers, D. L. Mendrick, R. S. Cotran & M. A. Gimbrone, Jr. 1987. Endothelial-dependent mechanisms of leukocyte adhesion: Regulation by interleukin 1 and tumor necrosis factor. *In* Leukocyte Emigration and Its Sequelae. H. Movat, Ed. 79–93. Karger, Basel.

23. Dunn, C. J. & W. E. Fleming. 1985. The role of interleukin 1 in the inflammatory response with particular reference to endothelial cell-leukocyte adhesion. *In* The Physiologic, Metabolic and Immunologic Actions of Interleukin 1. M. J. Kluger, J. J. Oppenheim & M. C. Powanda, Eds. 45–54. Alan R. Liss. New York, NY.

24. Schleimer, R. P. & B. K. Rutledge. 1986. Cultured human vascular endothelial cells acquire adhesiveness for neutrophils after stimulation with interleukin 1, endotoxin, and tumor-promoting phorbol diesters. J. Immunol. **136:** 649–654.

25. Gamble, J. R., J. M. Harlen, S. J. Klebanoff, A. F. Lopes & M. A. Vadas. 1985. Stimulation of the adherence of neutrophils to umbilical vein endothelium by human recombinant tumor necrosis factor. Proc. Nat. Acad. Sci. USA **82:** 8667–8671.

26. Pohlman, T. H., K. A. Stanness, P. G. Beatty, H. D. Ochs & J. M. Harlen. 1986. An endothelial cell surface factor(s) induced *in vitro* by lipopolysaccharide, interleukin 1, and tumor necrosis factor increases neutrophil adherence (in part) by a CDw18-dependent mechanism. J. Immunol. **136:** 4548–4553.

27. Cavender, D. E., D. O. Haskard, B. Joseph & M. Ziff. 1986. Interleukin 1 increases the binding of human B and T lymphocytes to endothelial cell monolayers. J. Immunol. **136:** 203–207.

28. Haskard, D., D. O. Cavender, P. Beatty, T. Springer & M. Ziff. 1986. T lymphocyte adhesion to endothelial cells: Mechanisms demonstrated by anti-LFA-1 monoclonal antibodies. J. Immunol. **137:** 2901–2906.

29. Pober, J. S., M. P. Bevilacqua, D. L. Mendrick, L. A. Lapierre, W. Fiers & M. A. Gimbrone, Jr. 1986. Two distinct monokines, interleukin 1 and tumor necrosis factor, each independently induce biosynthesis and transient expression of the same antigen on the surface of cultured human vascular endothelial cells. J. Immunol. **136:** 1680–1687.

30. Bevilacqua, M. P., J. S. Pober, D. L. Mendrick, R. S. Cotran & M. A. Gimbrone, Jr. 1987. Identification of an inducible endothelial-leukocyte adhesion molecule, ELAM-1. Proc. natl. Acad. Sci USA **84:** 9238–9242.

31. Bevilacqua, M. P., S. Stengelin, M. A. Gimbrone, Jr. & B. Seed. 1989. Endothelial leukocyte adhesion molecule 1: An inducible receptor for neutrophils related to complement regulatory proteins and lectins. Science **243:** 1160–1165.

32. Bevilacqua, M. P. & M. A. Gimbrone, Jr. 1990. Identification and characterization of

endothelial-leukocyte adhesion molecule 1. *In* Leukocyte Adhesion Molecules: Structure, Function and Regulation. T. Springer, D. Anderson, R. Rosenthal & T. Rothlein, Eds. 215–223. Springer-Verlag. New York, NY.

33. POBER, J. S., M. A. GIMBRONE, JR., L. A. LAPIERRE, D. L. MENDRICK, W. FIERS, R. ROTHLEIN & T. A. SPRINGER. 1986. Overlapping patterns of activation of human endothelial cells by interleukin 1, tumor necrosis factor and immune interferon. J. Immunol. **137:** 1893–1896.

34. POBER, J. S., T. COLLINS, M. A. GIMBRONE, JR., R. S. COTRAN, J. GITLIN, W. FIERS, C. CLAYBERGER, A. KRENSKY, S. J. BURAKOFF & C. S. REISS. 1983. Lymphocytes recognize human vascular endothelial and dermal fibroblast Ia antigens induced by recombinant immune interferon. Nature **305:** 726–729.

35. ARUFFO, A. & B. SEED. 1987. Molecular cloning of a CD28 cDNA by a high-efficiency COS cell expression system. Proc. Natl. Acad. Sci. USA **84:** 8573–8577.

36. SIEGELMAN, M. H., VAN DE RIJU & I. L. WEISSMAN. 1989. Mouse lymph node and homing receptor cDNA clone encodes a glycoprotein revealing tandem interaction domains. Science **243:** 1165–1172.

37. LASKY, L. A., M. S. SINGER, T. A. YEDROCK, D. DOWBENKO, C. FENNIE, H. RODRIGUEZ, T. NGUYEN. S. STACHEL & S. D. ROSEN. 1989. Cloning of a lymphocyte homing receptor reveals a lectin domain. Cell **56:** 1045–1055.

38. JOHNSTON, G. I., R. I. COOK & R. P. MCEVER. 1989. Cloning of GMP-140, a granule membrane protein of platelets and endothelium: sequence similarity to proteins involved in cell adhesion and inflammation. Cell **56:** 1033–1044.

39. LARSEN, E., A. CELI, G. E. GILBERT, B. C. FURIE, J. K. ERBAN, R. BONFANTI, D. WAGNER & B. FURIE. 1989. PADGEM Protein: A receptor that mediates the interaction of activated platelets with neutrophils and monocytes. Cell **59:** 305–312.

40. BEVILACQUA, M. P. 1989. Endothelial leukocyte adhesion molecule 1: An inducible receptor for neutrophils related to complement regulatory proteins and lectins. Circulation (Suppl) **80(4):** II–I.

41. COTRAN, R. S., M. A. GIMBRONE, JR., M. P. BEVILACQUA, D. L. MENDRICK & J. S. POBER. 1986. Induction and detection of human endothelial activation antigen *in vivo*. J. Exp. Med. **164(2):** 661–666.

42. COTRAN, R. S. & J. S. POBER. 1988. Endothelial activation: Its role in inflammatory and immune reactions. *In* Endothelial Cell Biology. N. Simionescu & M. Simionescu, Eds. 335–347. Plenum Publishing, New York, NY.

43. KLEIN, L. M., R. M. LAVKER, W. L. MATIS & G. F. MURPHY. 1989. Degranulation of human mast cells induces an endothelial antigen central to leukocyte adhesion. Proc. Natl. Acad. Sci. USA **86:** 8972–8976.

44. MESSADI, D. V., J. S. POBER, W. FIERS, M. A. GIMBRONE, JR. & G. F. MURPHY. 1987. Induction of an activation antigen on postcapillary venular endothelium in human skin organ cultures. J. Immunol. **139:** 1557–1562.

45. MUNRO, J. M., J. S. POBER & R. S. COTRAN. 1989. Tumor necrosis factor and interferon-gamma induce distinct patterns of endothelial activation and associated leukocyte accumulation in skin of *Papio Anubis*. Am. J. Pathol. **135:** 121–133.

46. CYBULSKY, M. I. & M. A. GIMBRONE, JR. 1989. Endotoxin-stimulated monocyte-selective adhesive mechanism in rabbit endothelium. FASEB J. **3(4):** A1319.

47. CYBULSKY, M. I. & M. A. GIMBRONE, JR. 1989. Expression of a monocyte-selective endothelial-leukocyte adhesion molecule (ATHERO-ELAM) in atherogenesis. Submitted.

48. LIBBY, P. 1987. The active roles of cells of the blood vessel wall in health and disease. *In* Molecular Aspects of Medicine. H. Baum, J. Gergely & B. L. Fanburg, Eds. Vol. **9(6):** 499–567. Pergamon Press. Oxford.

49. GERRITY, R. G., J. A. GOSS & L. SOBY. 1985. Control of monocyte recruitment by chemotactic factor(s) in lesion-prone areas of swine aorta. Arteriosclerosis **5:** 55–66.

50. JAUCHEM, J. R., M. LOPEZ, E. A. SPRAGUE & C. J. SCHWARTZ. 1982. Mononuclear cell chemoattractant activity from cultured arterial smooth muscle cells. Exp. Mol. Pathol **37:** 166–174.

51. VALENTE, A. J., S. R. FOWLER, E. A. SPRAGUE, J. L. KELLEY, C. A. SUENRAM & C. J.

SCHWARTZ. 1984. Initial characterization of a peripheral blood mononuclear cell chemoattractant derived from cultured arterial smooth muscle cells. Am. J. Pathol. **117:** 409–417.

52. MAZZONE, T., M. JENSEN & A. CHAIT. 1983. Human arterial wall cells secrete factors that are chemotactic for monocytes. Proc. Natl. Acad. Sci. USA **80:** 5094–5097.

53. DENHOLM, E. M. & J. C. LEWIS. 1987. Monocyte chemoattractants in pigeon aortic atherosclerosis. Am. J. Pathol. **126:** 464–475.

54. BERLINER, J. A., M. TERRITO, L. ALMADA, A. CARTER, E. SHAFONSKY & A. M. FOGELMAN. 1986. Monocyte chemotactic factor produced by large vessel endothelial cells *in vitro.* Arteriosclerosis **6:** 254–258.

55. VALENTE, A. J., D. T. GRAVES, C. E. VIALLE-VALENTIN, R. DELGADO & C. J. SCHWARTZ. 1988. Purification of a monocyte chemotactic factor secreted by non-human primate vascular cells in culture. Biochemistry **27:** 4162–4168.

56. QUINN, M. T., S. PARTHASARATHY & D. STEINBERG. 1988. Lysophosphatidylcholine: a chemotactic factor for human monocytes and its potential role in atherogenesis. Proc. Natl. Acad. Sci. USA **85:** 2805–2809.

57. WHEELER, M. E., F. W. LUSCINSKAS, M. P. BEVILACQUA & M. A. GIMBRONE, JR. 1988. Cultured human endothelial cells stimulated with cytokines or endotoxin produce an inhibitor of leukocyte adhesion. J. Clin. Invest. **82:** 1211–1218.

58. GIMBRONE, M. A., JR., M. S. OBIN, A. F. BROCK, E. A. LUIS, P. E. HASS, C. A. HEBERT, Y. K. YIP, D. W. LEUNG, D. G. LOWE, W. J. KOHR, K. B. DARBONNE, K. B. BECHTOL & J. B. BAKER. 1989. Endothelial-interleukin-8: A novel inhibitor of leukocyte-endothelial interactions. Science. **246:** 1601–1603.

59. BAGGIOLINI, M., A. WALZ & S. L. KUNKEL. 1989. Neutrophil-activating peptide-1/interleukin 8, a novel cytokine that activates neutrophils. J. Clin. Invest. **84(4):** 1045–1049.

60. HANSSON, G. K., L. JONASSON, P. S. SEIFERT & S. STEMME. 1989. Immune mechanisms in atherosclerosis (review). Arteriosclerosis **9:** 567–578.

Experimental Production of Intramural Hemorrhage by Induced Coronary Artery Spasm in Atherosclerotic Miniature Swine

Experimental Proof on the Roles of Spasm in Cardiac Events of Ischemic Heart Disease[a]

MOTOOMI NAKAMURA

Research Institute of Angiocardiology
and
Cardiovascular Clinic
Kyushu University Medical School
Fukuoka, Japan 812

INTRODUCTION

From a clinical standpoint in order to prevent the sudden occurrence of ischemic cardiac events it is important to clarify the mechanisms of sudden occurrence of spontaneous angina, unstable angina, sudden ischemic cardiac death, and acute myocardial infarction. However, no experimental animal model based on atherosclerosis for these ischemic cardiac events in coronary heart disease has been systematically attempted and accomplished, except for our animal model for coronary artery spasm.[1]

Controversy exists with respect to the pathogenesis of unstable angina and acute myocardial infarction. Maseri *et al.* observed that coronary spasm may be precipitate crescendos angina and possibly acute myocardial infarction,[2,3] whereas Moise *et al.* suggested that unstable angina was due to progression in the extent and severity of coronary atherosclerosis.[4] However, the link between coronary spasm and progression of organic stenosis, including sudden occlusion, is still completely missing.

Pathologically, the following lesions of coronary atherosclerosis are suggested as the potential causes of coronary occlusion: 1) progressive luminal narrowing, 2) with thrombosis at the presence of breaks of atheroma, 3) with hemorrhage in the atheromatous plaque, and 4) coronary artery spasm. However, none of these lesions has hitherto been experimentally demonstrated.

Experimental Production of Intramural Hemorrhage in Atheroma by Induced Coronary Spasm in Atherosclerotic Miniature Swine

History of Our Attempts to Develop Animal Models for Cardiac Events of Ischemic Heart Disease

In order to elucidate the mechanisms and roles of coronary artery spasm in the series of ischemic cardiac events, since the late 1970s, we have attempted to design an animal

[a]The author acknowledges grant support from the Ministry of Education, Science, and Culture of Japan.

model in which coronary spasm similar to that in patients with the variant type of angina pectoris can be produced repeatedly in experimental animals.

In the first attempt, we demonstrated that alpha-adrenergic stimulation after beta-blocking in normal dogs caused about a 3% reduction of the epicardial coronary artery diameter despite the rise of systemic blood pressure.[5] In the second attempt, we performed localized endothelial denudation of the epicardial coronary artery in dogs that were maintained on a high cholesterol diet for several months. And a significant augmentation of the vasoconstriction was noted after administration of ergonovine along the denuded site, but this hyperconstriction of the coronary artery was insufficient to produce acute myocardial ischemia.[6] Thus, we decided to change from dogs to swine, because development of hypercholesterolemia as well as atherosclerotic lesion is known to be much easier and faster in swine than in dogs. In 1983, we succeeded in provoking coronary spasm by giving histamine or serotonin intracoronarily or intravenously to the atherosclerotic miniature swine, Göttingen type, similar to those seen angiographically in patients with variant angina.[1] A close topologic correlation was noted between the site of intimal thickening and the loci of coronary spasm.[7] Since then we have improved our experimental protocols and presently have succeeded in producing severe coronary spasm easily by giving 1 μg of serotonin or 10 μg of ergonovine per kg of body weight intracoronarily at the presence of various degrees of coronary atherosclerosis. The details of these improvements in experimental protocol will be published elsewhere.[8]

Experimental Provocation of Intramural Hemorrhage in Coronary Atheroma Associated with Sudden Progression of Fixed Organic Coronary Stenosis

Here, I shall discuss the experimental production of the intramural hemorrhage that was provoked by coronary spasm at the mild to moderate degree of atheroma in atherosclerotic miniature swine. In order to elucidate the effects of coronary spasm on the structure of the epicardial coronary lesion, we conducted the following experiment, the details of which have been recently published.[9] Briefly, Göttingen type of miniature swine were fed a semisynthetic diet containing 2% cholesterol and 1.1% sodium cholate for six months. One month after starting high cholesterol feeding, the intima of the left epicardial coronary artery was injured by balloon catheter, and then X-ray irradiation in a dose of 1500 rad was given twice selectively to the area of the injured coronary artery, after 4 and 5 months of cholesterol feeding. Six months after being on the high cholesterol diet (FIG. 1) transient (group A) and repetitive episodes (group B) of coronary spasm were provoked every 5 minutes by a single or a fivefold intracoronary injection of serotonin in amount of 10 μg/kg, respectively. The angiographic extent of coronary spasm (FIG. 1) measured by selective coronary arteriography as dynamic percent narrowing of injured coronary artery was 84 ± 4 (n = 4) and $90 \pm 5\%$ (n = 6) in groups A and B, respectively, which was not significantly different between the two groups. Ventricular fibrillation due to acute myocardial ischemia after provoked spasm was found. Forty min after the final administration of serotonin, the spasm of the coronary artery was relieved by intracoronary administration of nitroglycerin and then the heart was isolated and perfusion fixed.

The main branch of the coronary artery including a spastic segment was divided into three parts, 5–10 mm proximal and distal to the spastic site and the spastic segment. The nonspastic other branches of the left coronary artery were taken as the control segments. Light and electron microscopic studies were performed. In the control coronary cinearteriography, the injured and X-ray irradiated site showed normal or wall irregularity. After serotonin, transient luminal reduction at the spastic site was always over 75% and

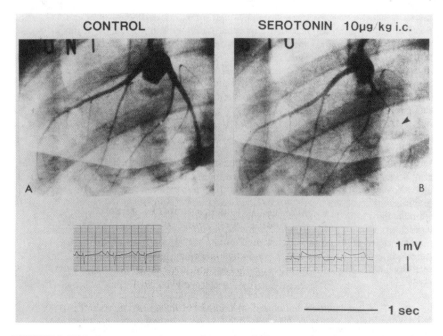

FIGURE 1. (**A**) Left coronary angiograms of control and (**B**) provocation of serotonin-induced (10 μg/kg i.c.) coronary spasm. *Arrowhead* indicates the severe spasm. (From Nagasawa *et al.*[9] Reprinted by permission from the American Heart Association.)

often 99% stenosis associated with ischemic ECG changes, but that at the nonspastic site was around 30 to 35% in both group A and B.

However, microscopic changes were different between group A and B. Namely, intramural hemorrhage (as shown in FIG. 2) was noted at the spastic site of all 6 pigs in group B, but none in 4 pigs of group A, although the newly developed capillaries in the atherosclerotic lesions were observed in all pigs of group A and B. Intramural hemorrhage was present inside the thickened intima and sometimes extended into the media, but there was no connection between hemorrhagic mass and the lumen. The intima of the non-spastic site was somewhat thickened but no capillary formation was observed. The luminal stenosis measured histologically, on cross section, was 13 to 16% at the proximal and/or distal site of spastic arteries in both group A and B, but 23 ± 5 and 56 ± 7% at the spastic site in group A and B, respectively. This increase in organic stenosis at the spastic site in group B was statistically significant ($P < 0.01$). These results may suggest that severe spasm for 30 min may damage the newly developed fragile capillaries causing hemorrhage which may increase the volume of intraplaque pressure of atheroma and result in progression of organic coronary stenosis. Electron microscopy of the luminal surface of the coronary arteries, demonstrated intercellular bridges of the endothelial cells at the spastic sites in both group A and B but not at the control site. The endothelial cells at the spastic site in group B were squeezed and its nuclei were moved toward the protruded site of cytoplasm. However, no focal detachment of endothelial cells from the underlying tissues, or platelet adhesion was observed. Only leukocytes adhered to the endothelium and their number was significantly larger at the spastic site in group B than at that in group A or at the nonspastic site in group B ($P < 0.01$). The present observations concerning leukocyte adhesion preferential to the endotherial gap along the repeated spastic site suggest that coronary spasm may cause leukocyte adherence as a result of alteration of the endothelial cells. Further studies on chronological observations of the endothelial lining and blood cell adherence after intramural hemorrhage and also on leukocyte-endothelial interactions have to be made. Recently, intramural hemorrhage not only in the thickened intima but also in the subendothelial space has been noted sometimes even in a single provocation of severe coronary spasm, and progression of organic stenosis has been found angiographically. Also, a 120-min duration of severe coronary spasm can produce acute myocardial infarction as evidenced by left ventriculography and serial changes in ECG. The details of these preliminary observations will be published elsewhere.[8]

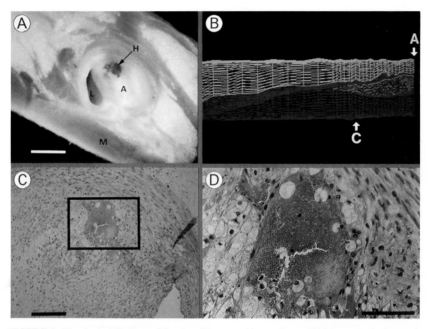

FIGURE 2. Histological findings of the site of intramural hemorrhage. **(A)** Macroscopic view at the hemorrhagic site of the left circumflex coronary artery. *Arrow* indicates the site of intramural hemorrhage. Abbreviations: L = lumen; A = atheroma; M = myocardium; H = hemorrhage. Bar represents 1 mm. **(B)** Computer-aided reconstruction of serial histological sections of the vessel shown in panel (A). Vascular lumen, internal elastic laminae, and external elastic laminae were traced by a joy stick during monitoring of the microscope on each section which was taken serially every 30 μm. Digitized data on these frames were stored in random access memory. Then, the vessel was reconstructed using a wire frame model and is presented as a two-dimensional view, staining the vascular lumen, intima, and hemorrhagic sites with white, blue, and red, respectively. This graphic representation was processed with the aid of the image software "Cosmozone" loaded on minicomputer. *Upward* (C) and *downward* (A) *arrows* indicate the sites of microscopical observation (panel C) and the surface shown in panel (A), respectively. **(C)** Microscopic features of the vessel in a low power magnification. Bar represents 200 μm. Intramural hemorrhage is located in the deeper site of thickened intima. *Inset* is further magnified and represented at (D). **(D)** High magnification of panel (C). Bar represents 50 μm. Red blood cells preserve their original shape. In this case, intramural hemorrhage is surrounded by foam cells. ((C) and (D) from Nagasawa *et al.*[9] Reprinted by permission from the American Heart Association.)

These serial experimental studies on coronary spasm suggested the close link of coronary spasm to development of acute myocardial ischemic events, such as spontaneous vasospastic angina, cardiac sudden death, progression of luminal narrowing of the coronary artery and possibly acute myocardial infarction.

ACKNOWLEDGMENTS

The author wishes to thank his co-workers, Drs. H. Tomoike, H. Ohtsubo, Y. Kikuchi, Y. Kawachi, Y. Maruoka, H. Shimokawa, S. Nabeyama, H. Yamamoto, H. Araki, Y. Nagata, K. Egashira, Y. Yamamoto, Y. Hayashi, A. Yamada, S. Sato, K. Nagasawa, J. Sadoshima, W. Mitsuoka, S. Egashira, T. Kuga, H. Tagawa, T. Yamamoto, and K. Tanaka.

REFERENCES

1. SHIMOKAWA, H., H. TOMOIKE, S. NABEYAMA, H. YAMAMOTO, H. ARAKI, M. NAKAMURA, Y. ISHII & K. TANAKA. 1983. Science **221:** 560–562.
2. MASERI, A., S. SEVERI, M. DE NES, A. L'ABBATE, S. CHIERCHIA., M. MARZILLI, A. M. BALLESTRA, O. PARODI, A. BIAGINI & A. DISTANTE. 1978. Am J Cardiol. **42:** 1019–1025.
3. Maseri, A., A. L'Abbate, G. Baroldi, S. Chierchia, M. Marzilli, A. M. Ballestra, S. Severi, O. Parodi, A. Biagini, A. Distante & A. PESOLA. 1978. N. Engl. J. Med. **229:** 1271–1277.
4. MOISE, A., P. THEROUX, Y. TAEYMANS, B. DESCOINGS, J. LESPERANCE, D. D. WATERS, G. B. PELLETIER & M. G. BOURRASSA. 1983. N. Engl. J. Med. **309:** 685–689.
5. NAKAMURA, M., H. TOMOIKE, H. OHTSUBO, K. SAKAI, K. NOGUCHI, A. TAKESHITA & Y. KIKUCHI. 1981. Basic Res. Cardiol. **76:** 498–502.
6. KAWACHI, Y., H. TOMOIKE, Y. MARUOKA, Y. KIKUCHI, H. ARAKI, Y. ISHII, K. TANAKA & M. NAKAMURA. 1984. Circulation **69:** 441–450.
7. EGASHIRA, K., H. TOMOIKE, Y. YAMAMOTO, A. YAMADA, Y. HAYASHI & M. NAKAMURA. 1986. Circulation **74:** 826–837.
8. In preparation.
9. NAGASAWA, K., H. TOMOIKE, Y. HAYASHI, A. YAMADA, T. YAMAMOTO & M. NAKAMURA. 1989. Circ. Res. **65:** 272–282.

Adrenaline and Noradrenaline as Possible Chemical Mediators in the Pathogenesis of Arteriosclerosis

W. H. HAUSS,[a] H.-J. BAUCH, AND H. SCHULTE

Institute of Arteriosclerosis Research
University of Münster
4400 Münster, Federal Republic of Germany

INTRODUCTION

Nowadays arteriosclerosis, the most important vascular disease, is the main cause of death in western industrialized countries. In these countries even more people die from arteriosclerosis than from malignant neoplasia.[1] Arteriosclerosis often causes thrombotic complications, the most prominent being myocardial infarction or stroke (brain infarction).[2] The causes of arteriosclerosis are still largely unknown. However, the occurrence of arteriosclerosis is strongly associated with exposure to certain atherogenic risk factors like smoking, hypertension, diabetes mellitus, hypercholesterolemia or mental stress.[3] These risk factors cause an activation of the mesenchymal cells involved in the pathogenesis of arteriosclerosis.[4, 5] Such mesenchymal cells are comprised of vascular wall cells, like endothelial and smooth muscle cells, as well as circulating blood cells, like platelets and monocytes/macrophages.[6] The activation of the mesenchymal cells, summarized in 1961 by Hauss under the term *"unspecific mesenchymal reaction (UMR)*,[7] characterizes the initial events in the pathogenesis of arteriosclerosis.[4-6] Thus, a very heterogeneous group of risk factors causes similar cell biological reactions. Therefore, it was our working hypothesis that these risk factors exhibit their biological activity in atherogenesis via substances which can be called "chemical mediators." Such chemical mediators should be substances which exert high biological activity. These substances might be hormones which would be capable of triggering cell biological reactions, notably the UMR, during early atherogenesis.

More recently, the catecholamines, adrenaline and/or noradrenaline, have been considered to play an important role in atherogenesis and the subsequent complications of arteriosclerosis. Raab *et al.* and Constantinides *et al.* have already indicated that catecholamines foster injury and increased permeability in the vascular endothelium.[8, 9] Moreover, it has been shown in several experiments that the application of adrenaline or noradrenaline induces atherosclerosis in rabbits[10, 11] or causes aggravation of aortic and coronary atherosclerosis in cholesterol-fed monkeys.[12] The infusion of noradrenaline in atherosclerotic and normal rhesus monkeys leads to the development of vascular thrombosis and even myocardial infarction, particularly in atherosclerotic animals.[13] In man extremely high plasma catecholamine levels are found in patients suffering from pheochromocytoma, a tumor of the adrenal medulla.[14] Generalized arteriosclerosis and arteriolosclerosis have been described even in young children with pheochromocytomas. Coronary sclerosis and myocardial infarction have been observed in pheochromocytoma

---

[a]Address for correspondence: Institut für Arterioskleroseforschung an der Universität, 4400 Münster, Domagkstr. 3, FRG.

patients as young as ten years of age.[15] Both vascular diseases are commonly found in adults. From these data it can be concluded that adrenaline and/or noradrenaline exhibit a strong atherogenic potency and thus may well contribute to the development of arteriosclerotic vascular lesions.

Thus, the available data favor the hypothesis that catecholamines could act as chemical mediators in the pathogenesis of arteriosclerosis. If these compounds were to act as chemical mediators during the pathogenesis of the disease in man, they should at least fulfill the following four criteria. I. They should trigger metabolic dysfunctions (*i.e.*, UMR) in mesenchymal cells, vascular wall cells and circulating blood cells involved in the pathogenesis of arteriosclerosis. II. Certain atherogenic risk factors should be associated with elevated plasma concentrations of adrenaline and/or noradrenaline. III. Plasma concentrations of catecholamines should also be correlated with different stages or activities of arteriosclerosis in man. IV. Severe persisting arteriosclerotic vascular diseases giving rise to thrombotic complications like myocardial infarction and stroke should be accompanied by elevated plasma levels of adrenaline and/or noradrenaline.

The present investigations were aimed at determining whether the catecholamines, adrenaline and noradrenaline, fulfil the above mentioned criteria.

PATIENTS, MATERIALS AND METHODS

Cell Cultures

Cell cultures from rat aortic smooth muscle cells and human umbilical vein endothelial cells were established and kept as described previously.[16-19] The influence of catecholamines on these cell cultures was studied using the same conditions as already published.[20]

Collection of Blood Samples and Quantitative Determination of Plasma Catecholamine Levels

Plasma catecholamine concentrations were determined using high performance liquid chromatography with electrochemical detection (HPLC-ECD).[21, 22] Plasma samples were collected and stored as described earlier.[21, 22]

Volunteers and Patients

Dialysis patients (n = 51) treated under limited care at the Institute for Nephrology were selected for the study. Clinical criteria from the Framingham Study[23] were employed to classify dialysis patients with respect to the existence of arteriosclerotic vascular changes, and their plasma catecholamine levels were monitored. Patients subjected to atherogenic risk factors and patients suffering from myocardial infarction (MI) or stroke were recruited from outpatients of the university hospital. For more detailed information refer to the literature.[24-27]

RESULTS

Influence of Adrenaline or Noradrenaline on the Proliferation of Cultured HUVEC and SMC

Cell biological studies of the behaviour of vascular wall cells during atherogenesis suggest that substances triggering the proliferation of vascular wall cells might be considered to exhibit a strong atherogenic potency.[28-33] We therefore studied the influence of adrenaline and noradrenaline on the proliferation of cultured human umbilical vein endothelial cells (HUVEC) and smooth muscle cells (SMC).

When 10^{-7} M adrenaline was added to the culture medium, endothelial cells from human umbilical veins were activated. The cells proliferated more rapidly than untreated control cells. SMC from rat aortas exposed to adrenaline or noradrenaline at a concentration of 10^{-7} M also exhibited enhanced proliferation. This reaction was time-dependent for both vascular wall cells. Maximal growth stimulation was observed when cell cultures reached the stationary growth phase, usually 4 days after the first addition of the catecholamines. The mitogenic effect of the catecholamines then was statistically significant for both vascular wall cells (TABLE 1.)

Influence of Atherogenic Risk Factors on Plasma Catecholamine Levels

The aforementioned data indicate that plasma adrenaline and/or noradrenaline concentrations could be of clinical importance for the pathogenesis of arteriosclerosis in man if some of the widely accepted atherogenic risk factors like smoking, hypertension, diabetes mellitus, hypercholesterolemia or mental stress were associated with elevated plasma catecholamine levels. Therefore, plasma catecholamine concentrations in healthy control volunteers, smoking, hypertensive and diabetic individuals and in man exposed to mental stress were determined.

Statistical investigations on the influence of atherogenic risk factors on catecholamine metabolism in man clearly showed that plasma adrenaline levels are statistically significantly elevated in patients suffering from essential hypertension, smokers and individuals exposed to mental stress. The mean basal adrenaline concentration in blood of smokers was generally twice as high as in nonsmoking individuals indicating that smoking causes elevation of plasma adrenaline concentration in the blood. This statement is verified by the observation that 10 minutes after smoking three cigarettes, plasma adrenaline concentration in smokers was again remarkably increased compared with the basal level in these individuals. In patients suffering from diabetes mellitus the same mean plasma adrenaline and noradrenaline levels were found as in healthy controls. Plasma noradrenaline levels were only statistically significantly elevated in individuals exposed to mental stress. The noradrenaline concentration was enhanced in patients suffering from essential hypertension, but this elevation just barely failed to be significant ($P = 0.054$) in our group of patients (TABLE 2). In this context it should be noted that the calculations for the control group given in TABLE 2 are representative for such a group and that during our investigations for each group endangered by an atherogenic risk factor, a specific age and sex-matched control group was selected for statistical analysis.

Plasma Catecholamine Levels at Different Stages of Arteriosclerosis in Man

The data given above show that at least three important and well established atherogenic risk factors, like smoking, hypertension and mental stress, are closely related with elevated plasma adrenaline or noradrenaline levels. In dialysis patients, who often develop rapidly progressing arteriosclerosis,[34] efforts were made to investigate whether plasma catecholamine levels were correlated with certain stages or activities of arteriosclerosis. The results are shown in FIG. 1.

Plasma adrenaline and noradrenaline levels found in dialysis patients (HDP) were approximately the same as those found in patients with normal renal function.[21, 22, 35, 36] However, dialysis patients suffering from arteriosclerosis (HDP, AS) show statistically

TABLE 1. Statistical Analysis (Mann–Whitney Wilcoxon Test for Related Samples) of the Influence of Adrenaline and Noradrenaline on the Growth of Cultured Endothelial Cells from Human Umbilical Veins (HUVEC) and Smooth Muscle Cells (SMC) from Rat Aortas

Medium	HUVEC (Cells/Flask)						Rat Aortic SMC (Cells/Flask)					
	Mean	SD	Median	Min	Max	Significance[a]	Mean	SD	Median	Min	Max	Significance[a]
Control (n = 16)	634560	45333	647303	59852	682152	—	2215157	451665	2240000	1487500	2924832	—
Adrenaline (n = 16) (10^{-7} M)	758299	43762	769087	598390	873155	$p < 0.005$	2478714	222513	2433924	2034312	2912000	$p < 0.01$
Noradrenaline (n = 16) (10^{-7} M)	729993	31728	737993	687863	784316	$p < 0.01$	2416747	387925	2400144	1712500	3000000	$p < 0.005$

[a]Mann–Whitney Wilcoxon Test for related samples.

TABLE 2. Statistical Investigations (Mann-Whitney U-Test) on the Influence of Atherogenic Risk Factors on Catecholamine Metabolism in Man

Risk Factor	Adrenaline (pg/ml)						Noradrenaline (pg/ml)					
	Mean	SD	Median	Min	Max	Significance[a]	Mean	SD	Median	Min	Max	Significance[a]
Control group (n = 35)	33.5	14.6	31.0	12.0	79.0	—	400.0	186.2	353.0	158.0	887.0	—
Ess. hypertension RR syst. > 160 mm Hg RR diast. > 95 mm Hg (n = 20)	97.2	67.5	76.5	15.0	266.0	$p < 0.001$	477.8	173.0	455.5	231.0	750.0	$p\ 0.054$ (n. s.)
Smoking (>25 cigar./day, basal level) (n = 15)	63.0	21.2	60.0	32.0	116.0	$p < 0.001$	408.8	93.0	404.0	222.0	547.0	n. s.
Smoking (>25 cigar./day, after smoking 3 cigar.) (n = 15)	126.7	48.9	118.0	59.0	229.0	$p < 0.001$	391.4	99.9	345.0	253.0	539.0	n. s.
Mental stress (Wiener Determination Test) (n = 29)	109.2	42.9	94.3	51.0	218.0	$p < 0.001$	580.6	184.6	562.0	219.0	875.0	$p < 0.01$
Diabetes mellitus type I (n = 16)	38.7	21.4	31.5	13.0	97.0	n. s.	410.5	293.8	341.5	152.0	1406.0	n. s.

[a]Mann–Whitney U Test.

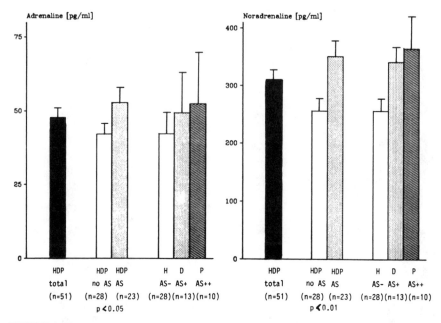

FIGURE 1. Plasma catecholamine levels (mean ± SD) in dialysis patients (HDP) and their relationship to arteriosclerosis (AS) and certain stages of this vascular disease (AS +; AS + +).

significantly elevated plasma adrenaline and noradrenaline concentrations compared to those of dialysis patients free from arteriosclerosis (HDP, no AS). Dialysis patients suffering from arteriosclerosis (HDP,AS) were subdivided into two subgroups, patients suffering from moderate arteriosclerosis (HDP, AS +) and patients suffering from severe arteriosclerosis (HDP, AS + +). Comparing these two subgroups with dialysis patients free from arteriosclerosis (HDP, AS−) clearly demonstrated that plasma adrenaline and plasma noradrenaline levels were positively correlated with the severity of the arteriosclerotic vascular disease. Thus, mean plasma catecholamine levels increase with the severity of the arteriosclerotic vascular disease (FIG. 1).

Plasma Catecholamine Levels in Patients Suffering from Persisting Arteriosclerotic Vascular Diseases

Myocardial infarction or stroke are closely connected with the occurrence of severe arteriosclerotic changes in the coronary or cerebral arteries. To investigate whether catecholamine metabolism plays a role in the pathogenesis of persisting arteriosclerotic vascular changes, respectively myocardial infarction or stroke, we therefore determined plasma catecholamine levels in patients having undergone such events.

Plasma catecholamine levels found in patients after having suffered from myocardial infarction or stroke at least one year ago and those found in age- and sex-matched healthy controls are shown in TABLE 3. The results show that even one year after infarction plasma adrenaline and noradrenaline concentrations were elevated in patients having suffered from myocardial infarction or stroke in comparison to plasma catecholamine levels from age and sex-matched healthy controls. The statistical analysis and the comparison of the groups using the Mann-Whitney U-Test clearly demonstrates that the observed elevations are statistically significant for both adrenaline and noradrenaline in patients having suffered from myocardial infarction. A statistically significant elevation of plasma adrenaline but not noradrenaline levels was observed in stroke patients. Plasma noradrenaline levels showed the same tendency, but did not reach significance in our group of patients.

The clinical and epidemiological importance of plasma adrenaline concentrations in patients following myocardial infarction or stroke is indicated in FIG. 2. This diagram shows the cumulative frequency of plasma adrenaline levels in patients having suffered from myocardial infarction or stroke and in healthy age- and sex-matched controls. As seen from the graph, plasma adrenaline levels from 15 to 60 pg/ml were typical for 98% of control individuals. Compared to these controls, about 70% of the patients who had had a myocardial infarction and 50% of the stroke patients had obviously elevated plasma adrenaline levels >60 pg/ml even one year after the event.

DISCUSSION

It was the aim of the present investigations to determine whether the catecholamines, adrenaline and/or noradrenaline, are substances that act as chemical mediators during the pathogenesis of arteriosclerosis in man and whether these substances contribute to the development and subsequent complications of this vascular disease.

To begin with, it has been shown that both catecholamines trigger the proliferation of cultured vascular wall cells, *i.e.*, endothelial and smooth muscle cells. Both cell types are strongly implicated in atherogenesis.[6, 28–33, 37, 38] Their activation, expressed as an increased cell proliferation, is a characteristic feature of the early phase in the development of arteriosclerotic vascular lesions.[4–6, 28–33] We have shown that cultured endothelial and smooth muscle cells exposed to adrenaline or noradrenaline exhibit increased proliferation. Thus, both catecholamines can trigger the activation of mesenchymal vascular wall cells. These findings agree with the results from other authors who also reported a stimulatory effect of catecholamines on cultured aortic endothelial[20, 39–41] and smooth muscle[20,42] cell proliferation.

Our investigations further show that at least the three important atherogenic risk factors, smoking, essential hypertension and mental stress are strongly associated with significantly elevated plasma catecholamine levels. These results are supported by find-

TABLE 3. Statistical Analysis (Mann-Whitney U-Test) on Plasma Adrenaline and Noradrenaline Levels in Patients One Year after Myocardial Infarction or Stroke

	Adrenaline (pg/ml)						Noradrenaline (pg/ml)					
Disease	Mean	SD	Median	Min	Max	Signif-icance[a]	Mean	SD	Median	Min	Max	Signif-icance[a]
Control group (n = 35)	33.5	14.6	31.0	12.0	79.0	—	400.0	186.2	353.0	158.0	887.0	—
Myocardial infarction (n = 35)	68.0	29.7	64.5	15.0	147.0	$p<$ 0.001	615.3	419.3	500.5	229.0	2436.0	$p<$ 0.01
Stroke (n = 35)	69.5	36.1	62.0	22.0	150.0	$p<$ 0.001	442.3	195.1	382.0	176.0	1030.0	n. s.

[a]Mann-Whitney U-Test.

ings from other authors who, using different methods, also reported elevated plasma catecholamine levels in hypertensive[43] and smoking[44] individuals and in persons exposed to mental stress.[45, 46] The above mentioned effects of catecholamines on vascular wall cells led us to speculate that, besides other effects, smoking, hypertension and mental stress exert chronic mitogenic stress on vascular wall cells within the scope of the UMR.

Dialysis patients represent a so-called high risk group, because in this group arterio-sclerosis develops often and progresses with great rapidity.[34] In this high risk group a positive correlation between plasma adrenaline and noradrenaline concentrations and different stages of arteriosclerosis is observed; plasma catecholamine levels increase with the severity of the vascular disease. This correlation can be compared to that between another well accepted risk factor, serum lipids, like cholesterol, LDL-cholesterol and HDL-cholesterol and their relationship to myocardial risk.[2, 47]

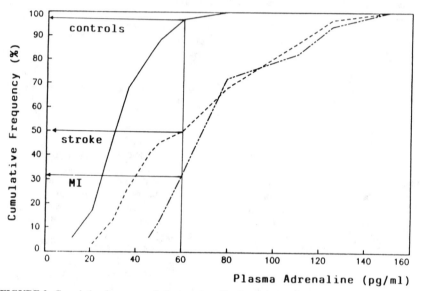

FIGURE 2. Cumulative frequency of plasma adrenaline levels in healthy controls (n = 35, ———) and in patients one year after myocardial infarction (n = 35, — - - — - -) or stroke (n = 35, - - - -).

That high catecholamine levels are linked to atherogenesis is further supported by the observation that persisting arteriosclerotic vascular changes in the coronary or cerebral arteries and concomitant thrombotic complications, myocardial infarction and stroke, are associated with elevated plasma adrenaline and/or noradrenaline levels even one year after infarction. Different epidemiological studies have shown that individual behavioural traits and social environmental conditions are risk factors for cardiovascular disease.[48-51] Other investigations done in our laboratory underline the importance of this risk factor, because during mental stress situations plasma catecholamine levels are significantly higher in patients suffering from coronary heart disease compared with controls.[24, 25]

The above mentioned results clearly show that adrenaline and noradrenaline fulfil important criteria making them putative chemical mediators in atherogenesis. Both com-pounds trigger the UMR in vascular wall cells, an important event in the pathogenesis of arteriosclerosis. Certain atherogenic risk factors are correlated with elevated plasma concentrations of these substances. Plasma concentrations of adrenaline and noradrenaline are also correlated with certain stages of arteriosclerosis in man. Furthermore, persisting arteriosclerotic vascular diseases are also associated with elevated plasma concentrations of adrenaline and noradrenaline. Thus, both compounds may well act as chemical mediators during the pathogenesis of arteriosclerosis in man.

The above mentioned hypothesis is supported by results from other authors who also studied the influence of catecholamines on other metabolic dysfunctions in mesenchymal cells important for the pathogenesis of arteriosclerosis. Sholley *et al.* found that endothelial cells could repopulate small denuded endothelial areas *in vitro* by migration alone.[52] Endothelial cell migration is considered to play an important role in the repair of vascular injuries.[52–55] Recently it has been shown by Bottaro *et al.* that migration of endothelial cells is significantly reduced by noradrenaline.[56] This indicates that at least noradrenaline could affect repair mechanisms of the vascular endothelium and thus might contribute to the manifestation of vascular injury leading to the formation of atherosclerotic lesions. Booyse *et al.*, studying platelet/endothelial cell interactions, found that platelet adherence to endothelial cells was significantly increased when these cells were preexposed to adrenaline.[57] Thus adrenaline may be considered as in injurious factor for the vascular endothelium. In clinical laboratories adrenaline is often used to induce platelet aggregation. It has been shown by Lande *et al.* that the elevation of plasma adrenaline levels causes enhanced platelet activation in man.[58] A significant increase of LDL-cholesterol uptake in the carotid arteries of rabbits caused by noradrenaline has also been reported.[59] Further, cultured pig aortic endothelial cells, pretreated with adrenaline or noradrenaline, exhibit a decreased prostacyclin synthesizing capacity.[60] All these phenomena are outstanding cell biological reactions during the pathogenesis of arteriosclerosis and all of them are triggered or at least influenced by adrenaline and/or noradrenaline. These findings underline the importance of both catecholamines in the development and subsequent complications of arteriosclerosis in man.

SUMMARY

We studied the relationships between adrenaline and noradrenaline and factors associated with arteriosclerosis to determine whether catecholamines contribute to the atherogenetic process. We investigated the effects of adrenaline and noradrenaline on cultures of vessel wall cells from rats and analyzed plasma catecholamine levels in humans exposed to atherogenic risk factors, undergoing hemodialysis treatment or following myocardial infarction or stroke.

I. Cultured endothelial and smooth muscle cells from vessel walls exhibited enhanced proliferation when exposed to adrenaline or noradrenaline. This indicates that catecholamines trigger the activation of vascular wall cells *in vitro*. Such activation, the unspecific mesenchymal reaction, is the predominant characteristic change in early atherogenesis.

II. In individuals subjected to the atherogenic risk factors smoking, essential hypertension and mental stress, plasma adrenaline concentrations were statistically significantly elevated. Mental stress also caused significantly elevated plasma noradrenaline levels. Plasma noradrenaline concentrations were also elevated in smoking and hypertensive individuals when compared with certain controls, but the differences failed to be statistically significant.

III. In dialysis patients, plasma adrenaline and noradrenaline concentrations showed a positive correlation with the activity of the sclerotic process; *i.e.*, plasma catecholamine concentrations increased with the severity of the disease.

IV. Patients with persisting arteriosclerotic vascular disease, *i.e.*, patients who had had a myocardial infarction or stroke, had significantly elevated plasma adrenaline and/or noradrenaline levels as late as one year after the event.

The results of our investigations suggest that adrenaline and noradrenaline may act as chemical mediators during atherogenesis in man, thus contributing to the development and subsequent complications of arteriosclerosis.

ACKNOWLEDGMENTS

The authors are indebted to Miss G. Börgeling and Miss M. Wieling for their skillful, excellent technical assistance, to Dr. D. Troyer for carefully reading the manuscript, and to G. Benning for typing the manuscript.

REFERENCES

1. WORLD HEALTH ORGANIZATION. 1985. World Statistics Annual. 250–254.
2. ASSMANN, G., Ed. 1982. Lipid Metabolism and Atherosclerosis. F. K. Schattauer Verlag. Stuttgart, FRG.
3. HAUSS, W. H., Ed. 1976. Koronarsklerose und Herzinfarkt. Thieme Verlag. Stuttgart, FRG.
4. HAUSS, W. H. 1976. Ann. N. Y. Acad. Sci. **275:** 286–301.
5. HAUSS, W. H. 1979. Cardiovasc. Res. Center Bull. **17:** 75–110.
6. ROSS, R. 1986. N. Engl. J. Med. **314:** 488–500.
7. HAUSS, W. H. & G. JUNGE-HÜLSING. 1961. Dtsch. med. Wschr. **86:** 763–768.
8. RAAB, W., E. STARK, W. H. MACMILLAN & W. R. GIGEE. 1961. Am. J. Cardiol. **8:** 203–211.
9. CONSTANTINIDES, P. & M. ROBINSON. 1969. Arch. Pathol. **88:** 106–112.
10. HELIN, P. I. LORENZEN, C. GARBARSCH & N. E. MATTHIESSEN. 1970. Atherosclerosis **12:** 125–132.
11. CAVALLERO, C., U. DITONDO, P. C. MINGAZZINE, P. C. PESANDO, & L. G. SPAGNOLI. 1973. Atherosclerosis **17:** 49–62.
12. KRUKEJA, R. S., B. N. DATTA & R. N. CHAKRAVARTI. 1981. Atherosclerosis **40:** 291–298.
13. BHATTACHARYA, S. K., R. N. CHAKRAVARTI & P. L. WAHI. 1974. Atherosclerosis **20:** 241–252.
14. BRAVO, E. L., R. C. TARAZI, R. W. GIFFORD & B. N. STEWART. 1979. N. Engl. J. Med. **301:** 682–686.
15. RAAB, W. 1953. Hormonal and Neurogenic Cardiovascular Disorders. Williams and Wilkins Co. Baltimore, MD.
16. ROSS, R. 1971. J. Cell Biol. **50:** 172–186.
17. HAUSS, W. H., J. MEY & H. SCHULTE. 1979. Atherosclerosis **34:** 119–143.
18. GRÜNWALD, J., H. ROBENEK, J. MEY & W. H. HAUSS. 1982. Exp. Mol. Pathol. **36:** 164–176.
19. JAFFE, E. A., R. L. NACHMAN, C. G. BECKER & C. R. MINICK. 1973. J. Clin. Invest. **52:** 2745–2756.
20. BAUCH, H.-J., J. GRÜNWALD, P. VISCHER, U. GERLACH & W. H. HAUSS. 1987. Exp. Pathol., **31:** 193–204.
21. BAUCH, H.-J., U. KELSCH & W. H. HAUSS. 1986. J. Clin. Chem. Clin. Biochem. **24:** 651–658.
22. BAUCH, H.-J., E. STRÜWER & U. KELSCH. 1989. Chromatographia **28:** 78–84.
23. KANNEL, W. B., P. A. WOLF & R. J. GARRISON. 1987. *In* The Framingham Study. NIH Publication No. 87-2284.
24. BAUCH, H.-J. & W. H. HAUSS. 1989. Chromatographia **28:** 69–77.
25. BAUCH, H.-J. & W. H. HAUSS. 1989. *In* Abh. d. Rhein-Westf. Akad. Wiss. W. H. Hauss, R. W. Wissler & H.-J. Bauch, Eds. Westdeutscher Verlag. Cologne & Opladen, FRG. In press.
26. BAUCH, H.-J., U. KELSCH, K.-H. GROTEMEYER, R. BUCHWALSKY & W. H. HAUSS. 1987. *In*

Frühveränderungen bei der Atherogenese. E. Betz, Ed. 147–155. W. Zuckschwerdt-Verlag. Munich, FRG.

27. BAUCH, H.-J., H. SCHULTE, E. SELHORST, U. KELSCH, R. BUCHWALSKY & W. H. HAUSS. 1988. *In* Die Anwendung aktueller Methoden in der Arteriosklerose-Forschung. E. Betz, Ed. 115–128. W. Kohlhammer Verlag. Stuttgart, FRG.

28. SCHMITT, G. H. KNOCHE, G. JUNGE-HÜLSING, R. KOCH & W. H. HAUSS. 1970. Z. Kreislaufforsch. **59:** 481–487.

29. SCHWARTZ, S. M. & E. P. BENDITT. 1977. Circ. Res. **41:** 248–255.

30. HAUSS, W. H., G. JUNGE-HÜLSING & U. GERLACH, Eds. 1968. Die unspezifische Mesenchymreaktion. Thieme Verlag. Stuttgart, FRG.

31. FLORENTIN, R. A., S. C. NAM, K. T. LEE & W. A. THOMAS. 1969. Arch. Pathol. **88:** 463–471.

32. ROSS, R. & J. A. GLOMSET. 1973. Science **180:** 1332–1339.

33. SCHWARTZ, S. M., C. M. GAJDUSEK & S. C. SELDEN. 1981. Arteriosclerosis **1:** 107–126.

34. WORLD HEALTH ORGANIZATION. 1978. Demographic Year Book, Genf.

35. BAUERSFELD, W., D. RATGE, E. KNOLL & H. WISSER. 1984. Fresenius Z. Anal. Chem. **317:** 679–680.

36. HJEMDAHL, P. 1984. Am. J. Physiol. **247:** 13–20.

37. GEER, J. C. & M. D. HAUST. 1972. *In* Monographs on Atherosclerosis. Vol. **2:** 4–27. Karger, Basel.

38. ROSS, R. & J. A. GLOMSET. 1976. N. Engl. J. Med. **295:** 369–377; 420–425.

39. D'AMORE, P. & D. SHEPRO. 1977. J. Cell Physiol. **92:** 177–184.

40. SHERLINE, P. & R. MASCARDO. 1984. J. Clin. Invest. **74:** 483–487.

41. BAUCH, H.-J., B. KEHREL, P. VISCHER, M. JOHN & W. H. HAUSS. 1987. *In* Frühveränderungen bei der Atherogenese. E. Betz, Ed. 46–56. W. Zuckschwerdt Verlag, Munich, FRG.

42. BLAES, N. & J. P. BOISSEL. 1983. J. CELL PHYSIOL. **116:** 167–172.

43. GOLDSTEIN, D. S. 1981. Hypertension **3:** 48–52.

44. CRYER, P. E., M. W. HAYMOND, G. V. SANTIAGO & S. D. SHAH. 1976. N. Engl. J. Med. **295:** 573–577.

45. KONES, R. J. 1979. Angiology **30:** 327–339.

46. DIEHL, K. L. & H. WERNZE. 1985. Herz-Kreislauf **3:** 113–121.

47. ASSMANN, G., Ed. 1989. Lipid Metabolism Disorders and Coronary Heart Disease. MMW Medizin Verlag. Munich, FRG.

48. ROSENMAN, R. H., R. J. BRAND, C. D. JENKINS, M. FRIEDMAN, R. STRAUS & M. WURM. 1975. J. Am. Med. Assoc. **233:** 872–877.

49. HAMBURG, D. A. & G. R. ELLIOTT. 1982. Arteriosclerosis **2:** 357–366.

50. FORSMAN, L. & L. E. LINDBLAD. 1983. Psychosom. Med. **45:** 435–445.

51. MANUCK, S. B., J. R. KAPLAN & K. A. MATTHEWS. 1986. Arteriosclerosis **6:** 2–14.

52. SHOLLEY, M. M., M. A. GIMBRONE & R. S. COTRAN. 1976. Lab. Invest. **36:** 18–25.

53. WALL, R. T., L. A. HARKER & G. E. STRIKER. 1978. Lab. Invest. **39:** 523–529.

54. HAUDENSCHILD, C. C. & S. M. SCHWARTZ. 1979. Lab. Invest. **41:** 407–418.

55. THORGEIRSSON, G., A. L. ROBERTSON & D. H. COWAN. 1979. Lab. Invest. **41:** 51–62.

56. BOTTARO, D., D. SHEPRO, S. PETERSON & H. B. HECHTMAN. 1985. Am. J. Physiol. **248:** C252–C257.

57. BOOYSE, F. M., S. BELL, B. SEDLAK & M. E. RAFELSON. 1975. Artery **1:** 518–539.

58. LANDE, K., K. GJESDAL, E. FONSTELIEN, S. E. KJELDSEN & I. EIDE. 1985. Thromb. Haemost. **54:** 450–453.

59. BORN, G. V. R. & S. SHAFFI. 1989. *In* Abh. d. Rhein.-Westf. Akad. Wiss. W. H. Hauss, R. W. Wissler & H.-J. Bauch, Eds. Westdeutscher Verlag, Cologne & Opladen, FRG. In press.

60. BAUCH, H.-J., P. VISCHER, B. KEHREL, J.GRÜNWALD, M. JOHN, W. STENZINGER & W. H. Hauss. 1987. *In* Prostaglandins in Clinical Research. H. Sinzinger & K. Schrör, Eds. 329–336. Alan R. Liss, Inc. New York, NY.

Cellular Interactions, Growth Factors, and Smooth Muscle Proliferation in Atherogenesis[a]

R. ROSS,[b] J. MASUDA,[c] AND E. W. RAINES[b]

bDepartment of Pathology
University of Washington
Seattle, Washington 98195
and
cNational Cardiovascular Center
Research Institute
5-7-1 Fujishiro-dai, Suita
Osaka 565, Japan

INTRODUCTION

Although it has been known for over a century that intimal lesions of atherosclerosis can lead to occlusion of critical arteries, we have only recently begun to understand the cellular interactions that precede the formation of these smooth muscle proliferative lesions. Predictions of some of the earliest changes that may occur in the arterial endothelium were made by John French[1] and by Poole and Florey.[2] Even earlier, Leary[3] had predicted that macrophages would also play a key role in these events. Many of these predictions have been confirmed by studies of lesion initiation and progression in experimentally induced atherosclerosis.

As McGill[4] has pointed out, the lesions of atherosclerosis probably represent a continuum from the fatty streak through the intermediate (fibrofatty) lesion to the fibrous plaque (advanced) lesions of atherosclerosis. The geographic pathology study of atherosclerosis[5] indicated that fatty streaks are ubiquitous at all ages and that they either progress through the three stages of atherogenesis to become fibrous plaques, remain unchanged as fatty streaks throughout life, or regress and disappear, depending upon the genetic makeup of the individual, the risk factors with which the individual is associated, and other factors that may alter individual susceptibility to the process of atherogenesis.

The following overview briefly outlines our current understanding of the cellular changes observed in hypercholesterolemic animal models of atherosclerosis. These studies support the concept that the earliest phases of atherosclerosis represent a specialized form of inflammation,[6,7] and that growth regulatory molecules produced by platelets, macrophages, and possibly smooth muscle and endothelial cells are responsible for the smooth muscle proliferative events.

Studies in Nonhuman Primates

To determine the cellular interactions that occur in the nonhuman primate under one set of circumstances known to induce atherogenesis, *i.e.*, chronic hypercholesterolemia,

[a]This work was supported in part by National Heart, Lung, and Blood Institute Grant HL-18645 to RR, and National Institutes of Health Grant RR-00166 to the Northwest Regional Primate Center.

two studies have investigated the nature of the cells involved, the anatomic sites at which this involvement occurs, and substances that may be released by these cells in inducing the intimal smooth muscle hyperplastic response of atherosclerosis.

The first of these was pursued in nonhuman primates by Faggiotto *et al.*,[8,9] who examined a series of pigtail monkeys (Macaca nemestrina) that were made hypercholesterolemic at high levels analogous to those observed in humans with the hereditary disease homozygous familial hypercholesterolemia (FH). A subsequent series of studies has recently been completed by Masuda and Ross[10] using the same genus of monkey, in which hypercholesterolemia was induced at levels closer to those found in humans afflicted with common hypercholesterolemia, namely, 200–400 mg/dL plasma cholesterol.

In both of these studies, the cellular interactions that take place, the anatomic sites at which they occur, and the changes that are associated with each of the different cell types are identical, although the time frames in which they take place are strikingly different; it takes longer in animals with low-level hypercholesterolemia for the same cellular changes to be observed. One additional difference observed by Masuda and Ross, who studied the animals over a period of 3½ to 4 years, as compared with Faggiotto *et al.*,[8,9] who studied the animals at monthly intervals for 13 months, was that the advanced lesions that form during relatively low-level hypercholesterolemia have much more fibrous connective tissue within the lesions than is found in lesions that form in animals with higher levels of plasma cholesterol for shorter intervals of time.

Leukocyte Adhesion and Formation of Early Lesions

One of the first changes that takes place in hypercholesterolemia, which appears to result from increased permeability of the endothelium, is the accumulation of lipid droplets and particulates in the subendothelial space, as described by Simionescu *et al.*[11] It is presumed that functional changes occur in the endothelial cells and that these changes are due to subtle alterations in cell junctions and other cell components. In hypercholesterolemia, this may result from exposure to chronic elevated levels of plasma lipoproteins, and perhaps, as suggested by Carew *et al.*,[12] to oxidized lipoproteins. These changes include increased adherence of monocytes and lymphocytes to the endothelial cells at sites throughout the arterial tree, particularly at branches and bifurcations (FIG. 1). This increased leukocyte attachment is presumably due to alterations in cell-surface constituents of both the leukocytes and the endothelial cells, and is associated with the formation of chemotactic substances by either the endothelium or by cells in the subendothelial space. These chemoattractants result in directed migration of the attached lymphocytes and monocytes between the endothelial cells into the subendothelial space, where many of the monocytes become converted to macrophages. Some of the macrophages take up the lipoprotein particles (many of which may be modified or oxidized lipoproteins) and become lipid-rich foam cells. The presence of these foam cells creates the first recognizable lesion of atherosclerosis, the fatty streak (FIG. 2a). Fatty streaks expand by continued adherence and migration of monocytes and lymphocytes into the lesions. In addition, there is replication of macrophages within the lesions.[13] Histochemical analysis of fatty streaks using cell-specific monoclonal antibodies has demonstrated both CD8-positive and CD4-positive T-lymphocytes together with the ubiquitous macrophages (FIG. 2b,c,d and FIG. 3).

As the fatty streaks expand, a third cell appears, the smooth muscle cell. These cells are derived either from preexisting intimal accumulations of smooth muscle cells that form during development[14] or from smooth muscle cells that migrate from the media into the intima, presumably due to the formation of chemoattractants (in this case by either the

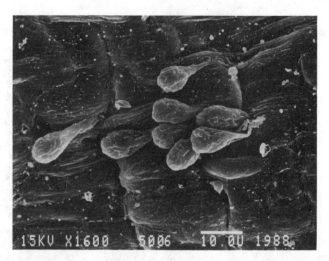

FIGURE 1. This scanning electron micrograph demonstrates numerous mononuclear cells attached to the surface of a fatty streak in a monkey that had been hypercholesterolemic at low levels for six months. The morphology of the cells is typical of what is seen prior to their migration between endothelial cells and entry into the subendothelial space.

activated macrophages, the overlying endothelial cells, or both). Thus the fatty streak begins as a pure macrophage-lymphocyte lesion and becomes a mixture of macrophages, lymphocytes, and smooth muscle cells. With time and lesion progression, such fatty streaks expand and become a complicated mixture of these cells and are called intermediate or fibrofatty lesions (FIG. 4).

Lesion Progression

The fatty streaks and fibrofatty lesions may progress to become fibrous plaques, depending on the conditions and their particular anatomic locations. Numerous cellular changes have been observed in association with the formation of fibrous plaques. Included in these changes are disruptions in endothelial-cell junctions overlying many of the lipid-laden foam cells, which may then protrude between the endothelial cells into the lumen of the artery (FIG. 5). In some instances, these exposed subendothelial foam cells act as thrombogenic sties, and platelet microthrombi form on their exposed surfaces (FIG. 6). This latter event is particularly prominent at branches and bifurcations in the arterial tree, where rheological forces may play a role in inducing increased platelet adherence to the exposed macrophages. Associated with these changes, the fatty streaks and fibrofatty lesions take on a progressively altered appearance, as numerous additional smooth muscle cells migrate in and proliferate both deep and near the lumen of the lesion to form a fibrous cap (FIG. 7). This fibrous cap consists of smooth muscle intermixed with connective tissue and numerous macrophages, and covers a deeper layer of lipid-filled macrophages intermixed with T-lymphocytes, which overlies a still deeper layer of proliferating smooth muscle cells. Most of the proliferative activity appears to occur near the shoulder of these enlarging lesions as observed by Rosenfeld and Ross,[13] as well as deep within the lesions, so that ultimately a massive intimal smooth-muscle-proliferative lesion forms, which contains macrophages and T-lymphocytes and takes the final appearance of the advanced, or complicated, occlusive lesion of atherosclerosis.

It has been suggested that numerous growth regulatory molecules, and in particular platelet-derived growth factor (PDGF), may be responsible for the migration, proliferation, and formation of connective tissue by the smooth muscle cells. These growth regulatory molecules also modulate angiogenesis, cell-cell adhesion, and cell metabolism, including lipid uptake.

Platelet-Derived Growth Factor

Platelet-derived growth factor was originally discovered in 1974 as one of the principal sources of mitogenic activity present in whole blood serum and missing in plasma.[15,16] A great deal has been learned about this molecule since that time. Mature PDGF derived from human platelets is a disulfide-bonded dimer of 28,000–35,000 daltons.[17] It consists of two peptide chains, termed A and B, which bear a 60% amino acid sequence homology with one another.[18-20] Each of these chains is coded for on separate chromosomes, and all three possible dimeric configurations of PDGF have been observed; namely, AB, BB, and AA.[21,22] Human platelet PDGF consists of approximately 40% AB heterodimer and approximately 30% each of the AA and BB homodimers.[23] All three forms of PDGF are mitogenic for mesenchymal connective tissue cells such as smooth muscle, fibroblasts, astrocytes, chondrocytes, and osteoblasts.[21,22]

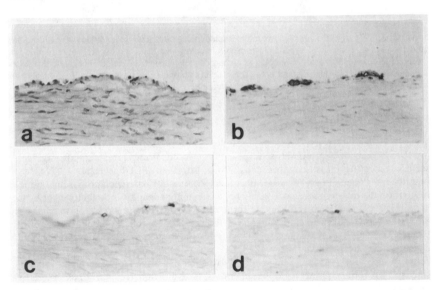

FIGURE 2. This composite of four micrographs demonstrates the cells that comprise a fatty streak from a six-month low-level hypercholesterolemic monkey. (**a**) is stained with hematoxylin and eosin. (**b**) is an immunoperoxidase preparation using monoclonal antibody HAM-56, demonstrating the localization of monocyte-derived macrophages. (**c**) uses monoclonal antibody OKT-4A to demonstrate CD4-positive lymphocytes. (**d**) uses monoclonal antibody G10.1 to demonstrate CD8-positive T-lymphocytes. Thus, as in human lesions, the early fatty streak consists of mixtures of monocyte-derived macrophages and T-lymphocytes.

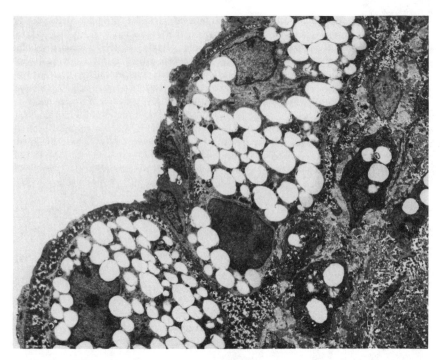

FIGURE 3. This transmission electron micrograph demonstrates a portion of a fatty streak from the thoracic aorta of a low-level hypercholesterolemic monkey that had been hypercholesterolemic for six months. Foam cells that are macrophages lie immediately beneath the endothelium. There are also accumulations of lipid deposits and other dense debris among and between the cells. Beneath the macrophages are several smooth muscle cells containing 2-3 lipid droplets. Magnification X 3000.

PDGF induces a proliferative response by binding to specific high-affinity, cell-surface receptors on susceptible cells. Two forms of PDGF receptors have been described,[24,25] and dimers of two distinct receptor subunits have been proposed to dimerize to form the different receptors.[26,27] The two receptor subunits, brought together by the appropriate covalently linked dimeric form of PDGF, depend upon the form of PDGF presented to the cell. The alpha subunit of the receptor can bind to either the A- or the B-chain of PDGF, whereas the beta subunit can bind to only the B-chain of PDGF. As a consequence, the BB homodimer of PDGF is a universal mitogen for PDGF receptive cells, whereas the AA form will bind only to cells that have sufficient alpha subunits, since the AA form requires two alpha subunits to form a mature receptor. Thus the relative mitogenicity of PDGF depends both upon the isoform of PDGF presented to the cells and the relative numbers of α and β receptor subunits on the cells.[27] Much remains to be learned about the two forms of the PDGF receptor; however, all three isoforms of PDGF and all three dimeric forms of the receptor appear to be capable of inducing both mitogenesis[27–29] and chemotaxis.[30] Whether all of the other known biological responses to PDGF can be transmitted by all of the appropriate combinations of receptor and ligand remains to be determined.

PDGF can be formed by many diploid cells. However, as with the platelet, the expression and secretion of PDGF in normal cells is tightly regulated. In arterial cells, it has been demonstrated that activated macrophages, endothelial cells, and smooth muscle cells and fibroblasts can all synthesize and secrete the different dimeric forms of PDGF.[22] Thus these cells may interact with one another in either a paracrine or an autocrine fashion if they are appropriately stimulated to form PDGF molecules. The biological activity of PDGF is dependent on the expression and secretion of both the growth factor and its receptor. PDGF receptor expression is also tightly regulated. *In vivo*, the β-subunit of the PDGF receptor is expressed at low levels in normal vessels, but is increased in arterial lesions.[31] We have recently demonstrated the presence of PDGF B-chain protein within a subset of macrophages observed in all stages of lesion development in both human and nonhuman primate lesions.[32] Thus the macrophage may play a critical role in providing PDGF, and consequently in the initiation and progression of this disease process.

The Possible Role of Other Growth Factors

Because the different cells associated with the lesions of atherosclerosis have the capacity to form numerous growth regulatory molecules in addition to PDGF, including molecules that stimulate cell proliferation as well as those that can inhibit cell proliferation, it will be important to determine the nature of the different molecules formed by

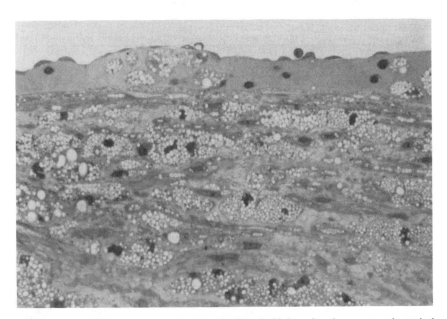

FIGURE 4. This light micrograph of a 1-μ plastic-embedded section demonstrates the typical appearance of a fibrofatty lesion that contains a mixture of lipid-laden macrophages and lipid-laden smooth muscle cells together with accumulations of connective tissue. Numerous foam cells can be seen throughout the lesion. It is difficult at this magnification to separate smooth muscle cells from macrophages; however, the relatively thin, elongated cells with smaller numbers of lipid droplets tend generally to be smooth muscle cells.

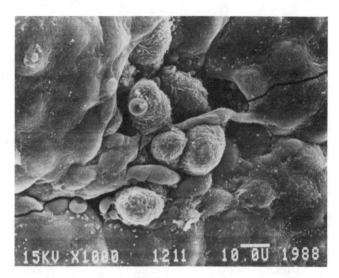

FIGURE 5. This scanning electron micrograph demonstrates the surface appearance of a fatty streak from the thoracic aorta near a branch of a low-level hypercholesterolemic animal that had been on the diet for one year. Endothelial retraction has exposed numerous foam cells within the fatty streak, and a number of endothelial cells appear to have migrated, possibly in an attempt to regenerate and re-cover the exposed lesion. Such areas of foam cell exposure are commonly seen at branches and bifurcations after prolonged duration of chronic hypercholesterolemia.

each of the cells and the circumstances under which the different genes for each of these molecules are expressed during lesion formation and progression.

As an example of the potential complexity of these interactions, transforming growth factor-beta (TGFβ) has been characterized as growth inhibitory for cells such as endothelium, fibroblasts, and, in most cases, smooth muscle; whereas interleukin-1 (IL-1) and tumor necrosis factor-alpha (TNFα) have been reported to have varying activities, depending upon the cells on which they act. IL-1 has been described as mitogenic for fibroblasts and smooth muscle. Recently it has been found that the mitogenic activity previously ascribed to IL-1 is due to the fact that IL-1 induces PDGF A-chain gene expression in smooth muscle cells, which then go on to synthesize and secrete PDGF-AA, and stimulate themselves.[33] In a similar fashion, TNFα can induce PDGF B-chain expression by arterial endothelial cells, which can affect surrounding cells in a paracrine manner.[34] Thus the composition of the lesions of atherosclerosis is complex in terms of its cellular makeup, the potential genes expressed, and the various growth activators and growth inhibitors that may be synthesized and secreted by each of the cells involved in atherogenesis.

Response to Injury Hypothesis of Atherosclerosis

The Response to Injury Hypothesis of Atherosclerosis[6] takes into account most of the cellular observations described above and the various growth regulatory molecules that can be formed by the cells as they interact in the complex microenvironment within the artery wall. This hypothesis is constantly being tested and reformulated as different components are examined, modified, disproved, or withstand the test of time. It suggests that some form of "injury" occurs to the endothelium at particular sites in the arterial tree. Endothelial dysfunction may result, dependent upon the factors involved in hypercholesterolemia, hypertension, cigarette smoking, diabetes, etc. The resultant endothelial changes stimulate a specialized form of chronic inflammation involving adherence of monocyte/macrophages and T-lymphocytes and their migration into the intima due to local elaboration of chemotactic factors. The macrophages then become activated and form growth regulatory molecules (including PDGF) that stimulate smooth muscle migration, proliferation, and connective tissue formation. In hyperlipidemic individuals, foam cells may form at this stage. If the "injury" persists, the cellular interactions among the lymphocytes, macrophages, and smooth muscle cells eventually lead to lesion progression and enlargement and ultimate occlusion of the artery, the surface of which may be prone to thrombosis. This hypothesis has permitted the development of new experimental approaches to questions concerning the role each cell type plays in atherogenesis and how cellular interactions relate to the different risk factors that have been epidemiologically associated with increased incidence of atherosclerosis. The elucidation of the roles of these cells and of the growth regulatory molecules they form and respond to will ultimately determine our approaches to diagnosis, treatment, and prevention of this disease process.

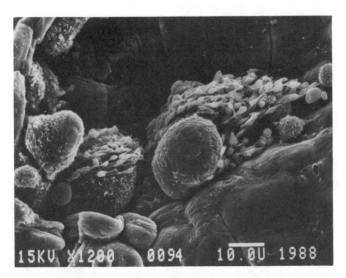

FIGURE 6. This scanning electron micrograph demonstrates the appearance at a branch in the abdominal aorta of the surface of a fatty streak from a monkey that had been on a low-level hypercholesterolemic diet for six months. Exposure of foam cells and microthrombi attached to several of the exposed foam cells is apparent in this scanning electron micrograph. Microthrombi attached to exposed foam cells in fatty streaks were found at branches and bifurcations in every animal in the studies of low-level and high-level hypercholesterolemia.

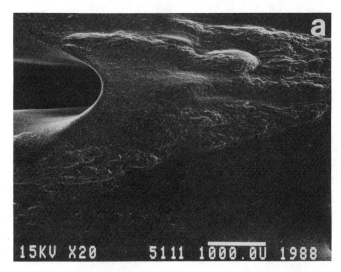

FIGURE 7. (a) is a low-magnifcation scanning electron micrograph of the surface of a fibrous plaque in the abdominal aorta in the outflow tract of an animal that had been hypercholesterolemic for two years at a low level. The raised, irregular appearance of this lesion can be readily seen in this micrograph.

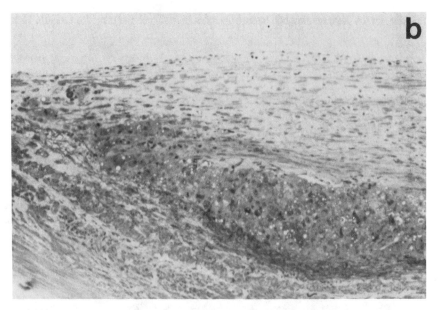

FIGURE 7. (b) is a 1-μ plastic-embedded section of a fibrous plaque from a portion of the iliac artery of a low-level hypercholesterolemic monkey that had been on the diet for two years. The fibrous cap, which covers an accumulation of lipid-containing cells deep within the core of the lesion, and which overlies a large number of smooth muscle cells and gives the discrete appearance of a fibrous plaque, can be readily seen in this very low-power light micrograph.

REFERENCES

1. FRENCH, J. E. 1966. Atherosclerosis in relation to the structure and function of the arterial intima, with special reference to the endothelium. Int. Rev. Exp. Pathol. **5:** 253–353.
2. POOLE, J. C. F. & H. W. FLOREY. 1958. Changes in the endothelium of the aorta and the behaviour of macrophages in experimental atheroma of rabbits. J. Pathol. Bacteriol. **75:** 245–253.
3. LEARY, T. 1941. The genesis of atherosclerosis. Arch. Pathol. **32:** 507–555.
4. MCGILL, H. C., JR. 1984. Persistent problems in the pathogenesis of atherosclerosis. Arteriosclerosis **4:** 443–451.
5. MCGILL, H. C., Jr., Ed. 1968. The Geographic Pathology of Atherosclerosis. Williams and Wilkins. Baltimore, MD.
6. ROSS, R. 1986. The pathogenesis of atherosclerosis—an update. N. Engl. J. Med. **314:** 488–500.
7. MUNRO, J. M. & R. S. COTRAN. 1988. Biology of disease. The pathogenesis of atherosclerosis: Atherogenesis and inflammation. Lab. Invest. **58:** 249–261.
8. FAGGIOTTO, A., R. ROSS & L. HARKER. 1984. Studies of hypercholesterolemia in the nonhuman primate. I. Changes that lead to fatty streak formation. Arteriosclerosis **4:** 323–340.
9. FAGGIOTTO, A. & R. ROSS. 1984. Studies of hypercholesterolemia in the nonhuman primate. II. Fatty streak conversion to fibrous plaque. Arteriosclerosis **4:** 341–356.
10. MASUDA, J. & ROSS, R. 1990. Atherogenesis during low-level hypercholesterolemia in the nonhuman primate. I. Fatty streak formation. Arteriosclerosis **10:** 164–177.
11. SIMIONESCU, N., E. VASILE, F. LUPU, G. POPESCU & M. SIMIONESCU. 1986. Prelesional events in atherogenesis. Accumulation of extracellular cholesterol-rich liposomes in the arterial intima and cardiac valves of the hyperlipidemic rabbit. Am. J. Pathol. **123:** 109–125.
12. CAREW, T. E., D. C. SCHWENKE & D. STEINBERG. 1987. Antiatherogenic effect of probucol unrelated to its hypercholesterolemic effect: Evidence that antioxidants *in vivo* can selectively inhibit low density lipoprotein degradation in macrophage-rich fatty streaks and slow the progression of atherosclerosis in the Watanabe heritable hyperlipidemic rabbit. Proc. Natl. Acad. Sci. USA **84:** 7725–7729.
13. ROSENFELD, M. E. & R. ROSS. Macrophage and smooth muscle cell proliferation in atherosclerotic lesions of WHHL and comparably hypercholesterolemic fat-fed rabbits. Arteriosclerosis. In press.
14. FLORENTIN, R. A., S. C. NAM, A. S. DAOUD, R. JONES, R. F. SCOTT, E. S. MORRISON, D. N. KIM, K. T. LEE, W. A. THOMAS, W. J. DODDS & K. D. MILLER. 1968. Dietary-induced atherosclerosis in miniature swine, I-V. Exp. Mol. Pathol. **8:** 263–301.
15. KOHLER, N. & A. LIPTON. 1974. Platelets as a source of fibroblast growth-promoting activity. Exp. Cell Res. **87:** 297–301.
16. ROSS, R., J. GLOMSET, B., KARIYA & L. HARKER. 1974. A platelet-dependent serum factor that stimulates the proliferation of arterial smooth muscle cells *in vitro*. Proc. Natl. Acad. Sci. USA **71:** 1207–1210.
17. RAINES, E. W. & R. ROSS. 1982. Platelet-derived growth factor. I. High yield purification and evidence for multiple forms. J. Biol. Chem. **257:** 5154–5160.
18. ANTONIADES, H. N. & M. W. HUNKAPILLER. 1983. Human platelet-derived growth factor (PDGF): Amino-terminal amino acid sequence. Science **220:** 963–965.
19. WATERFIELD, M. D., G. T. SCRACE, N. WHITTLE, P. STROOBANT, A. JOHNSSON, A. WASTESON, B. WESTERMARK, C.-H. HELDIN, J. S. HUANG & T. F. DEUEL. 1983. Platelet-derived growth factor is structurally related to the putative transforming protein p28^{sis} of simian sarcoma virus. Nature **304:** 35–39.
20. JOHNSSON, A., C.-H. HELDIN, A. WASTESON, B. WESTERMARK, T. F. DEUEL, J. S. HUANG, P. H. SEEBURG, A. GRAY, A. ULLRICH, G. SCRACE, P. STROOBANT & M. D. WATERFIELD. 1984. The c-sis gene encodes a precursor of the B chain of platelet-derived growth factor. EMBO J. **3:** 921–928.
21. ROSS, R., E. W. RAINES & D. F. BOWEN-POPE. 1986. The biology of platelet-derived growth factor. Cell **46:** 155–169.
22. RAINES, E. W., D. F. BOWEN-POPE & R. ROSS. 1990. Platelet-derived growth factor. *In* Handbook of Experimental Pharmacology: Peptide Growth Factors and their Receptors. M. B. Sporn & A. B. Roberts, Eds. Vol. **95I:** 173–262. Springer-Verlag. New York, NY.

23. HART, C. E., M. BAILEY, D. A. CURTIS, S. OSBORN, E. RAINES, R. ROSS & J. W. FORSTROM. 1990. Purification of PDGF-AB and PDGF-BB from human platelet extracts and the identification of all three PDGF dimers in human platelets. Biochemistry **29:** 166–172.

24. HART, C. E., J. W. FORSTROM, J. D. KELLY, R. A. SEIFERT, R. A. SMITH, R. ROSS, M. J. MURRAY & D. F. BOWEN-POPE. 1988. Two classes of PDGF receptor recognize different isoforms of PDGF. Science **240:** 1529–1531.

25. HELDIN, C.-H., G. BACKSTROM, A. OSTMAN, A. HAMMACHER, L. RONNSTRAND, K. RUBIN, M. NISTER & B. WESTERMARK. 1988. Binding of different dimeric forms of PDGF to human fibroblasts: evidence for two separate receptor types. EMBO J. **7:** 1387–1393.

26. HELDIN, C.-H., A. ERNLUND, C. RORSMAN & L. RONNSTRAND. 1989. Dimerization of B-type platelet-derived growth factor receptors occurs after ligand binding and is closely associated with receptor kinase activation. J. Biol. Chem. **264:** 8905–8912.

27. SEIFERT, R. A., C. E. HART, P. E. PHILLIPS, J. W. FORSTROM, R. ROSS, M. J. MURRAY & D. F. BOWEN-POPE. 1989. Two different subunits associate to create isoform-specific platelet-derived growth factor receptors. J. Biol. Chem. **264:** 8771–8778.

28. YARDEN, Y., J. A. ESCOBEDO, W.-J. KUANG, T. L. YANG-FENG, T. O. DANIEL, P. M. TREMBLE, E. Y. CHEN, M. E. ANDO, R. N. HARKINS, U. FRANCKE, V. A. FRIED, A. ULLRICH & L. T. WILLIAMS. 1986. Structure of the receptor for platelet-derived growth factor helps define a family of closely related growth factor receptors. Nature **323:** 226–232.

29. MATSUI, T., M. HEIDARAN, T. MIKI, N. POPESCU, W. LA ROCHELLE, M. KRAUS, J. PIERCE & S. AARONSON. 1989. Isolation of a novel receptor cDNA establishes the existence of two PDGF receptor genes. Science **243:** 800–804.

30. FERNS, G., M. REIDY & R. ROSS. Vascular effects of cyclosporin A *in vivo* and *in vitro*. Am. J. Pathol. In press.

31. RUBIN, K., G. K. HANSSON, L. RONNSTRAND, L. CLAESSON-WELSH, B. FELLSTROM, A. TINGSTROM, E. LARSSON, L. KLARESKOG, C.-H. HELDIN & L. TERRACIO. 1988. Induction of B-type receptors for platelet-derived growth factor in vascular inflammation: possible implications for development of vascular proliferative lesions. Lancet June 18, **i:** 1353–1356.

32. ROSS, R., J. MASUDA, E. W. RAINES, A. M. GOWN, S. KATSUDA, M. SASAHARA, L. T. MALDEN, M. HIDEYUKI & H. SATO. Localization of PDGF-B protein in macrophages in all phases of atherogenesis. Science. In press.

33. RAINES, E. W., S. K. DOWER & R. ROSS. 1989. IL-1 mitogenic activity for fibroblasts and smooth muscle cells is due to PDGF-AA. Science **243:** 393–396.

34. HAJJAR, K. A., D. P. HAJJAR, R. L. SILVERSTEIN & R. L. NACHMAN. 1987. Tumor necrosis factor-mediated release of platelet-derived growth factor from cultured endothelial cells. J. Exp. Med. **166:** 235–245.

Electron Microscopic Exploration of Human Endothelium in Step-Serial Sections of Early and Advanced Atherosclerotic Lesions

PARIS CONSTANTINIDES AND MARTHA HARKEY

Pathology Department
Louisiana State University Medical School
P.O. Box 33932
Shreveport, Louisana 71130-3932

INTRODUCTION

In the late 1950s we were able to confirm the earlier observations of Anitschow[1] and Ssolowjew[2] that in cholesterol-fed rabbits lipids deposit at the sites of arterial injury, and, in addition, we found that (a) injury increased the *amount* of lipid deposition, and (b) it stimulated a very rapid arterial (smooth muscle) cell proliferation.[3] During the subsequent 30 years strong experimental evidence accumulated that injury can promote both lipid deposition and smooth muscle proliferation by increasing the permeability of the endothelium for plasma lipoproteins and for various mitogens.

Most of the insults that commonly act on human arteries seem to increase endothelial permeability functionally, by changing endothelial structure, or by opening endothelial junctions, as, *e.g.,* has been found to be the case for angiotensin,[4] hypertension,[5] and prolonged hyperlipemia.[6] A complete endothelial denudation with massive platelet aggregation over the denuded arterial surface, such as produced experimentally by balloon catheterisation,[7] does not seem to be induced by most of the naturally and commonly occurring insults that we know so far. And yet, because the platelet-derived growth factor (PDGF) released in balloon experiments triggers an extremely rapid smooth muscle proliferation, many investigators today assume—without real evidence—that endothelial denudation and platelet aggregation is a main initiating event in human atherogenesis. To find out whether such events occur at any stage of human atherosclerosis we recently undertook this electron microscopic study of early and advanced human lesions.

MATERIALS AND METHODS

We first examined light microscopically toluidine blue stained 1-μ thick (semi-thin) sections from 597 tissue blocks taken step-serially every mm from 26 normal arterial wall segments, 49 early myoproliferative lesions, and 48 advanced plaques with cap and gruel. All of these specimens were obtained from 17 popliteal arteries taken immediately after amputation surgery on persons 52–101 years old, and from 39 coronary arteries and thoracic and abdominal aortae taken from 16 autopsies of 1–79-year-old persons. Twelve of the 16 autopsies were performed between 1 and 5 hours, and the remaining 4 between 5 and 8 ½ hours after death.

We then examined with the transmission electron microscope ultra-thin sections of the 102 most interesting of the above 597 blocks, all of which were about 1 mm thick (from

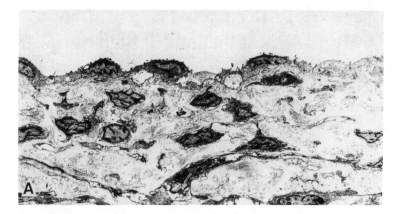

FIGURE 1. (A) Typical continuous endothelium lining a focus of intimal muscular proliferation (early lesion) in a baby common iliac artery. Note the high frequency of nonsyncytial endothelial nuclei and the variable cytoplasmic electron density, 1400.

luminal surface towards the adventitia of the artery) thus usually encompassing the entire thickness of a myoproliferative lesion and most or all of the thickness of the cap of an advanced plaque.

The general processing of the arterial material can be summarized as follows: The 1–3-cm-long arterial cylinders were immersed unopened into neutral formalin fixative to avoid artificial loss from air-drying, rinsing, and touching of the unfixed endothelium, *i.e.*, from manipulations that damage it. After formalin fixation for several days the arterial cylinders were opened with instruments, and their lesions were identified and cut step-serially into 1-mm-wide blocks that were post-fixed in glutaraldehyde-osmic acid and

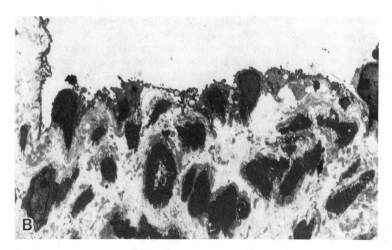

FIGURE 1. (B) Continuous endothelium lining a focus of muscular proliferation in a popliteal artery. Note its focally extreme thiness, 2200×.

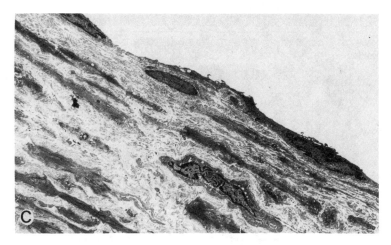

FIGURE 1. (C) Continuous endothelium lining a focus of intimal muscular proliferation in the abdominal aorta of a kidney donor, 2200 × .

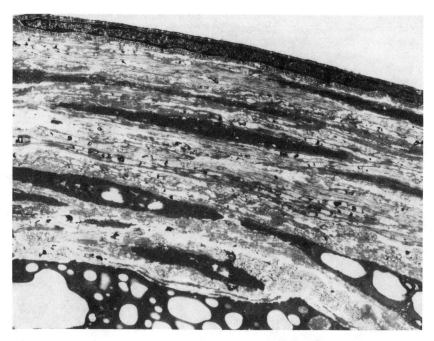

FIGURE 2. Typical continuous thin endothelium lining the nonnecrotic fibrous cap of an advanced plaque with several layers of collagen-producing myocytes, some of which have picked up lipid in the deeper cap layer, 8800 × .

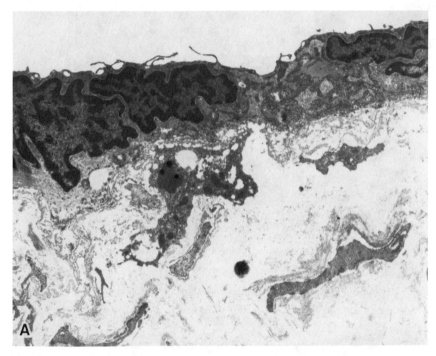

FIGURE 3. (A) Endothelial syncytium over an early myoproliferative lesion. Note also the development of microvilli on the luminal endothelial surface and the proliferation and dilatation of the rough endoplasmic reticulum sacs that are filled with proteinaceous fluid, 8800 ×.

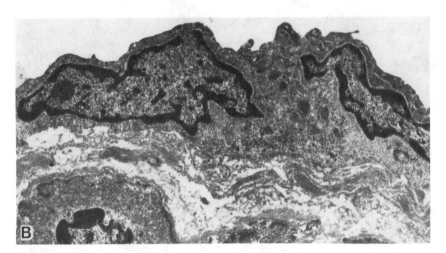

FIGURE 3. (B) Endothelial syncytium over the cap of an advanced plaque, 14000 ×.

processed through dehydration into epon embedding for semi-thin and ultra-thin sectioning.

Nine advanced lesions with calcifications were decalcified effectively in 1% formic acid for 1 day after formalin and before glutaraldehyde fixation.

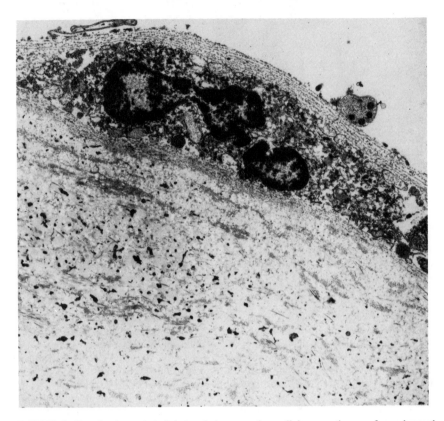

FIGURE 4. True *in vivo* endothelial denudation over the acellular necrotic cap of an advanced plaque, with a necrotic cap cell in the process of disintegration. One platelet adheres to the de-endothelialised surface, 6000×.

RESULTS

We obtained the following results in this study.

(1) No endothelial denudation with platelet aggregation was seen over any normal arterial segment, any of the 49 early myoproliferative lesions, or most of the 48 advanced plaques whose cap was not necrotic (FIGS. 1, 2). The endothelium was continuous in all the above specimens except for some stretches of artifactual losses that were obviously due to postmortem autolysis mainly in the 4 autopsies done between 5 and 8 ½ hours after death.

(2) The continuous endothelium was often syncytial mostly over advanced plaques (in

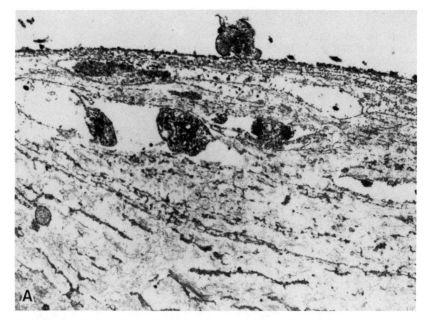

FIGURE 5. (A) True *in vivo* endothelial denudation over the acellular, fluid-soaked necrotic cap of an advanced plaque, showing one platelet that adheres to the de-endothelialised surface and three platelets that have penetrated into the upper cap, 6000×.

16 of the 48 specimens) with 2 or more nuclei contained in the same cytoplasm (FIG. 3). No centrioles were observed in any of the sections of these syncytial endothelial cells.

(3) We saw short stretches of true *in vivo* endothelial denudation with platelet adherence and aggregation only over the surface of 9 of the 48 advanced plaques whose caps showed destructive changes in the form of acellularity (almost complete disappearance of living smooth muscle cells) in 6 of the lesions, necrosis and beginning disintegration of muscle cells in 4 of the lesions, and microhemorrhages in the inner cap of 2 of the lesions (FIGS. 4,5). In 2 of the above plaques, some platelets had also penetrated into the superficial layers of the cap.

(4) Three types of endothelial changes were frequently seen over both early and advanced lesions, namely, (a) opened interendothelial junctions (FIGS. 6,7), (b) endothelial lipid inclusions of electron dense and mixed types (FIG. 8), and (c) numerous dilated endoplasmic reticulum sacs, filled with proteinaceous fluid (FIG. 9). In addition, autolytic changes in the form of water swelling of whole endothelial cells and their intracellular sacs were sometimes seen in lesions from the 4 autopsies done between 5 and 8 ½ hours after death.

(5) Underneath the endothelium, the foam cells in the caps of all advanced lesions were a mixed population of dual origin, some myocytic and some monocytic, and many of the ones maximally filled with lipid in the deeper cap were disintegrating, adding their lipid contents to the extracellular lipid pool of their plaque. Also, myocytes of the synthetic type (with prominent rough endoplasmic reticulum) and binucleate myocytes, along with fresh immigrant cells from the blood such as lymphocytes and lipid-free monocytes were occasionally seen in the advanced plaque caps.

CONCLUSIONS AND DISCUSSION

We have drawn the following conclusions from our results:

(1) Endothelial denudation does not seem to be a common initiating event in human atherogenesis, since we did not find it over any early purely myoproliferative lesions. Our transmission electron microscopic findings thus agree on this point with the results obtained by Repin *et al.* with the scanning electron microscope[8] and by Massman and Papamichael in their light microscopic studies of Häutchen preparations.[9]

(2) True *in vivo* endothelial denudation accompanied by platelet adherence and aggregation can occur over some advanced human plaques with largely necrotic caps as a prelude to mural thrombosis over the disintegrating surface of such lesions. It thus seems to develop occasionally as a *late* complication—not an early initiating event—in human atherosclerosis, in line with our light microscopic findings of 25 years ago that thrombosis in human atherosclerotic arteries is always initiated by a breakdown of the mostly necrotic caps of advanced lesions that leads to tears and frequently hemorrhages into such plaques.[10,11] The necrosis of endothelium and underlying cap cells in advanced lesions could be caused not only by chemical, metabolic, or immune insults coming from the blood (and attacking from the lumen) but also by toxic degradation products of atheroma lipids that could diffuse to the surface of an advanced plaque from its deeper lipid mass

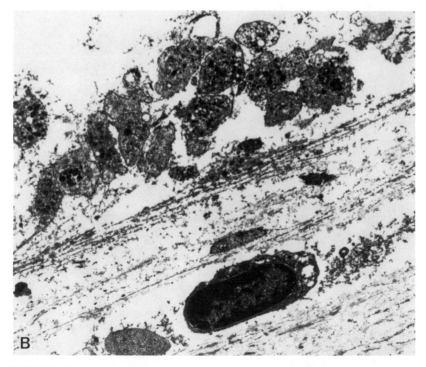

FIGURE 5. (B) True *in vivo* endothelial denudation over the almost entirely acellular necrotic cap of another advanced plaque, showing a platelet aggregate that developed over the raw surface and again the penetration of some platelets into the upper cap zone, 6000×.

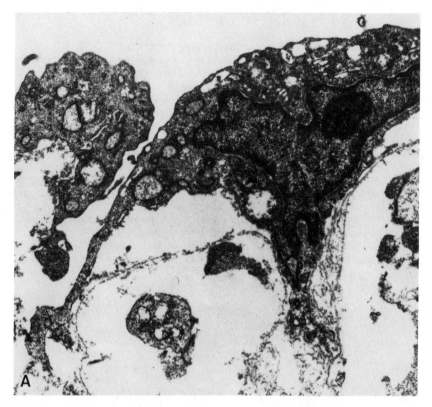

FIGURE 6. (A) Narrowly opened junction between two endothelial cells with significant swelling of intracytoplasmic sacs, 14000 × .

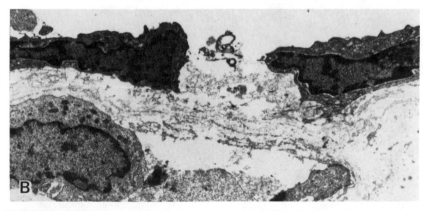

FIGURE 6. (B) Widely opened junction between two endothelial cells that are free of other structural abnormalities, 6000 × .

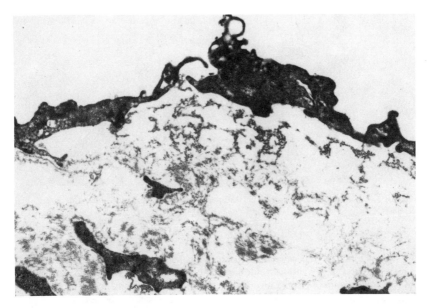

FIGURE 7. Beginning opening of an endothelial junction, 14000 ×.

(gruel)—a theoretical possibility that to date has been totally unexplored and yet deserves future study.

(3) The opened endothelial junctions frequently seen over both early and advanced human lesions are similar to ultrastructural endothelial changes produced experimentally by several naturally occurring injurious agents, including hypertension, angiotensin, hypercalcemia, and chronic hyperlipemia,[12] and they clearly show that the endothelium over

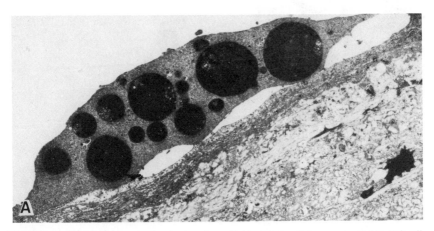

FIGURE 8. (A) Many completely electron-dense lipid globules filling up an endothelial cell, 6000 ×.

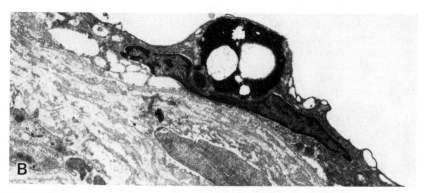

FIGURE 8. (B) A large partly translucent and partly electron-dense lipid globule in an endothelial cell, 8800×.

all lesions is much more permeable to plasma constituents than that over the normal wall. Such an increased permeability would inevitably promote a flooding of the inner arterial wall by a whole soup of plasma macromolecules, *i.e.*, lipoproteins, proteins, and various circulating mitogens,[12] including soluble PDGF that has recently been found to circulate in the blood at all times.[13] Thus platelet-derived mitogens—along with several other mitogens—could participate in the stimulation of myocytic proliferation under a hyperpermeable endothelium, without a platelet aggregation on de-endothelialised surfaces.

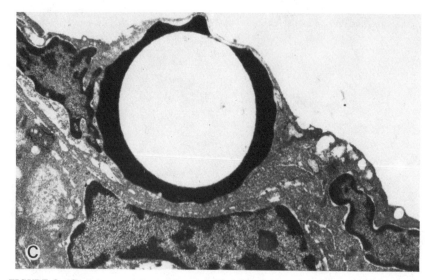

FIGURE 8. (C) A huge mostly translucent lipid globule with a dense rim in the endothelium, 14000×.

(4) The very frequent and massive endothelial lipid inclusions that were observed at all stages of human atherosclerosis—but not in normal wall—strikingly parallel those produced experimentally in the endothelium of animals by chronic hyperlipemia[6] and certainly provide a powerful new histological argument for the key role of hyperlipemia in human atherogenesis.

Further research is necessary to identify the nature of the dense and lucent components of these lipid inclusions and to find out whether the lipids first enter the endothelial cells as electron-dense and are later turned into electron-lucent material through enzymatic action, or vice versa.

(5) The striking proliferation of the rough endoplasmic reticulum sacs and the filling of the sacs with proteinaceous fluid in several endothelial cells that gave them a plasma

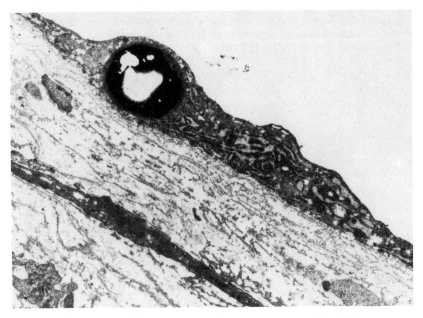

FIGURE 9. An activated (synthetic-type) endothelial cell with a lipid inclusion and markedly proliferated rough endoplasmic reticulum sacs that are filled with a proteinaceous fluid, 8800×.

cell-like ("synthetic cell-like") appearance most probably represented a marked activation of the enzyme-producing apparatus in some lining cells in reaction to plasma-derived insults. Further research is needed for the identification of such possibly reactive products which might represent endothelial lipo-oxygenases[14] and (or) other lipid-handling enzymes.

The considerable frequency of syncytial endothelial nuclei that we observed mostly over advanced human plaques agrees with the findings of others.[8,9] These syncytia could express either a rapid endothelial mitosis to replace injured lining cells (with the nuclei dividing faster than the cytoplasm) *or* a fusion of two or more endothelial cells (perhaps caused by a propylene glycol-like membrane fusing effect of lipoproteins or viruses). Our failure to find any centrioles in a good number of serial ultra-thin sections through 12 of these syncytial endothelial cells favors—but does not yet prove—the latter alternative.

SUMMARY

A transmission electron microscopic study of step-serial sections of numerous human early and advanced atherosclerotic lesions obtained under conditions preventing artificial endothelial loss was undertaken. It was found that (1) *no* endothelial denudation with platelet aggregation occurred over any early myoproliferative lesions, (2) endothelial denudation with platelet aggregation had developed *only* over the mostly necrotic caps of some advanced end-stage lesions, and (3) *all* stages of atherosclerosis showed endothelial changes that indicated increased permeability of the endothelium over plaques for plasma constituents, namely, opened interendothelial junctions and endothelial lipid inclusions.

These results suggest that endothelial denudation and platelet aggregation is *not* an initiating event in human atherogenesis but something that happens late over the disintegrating surface of some end-stage lesions as a prelude to supra-plaque thrombosis—in agreement with our light microscopic findings of 25 years ago that thrombosis in human atherosclerotic arteries is usually triggered by a breakdown of the mostly necrotic caps of advanced plaques.

REFERENCES

1. ANITSCHKOW, N. 1933. Experimental arteriosclerosis in animals. *In* Arteriosclerosis—A Survey of the Problem. E. V. Cowdry, Ed. 271–322. Macmillan Publ. New York.
2. SSOLOWJEW, A. 1929. Zeitschr. f.d. exper. Med. **69:** 94–97.
3. CONSTANTINIDES, P., N. GUTMANN-AUERSPERG & D. HOSPES. 1958. AMA Arch. Pathol. **66:** 247–254.
4. CONSTANTINIDES, P. 1971. Endothelial injury in the pathogenesis of arteriosclerosis. Opening Address to the Lindau International Symposium of April 1970 on The Artery and the Process of Arteriosclerosis, Pathogenesis I—Advances in Experimental Medicine and Biology. Vol. 16A: 185–212. Plenum Press Publ. New York and London.
5. SUZUKI, K., S. OOKAWARA & G. OONEDA. 1971. Exp. Mol. Pathol. **15:** 198–208.
6. CONSTANTINIDES, P. & K. D. WIGGERS. 1974. Virchow's Arch. A **362:** 291–310.
7. ROSS, R. 1976. Triangle **15:** 45–51.
8. REPIN, V. S., V. V. DOLGOV, O. E. ZAIKINA, I. D. NOVILOV, A. S. ANTONOV, M. A. NIKOLAEVA & V. N. SMIRNOV. 1984. Atherosclerosis **50:** 35–52.
9. MASSMANN, J. & G. PAPAMICHAEL. 1984. Zbl.allg. Pathol. pathol. Anat. **129:** 487.
10. CONSTANTINIDES, P. 1964. J. Am. Med. Assoc. **188**(6): (News Section) 35–36.
11. CONSTANTINIDES, P. 1966. J. Atheroscler. Res. **6:** 1–17.
12. CONSTANTINIDES, P. 1984. Ultrastructural Pathobiology. 99–134. Elsevier Publ. Amsterdam, New York, and Oxford.
13. NILSSON, J., J. SVENSSON, A. HAMSTEN & U. DE FAIRE. 1986. Atherosclerosis **61:** 237–243.
14. STEINBERG, D., S. PARTHASARATHY, T. E., CAREW, J. C. KHOO & M. L. WITZTUM. 1989. N. Engl. J. Med. **320:** 915–924.

Arterial Metabolism of Lipoproteins in Relation to Atherogenesis

DANIEL STEINBERG

Department of Medicine
University of California, San Diego
La Jolla, California 92093-0613

The Atheroscleroses

It is clear that hyperlipoproteinemia in some fashion plays a causative role in atherosclerosis; it is equally clear that hyperlipoproteinemia is by no means the only causative factor. Indeed, as we become more sophisticated in our understanding of the atherogenic process and as we elucidate the pathogenetic factors, we will probably "split" atherosclerosis into more and more subcategories just as we have "split" gout and many other metabolic disturbances into subcategories. The subcategory with which we shall be concerned here is the category of what I suggest we call "lipoprotein-induced atherosclerosis." By that I mean any form of atherosclerosis in which hyperlipoproteinemia is the *dominant* causative factor (albeit not necessarily the *only* causative factor). Other likely categories that may be defined as we learn more about their pathogenesis would include "cigarette smoking-induced atherosclerosis," "hypertension-induced atherosclerosis" and so on. We already know that coronary heart disease risk attributable to these and other factors tends to be additive. But we are still very much in the dark with regard to detailed mechanisms.

It is generally accepted now that low density lipoprotein (LDL) and β-very low density lipoprotein (β-VLDL) are atherogenic lipoproteins and that high density lipoprotein (HDL), or at least some subfraction of it, is "antiatherogenic." The issue with regard to the triglyceride-rich lipoproteins is less clear. In this paper we shall confine our discussion to the LDL and β-VLDL fractions primarily, *i.e.,* "LDL-induced atherosclerosis" and "β-VLDL-induced atherosclerosis." The focus of this paper is even narrower. We shall confine our considerations to the earliest stages of atherogenesis, namely, the genesis of the fatty streak lesion. The justification for that focus is the presumption that the fatty streak is the precursor of the fibrous plaque and the more complicated lesions. Evidence supporting that presumption has been presented both in experimental animals and in man.[1,2] If we can elucidate the cellular and molecular mechanisms underlying the initiation of the fatty streak lesion, we might be in a better position to design interventions that would arrest the process early on. This is not at all to gainsay the importance of studying the later lesions as well. After all, those are the lesions that are clinically significant and we already know it is possible to intervene effectively at the later stages so as to arrest or even reverse later lesions. The fatty streak lesion is, in contrast, a silent, asymptomatic lesion. On the other hand, if it is the starting point for the clinically threatening lesions, there would obviously be virtue in limiting its development and, hopefully, "nipping things in the bud."

Role of the Monocyte/Macrophage

The fatty streak lesion, both in experimental animals and in man, is characterized by an accumulation in the subendothelial space of large, fat-loaded "foam cells" derived

125

mainly from circulating monocytes that have taken up residence beneath the endo-thelium.[3,4] Some are derived also from smooth muscle cells but these constitute a small proportion in the early lesions. Consequently, there has been a great deal of interest in the mechanisms by which the monocyte/macrophage takes up lipoproteins and becomes loaded with cholesteryl esters and other lipids.

Goldstein et al.[5] were the first to call attention to the paradoxical fact that in vitro incubation of monocyte/macrophages with native LDL, even at high concentrations, failed to generate foam cells. They then looked for modifications of LDL that might enhance its uptake and found that chemical acetylation did just that. Incubation of mouse peritoneal macrophages with acetylated LDL did lead to foam cell formation and, im-portantly, this uptake was saturable and specific, attributable to what they termed the "acetyl LDL receptor.[6] There was, however, no evidence that acetylation occurred at any significant rate in vivo and a search began for biological equivalents of acetylation. Henriksen, Mahoney, and Steinberg[7] demonstrated that incubation of LDL with cultured endothelial cells induced a number of dramatic changes in the structure of the LDL. The product was taken up in part by the same receptor that takes up acetylated LDL, and taken up rapidly enough to generate foam cells.[8,9] The modification induced by the cells was brought about by oxidation[10,11] and this process has been intensively studied in recent years. All three of the major cell types in an atherosclerotic lesion (endothelial cells, smooth muscle cells, and macrophages) are capable of inducing oxidative modification of LDL and there is now considerable evidence to suggest that the process also occurs in vivo. The evidence for the in vivo occurrence of oxidative modification of LDL and for its potential importance in atherogenesis has recently been reviewed by Steinberg et al.[12]

In the present paper we would like to call particular attention to the fact that other modifications of LDL may also be of importance in favoring foam cell formation through receptor-mediated uptake. At least four different receptors are now recognized that can take up LDL or modified forms of LDL rapidly enough to lead to foam cell formation. These are listed in TABLE 1 along with the forms of LDL that they can take up at a sufficiently rapid rate to be potentially relevant to fatty streak formation.

The Receptor for Native LDL

Even in the total absence of functional LDL receptors (as in patients with receptor-negative familial hypercholesterolemia of the homozygous type) or in experimental ani-mals with a near-complete deficiency of LDL receptors (the Watanabe Heritable Hyper-lipidemic (WHHL) rabbit), foam cells develop and atherosclerosis proceeds at a rapid rate. Thus, the presence of the LDL receptor is not a necessary condition for foam cell formation. However, it does not follow that the presence of LDL receptors—in those animals that do express them—is necessarily irrelevant to their atherogenic process. The first point that should be made is that the time scale of in vitro experiments on foam cell formation is highly compressed. Most studies extend over only a few days whereas the genesis af atherosclerotic lesions in animals extends over many months and in man over many years. It would be a mistake to conclude that the inability to generate a foam cell by 72 hours of exposure to native LDL in a cell culture dish rules out a role for the LDL receptor in a process that may take ten years in vivo! The second point is that even though native LDL does not itself lead to foam cell formation, variations of LDL that might still be recognized by the LDL receptor could play a role. In fact, Khoo and co-workers have recently described just such a situation.[13]

The history behind these latter studies is of interest. Dr. Khoo was carrying out a series of studies on the ability of cholesterol-loaded macrophages to mobilize their stored cholesteryl esters. In the course of that work, he noted that LDL preparations that had been stored in the refrigerator for long periods of time were more useful for loading up the cells with cholesterol than was fresh LDL. As everyone who works with lipoproteins knows, stored preparations tend to accumulate a sediment and Dr. Khoo speculated that some sort of aggregation might be involved. He was able to mimic this by simply putting fresh preparations of LDL in a conical centrifuge tube and subjecting them to vortexing, *i.e.*, putting them on the ordinary lab-top vortexing machine to swirl the preparation vigorously. This led to an immediate appearance of opalescence and that opalescence increased rapidly as a function of the number of seconds of vortexing. There were no other proteins present in the medium and so these aggregates represent LDL *self*-aggregation. The rate of uptake of the aggregates into macrophages was far greater than that of native LDL and led to massive accumulation of cholesteryl esters. Special care was taken to prevent oxidation of the LDL during the vortexing and examination of the aggregated LDL showed no increase in thiobarbituric acid-reactive substances. Unlabeled acetylated LDL did not compete for uptake.

Several lines of evidence indicated that these LDL self-aggregates are taken up by way of the LDL receptor (the B/E receptor of Brown and Goldstein) and that they are taken up not by pinocytosis but largely by phagocytosis:

TABLE 1. Monocyte/Macrophage Receptors That May Play a Role in the Generation of Foam Cells

Receptors	Effective Ligands
1. LDL receptor (B/E receptor)	a. Aggregates of LDL with itself b. ? Aggregates of LDL with other macromolecules (*NOT* native LDL itself)
2. Acetyl LDL receptor	a. Chemically modified forms of LDL (acetyl-, acetoacetyl-, MDA-LDL) b. Oxidatively modified LDL
3. Oxidized LDL receptor(s)	a. Oxidatively modified LDL b. ? Acetyl LDL
4. F_c receptor	a. Immune complexes of oxidized LDL and autoantibodies against it b. Immune complexes of glycated LDL and autoantibodies against it c. Other lipoprotein-antibody complexes

1. Reductively methylated LDL, which is not recognized by the B/E receptor, aggregated to an extent comparable to that of untreated LDL but the aggregates were taken up much less avidly than aggregates of native LDL.
2. High concentrations of native LDL (but not acetylated LDL) competed with aggregates for uptake.
3. A monoclonal antibody directed against the LDL receptor (mAbC7) strongly inhibited the uptake of LDL aggregates but did not inhibit the uptake of acetylated LDL.
4. Cytochalasin B, which inhibits phagocytosis, strongly inhibited the uptake of aggregated LDL but did not inhibit the uptake of acetylated LDL. Consequently, it is proposed that the uptake of LDL aggregates occurs as a result of interactions with the LDL receptor by a zipper mechanism like that proposed for the uptake of imune complexes.[14]

More recent studies by Khoo et al.[15] have led to a postulated mechanism for this aggregation. HDL or purified HDL apoproteins (including apo A-I, apo C, and apo E) can inhibit the aggregation. Since HDL and these apoproteins do not form complexes with LDL, the basis for the inhibiton was unclear. Suits et al.[16] confirmed and extended the results of Khoo et al., showing that LDL self-aggregates induced by treatment with phospholipase C behave much like those induced by vortexing. Further studies by Khoo et al.[15] showed that HDL could also prevent aggregation of LDL induced by treatment with phospholipase C and that induced by heating. The results suggested that the mechanism involved in these three different kinds of aggregation might have something in common. What Khoo et al.[15] propose is that hydrophobic domains of LDL are intermittently exposed and this provides intermittent opportunities for hydrophobic LDL-LDL interaction to occur. The frequency with which such exposure of hydrophobic domains occurs may very well be increased during vortexing (perhaps because of the creation of a larger surface area) or by breakdown of the phospholipid shell by phospholipases or during heating. Apo a-I, by virtue of its amphipathic helical structure, may bind to such exposed hydrophobic domains and thus block LDL-LDL interactions.

Does anything analogous occur in vivo? To the extent that LDL is exposed to large surfaces of connective tissue matrix in the subendothelial space and to the extent that it is subject to enzymatic attack under some conditions in that space, the development of aggregates is at least a possibility. Recently, Frank and Fogelman,[17] using a novel electron microscopic technique, have described large aggregates in the subendothelial space with dimensions that could represent LDL aggregates. However, it remains to be determined whether they do in fact arise from LDL. Polacek et al.[18] noted several years ago that incubation of LDL with neutrophils generated a modified form. Subsequent studies showed that the change was probably due to secreted elastase and that the treated LDL formed dimers taken up more rapidly by macrophages.[19] These "mini-aggregates" are taken up via the LDL receptor.

Before leaving this topic, we would like to venture a highly speculative suggestion. The mechanisms by which a high level of HDL protects against atherosclerosis has not been fully established, although the most plausible and attractive hypothesis is that it is through facilitation of reverse cholesterol transport. Should the self-aggregation of LDL be shown by further studies to contribute to foam cell formation in vivo, then the ability of HDL to interfere with that process could afford an alternative (or at least an additional) mechanism.

In cholesterol-fed animals and in patients with type III hyperlipoproteinemia, there is an accumulation of VLDL molecules enriched in cholesteryl esters.[20] These have the flotation properties of VLDL but the electrophoretic mobility of LDL—the so-called β-VLDL. This species of lipoprotein has a very high affinity for the LDL receptor, probably because of its enrichment in apo E, and it is taken up avidly by macrophages, giving rise to foam cells. It was first proposed that this uptake was referable to a special receptor because LDL appeared not to compete with β-VLDL[21] for uptake and because cells from a patient deficient in LDL receptors appeared to be fully competent in the uptake and degradation of β-VLDL.[22] More recent findings, however, show that the apparent failure of LDL to compete is due to the much higher affinity of β-VLDL. The early studies had not been carried out at sufficiently high ratios of LDL to β-VLDL. The apparent ability of the receptor-deficient WHHL cells to take up β-VLDL is, in retrospect, due to the presence of a small number of LDL receptors in the WHHL rabbit. When cells from bona fide LDL receptor-negative patients are used, β-VLDL is not taken up.[23] As mentioned, uptake of β-VLDL leads to foam cell formation and massive cholesteryl ester accumulation in cell culture. This is rather paradoxical in that the uptake of cholesterol in the form of LDL causes downregulation of the LDL receptor whereas uptake of β-VLDL does not appear to downregulate. The explanation for this must reside in some different handling of β-VLDL relative to the handling of LDL. Whatever the mechanisms involved, it now appears that uptake of β-VLDL by way of the native B/E receptor is effective in generating foam cells. Thus, in summary of this section, the LDL receptor indeed can and probably does play a role in foam cell formation but not through the uptake of LDL itself. Aggregates of LDL or β-VLDL are legitimate ligands for the receptor and they can cause foam cell formation. It is quite possible that other aggregates of LDL— aggregates of LDL with other macromolecules such as proteoglycans, elastin, collagen, etc.—may under some circumstances also be ligands for the LDL receptor and be taken up by phagocytosis in a fashion analogous to the uptake of LDL self-aggregates. Further research along these lines is obviously needed.

Acetyl LDL Receptor

As discussed above, macrophages express a receptor that does not recognize native LDL but recognizes chemically acetylated LDL.[5,6] It also recognizes acetoacetylated LDL[24] or malondialdehyde-conjugated LDL.[25] Incubation of macrophages with these chemically modified forms of LDL can generate foam cells whereas incubation with native LDL cannot. However, these chemically modified forms of LDL are not known to occur *in vivo*. Oxidation of LDL, whether induced by cells or by incubation with metal catalysts, can generate a form of LDL recognized by the same receptor that recognizes these chemically modified forms of LDL.[7–12] At first this sharing of the same receptor seemed puzzling but we now can see the probable reason. During oxidation of LDL, the polyunsaturated fatty acids are degraded to yield an array of lower molecular weight fragments, many of them in the form of aldehydes.[26] These range from a 3-carbon fragment (malondialdehyde) up to a 9-carbon fragment (4-hydroxynonenal) and all have the potential of reacting with free amino groups on the lysine side chains of apo B or with other free amino groups in the LDL molecule. This is exactly what happens with chemical treatments of the kind listed above, *i.e.*, the epsilon amino groups of lysine residues are conjugated with malondialdehyde or with acetoacetic acid, etc. Thus there is an analogy but we still do not know exactly how these chemical modifications or oxidation of LDL generate the new "epitope(s)" recognized by the acetyl LDL receptor. At any rate, the uptake of oxidized LDL can lead to cholesterol accumulation in cultured macrophages and could then contribute to foam cell formation *in vivo*. Before going on, it should be mentioned that the uptake of oxidized LDL is not entirely accounted for by uptake via the acetyl LDL receptor (see below).

What is the available evidence that oxidation of LDL occurs under *in vivo* conditions? Four different lines of evidence have been presented:

1. *Treatment of LDL receptor-deficient rabbits (WHHL rabbits) with an antioxidant compound slows the progression of their atherosclerosis and reduces the rate of uptake and degradation of native LDL by their arterial macrophages.*

If oxidation of LDL is a prerequisite for rapid uptake of LDL into macrophages, prevention of that oxidation should slow the uptake of injected native LDL into arterial macrophages and possibly even slow the progression of lesions. Both of these have been demonstrated in the studies of Carew, Schwenke, and Steinberg.[27] Kita *et al.*[28] independently demonstrated an inhibition of the progression of lesions in WHHL rabbits. The antioxidant used in both studies was probucol, a compound that has been clinically used to lower cholesterol levels. However, the effects in the rabbit studies occurred despite the fact that plasma cholesterols in the treated and control groups were deliberately held at the same level.

2. *Antibodies directed against oxidized LDL or "models" of oxidized LDL react with materials in arterial lesions.*

As discussed briefly above, the oxidation of LDL is accompanied by the generation of lower molecular weight fragments of polyunsaturated fatty acids and these fragments can covalently react with the LDL protein or with free amino groups of LDL lipids. Malondialdehyde is one such fragment. Haberland and co-workers[29] showed that lesions of WHHL rabbits stain positively with an antibody directed against malondialdehyde-conjugated LDL. This work was confirmed and extended in the studies of Palinski et al.[30] and Rosenfeld et al.[31] using antisera against MDA-LDL and against 4-HNE-LDL and also a monoclonal antibody against oxidized LDL (reactive epitope not yet identified). These immunostaining studies demonstrated reactive material both extracellularly and intracellularly. The macrophages were notably rich in reactive materials that were present throughout the cell and coincided with lipid storage vesicles. It seems unlikely that much, if any, of this can represent intact oxidized LDL. It seems more likely that the epitope being recognized persists even after the LDL has undergone degradation and that this accounts for its appearance intracellularly. Mitchinson and co-workers have previously described the presence of ceroid in arterial lesions, some of it in the form of rings.[32] The staining pattern in the studies of Rosenfeld et al. was in many instances reminiscent of this pattern of ceroid distribution. In addition to this heavy staining of macrophages, there was some extracellular reactive material but the former was decidedly more striking. The macrophages did not react with antibody directed against intact apo B-100, again suggesting that what is being stained within the macrophage represents degraded LDL apoprotein.

It should be stressed that demonstration of a reactive material in a tissue section cannot identify it necessarily as "oxidized LDL." As shown by the work of Witztum and co-workers,[33] antibodies generated against modified forms of LDL may recognize and react with a very narrowly defined epitope. For example, antibodies against MDA-LDL will react with MDA-conjugated polylysine (although with low affinity) and with a number of MDA-protein conjugates. Consequently, the reactivity of materials with such an antibody could reflect the presence of the MDA-lysine structure in *any* protein or fragment derived from proteins. Thus, these studies utilizing immunostaining are *compatible* with the presence of oxidized LDL or its fragments in the arterial lesions but do not necessarily establish it. The studies described in the next section, however, show that *some* oxidized LDL is indeed present.

3. *Isolation and characterization of oxidized LDL from human and rabbit arterial lesions.*

Ylä-Herttuala and co-workers[34] have developed and utilized a kinder, gentler method for isolating LDL from arterial tissue. The method involves no homogenization and no exposure to conditions that might themselves damage LDL or generate lipid artifacts. The tissue is minced and gently incubated overnight with physiologic buffers to elute that fraction of tissue LDL that can be gently eluted. Dr. Ylä-Herttuala, during a stay in La Jolla as a Fogarty International Fellow, has applied this technique and demonstrated the presence of oxidized LDL both in human lesions and in lesions of the WHHL rabbit.[30,35] He was able to show that the LDL fraction included material with physical and chemical properties like those of oxidized LDL. It showed an increased electrophoretic mobility, an increased hydrated density and was degraded at a much higher rate than native LDL by macrophages in culture. Most important, Western blots showed that this LDL reacted with antibodies against MDA-LDL and against 4-HNE-LDL. Both the intact apo B-100 and several of the lower molecular weight fragments derived from it (presumably the result of oxidative damage) reacted with the antibodies. These studies do not establish just how much of the LDL in the artery wall is in the oxidized form but they do at least demonstrate that the suspected oxidized species is present. Oxidized LDL could not be demonstrated in normal sections of artery but the yield of LDL from such normal areas is very low and the negative result is not readily interpreted.

4. *Demonstration of the presence of autoantibodies against oxidized LDL.*

Palinski *et al.*[30] demonstrated that both human serum and rabbit serum contain autoantibodies reactive with MDA-LDL [and with other "models" of oxidized LDL]. Although of low titer, these autoantibodies were present at significant levels both in normal subjects and patients with established coronary heart disease. They were also present both in wild-type New Zealand White rabbits and in WHHL rabbits. Obviously the presence of such autoantibodies implies the presence of the appropriate antigen. However, one cannot say with certainty that the antigen is oxidized LDL itself. For reasons discussed above, the antigen could conceivably be some other protein-lipid complex in which the MDA-lysine conjugate is present and this need not be LDL. On the other hand, we know from the work of Witztum and coworkers that MDA-LDL and other "models" of LDL are much better antigens than MDA-conjugates of other proteins.[33] We also now know that oxidized LDL is in fact present. Thus, these findings add further strength to the supposition that oxidation of LDL does take place and that this occurs in man as well as in rabbits.

In summary, a number of different lines of evidence, including *in vivo* evidence now, support the presumption that oxidation of LDL does take place *in vivo* and that that oxidation enhances the rate of progression of atherosclerotic lesions. Below we will mention additional mechanisms by which oxidized LDL may be contributing to the atherogenic process over and above the effect on foam cell formation.

Additional Receptor(s) for Oxidized LDL

The early studies of Henriksen *et al.* showed that endothelial cell-modified LDL was taken up in part by way of the acetyl LDL receptor.[7–9] However, unlabeled acetyl LDL competition was incomplete, often decreasing the uptake of modified LDL by only about 50 or 60%. Sparrow *et al.*[36] reinvestigated this in a more formal manner. They showed that unlabeled oxidized LDL could inhibit essentially all of the uptake of labeled oxidized LDL, indicating that most of the uptake was via a saturable mechanism. However, unlabeled acetyl LDL only partially inhibited both binding and uptake of oxidized LDL. Unlabeled oxidized LDL, on the other hand, was able to inhibit the binding and uptake of labeled acetyl LDL almost completely. They concluded that the mouse peritoneal macrophage must have at least one additional receptor recognizing oxidized LDL but not acetyl LDL. The findings were equally compatible with the presence of a single receptor of complex structure and with several binding sites. Arai and co-workers[37] have also reexamined the binding and uptake of oxidized LDL in a similar fashion. From their results they suggest the presence of three receptors: a receptor that recognizes both acetyl LDL and oxidized LDL; a receptor that recognizes only acetyl LDL; and a receptor that recognizes only oxidized LDL.

F_c Receptor

Immune complexes of any type can be taken up avidly by macrophages via the F_c receptors. This was recognized by Brown and Goldstein in their early studies on foam cell formation.[6] The possibility that an immune mechanism of this type may be significant has been increased by the demonstration of autoantibodies against modified forms of LDL. Witztum and co-workers showed that even very minor modifications in the structure of LDL render it immunogenic.[33] We now know that oxidized LDL is generated *in vivo* and that autoantibodies against oxidized LDL can be demonstrated.[12] If immune complexes were generated in the plasma compartment, one might anticipate their removal preferentially in liver and spleen but immune complexes formed within the artery wall would be fair game for the macrophages. In other words, if immune globulins enter the artery wall and react with modified forms of LDL in the intima, such complexes could contribute importantly to foam cell formation. Thus, modifications of LDL such as oxidation would have the potential of enhancing foam cell formation in two different ways: 1) through uptake via special receptors recognizing oxidized LDL itself; and 2) by uptake of immune complexes via the F_c receptor.

What is the "Normal" Function of the Acetyl LDL Receptor and the Oxidized LDL Receptor(s)?

Unless the acetyl LDL receptor and the oxidized LDL receptor are vestigial receptors (analogous to the vermiform appendix) they must have some survival value to justify their existence. Promoting atherosclerosis would obviously not have survival value! In any case, protecting against atherosclerosis (even if it did that) would not explain its persistence through evolution because atherosclerosis only takes a significant toll after the childbearing period is over. It seems reasonable to suggest that the true function of these

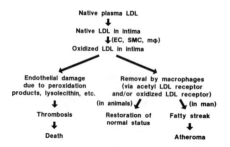

FIGURE 1. Schematic representation of an hypothesis that could account for the selective advantage conferred by the acetyl LDL or "scavenger" receptor. (See text for discussion.)

receptors, like that of most of the receptors on macrophages, is to remove potentially harmful materials. Macrophages are provided with receptors that help it identify and remove bacteria, cell debris, redundant connective tissue and so on. When Brown and Goldstein assigned the name of scavenger receptor, they actually used the term to refer to "scavenging" of LDL that was not taken up by way of the LDL receptor pathway. They may have chosen a more appropriate name than was apparent at the time. We now know that oxidized LDL is cytotoxic[10] and that oxidized fatty acids generated in membranous structures are likely also to be cytotoxic. From the work of Chisholm and his co-workers in Cleveland, it is clear that even relatively low concentrations of oxidized LDL can be highly cytotoxic to cells, at least in culture. Now, damage to endothelial cells in even a young animal could predispose to thrombosis. Such thrombosis could be crippling or even fatal and this would be very good thing for evolution to select *against*. A case can be made, then, that clearance of oxidized LDL by way of the acetyl LDL receptor and/or the oxidized LDL receptor is a way to prevent premature death in young animals (see FIG. 1). In this way, we can understand how the receptors in question would confer selective advantage. The implication of this hypothesis is that there is a continuous, on-going surveillance system by which monocyte/macrophages "clear" the vessel wall of potentially cytotoxic materials, including oxidized LDL. When, however, there is concurrent hypercholesterolemia and the animal (man) lives long enough, the system becomes overburdened. Foam cells accumulate and, eventually, the resultant fatty streaks go on to evolve into clinically threatening lesions.[38]

We suggest further that more than removal of oxidized LDL may be involved here. Tissue damage of almost any kind can be associated with generation of free radical oxygen and activation of phospholipases, suggesting some commonality with oxidation of LDL. Thus, the receptors under discussion may also be involved importantly in the clearance of cell debris at sites of *any* tissue damage, not just damage to LDL in the artery wall.

SUMMARY

In this short review we have concentrated on the ways in which modification of LDL structure may account for foam cell formation. We have presented *in vivo* evidence as well as *in vitro* evidence supporting the proposition that modification of native LDL is a prerequisite for foam cell formation and atherogenesis. Actually, oxidized LDL can contribute to atherogenesis in other ways as well. Oxidized LDL is chemotactic for circulating monocytes, yet inhibits the motility of the tissue macrophage as shown by Quinn *et al.*[39] Also, oxidized LDL is cytotoxic as discussed above and this could play a crucial role in the transition from the fatty streak lesion to the clinically more consequential fibrous plaque and complicated lesion. If further research supports the importance of LDL modification in atherogenesis, a whole new array of possibilities opens itself to us for intervention. Anything that interferes with the relevant modifications of the LDL structure would presumably be additive to interventions lowering the plasma concentration of LDL. At the moment, the only such intervention that appears to be feasible is prevention of LDL oxidation. Possibly we may find ways to interfere with immune mechanisms that are involved in some patients; conceivably we might be able to interfere with the aggregation of LDL with itself or with other complexes in the artery wall that appear also to favor initiation of the atherogenic process.

REFERENCES

1. STRONG, J. P. & H. C. MCGILL, JR. 1961. The natural history of coronary atherosclerosis. Am. J. Path. **40:** 37–49.

2. STARY, H. L. 1987. Evolution and progression of atherosclerosis in the coronary arteries of children and adults. *In* Atherogenesis and Aging. S. R. Bates & E. C. Giangloff, Eds. Springer-Verlag. New York, NY.

3. AQEL, N. M., R. Y. BALL, H. WALDMAN & M. J. MITCHINSON, 1984. Monocytic origin of foam cells in human atherosclerotic plaques. Atherosclerosis **53:** 265–271.

4. ROSENFELD, M. E., T. TSUKADA, A. M. GOWN & R. ROSS. 1987. Fatty streak initiation in the WHHL and comparably hypercholesterolemic fat-fed rabbits. Arteriosclerosis **1:** 9–23.

5. GOLDSTEIN, J. L., Y. K. HO, S. K. BASU & M. S. BROWN. 1979. Binding site on macrophages that mediates uptake and degradation of acetylated low density lipoprotein, producing massive cholesterol deposition. Proc. Natl. Acad. Sci. USA **76:** 333–337.

6. BROWN, M. S. & J.L. GOLDSTEIN. 1983. Lipoprotein metabolism in the macrophage: Implications for cholesterol deposition in atherosclerosis. Ann. Rev. Biochem. **52:** 223–262.

7. HENRIKSEN, T., E. M. MAHONEY & D. STEINBERG. 1981. Enhanced macrophage degradation of low density lipoprotein previously incubated with cultured endothelial cells: Recognition by the receptor for acetylated low density lipoproteins. Proc. Natl. Acad. Sci. USA **78:** 6499–6503.

8. HENRIKSEN, T., E. M. MAHONEY & D. STEINBERG. 1983. Enhanced macrophage degradation of biologically modified low density lipoprotein. Arteriosclerosis **3:** 149–159.

9. HENRIKSEN, T., E.M. MAHONEY & D. STEINBERG. 1983. Enhanced macrophage degradation
    of biologically modified low density lipoprotein. Arteriosclerosis **3:** 149–159.
10. MOREL, D. W., P. E. DiCORLETO & G. M. CHISOLM. 1984. Endothelial and smooth muscle
    cells alter low density lipoprotein *in vitro* by free radical oxidation. Arteriosclerosis **4:** 357–
    364.
11. STEINBRECHER, U. P., S. PARTHASARATHY, D. S. LEAKE, J. L. WITZTUM & D. STEINBERG.
    1984. Modification of low density lipoprotein by endothelial cells involves lipid peroxidation
    and degradation of low density lipoprotein phospholipids. Proc. Natl. Acad. Sci. USA **83:**
    3883–3887.
12. STEINBERG, D., S. PARTHASARATHY, T. E. CAREW, J. C. KHOO & J. L. WITZTUM. 1989.
    Beyond cholesterol: Modifications of low density lipoprotein that increase its atherogenicity.
    N. Engl. J. Med. **320:** 915–924.
13. KHOO, J. C., E. MILLER, P. MCLOUGHLIN & D. STEINBERG. 1988. Enhanced macrophage
    uptake of low density lipoprotein after self-aggregation. Arteriosclerosis **8:** 348–358.
14. GRIFFIN, F. M., JR., J. A. GRIFFIN & S. C. SILVERSTEIN. 1976. Studies on the mechanism of
    phagocytosis. II. The interaction of macrophages with antiimmunoglobulin IgG-coated bone
    marrow-derived lymphocytes. J. Exp. Med. **144:** 788–809.
15. KHOO, J. C., E. MILLER, P. MCLOUGHLIN & D. STEINBERG. 1990. Prevention of low density
    lipoprotein aggregation by high density lipoprotein and apolipoprotein A-I. J. Lipid Res. In
    press.
16. SUITS, A. G., A. CHAIT, M. AVIRAM & J. W. HEINECKE. 1989. Phagocytosis of aggregated
    lipoprotein by macrophages: Low density lipoprotein receptor-dependent foam-cell forma-
    tion. Proc. Natl. Acad. Sci. USA **86:** 2713–2717.
17. FRANK, J. S. & A. M. FOGELMAN. 1989. Ultrastructure of the intima in WHHL and choles-
    terol-fed rabbit aortas prepared by ultra-rapid freezing and freeze-etching. J. Lipid Res.
    30: 967–978.
18. POLACEK, D., R. E. BYRNE, G. M. FLESS & M. SCANU. 1986. *In vitro* proteolysis of human
    plasma low density lipoproteins by an elastase released from human polymorphonuclear cells.
    J. Biol. Chem. **261:** 2057–2063.
19. POLACEK, D., R. E. BYRNE & A. M. SCANU. 1988. Modification of low density lipoproteins
    by polymorphonuclear cell elastase leads to enhanced uptake by human monocyte-derived
    macrophages via the low density lipoprotein receptor pathway. J. Lipid Res. **29:** 797–808.
20. MAHLEY, R. W. 1983. Development of accelerated atherosclerosis. Concepts derived from cell
    biology and animal model studies. Arch. Pathol. Lab. Med. **107:** 393–398.
21. GOLDSTEIN, J. L., Y. K. HO, M. S. BROWN, T. L. INNERARITY & R. W. MAHLEY. 1980.
    Cholesteryl ester accumulations in macrophages resulting from receptor-mediated uptake and
    degradation of hypercholesterolemic canine very low density lipoproteins. J. Biol. Chem.
    255: 1839–1848.
22. VAN LENTEN, B. J., A. M. FOGELMAN, M. M. HOKOM, L. BENSON, M. E. HABERLAND &
    P.A. EDWARDS. 1983. Regulation of the uptake and degradation of β-very low density
    lipoprotein in human monocyte macrophages. J. Biol. Chem. **258:** 5151–5157.
23. KOO, C., M. E. WERNETTE-HAMMOND & T. L. INNERARITY. 1986. Uptake of canine β-very
    low density lipoproteins by mouse peritoneal macrophages is mediated by a low density
    lipoprotein receptor. J. Biol. Chem. **261:** 194–201.
24. MAHLEY, R. W., T. L. INNERARITY, K. H. WEISGRABER & S. Y. OH. 1979. Altered metab-
    olism *(in vivo* and *vitro)* of plasma lipoprotein after selective chemical modification of lysine
    residues of the apoproteins. J. Clin. Invest. **64:** 743–750.
25. FOGELMAN, A. M., I. SCHECHTER, J. SEAGER, M. HOKUM, CHILD, J. S. & P. E. EDWARDS.
    1980. Malondialdehyde alteration of low density lipoprotein leads to cholesterol accumulation
    in human monocyte-macrophages. Proc. Natl. Acad. Sci. USA **74:** 2214–2218.
26. ESTERBAUER, H., G. JURGENS, O. QUEHENBERGER & E. KELLER. 1987. Autooxidation of
    human low density lipoprotein: Loss of polyunsaturated fatty acids and vitamin E and gen-
    eration of aldehyde. J. Lipid Res. **28:** 495–509.
27. CAREW, T. E., D. C. SCHWANKE & D. STEINBERG. 1987. Antiatherogenic effect of probucol
    unrelated to its hypocholesterolemic effect: Evidence that antioxidants *in vivo* can selectively
    inhibit low density lipoprotein degradation in macrophage-rich fatty streaks slowing the

progression of atherosclerosis in the WHHL rabbit. Proc. Natl. Acad. Sci. USA **84:** 7725–7729.

28. KITA, T., Y. NAGANO, M. YOKODE, K. ISHII, N. KUME, A. OOSHIMA, H. YOSHIDA & C. KAWAI. 1987. Probucol prevents the progression of atherosclerosis in Watanabe heritable hyperlipidemic rabbit, an animal model for familial hypercholesterolemia. Proc. Natl. Acad. Sci. USA **84:** 5928–5931.

29. HABERLAND, M. E., D. FONG & L. CHENG. 1988. Malondialdehyde-altered protein occurs in atheroma of Watanabe heritable hyperlipidemic rabbits. Science **241:** 215–218.

30. PALINSKI, W., M. E. ROSENFELD, S. YLÄ-HERTTUALA, G. C. GURTNER, S. S. SOCHER, S. W. BUTLER, S. PARTHASARATHY, T. E. CAREW, D. STEINBERG & J. L. WITZTUM. 1989. Low density lipoprotein undergoes oxidative modification *in vivo*. Proc. Natl. Acad. Sci. USA **86:** 1372–1376.

31. ROSENFELD, M. E., W. PALINSKI, S. YLÄ-HERTTUALA, S. BUTLER & J. L. WITZTUM. 1989. Distribution of oxidized proteins and apolipoprotein B in atherosclerotic lesions of varying severity from WHHL rabbits: Immunocytochemical analysis using antibodies generated against modified and native LDL. Arteriosclerosis. In press.

32. MITCHINSON, M. J., R. Y. BALL, K. L. H. CARPENTER & D. V. PARUMS. 1988. Macrophages and ceroid in atherosclerosis. *In* Hyperlipidaemia and Atherosclerosis. K. E. Suckling & P. H. E. Groat, Eds. 117–134. Academic Press. London.

33. STEINBRECHER, U. P., M. FISHER, J. L. WITZTUM & L. K. CURTISS. 1984. Immunogenicity of homologous low density lipoprotein after methylation, ethylation, acetylation or carbamylation: Generation of antibodies specific for derivatized lysine. J. Lipid Res. **25:** 1109–1116.

34. YLÄ-HERTTUALA, S., O. JAAKKOLA, C. EHNHOLM, M. J. TIKKANEN, T. SOLAKIVI, T. SÄRKIOJA & T. NIKKARI. 1988. Characterization of two lipoproteins containing apolipoproteins B and E from lesion-free human aortic intima. J. Lipid Res. **29:** 563–572.

35. YLÄ-HERTTUALA, S., W. PALINSKI, M. E. ROSENFELD, S. PARTHASARATHY, R. E. CAREW, S. BUTLER, J. L. WITZTUM & D. STEINBERG. 1989. Evidence for the presence of oxidatively modified low density lipoprotein in atherosclerotic lesions of rabbit and man. J. Clin. Invest. **84:** 1086–1095.

36. SPARROW, C. P., S. PARTHASARATHY & D. STEINBERG. 1989. A macrophage receptor that recognizes oxidized LDL but not acetylated LDL. J. Biol. Chem. **264:** 599–2604.

37. ARAI, H., T. KITA, M. YOKODE, S. NARUMIYA & C. KAWAI. 1989. Multiple receptors for modified low density lipoproteins in mouse peritoneal macrophages: Different uptake mechanisms for acetylated and oxidized low density lipoproteins. Biochem. Biophys. Res. Commun. **159:** 1375–1382.

38. STEINBERG, D. 1988. Metabolism of lipoproteins and their role in the pathogenesis of atherosclerosis. Atherosclerosis Rev. **18:** 1–24.

39. QUINN, M. T., S. PARTHASARATHY & D. STEINBERG. 1985. Endothelial cell-derived chemotactic activity for mouse peritoneal macrophages and the effects of modified forms of low density lipoprotein. Proc. Natl. Acad. Sci. USA **82:** 5949–5953.

Peroxidized Lipoproteins Recognized by a New Monoclonal Antibody (DLR1a/104G) in Atherosclerotic Lesions[a]

TATSUYA TAKANO AND HIRO-OMI MOWRI

Department of Microbiology and Molecular Pathology
Faculty of Pharmaceutical Sciences
Teikyo University
Sagamiko, Kanagawa 199-01, Japan

INTRODUCTION

It is considered that peroxidized lipoproteins, one of the modified classes of lipoproteins, are involved in the development of atherosclerosis. However, it has not yet been clarified what kinds of peroxidized lipoproteins exist *in vivo* and how these peroxidized lipoproteins are involved in the pathogenesis.

In a previous study,[1] we demonstrated the presence of peroxidized lipids such as 13-hydroxyoctadecadienoic acid in accumulated lipids of atherosclerotic aortas of WHHL (Watanabe-heritable hyperlipidemic) rabbits. Harland *et al.*[2] also detected similar peroxidized fatty acids in human atherosclerotic aortas. It has been proposed[3] that the peroxidation of LDL may occur through the interaction of LDL with endothelial cells, macrophages, or smooth muscle cells. Peroxidized lipids may be accumulated in extracellular lipids which are partly derived from disrupted foam cells.[4]

In this study, to examine the involvement of peroxidized lipoproteins in atherogenesis, attempts were made to prepare a monoclonal antibody that recognizes peroxidized lipoproteins through immunization with the float-up fraction prepared from atherosclerotic aortas. We obtained a novel monoclonal antibody[5] that is different in specificity from those prepared, using MDA-LDL as an immunogen, by Gonen *et al.*[6] and Salmon *et al.*[7] and that recognizes peroxidized lipoproteins existing in atherosclerotic lesions.

MATERIALS AND METHODS

Preparation of Immunogen

Thoracic atherosclerotic aortas of female homozygous WHHL rabbits (2 years old; raised in our laboratory) were cut into pieces with scissors in 10 vol. (v/w) of ice-cold 0.25 M sucrose, 1 mM versene, and 0.1% ethanol (pH 7.4), and then squeezed through four layers of gauze. A one-fifth volume of 1 mM versene and 0.1% ethanol (pH 7.4) was layered over the filtrate, followed by centrifugation at 1000 × g for 30 min at 4°C under argon gas. The float-up fraction was recovered in the 1 mM versene and 0.1% ethanol

[a]This work was supported in part by grants from the Naito Foundation and the Ministry of Education, Science, and Culture of Japan.

layer, and then mixed with an equal volume of Freund's adjuvant to obtain an antigen solution.

Immunization Procedure and Preparation of the Monoclonal Antibody

Female BALB/c mice were immunized three times with the antigen solution over a period of 2 months (with the complete adjuvant, the incomplete adjuvant, and no adjuvant, respectively). Spleen cells were removed 4 days after the final injection. These cells were fused with myeloma P3/U1 cells, followed by culturing in HAT (hypoxanthine, aminopterin, and thymidine) selection medium. Hybridomas were selected by ELISA using peroxidized and native LDLs.

RESULTS

Establishment of a Hybridoma-Producing Antibody against Peroxidized LDL

BALB/c mice were immunized with the float-up fraction prepared from atherosclerotic aortas. To select hybridomas that produce antibodies recognizing peroxidized LDL, ELISA was performed for screening of the hybridoma culture media. Seven hybridoma clones producing antibodies highly reactive to peroxidized LDL, but negative as to native LDL, were obtained from 298 wells on the first screening. Three of them were subjected to limiting dilution, and a stable and rapidly growing hybridoma, DLR1a/104G, was obtained. The class of the monoclonal antibody was determined to be IgM by Ouchterlony analysis.

Immunoreactivity of the DLR1a/104G Antibody with Modified LDLs

By means of the ELISA and immunoblotting technique, it was demonstrated that the monoclonal antibody strongly reacted with peroxidized LDL but negatively with native LDL and acetyl LDL.

On ELISA with modified and native LDLs, the reactivity of the antibody with peroxidized LDL increased in a dose-dependent manner at concentrations between 1 and 10 μg of protein per ml. The value with peroxidized LDL at a concentration of 10 μg protein/ml was about 30-times higher than those with native and the other modified LDLs (FIG. 1).

On agarose gel electrophoresis of the modified and native LDLs (FIG. 2), peroxidized LDL gave a broad protein band exhibiting greater mobility than that of native LDL. Both acetyl- and MDA-LDL also showed greater mobility than native LDL. Immunoblotting with the DLR1a/104G antibody to peroxidized LDL gave a broad immunostained band corresponding to the protein band. The native, acetyl- and MDA-LDLs did not react with the antibody. These results were almost the same as those obtained by the ELISA.

Characteristics of Antigenicity in the Case of Peroxidized LDL

The reactivity of the antibody with peroxidized LDL at various concentrations, as judged on ELISA, did not decrease on extraction of lipids with hexane/isopropanol (FIG. 3). This result suggests that the antigenic material in peroxidized LDL exists in the unextracted fraction.

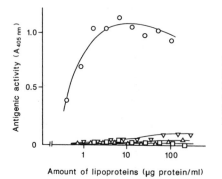

Amount of lipoproteins (μg protein/ml)

FIGURE 1. Reactivity of the monoclonal DLR1a/104G antibody with modified and native LDLs as determined by ELISA. Microtiter plates were coated with modified and native LDLs (0.4–200 μg protein per ml). $\bigcirc$, peroxidized LDL; $\triangledown$, MDA-LDL; $\triangle$, acetyl LDL; and $\square$, native LDL.

Correlation between the antigenic activity and fluorescent substances (E_{350}, F_{430}), which may be produced through the conjugation of peroxidized lipids with the amino groups of proteins, was observed in the process of peroxidation of LDL with $CuSO_4$. As shown in FIGURE 4A, the antigenic activity of LDL increased with incubation time with 10 μm $CuSO_4$ at 37°C. The amount of the fluorescent substances formed in the protein fraction increased in parallel with the antigenic activity. At 4°C, neither antigenicity nor the fluorescent substance was detected. This result suggests that the antigenic material is related to the fluorescent substance formed in the protein fraction.

The band of protein derived from peroxidized LDL was mainly detected at the top of the gel, which is different from the case of the intact apolipoprotein B band, on SDS-polyacrylamide gel electrophoresis (FIG. 5A). On Western blotting developed with the DLR1a/104G antibody, an immunostained band was detected at almost the same position as the protein band of peroxidized LDL, as can be seen in the left lane of FIGURE 5B. The antibody, however, did not react with intact apolipoprotein B of LDL, as can be seen in the right lane of FIGURE 5B.

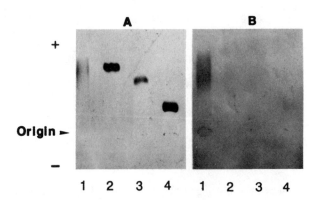

FIGURE 2. Reactivity of the monoclonal DLR1a/104G antibody with modified and native LDLs as determined by immunoblotting. (**A**) Modified and native LDLs (2 μg total cholesterol eqv.) were submitted to 1% agarose gel electrophoresis. Proteins on the gel were stained with Coomassie blue. (**B**) After electrophoresis, the proteins were transferred to nitrocellulose and then immunostained. *Lanes*: 1, peroxidized LDL; 2, MDA-LDL; 3, acetyl LDL: and 4, native LDL.

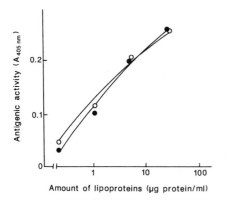

FIGURE 3. Antigenic activity of peroxidized LDL extracted with hexane/isopropanol. Plates were coated with peroxidized LDL (0.2–27 μg protein per ml). Lipids of peroxidized LDL in the wells were extracted with hexane/isopropanol (3:2, v/v) at 4°C overnight. Antigenic activity was measured by ELISA (●). As a control, antigenic activity of peroxidized LDL without organic solvent treatment was also determined (○).

Cross-Reactivity of the DLR1a/104G Antibody with the Float-Up Fraction Prepared from Atherosclerotic Aortas

The inhibitory effect of the float-up fraction on the reactivity of the antibody with $CuSO_4$-peroxidized LDL was examined by ELISA (Fig. 6). The monoclonal antibody used for this particular experiment was purified on a Sephacryl S-300 column. The reactivity was strongly inhibited by peroxidized LDL, which was used as a positive control. The amount of peroxidized LDL required for 50% inhibition was about 5 μg protein per ml. MDA-LDL slightly affected the reactivity at higher concentrations. Native and acetyl-LDL did not inhibit the reactivity at all. The float-up fraction inhibited the reactivity significantly, and the effect was observed at concentrations no higher than 10 μg protein per ml. The amount of the float-up fraction required for 50% inhibition was 70 μg protein per ml. This result suggests that an antigenic determinant which is the same as that for peroxidized LDL exists in atherosclerotic lesions.

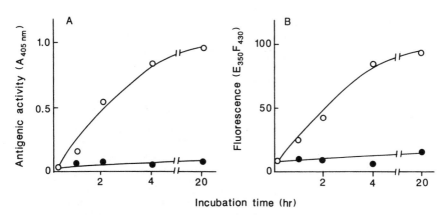

FIGURE 4. Correlation of the antigenic activity and the fluorescent substances formed in the process of LDL peroxidation. LDL (50 μg total cholesterol per ml) was incubated with 10 μM $CuSO_4$ at 37°C (○) or 4°C (●) in D'PBS(−). After the addition of 1 mM dibutylhydroxytoluene, the antigenic activity was determined by ELISA **(A)** and the fluorescence at E_{350} and F_{430} was measured as described under Materials and Methods **(B)**.

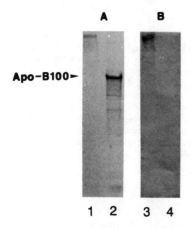

FIGURE 5. SDS-polyacrylamide gel electrophoresis and immunoblotting of peroxidized and native LDLs. Peroxidized LDL and native LDL (10 μg total cholesterol eqv.) were submitted to 2% SDS, 3–15% polyacrylamide gradient slab gel electrophoresis. **(A)** The proteins on the gel were stained with Coomassie blue, and **(B)** the proteins transferred to nitrocellulose were determined by immunoblotting. *Lanes* 1 and 3, peroxidized LDL; *lanes* 2 and 4, native LDL.

DISCUSSION

There is indirect evidence suggesting that peroxidized lipoproteins exist in atherosclerotic aortas.[1] This study was undertaken to prepare a monoclonal antibody that recognizes peroxidized lipoproteins in order to demonstrate the existence of peroxidized lipoproteins in atherosclerotic aortas. We succeeded in establishing a clone (DLR1a/104G) that produces a novel monoclonal antibody, which recognizes peroxidized lipoproteins, using the float-up fraction prepared from an atherosclerotic arterial homogenate as an immunogen.[5] The antibody produced by DLR1a/104G was highly reactive with peroxidized LDL prepared by $CuSO_4$-catalyzed peroxidation.

ELISA and immunoblotting demonstrated that the DLR1a/104G monoclonal antibody reacts with peroxidized lipoproteins in a specific way (FIGS. 1, 2, 5, and 6). The antigenic determinant may be associated with peroxidized LDL particles, since the immunostained band recognized by the DLR1a/104G antibody migrated together with that of protein after peroxidation with $CuSO_4$ (FIG. 2). The antigenicity of peroxidized LDL may be associated with a substance in the protein fraction, because the antigenic activity of peroxidized LDL did not decrease on extraction with hexane/isopropanol (FIG. 3), and because the immunostained band coincided with that of protein after peroxidation with $CuSO_4$ on

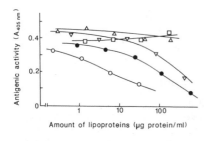

Amount of lipoproteins (μg protein/ml)

FIGURE 6. Cross-reactivity of the monoclonal DLR1a/104G antibody with the float-up fraction prepared from atherosclerotic aortas. The purified DLR1a/104G IgM antibody (0.3 μg protein/ml) was incubated with various concentrations of the float-up fraction, and modified and native LDLs at 4°C overnight. The mixtures were added to the wells, which had been previously coated with peroxidized LDL (1 μg total cholesterol eqv./ml) followed by blocking. The reactivity of the float-up fraction, and the modified and native LDLs was determined as the inhibition of the reactivity of the antibody with peroxidized LDL by ELISA. ●, float-up fraction; ○, peroxidized LDL; ▽, MDA-LDL; △, acetyl-LDL; and □, native LDL.

SDS-polyacrylamide gel electrophoresis (FIG. 5). Furthermore, the antigenic determinant may be related to the fluorescent substance in the protein fraction of peroxidized LDL, as suggested by the correlation of the antigenic activity with the fluorescence (FIG. 4). The DLR1a/104G antibody may recognize a modified form of apolipoprotein B, since the peroxidation of LDL results in formation of the fluorescent substance which is due to the derivatization of apolipoprotein B by peroxidized lipids.[8]

Gonen et al. recently prepared monoclonal EB-3 antibody using MDA-LDL as an immunogen.[6] They demonstrated that the EB-3 antibody reacts strongly with MDA-LDL but not significantly with native LDL or other modified LDLs (acetylated, carbamylated, and glycosylated LDLs). However, the reactivity of the antibody with peroxidized LDL was not mentioned. According to their results, the lipoprotein fraction prepared from the media or intima failed to react with the EB-3 antibody. Our results showed that float-up fraction prepared from atherosclerotic aortas reacted with the DLR1a/104G antibody. These results support the view that peroxidized lipoproteins, which have an antigenic determinant in common with peroxidized LDL, exist in atherosclerotic lesions.

As to peroxidized lipoproteins in atherosclerotic lesions, antigenic activity in the float-up fraction could not be detected by ELISA or immunoblotting, although an inhibitory effect of the float-up fraction on the reactivity of the antibody with peroxidized LDL was observed (FIG. 6). One possible reason is that the large amount of lipids in this fraction prevents the detection of the activity by these methods.

This is the first report suggesting the existence of peroxidized lipoproteins in atherosclerotic lesions, as judged using monoclonal DLR1a/104G antibody, which recognized peroxidized lipoproteins in atherosclerotic aortas as well as peroxidized LDL prepared by $CuSO_4$-catalyzed peroxidation.

SUMMARY

Monoclonal DLR1a/104G antibody, which recognizes peroxidized lipoproteins, was raised. Mice were immunized with the float-up fraction of the atherosclerotic arterial homogenate from WHHL rabbits. Sensitized spleen cells were fused with myeloma cells (3P/U1). Hybridoma clones were selected using peroxidized LDL prepared by $CuSO_4$-catalyzed peroxidation and native LDL as positive and negative standards, respectively. The monoclonal DLR1a/104G antibody was highly reactive with peroxidized LDL, slightly with LDL modified with malondialdehyde, but not significantly with acetyl- or native LDL. The antigenicity in the case of peroxidized LDL did not decrease on extraction with hexane/isopropanol (3:2). The antigenicity coincided with the fluorescence (E_{350}, F_{430}) of the protein fraction of LDL peroxidized with $CuSO_4$. These results suggest that an antigenic determinant exists in atherosclerotic lesions, which is the same as that for lipoproteins peroxidized with $CuSO_4$.

ACKNOWLEDGMENTS

We are grateful to Drs. Yoshio Watanabe and Kazushi Hirohata (Kobe University) for providing us with the WHHL rabbits and for advice as to their maintenance.

REFERENCES

1. MOWRI, H., K. CHINEN, S. OHKUMA & T. TAKANO. 1986. Peroxidized lipids isolated by HPLC from atherosclerotic aorta. Biochem. Int. **12:** 347–352.

2. HARLAND, W. A., J. D. GILBERT & C. J. W. BROOKS. 1973. Lipids of human atheroma. VIII. Oxidised derivatives of cholesteryl linoleate. Biochim. Biophys. Acta **316:** 378–385.
3. STEINBRECHER, U. P., S. PARTHASARATHY, D. S. LEAKE, J. L. WITZTUM & D. STEINBERG. 1984. Modification of low density lipoprotein by endothelial cells involves lipid peroxidation and degradation of low density lipoprotein phospholipids. Proc. Natl. Acad. Sci. USA **81:** 3883–3887.
4. AMANUMA, K., T. KANASEKI, Y. IKEUCHI, S. OHKUMA & T. TAKANO. 1986. Studies on fine structure and location of lipids in quick-freeze replicas of atherosclerotic aorta of WHHL rabbits. Virchows Arch. A **410:** 231–238.
5. MOWRI, H., S. OHKUMA & T. TAKANO. 1988. Monoclonal DLR1a/104G antibody recognizing peroxidized lipoproteins in atherosclerotic lesions. Biochim. Biophys. Acta **963:** 208–214.
6. GONEN, B., J. J. FALLON & S. A. BAKER. 1987. Immunogenicity of malondialdehyde-modified low density lipoproteins. Studies with monoclonal antibodies. Atherosclerosis **65:** 265–272.
7. SALMON, S., C. MAZIERE, L. THERON, I. BEUCLER, M. AYRAULT-JARRIER, S. GOLDSTEIN & J. POLONOVSKI. 1987. Immunological detection of low-density lipoproteins modified by malondialdehyde *in vitro* or *in vivo*. Biochim. Biophys. Acta **920:** 215–220.
8. STEINBRECHER, U. P. 1987. Oxidation of human low density lipoprotein results in derivatization of lysine residues of apolipoprotein B by lipid peroxide decomposition products. J. Biol. Chem. **262:** 3603–3608.

The Phenotypes of Smooth Muscle Expressed in Human Atheroma[a]

G. R. CAMPBELL[b] AND J. H. CAMPBELL[c]

[b]Department of Anatomy
University of Melbourne
Grattan Street
Parkville, Victoria, 3052 Australia
and
[c]Baker Medical Research Institute
Commercial Road
Prahran, Victoria, 3181 Australia

INTRODUCTION

In 1866 Langhans described a population of subendothelial cells which he regarded as fibroblasts or fibrocytes.[1] Since then, these cells have been described as modified smooth muscle cells (see REF. 2), multifunctional mesenchymal cells,[3] differentiating or dedifferentiating smooth muscle cells,[4] intermediate smooth muscle cells,[5] or mesenchymal appearing.[6] Ultrastructural studies indicated that these cells are smooth muscle of altered phenotypic state[2,7,8] and in recent years a wide variety of techniques has been used to demonstrate further structural and functional differences between medial smooth muscle cells and those in or around human atheromatous lesions (see TABLE 1). Thus there is now overwhelming evidence that populations of smooth muscle cells in an atherosclerotic plaque (and involved in atherogenesis) express different phenotypes from those of the normal media.

This article describes some of the different phenotypes expressed by smooth muscle cells in atheroma and discusses two experimental models in which many of these phenotypic populations can be reproduced.

Phenotypic Expression of Smooth Muscle in Atheroma

Cell Shape

An innovative approach—alcoholic alkaline dissociation of fixed specimens—has allowed quantitation of the cell population of normal and atherosclerotic human aortic intima. Apart from the cells of hematogenous origin, the population can be divided into four different groups on the basis of shape: elongated bipolar cells, elongated cells with side processes, stellate cells, and irregularly shaped cells.[9,10] These four groups all appear to be differing phenotypes of smooth muscle.[10,15,25] Alterations in the numbers of cells within a particular category varies with specific parameters related to atherosclerosis. For example, there is a high positive correlation between increases in numbers of stellate

[a]This work was supported by grants from the National Heart Foundation of Australia and the National Health and Medical Research Council.

143

TABLE 1. Smooth Muscle Phenotypic Changes in Human Atheroma

Feature	Aortic Media	Aortic Intima Associated with Atheroma	Reference
Cell shape	Largely spindle or bipolar	up to 40% stellate in shape	9,10
$V_V$myo	77%	52%	11,12
Actin	47.58 pg/cell	21.39 pg/cell	13
α-SM-actin	62%	10%	14
β-actin	31%	70%	14
γ-actin	—	20%	14
Myosin			
Human uterine	+	+ − (5–33% of total)	15
Chicken gizzard	+	few	16
Bovine aortic	+	some	17
Human platelet	few	+	17
Tropomyosin	13.08 pg/cell	4.92 pg/cell	13
Intermediate filaments			
Vimentin	6.07 pg/cell	16.49 pg/cell	13
D+V+	most	few	18
D−V+	few	almost all	18
Meta-vinculin	39%	18%	19
Caldesmon (150 KDa)	79%	50%	19
Cyclic nucleotides		cyclic GMP ↑ 1.5–2-fold	20
		cyclic AMP ↓ 2–8-fold	20
90-Kd surface antigen	−	+	21
Fibronectin (extra domain A)	−	+	22
MHC antigens			
HLA-DR	−	+ (up to 33% of cells)	23
HLA-DQ	−	+	23
Decay-accelerating factor	−	+	24
PDGF mRNA			
A-chain	3.9% (of positive cells)	85.1% (of positive cells)	6
B-chain	0.9% (of positive cells)	75% (of positive cells)	6

shaped cells within the intima and increases in intimal thickening, deposition of lipid, and collagen synthesis.[10]

Volume Fraction of Myofilaments ($V_V$myo)

The $V_V$myo of smooth muscle cells in diffuse intimal thickenings of human carotid artery adjacent to atheromatous plaques differs from that in atherosclerosis-free areas of intima (52% and 75% respectively). Also, adjacent to the plaque the $V_V$myo of the intimal cells is significantly lower than that of the subjacent medial cells (52% and 77% respectively),[11] but in atherosclerosis-free areas the $V_V$myo in smooth muscle cells from the diffuse intimal thickening is not significantly different from that of the media (75% and 79% respectively).[12]

Actin

Six actin isoforms have been described in mammals, four of which are specific for muscle tissues, the remaining two, called cytoplasmic (β and γ), are found in practically all cells. The four muscle actin isoforms: α-skeletal, α-cardiac, and α- and γ-smooth muscle are specific for skeletal, cardiac, and smooth muscle tissues respectively.[25] Not only is there a dramatic drop in the amount of actin present in smooth muscle cells of human aortic fibrous plaque when compared with cells of the media (21.39 pg/cell plaque-47.58 pg/cell media)[13] but there are changes in the actin isoforms expressed by the cells. Smooth muscle of the media contains 62% of its actin in the α-smooth muscle form and 31% of the β-nonmuscle form. Smooth muscle of the plaque contains 10% α-smooth muscle actin, 70% β-actin and 20% γ-actin.[14]

Myosin

Different myosin isoforms exist in smooth muscle[27-31] and these can be differentially expressed under specific conditions.[32-35] Polyclonal antibodies to human uterine myosin,[15] chicken gizzard myosin,[16] and bovine aortic myosin[17] stain aortic smooth muscle cells, but only a limited number of smooth muscle cells in the human fibrous plaque stain with chicken gizzard and bovine aortic myosin, while human uterine myosin antibodies do not stain a population of 5–33% of the smooth muscle cells. Antibodies to human platelets stain a few cells in the media and most of the cells in the fibrous plaque.[17] These data indicate that different isoforms of myosin are expressed in smooth muscle cells of the atheromatous plaque.

Tropomyosin

Smooth muscle cells of the human aortic fibrous plaque contain less than half (13.08 pg/cell cf 4.92 pg/cell) the amount of tropomyosin than cells of the media.[13]

Intermediate Filaments

The intermediate filaments of vascular smooth muscle cells can contain both desmin and vimentin (*i.e.,* D+ V+) or contain vimentin only (*i.e.,* D−V+). The media of the human aorta contains few smooth muscle cells which are D−V+ and most cells are D+V+. However, smooth muscle cells within the fibrous plaque are almost all D−V+, only a few being D+V+.[8] There is almost a threefold increase in the amount of vimentin present in cells of fibrous plaques when compared with cells of the aortic media.[13]

Vinculin/Meta-Vinculin

Vinculin is a 130,000-dalton cytoskeleton protein which is associated with microfilament-membrane association sites, including cell-cell and cell-matrix contact areas.[36] It has been postulated that it plays a key role in microfilament-membrane linkage and has been detected in many different cell types.[37] Four isoforms have been detected (α, α¹, β and γ).[38]

Meta-vinculin is a 150,000-dalton cytoskeleton protein which shares similar properties to vinculin.[39] It is located in F-actin-membrane attachment sites or dense bodies and appears to be specific for smooth muscle.[40] Meta-vinculin can exist in two isoforms, α- and β-meta-vinculin.[38]

In the media of normal aorta, meta-vinculin accounts for 41% of total immunoreactive vinculin (meta-vinculin + vinculin), while the total fractional meta-vinculin content of normal total intima is 39%. However, in the total intima containing atheroma the fractional meta-vinculin content drops to 17.9%.[19]

Caldesmon

Caldesmon is a major component of the contractile apparatus of smooth muscle. It is believed to be involved in a Ca^{++}-dependent control mechanism modulating actin-myosin interaction, and thus contraction.[41] It is present on some of the thin filaments of smooth muscle[42] and binds to myosin.[43] Two different species of caldesmon exist, and in vascular smooth muscle a 150 KDa is the predominant form.[41] Platelets, lymphocytes, and peritoneal macrophages contain a lower molecular weight form of about 70 KDa.[44]

In normal aortic media 150 KDa caldesmon constitutes 79% of the total caldesmon and 75% of the normal total intima. However, in intima containing atheroma 150 KDa caldesmon constitutes only 50.5% of the total caldesmon.[19]

Cyclic Nucleotides

Cyclic nucleotides play important regulatory roles in mediating hormonal effects on cells. Cyclic AMP content in fatty streaks and atherosclerotic plaques is 3–5-fold lower than uninvolved human aortic intima. Cyclic GMP levels in atherosclerotic plaques are 3-fold higher than in grossly normal areas. Basal activity of adenylate cyclase in fatty streaks and plaques is 2–6-fold lower than in unaffected intima.[20,45]

Fibronectin

Fibronectin is a 500-KDa glycoprotein found in extracellular matrix and blood plasma. It consists of two subunit chains linked by disulphide bonds. Each subunit is divided into domains which specifically bind cell surface components, collagen, heparin, and fibrinogen/fibrin.[46] Thus, by means of these domains, fibronectin mediates the attachment and spreading of cells on a variety of substrata and influences their migration, growth, and differentiation.[47] The differences in the primary structures of fibronectin synthesized by various cells are due to alternative splicing of the RNA transcript of a single fibronectin gene. Sequence variations in humans can occur at three different points of the fibronectin subunit: extra domain A, extra domain B and IIICS.[46] Extra domain A fibronectin is not present in the tunica media of the human aorta. However, it is present in diffuse intimal thickenings and atherosclerotic plaques of human aorta.[22]

Class II Antigens of the Major Histocompatibility Complex (MHC)

The class II MHC antigens are involved in communication between cells which regulate the immune response. Functionally, these antigens, termed HLA-DR, HLA-DP, and HLA-DQ, participate in the presentation of foreign antigens to T-lymphocytes,[23] and therefore, are normally only expressed by cells of the immune system. However, many smooth muscle cells of the human atherosclerotic plaque express HLA-DR and HLA-

DQ[23,48], demonstrating another form of phenotypic expression of smooth muscle in lesions.

Platelet Derived Growth Factor (PDGF)

PDGF can be produced by many cell types, including macrophages, endothelial cells, and arterial smooth muscle cells *in vitro*.[49] Smooth muscle cells *in situ* within the human aortic media produce little PDGF A or B chain, but do produce significant amounts within atherosclerotic plaques.[6,50]

Models to Examine Different Phenotypes of Smooth Muscle

Two models are widely used to examine changes in smooth muscle phenotype: the arterial denudation–response to injury model, and the growth of arterial smooth muscle cells in culture. In both of these models smooth muscle can express, under ceratin conditions, many of the phenotypes observed in human atheroma. They therefore provide powerful tools to help us understand the significance of the structural and functional changes in the cells and how these relate to the disease process.

A. Arterial Denudation–Response to Injury

In this model, injury to the endothelium has been caused by a variety of traumata (see REF. 51). Regardless of the mode of injury, if the damage is of sufficient size smooth muscle cells from the media migrate to the intima where they subsequently proliferate forming a neo-intima of largely longitudinally orientated smooth muscle cells. Proliferation reaches a maximum in the neo-intima during the first week following endothelial denudation and returns to baseline by 8 weeks when the intima is re-endothelialized.[52] The interesting feature of this *in vivo* model is that, as can be seen in TABLE 2, many of the smooth muscle phenotypic changes appear reversible. This raises the question as to whether any of the phenotypes of smooth muscle expressed in human atheroma can revert to normal with changing conditions.

$V_V$myo Changes in Endothelial Denuded Vessels

Dramatic reversible changes in $V_V$myo occur over an 18-week period in smooth muscle cells of the neo-intima following balloon catheter injury (FIG. 1).[53]

Actin

Neo-intimal smooth muscle cells contain significantly less α-smooth muscle actin (determined by mRNA) than medial cells at 5 days and 15 days following injury. However, by 60 days the levels have returned to those of the media. Concomitant with the decrease in α-smooth muscle actin there is an increase in β- and γ-actin at 5 and 15 days, also returning to normal medial cell levels by 60 days post-injury.[55,56] The amount of actin per cell also decreases significantly in the 15-day post-injury neo-intimal smooth muscle cell compared to those of the media, with a return to similar levels by 75 days.[54]

TABLE 2. Smooth Muscle Phenotypic Changes in Experimental Intimal Thickening

Feature	Normal Media	Short-Term Neo-Intima	Long-Term Neo-Intima	Reference
$V_V$myo	68%	37% (2 weeks)	62% (18 weeks)	53
Actin	20.79 pg/cell	13.62 pg/cell (15 days)	18.06 pg/cell (75 days)	54
α-SM actin mRNA	81.2% (of total actin)	45% (5 days)		55
β-actin mRNA	13.9%	39.3% (5 days)		55
γ-actin mRNA	4.9%	15.7% (5 days)		55
α-SM actin mRNA	33.2% (of total actin)	10.7% (15 days)	35.2% (60 days)	56
β-actin mRNA	51.3%	71.1% (15 days)	51.9% (60 days)	56
γ-actin mRNA	15.5%	18.2% (15 days)	12.9% (60 days)	56
Myosin				
Bovine aortic	+	few (15 days)		17
Human platelet	few	+ (15 days)		17
Chicken gizzard	+	few (14 days)	+ (6 weeks)	16
Intermediate filaments				
D− V+	51%	79% (15 days)	50% (75 days)	54
D+ V+	48%	21% (15 days)	50% (75 days)	54
D+ V−	1%	0% (15 days)	0% (75 days)	54
Fibronectin (extra domain A)	−	+ (14 days)		22
MHC antigens				
I-A	−	8.4% (14 days)	1.8% (12 weeks)	57
I-E	−	5.9% (14 days)	0.5% (12 weeks)	57

Myosin

Smooth muscle cells which have migrated into the intima and proliferated contain less smooth muscle myosin than cells of the media.[16,17] The levels return by 6 weeks post-injury.[16] Antibodies to nonmuscle platelet myosin stain few smooth muscle cells in the media, but most neo-intimal cells 15 days post-injury.[17]

Intermediate Filaments

Fifty-one percent of the smooth muscle cells of the normal rat aortic media show a positive stain for vimentin alone, 48% are positive for both vimentin and desmin, and 1% are positive for desmin alone. Fifteen days after injury, 79% of the cells from the neo-intima are positive for vimentin alone, 21% for both vimentin and desmin, and none for desmin alone. Seventy-five days post-injury 50% of the neo-intimal cells stain for vimentin alone and 50% for both vimentin and desmin. None stain for desmin alone.[54]

Fibronectin

Fourteen days after balloon catheter injury to the rat aorta, extra domain A fibronectin staining is found in the neo-intima but not in the media.[22]

MHC Antigens

The rat class II MHC antigens are designated I-A and I-E. No I-A or I-E staining smooth muscle cells are normally found in the rat carotid artery media. Two weeks after balloon catheter injury maximum expression of I-A (8.4%) and I-E (5.9%) is found in quiescent cells. The expression of these antigens then declines to 1.8% I-A and 0.5% I-E by 12 weeks post-injury.[57]

B. Smooth Muscle Cell Culture

Smooth muscle cells expressing different phenotypic characteristics can be observed in culture, some of which are listed in TABLE 3. Two different culture techniques are in widespread usage: primary cell culture and explant outgrowth followed by subculture.[59] These and other variations in culturing conditions often provide variations in phenotype, consequently this article will only concentrate on some of the phenotypic changes (structural and functional) in primary cultured rabbit aortic smooth muscle cells.

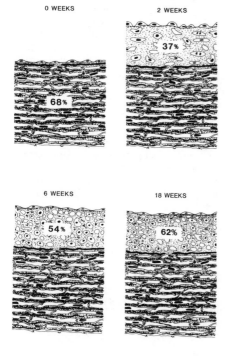

FIGURE 1. Volume fraction of myofilaments ($V_V$myo), expressed as a percentage of cytoplasmic volume, in smooth muscle cells in media (0 weeks) and neo-intima of rabbit carotid artery 2, 6, and 18 weeks after endothelial denudation (see REF. 53).

TABLE 3. Some Phenotypic Changes of Smooth Muscle Cells in Culture

	Reference
1. Changes in $V_V$myo and amount of myofilaments	58, 59, 60, 61
2. Alteration in the pattern of actin isoforms expressed	14, 61, 62, 63
3. Alteration in the pattern of myosin heavy chains present	64, 65, 66, 67, 68
4. Increase in cells containing vimentin only; decrease in vimentin plus desmin containing cells	69
5. Decreases in the amounts of γ-vinculin and meta-vinculin expressed	38, 70, 71
6. Alteration in the form of caldesmon expressed	19, 72, 73
7. Different forms of fibronectin expressed	22
8. Class II MHC gene expression stimulated by interferon γ	74, 75
9. PDGF-A and PDGF-B genes expressed	76, 77, 78, 79

$V_V$myo and Myofilaments

When examined by ultrastructural morphometry smooth muscle cells in the aorta of the 9-week-old rabbits have a $V_V$myo of 39.5 ± 1.2% (FIG. 2). When the aorta is dispersed by enzyme digestion into single cells[61] then pelleted by centrifugation, the $V_V$myo falls to 35.4 ± 1.5% (these cells are termed contractile). When these cells are seeded in primary culture at 3.03 ± 0.09 × 10⁵ cells/dish (mean ± standard deviation) they have a seeding efficiency of 72% leaving 2.18 ± 0.08 × 10⁵ cells attached to each dish on day 1. The $V_V$myo of these cells is 34.6 ± 2.3%. This decreases gradually over day 2 (30.3 ± 0.8%), day 3 (26.9 ± 2.8%), and day 4 (22.5 ± 2.3%), falling sharply to 11.5 ± 1.6% on day 5, one day prior to the onset of logarithmic growth (these cells are termed reversible synthetic). The $V_V$myo remains low over the next 2 or 3 days, then begins to rise once confluency (7.80 ± 0.29 × 10⁵ cells/dish) is reached on day 9 (21.9 ± 1.2%). Two days after confluency (day 11), the $V_V$myo increases to 30.6 ± 0.6% and on day 12 is 32.0 ± 2.5%, indicating that the cells have almost regained their original complement of myofilaments. Thus at this seeding density the cells show a reversible change in phenotype.[61]

When the rabbit aortic smooth muscle cells are seeded sparsely in primary culture at 0.30 ± 0.02 × 10⁵ cells/dish they have a seeding efficiency of 66% leaving 0.20 ± 0.02 × 10⁵ cells/dish on day 1. Logarithmic growth commences on day 6 and continues until confluency on day 19 (7.70 ± 0.42 × 10⁵ cells/dish), after which the cell number remains constant (day 24: 8.26 ± 0.36 × 10⁵ cells/dish). The $V_V$myo of this population

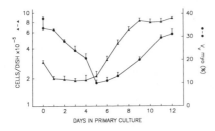

FIGURE 2. Aortic smooth muscle cells from 9-week-old rabbit enzymatically dispersed and seeded into primary culture at 3.03 ± 0.09 × 10⁵ cells/30 mm dish (moderate seeding density) and grown for 12 days. Growth curve (▲—▲). $V_V$myo of smooth muscle cells (●—●) in intact tissue *(top point)* and freshly dispersed cells *(lower point)* on day 0 and on days indicated in culture (see REF. 61).

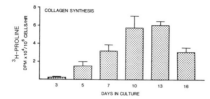

FIGURE 3. Aortic smooth muscle cells from 9-week-old rabbit enzymatically dispersed and seeded into primary culture. These cultures were labelled with [5-³H] proline for 4 hours and synthesis of collagen determined by the collagenase-susceptible protein assay.[80]

of cells decreases to 10.3 ± 0.2% on day 5, then remains low throughout the culture period, including 5 days after confluency (day 24) when the $V_V$myo is 8.1 ± 1.2% (these cells are termed irreversible synthetic because they never return to the contractile state, even after confluency).[61]

Collagen Synthesis

Synthesis of collagen was determined by bacterial collagenase digestion[80] at days 3, 5, 7, 10, 13, and 16 in primary culture of 9-week rabbit aortic media. Day 5 synthetic cells synthesize collagen at a rate which is approximately 7-times ($p < 0.01$) that of day 3 cells (FIG. 3). Consequently the relative rate of collagen synthesis is not significantly altered between day 3 and 5 when smooth muscle cells have modulated to the synthetic phenotype. However, between day 5 and day 10 there is an increase in the relative rate of collagen synthesis due to a 40-fold increase ($p < 0.001$) in collagen production.

The level of collagen synthesis on day 13 is not significantly different from the

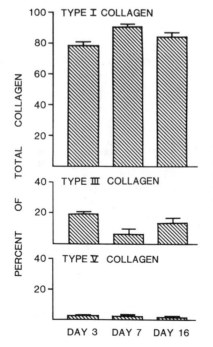

FIGURE 4. Cell cultures as in FIGURE 3 were labelled with [5-³H] proline for 4 hours and pepsin-digested collagens analysed by electrophoresis. The proportions of collagen were determined by excision of the collagenous bands, digestion with Protosol and scintillation counting.[80]

respective level of day 10 when the culture is confluent. However, when the cells have reverted to the contractile phenotype on day 16, collagen synthesis declines to half of the day-13 level (p <0.001).

Electrophoretic analysis of pepsin-resistant radiolabelled protein has been used to determine the relative distribution of type I, III, and V collagens as the smooth muscle cells alter phenotype.[80] Day-3 contractile cells synthesize 78.1% ± 3.5% (mean ± SD) type I collagen, which increases to 90.3% ± 2.0% (p <0.001) on day 7 when the cells are synthetically active. This is accompanied by a decrease in the relative proportion of type III collagen from 17.5% ± 4.7% to 5.8% ± 1.8% (p <0.001). The enrichment of type I collagen (and concomitant reduction in type III) is significantly reversed (p <0.005) at day 16 when the cells return to the contractile state, with 83.3% ± 2.8% type I collagen and 13.1% ± 2.8% type III collagen produced (FIG. 4). Although there is enrichment of type I collagen as smooth muscle cells modulate to the synthetic state, the predominant collagen species synthesized by smooth muscle cells (irrespective of phenotype), is always type I collagen. Type V collagen constitutes only 3–5% and is not significantly altered by the phenotypic state of the smooth muscle cells (FIG. 4).[80]

Lipoprotein Metabolism

The ability of rabbit aortic smooth muscle cells in the three different phenotypes; contractile, reversible synthetic, and irreversible synthetic, to metabolise β-VLDL, VLDL and LDL has been examined in culture.[81] The data, measured as cell-associated radioactivity at 4°C and expressed as ng lipoprotein protein bound per 10^6 cells, shows highly consistent differences between the three cell phenotypes (FIG. 5). The binding of LDL to the three phenotypes is about equally specific (displacable by excess unlabelled

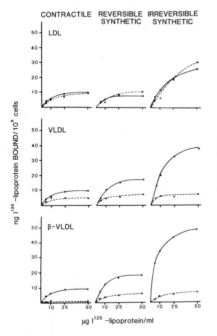

FIGURE 5. Specific (●—●) and nonspecific (●--●) binding of ^{125}I-labelled lipoproteins (β-VLDL, VLDL, and LDL) to rabbit aortic smooth muscle cells in three different phenotypes in culture.[81]

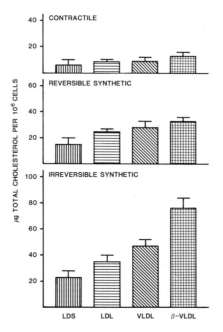

FIGURE 6. Mass of total cholesterol in 9-week rabbit aortic medial smooth muscle in culture in three different phenotypes following 24-hour incubations in 5% lipoprotein-deficient serum alone or with 75 μg/ml lipoprotein (β-VLDL, VLDL, and LDL).[81]

lipoprotein) and nonspecific, suggesting substantial non-receptor-mediated binding of LDL. By contrast, the binding of both normal VLDL and of β-VLDL is predominantly specific and saturable over the concentrations tested (5–50 μg protein/ml medium).

The mass of total cholesterol in cells of the three phenotypes following 24-hour incubations with 5% LDS alone or with 5% LDS plus LDL, normal VLDL, or β-VLDL (at 75 μg protein/ml) are shown in FIGURE 6. The larger cell size and the greater content of membranous organelles are reflected in the greater cholesterol mass in the synthetic, compared with the contractile, phenotypes (see the lipoprotein-free incubations). The addition of LDL fails to increase the cellular cholesterol over that in lipoprotein-free incubations while incubation with β-VLDL doubles the cholesterol mass of the reversible-synthetic cells and more than triples that in the irreversible-synthetic cells. The amount of triglyceride rises in parallel with cholesterol, with the greatest levels in irreversible-synthetic state cells incubated with β-VLDL (56 ± 2 μg/10^6 cells) compared with 28 ± 5 μg/10^6 cells in lipoprotein-free incubations.[81]

CONCLUSION

Smooth muscle cells in the human atherosclerotic plaque express a range of different phenotypes, reflected in changes in cell shape, $V_V$myo, actin isoforms, myosin isoforms, tropomyosin levels, type of intermediate filament, amounts of meta-vinculin and caldesmon, levels of cyclic nucleotides, type of fibronectin produced, MHC antigen expression, decay activating factor expression, and gene expression for PDGF.

Similar expressions of phenotype can be found in smooth muscle cells of the neo-intima of an endothelial-denuded artery, and in cell culture.

Primary cell culture is a useful model system to examine changes in phenotype of smooth muscle since the cells under these conditions show many of the functional changes characteristic of atheroma including an increased ability to proliferate, an increased ability to synthesize extracellular matrix (in particular collagen type I) and increased binding of lipoproteins and accumulation of lipid.

ACKNOWLEDGMENTS

The authors extend their gratitude to Ms Ann Best, Simone Young, and Julie Safstrom for aid in the preparation of the manuscript.

REFERENCES

1. LANGHANS, TH. 1866. Beiträge zur normalen und pathologischen Anatomie der Arterien. Arch. Pathol. Anat. Physiol. Klin. Med. **36:** 187–226.
2. GEER, J. C. & M. D. HAUST. 1972. Identification of cells in atherosclerotic lesions: A historical review. *In* Smooth Muscle Cells in Atherosclerosis. Monographs on Atherosclerosis. Vol. **2:** 4–26. Karger. Basel, Switzerland.
3. WISSLER, R. W. 1968. The arterial medial cells, smooth muscle or multifunctional mesenchyme? J. Atheroscler. Res. **8:** 201–213.
4. GEER, J. C. 1965. Fine structure of human aortic intimal thickening and fatty streaks Lab. Invest. **14:** 1764–1783.
5. ALTSCHUL, R. 1950. Selected Studies on Arteriosclerosis. Charles C. Thomas. Springfield.
6. WILCOX, J. N., K. M. SMITH, L. T. WILLIAMS, S. M. SCHWARTZ & D. GORDON. 1988. Platelet-derived growth factor mRNA detected in human atherosclerotic plaques by in situ hybridisation. J. Clin. Invest. **82:** 1134–1143.
7. HAUST, M. D. 1983. Atherosclerosis-lesions and sequelae. *In* Cardiovascular Pathology. Vol. 1: 191–315. M. D. Silver, Ed. Churchill Livingstone. New York, NY.
8. ROSS, R., T. N. WIGHT, E. STRANDNESS & B. THIELE. 1984. Human atherosclerosis. I. Cell constitution and characteristics of advanced lesions of the superficial femoral artery. Am. J. Pathol. **114:** 79–93.
9. OREKHOV, A. M., I. I. KARPOVA, V. V. TERTOV, S. A. RUDCHENKO, E. R. ANDREEVA, A. V. KRUSHINSKY & V. N. SMIRNOV. 1984. Cellular composition of atherosclerotic and uninvolved human aortic subendothelial intima. Light microscopic study of dissociated aortic cells. Am. J. Pathol. **115:** 17–24.
10. OREKHOV, A. N., E. R. ANDREEVA, A. V. KRUSHINSKY, I. D. NOVIKOV, V. V. TERTOV, G. V. NESTAIKO, KH. A. KHASHIMOV, V. S. REPIN & V. N. SMIRNOV. 1986. Intimal cells and atherosclerosis. Relationship between the number of intimal cells and major manifestations of atherosclerosis in the human aorta. Am. J. Pathol. **125:** 402–415.
11. MOSSE, P. R. L., G. R. CAMPBELL, Z-L. WANG & J. H. CAMPBELL. 1985. Smooth muscle phenotypic expression in human carotid arteries. I. Comparison of cells from diffuse intimal thickenings adjacent to atheromatous plaques with those of the media. Lab. Invest. **53:** 555–562.
12. MOSSE, P. R. L., G. R. CAMPBELL & J. H. CAMPBELL. 1986. Smooth muscle phenotypic expression in human carotid arteries. II. Comparison of cells from areas of artherosclerosis-free diffuse intimal thickenings with those of the media. Arteriosclerosis **6:** 664–670.
13. KOCHER, O. & G. GABBIANI. 1986. Cytoskeletal features of normal and atheromatous human arterial smooth muscle cells. Hum. Pathol. **17:** 875–880.
14. GABBIANI, G., O. KOCHER, W. S. BLOOM, J. VANDEKERCKHOVE & K. WEBER. 1984. Actin expression in smooth muscle cells of rat aortic intimal thickening, human atheromatous plaque and cultured rat aortic media. J. Clin. Invest. **73:** 148–152.
15. Babaev, V. R., A. S. Antonov, O. S. Zacharova, Y. A. Romanov, A. V. Krushinsky, V. P. Tsibulsky, V. P. Shirinsky, V. S. Repin & V. N. SMIRNOV. 1988. Identification of intimal subendothelial cells from human aorta in primary culture. Atherosclerosis **71:** 45–56.
16. CAMPBELL, G. R. & J. H. CAMPBELL. 1987. Smooth muscle cells. *In* Atherosclerosis: Biology

and Clinical Science. A. G. Olsson, Ed. 105–115. Churchill Livingstone, Inc. New York, NY.

17. BENZONANA, G., O. SKALLI & G. GABBIANI. 1988. Correlation between the distribution of smooth muscle or non-muscle myosins and α-smooth muscle actin in normal and pathological soft tissues. Cell Motil. Cytoskeleton 11: 260–274.

18. OSBORN, M., J. CASELITZ, K. PÜSCHEL & K. WEBER. 1987. Intermediate filament expression in human vascular smooth muscle and in atherosclerotic plaques. Virchows Arc. A. 411: 449–458.

19. GLUKHOVA, M. A., A. E. KABAKOV, M. G. FRID, O. I. ORNATSKY, A. M. BELKIN, D. N. MUKHIN, A. N. OREKHOV, V. E. KOTELIANSKY & V. N. SMIRNOV. 1988. Modulation of human aorta smooth muscle cell phenotype: A study of muscle-specific variants of vinculin, caldesmon, and actin expression. Proc. Natl. Acad. Sci. USA 85: 9542–9546.

20. TERTOV, V. V., A. N. OREKHOV, G. YU. GRIGORIAN, G. S. KURENNAYA, S. A. KUDRYASHOV, V. A. TKACHUK & V. N. SMIRNOV. 1987. Disorders in the system of cyclic nucleotides in atherosclerosis: Cyclic AMP and cyclic GMP content and activity of related enzymes in human aorta. Tissue Cell 19: 21–28.

21. PRINTSEVA, O. JU., M. M. PECLO, A. V. TJURMIN, A. I. FAERMAN, S. M. DANILOV, V. S. REPIN & V. N. SMIRNOV. 1989. A 90-Kd surface antigen from a subpopulation of smooth muscle cells from human atherosclerotic lesions. Am. J. Pathol. 134: 305–313.

22. GLUKHOVA, M. A., M. G. FRID, B. V. SHEKHONIN, T. D. VASILEVSKAYA, J. GRÜNWALD, M. SAGINATI & V. E. KOTELIANSKY. 1989. Expression of extra domain A fibronectin sequence in vascular smooth muscle cells is phenotype dependent. J. Cell Biol. 109: 357–366.

23. HANSSON, G. K., L. JONASSON, J. HOLM & L. CLAESSON-WELSH. 1986. Class II MHC antigen expression in the atherosclerotic plaque: smooth muscle cells express HLA-DR, HLA-DQ and the invariant gamma chain. Clin. Exp. Immunol. 64: 261–268.

24. SEIFERT, R. & G. K. HANSSON. 1989. Decay-accelerating factor is expressed on vascular smooth muscle cells in human atherosclerotic lesions. J. Clin. Invest. 84: 597–604.

25. CHAZOV, E. I., V. S. REPIN, A. N. OREKHOV, A. S. ANTONOV, S. N. PREOBRAZHENSKY, E. L. SOBOLEVA & V. N. SMIRNOV. 1986. Atherosclerosis: What has been learned studying human arteries. Atheroscler. Rev. 14: 7–60.

26. VANDEKERKHOVE, J. & K. WEBER. 1978. At least six different actins are expressed in higher mammal: An analysis based on the amino acid sequence of the amino-terminal tryptic peptide. J. Mol. Biol. 126: 783–802.

27. BECKERS-BLEUKX, G. & G. MARÉCHAL. 1985. Detection and distribution of myosin isozymes in vertebrate smooth muscle. Eur. J. Biochem. 152: 207–211.

28. LEMA, M. J., E. D. PAGANI, R. SHEMIN & F. J. JULIAN. 1986. Myosin isozymes in rabbit and human smooth muscles. Circ. Res. 59: 115–123.

29. ROVNER, A. S., M. M. THOMPSON & R. A. MURPHY. 1986. Two different heavy chains are found in smooth muscle myosin. Am. J. Physiol. 250: C861–C870.

30. EDDINGER, T. J. & R. A. MURPHY. 1988. Two smooth muscle myosin heavy chains differ in their light meromyosin fragment. Biochemistry 27: 3807–3811.

31. NAGAI, R., M. KURO-O, P. BABIJ & M. PERIASAMY. 1989. Identification of two types of smooth muscle myosin heavy chain isoforms by cDNA cloning and immunoblot analysis. J. Biol. Chem. 264: 9734–9737.

32. LARSON, D. M., K. FUJIWARA, W. ALEXANDER & M. A. GIMBRONE, JR. 1984. Myosin in cultured vascular smooth muscle cells: Immunofluorescence and immunochemical studies of alterations in antigenic expression. J. Cell Biol. 99: 1582–1589.

33. ROVNER, A. S., R. A. MURPHY & G. K. OWENS. 1986. Expression of smooth muscle and non-muscle myosin heavy chains in cultured vascular smooth muscle cells. J. Biol. Chem. 261: 14740–14745.

34. SEIDEL, C. L., C. L. WALLACE, D. K. DENNISON & J. C. ALLEN. 1989. Vascular myosin expression during cytokinesis, attachment, and hypertrophy. Am. J. Physiol. 256: C793–C798.

35. KUMAR, C. C., S. R. MOHAN, P. J. ZAVODNY, S. K. NARULA & P. J. LEIBOWITZ. 1989. Characterization and differential expression of human vascular smooth muscle myosin light chain 2 isoform in non-muscle cells. Biochem. 28: 4027–4035.

36. GEIGER, B. 1979. A 130K protein from chicken gizzard: its localization at the termini of microfilament bundles in cultured chicken cells. Cell **18:** 193–205.

37. EVANS, R. R., R. M. ROBSON & M. H. STROMER. 1984. Properties of smooth muscle vinculin. J. Biol. Chem. **259:** 3916–3924.

38. BELKIN, A. M., O. I. ORNATSKY, A. E. KABAKOV, M. A. GLUKHOVA & V. E. KOTELIANSKY. 1988. Diversity of vinculin/meta-vinculin in human tissues and cultivated cells. Expression of muscle specific variants of vinculin in human aorta smooth muscle cells. J. Biol. Chem. **263:** 6631–6635.

39. SILICIANO, J. D. & S. W. CRAIG. 1987. Properties of smooth muscle meta-vinculin. J. Cell Biol. **104:** 473–482.

40. GLUKHOVA, M. A., A. E. KABAKOV, A. M. BELKIN, M. G. FRID, O. I. ORNATSKY, N. I. ZHIDKOVA & V. E. KOTELIANSKY. 1986. Meta-vinculin distribution in adult human tissues and cultured cells. FEBS Lett. **207:** 139–141.

41. FÜRST, D. O., R. A. CROSS, J. DEMAY & J. V. SMALL. 1986. Caldesmon is an elongated, flexible molecule localized in the actomyosin domain of smooth muscle. EMBO J. **5:** 251–257.

42. LEHMAN, W., A. SHELDON & W. MADONIA. 1987. Diversity in smooth muscle filament composition. Biochim. Biophys. Acta **914:** 35–39.

43. IKEBE, M. & S. REARDON. 1988. Binding of caldesmon to smooth muscle myosin. J. Biol. Chem. **263:** 3055–3058.

44. OWADA, M. K., A. HAKURA, K. IIDA, I. YAHARA, K. SOBUE & S. KAKIUCHI. 1984. Occurrence of caldesmon (a calmodulin-binding protein) in cultured cells: Comparison of normal and transformed cells. Proc. Natl. Acad. Sci. USA **81:** 3133–3137.

45. TERTOV, V. V., A. N. OREKHOV, S. A. KUDRYASHOV, A. L. KLIBANOV, N. N. IVANOV, V. P. TORCHILIN & V. N. SMIRNOV. 1987. Cyclic nucleotides and artherosclerosis: Studies in primary culture of human aortic cells. Exp. Mol. Pathol. **47:** 377–389.

46. HYNES, R. O. 1985. Molecular biology of fibronectin. Annu. Rev. Cell Biol. **1:** 67–90.

47. YAMADA, K. M., S. K. AKIYAMA, T. HASEGAWA, E. HASEGAWA, M . J. HUMPHRIES, D. W. KENNEDY, K. NAGATA, H. URUSHIHARA, K. OLDEN & W-T. CHEN. 1985. Recent advances in research on fibronectin and other cell attachment proteins. J. Cell Biochem. **28:** 79–97.

48. JONASSON, L., J. HOLM, O. SKALLI, G. GABBIANI & G. K. HANSSON. 1985. Expression of class II transplantation antigen on vascular smooth muscle cells in human artherosclerosis. J. Clin. Invest. **76:** 125–131.

49. ROSS, R. 1986. The pathogenesis of atherosclerosis—an update. N. Engl. J. Med. **314:** 488–500.

50. BARRETT, T. B. & E. P. BENDITT. 1988. Platelet-derived growth factor gene expression in human atherosclerotic plaques and normal artery wall. Proc. Natl. Acad. Sci. USA **85:** 2810–2814.

51. CAMPBELL, G. R. & J. H. CAMPBELL. 1985. Smooth muscle cell phenotypic changes in arterial wall homeostasis: Implications for the pathogenesis of atherosclerosis. Exp. Mol. Pathol. **42:** 139–162.

52. CLOWES, A. W., M. A. REIDY & M. M. CLOWES. 1983. Mechanisms of stenosis after arterial injury. Lab. Invest. **49:** 208–215.

53. MANDERSON, J. A., P. R. L. MOSSE, J. A. SAFSTROM, S. B. YOUNG & G. R. CAMPBELL. 1989. Balloon catheter injury to rabbit carotid artery. I. Changes in smooth muscle phenotype. Arteriosclerosis **9:** 289–298.

54. KOCHER, O., O. SKALLI, W. S. BLOOM & G. GABBIANI. 1984. Cytoskeleton of rat aortic smooth muscle cells. Normal conditions and experimental intimal thickening. Lab. Invest. **50:** 645–652.

55. CLOWES, A. W., M. M. CLOWES, O. KOCHER, P. ROPRAZ, C. CHAPONNIER & G. GABBIANI. 1988. Arterial smooth muscle cells in vivo: Relationship between actin isoform expression and mitogenesis and their modulation by heparin. J. Cell Biol. **107:** 1939–1945.

56. BARJA, F., C. COUGHLIN, D. BELIN & G. GABBIANI. 1986. Actin isoform synthesis and mRNA levels in quiescent and proliferating rat aortic smooth muscle cells in vivo and in vitro. Lab. Invest. **55:** 226–233.

57. JONASSON, L., J. HOLM & G. K. HANSSON. 1988. Smooth muscle cells express Ia antigens during arterial response to injury. Lab. Invest. **58:** 310–315.

58. CHAMLEY, J. H., G. R. CAMPBELL, J. D. McCONNELL & U. GRÖSCHEL-STEWART. 1977. Comparison of vascular smooth muscle cells from adult human, monkey and rabbit in primary culture and in subculture. Cell Tissue Res. **177:** 503–522.

59. CHAMLEY-CAMPBELL, J. H., G. R. CAMPBELL & R. ROSS. 1979. The smooth muscle cell in culture. Physiol. Rev. **59:** 1–61.

60. THYBERG, J., L. PALMBERG, J. NILSSON, T. KSIAZEK & M. SJÖLUND. 1983. Phenotype modulation in primary cultures of arterial smooth muscle cells. On the role of platelet derived growth factor. Differentation **25:** 156–167.

61. CAMPBELL, J. H., O. KOCHER, O. SKALLI, G. GABBIANI & G. R. CAMPBELL. 1989. Cyto-differentiation and expression of alpha-smooth muscle actin mRNA and protein during primary culture of aortic smooth muscle cells. Correlation with cell density and proliferative state. Arteriosclerosis **9:** 633–643.

62. OWENS, G. K., A. LOEB, D. GORDON & M. M. THOMPSON. 1986. Expression of smooth muscle-specific α-isoactin in cultured vascular smooth muscle cells: Relationship between growth and cytodifferentiation. J. Cell Biol. **102:** 343–352.

63. KOCHER, O. & G. GABBIANI. 1987. Analysis of α-smooth-muscle actin mRNA expression in rat aortic smooth-muscle cells using a specific cDNA probe. Differentiation **34:** 201–209.

64. GRÖSCHEL-STEWART, U., J. H. CHAMLEY, J. D. McCONNELL & G. BURNSTOCK. 1975. Comparison of the reaction of cultured smooth and cardiac muscle cells and fibroblasts to specific antibodies to myosin. Histochemistry **43:** 215–224.

65. LARSON, D. M., K. FUJIWARA, R. W. ALEXANDER & M. A. GIMBRONE, JR. 1984. Myosin in cultured vascular smooth muscle cells: Immunofluorescence and immunochemical studies of alterations in antigenic expression. J. Cell Biol. **99:** 1582–1589.

66. ROVNER, A. S., R. A. MURPHY & G. K. OWENS. 1986. Expression of smooth muscle and non-muscle myosin heavy chains in cultured vascular smooth muscle. J. Biol. Chem. **261:** 14740–14745.

67. KAWAMOTO, S. & R. S. ADELSTEIN. 1987. Characterization of myosin heavy chains in cultured aorta smooth muscle cells. A comparative study. J. Biol. Chem. **262:** 7282–7288.

68. SEIDEL, C. L., C. L. WALLACE, D. K. DENNISON & J. C. ALLEN. 1989. Vascular myosin expression during cytokinesis, attachment, and hypertrophy. Am. J. Physiol. **256:** C793–C798.

69. SKALLI, O., W. S. BLOOM, P. ROPRAZ, B. AZZARONE & G. GABBIANI. 1986. Cytoskeletal remodelling of rat aortic smooth muscle cells *in vitro:* relationships to culture conditions and analogies to *in vivo* situations. J. Submicrosc. Cytol. **18:** 481–493.

70. GLUKHOVA, M. A., A. E. KABAKOV, A. M. BELKIN, M. G. FRID, O. I. ORNATSKY, N. I. ZHIDKOVA & V. E. KOTELIANSKY. 1986. Meta-vinculin distribution in adult human tissues and cultured cells. FEBS Lett. **207:** 139–141.

71. HERMAN, B., M. W. ROE, C. HARRIS, B. WRAY & D. CLEMMONS. 1987. Platelet-derived growth factor-induced alterations in vinculin distribution in porcine vascular smooth muscle cells. Cell Motil. Cytoskel. **8:** 91–105.

72. GLUKHOVA, M. A., A. E. KABAKOV, O. I. ORNATSKY, T. D. VASILEVSKAYA, V. E. KOTE-LIANSKY & V. N. SMIRNOV. 1987. Immunoreactive forms of caldesmon in cultivated human vascular smooth muscle cells. FEBS Lett. **218:** 292–294.

73. UEKI, N., K. SOBUE, K. KANDA, T. HADA & K. HIGASHINO. 1987. Expression of high and low molecular weight caldesmons during phenotypic modulation of smooth muscle cells. Proc. Natl. Acad. Sci. USA **84:** 9049–9053.

74. HANSSON, G. K., L. JONASSON, J. HOLM, M. M. CLOWES & A. W. CLOWES. 1988. γ-Interferon regulates vascular smooth muscle proliferation and Ia antigen expression *in vitro* and *in vivo.* Circ. Res. **63:** 712–719.

75. WARNER, S. J. C., G. B. FRIEDMAN & P. LIBBY. 1989. Regulation of major histocompatibility gene expression in human vascular smooth muscle cells. Arteriosclerosis **9:** 279–288.

76. SJOLÜND, M., U. HEDIN, T. SEJERSEN, C-H. HELDIN & J. THYBERG. 1988. Arterial smooth muscle cells express platelet-derived growth factor (PDGF) A chain mRNA, secrete a PDGF-like mitogen, and bind exogenous PDGF in a phenotype- and growth state-dependent manner. J. Cell Biol. **106:** 403–413.

77. MAJESKY, M., E. P. BENDITT & S. M. SCHWARTZ. 1988. Expression and developmental

control of platelet-derived growth factor A-chain and B-chain/*Sis* genes in rat aortic smooth muscle cells. Proc. Natl. Acad. Sci. USA **85:** 1524–1528.

78. VALENTE, A. J., R. DELGADO, J. D. METTER, C. CHO, E. A. SPRAGUE, C. J. SCHWARTZ & D. T. GRAVES. 1988. Cultured primate aortic smooth muscle cells express both the PDGF-A and PDGF-B genes but do not secrete mitogenic activity or dimeric platelet-derived growth factor protein. J. Cell. Physiol. **136:** 479–485.

79. BIRINYI, L. K., S. J. C. WARNER, R. N. SALOMON, A. D. CALLOW & P. LIBBY. 1989. Observations on human smooth muscle cell cultures from hyperplastic lesions of prosthetic bypass grafts—Production of platelet-derived growth factor like mitogen and expression of a gene for a platelet-derived growth factor receptor—A preliminary study. J. Vasc. Surg. **10:** 157–165.

80. ANG, A. H., G. TACHAS, J. H. CAMPBELL, J. F. BATEMAN & G. R. CAMPBELL. 1990. Collagen synthesis by cultured rabbit aortic smooth muscle cells: alteration with phenotype. Biochem. J. **265:** 461–469.

81. CAMPBELL, J. H., M. F. REARDON, G. R. CAMPBELL & P. J. NESTEL. 1985. Metabolism of atherogenic lipoproteins by smooth muscle cells of different phenotype in culture. Arteriosclerosis **5:** 318–328.

Extracellular Matrix-Smooth Muscle Phenotype Modulation by Macrophages[a]

JULIE H. CAMPBELL,[b] SILVIA G. KALEVITCH,[b]
ROBYN E. RENNICK,[b,c] AND GORDON R. CAMPBELL[c]

[b]Cell Biology Laboratory
Baker Medical Research Institute
Commercial Road, Prahran
Victoria 3181, Australia
and
[c]Cardiovascular Research Unit
Department of Anatomy
University of Melbourne
Parkville 3052, Australia

Smooth Muscle Phenotype in Atheroma

Smooth muscle cells in the intima of human arteries involved in atherogenesis are phenotypically different from those of the underlying media, and amongst other features, have a decreased volume fraction of myofilaments ($V_v$myo).[1] In primary cell culture, medial smooth muscle cells which have been enzyme-dispersed and seeded at densities below confluence undergo a similar change in phenotypic expression during the first five days after isolation. This is accompanied by distinct alterations in biology, including the ability to proliferate logarithmically in response to mitogens, synthesis of 26–45-fold the amount of collagen (particularly type I) as cells with a high $V_v$myo, and accumulation of 7-fold the amount of lipid on exposure to β-VLDL.[2] Since these are all characteristic features of smooth muscle cells in atheroma, change in phenotype of smooth muscle cells may be an important initial event in the development of this disease. This raises the question, what determines the phenotypic expression of smooth muscle cells? That is, what determines whether a smooth muscle cell is contractile (high $V_v$myo) and unresponsive to atherogenic stimuli such as mitogens and certain lipoproteins, or whether it has a low $V_v$myo and is responsive to these agents?

Phenotype Is Controlled by Matrix

Studies in our laboratory implicate cell-matrix interactions in control of smooth muscle phenotype. In primary cell culture, a crude extract of glycosaminoglycans from the aortic intima plus inner media maintains sparsely-seeded smooth muscle with a high $V_v$myo. Treatment of this aortic extract with heparinase from Flavobacterium heparinum destroys the active factor, indicating that glycosaminoglycans of the heparan sulphate species are responsible; and indeed, addition of the closely related glycosaminoglycan heparin maintains sparsely-seeded smooth muscle in the contractile state.[3] This has recently been confirmed by Herbert et al.[4] who also found a similar effect with pentosan

[a]This work was supported by grants from the National Heart Foundation of Australia and the National Health and Medical Research Council of Australia.

159

polysulphate, a semi-synthetic sulphated polysaccharide. Smooth muscle cells in primary culture can also be maintained in the contractile state by seeding the freshly-dispersed cells at confluent density, or by placing sparsely-seeded cells with a spatially separated feeder layer of confluent contractile smooth muscle cells or endothelial cells[5] which produce large amounts of an antiproliferative heparan sulphate species.[6] It thus appears that the presence of heparin-like glycosaminoglycans is an important determinant of the phenotype that smooth muscle expresses, and that high levels of this glycosaminoglycan species maintain the cells in a contractile (high $V_v$myo) state. Any factor which removes this substance (*e.g.*, enzyme dispersion and dilution through sparse-seeding) may therefore induce the cells to undergo a change in phenotype to a low $V_v$myo. Smooth muscle cells which have been seeded sparsely onto a layer of type IV collagen or basement membrane Matrigel (a solubilised extract of EHS tumour basement membrane containing collagen type IV, laminin, heparan sulphate proteoglycan, and entactin) do not undergo a change in phenotype, nor do isolated smooth muscle cells which have been completely embedded in a gel of collagen type I.[7] Thus replacement of certain components of the basal lamina, or providing a microenvironment in which the basal lamina can be rapidly reconstituted, encourages maintenance of the contractile state.

Macrophages Induce Change in Phenotype

Peritoneal macrophages grown in co-culture with a confluent monolayer of high $V_v$myo smooth muscle cells induce a significant decrease in $V_v$myo after three days as compared with both the freshly isolated smooth muscle cells and those grown for three days in the absence of macrophages.[8] Since invasion of the artery wall by monocytes (which subsequently become macrophages) is one of the earliest cellular events in experimental atherogenesis,[9] it may be through the influence of these cells that smooth muscle phenotypic change is induced in the initial stages of the disease.

Do Macrophages Induce Change in Phenotype by Degrading Heparan Sulphate?

The aim of the present study was to determine whether macrophages initiate change in smooth muscle phenotypic expression through degradation of heparan sulphate proteoglycans on the smooth muscle cell surface. An assay for heparan sulphate-degrading enzymes was set up as described by Savion *et al.*[10] Bovine aortic endothelial cells were seeded sparsely into 30-mm plastic culture dishes in the presence of 40 μCi/ml $Na_2[^{35}S]O_4$. Five to 7 days after the cells had achieved confluency, the endothelial cells were removed by Triton X-100, leaving a layer of ^{35}S-labelled extracellular matrix on the bottom of the dish. About 70% of the incorporated ^{35}S was in the form of heparan sulphate, and 30% in chondroitin sulphate and dermatan sulphate. The factor to be tested for heparan sulphate-degrading activity was added to the washed matrix for 24 hours at 37°C at neutral pH, then an aliquot of the supernatant passed through a Sepharose 6B column and the fractions counted by liquid scintillation.

Firstly, as control, medium 199 without serum (1.5 ml, pH 7.0) was incubated with the thoroughly washed ^{35}S-labelled extracellular matrix. After gel filtration of the supernatant, all the radioactivity co-migrated with dextran blue ($M_r = 2 \times 10^6$ daltons) to elute at the void volume (V_0), indicating that only high molecular weight undegraded proteoglycans had been released into the medium. Free $[^{35}S]O_4^{2-}$ applied directly to the column eluted with a K_{av} of 0.86 (FIG. 1).

After incubation of the matrix with living mouse peritoneal macrophages or J774 macrophages (1 $\times$ 10^6 cells/ml), the peak at V_0 was small, and instead more than 80%

of the radioactivity eluted with a K_{av} of 0.84, indicating that most of the ^{35}S-labelled glycosaminoglycan chains of the proteoglycans had been completely degraded (FIG. 2). When 10 μg/ml sodium heparin was added to the incubation with living macrophages, the size of the K_{av} 0.84 peak was decreased, and the peak at V_0 increased. As well, a number of small peaks appeared at K_{av} 0.5 or less. When macrophages were lysed and a 100-μl aliquot incubated in 1.4 ml medium 199 without serum with the ^{35}S-labelled matrix, most of the degradation products eluted with a K_{av} of 0.60, with smaller peaks at V_0 and at K_{av} of 0.84 (FIG. 2). Based on a comparison of the experimental K_{av} values on Sepharose 6B columns with those determined for chondroitin sulphate fractions of known molecular weight, it was estimated that the degradation fragments at K_{av} 0.60 had a molecular weight of about 10,000 daltons.

When fresh macrophage-conditioned medium (4×10^6 cells/ml serum-free medium for 24 hours at 37°C) was incubated with ^{35}S-labelled matrix, most of the released radioactivity eluted at V_0, similar to that observed with fresh medium 199 without serum, with minor peaks at K_{av} 0.60 and 0.84. Addition of an equal volume of the macrophage-conditioned medium and fresh medium to confluent 30 mm dishes of high $V_v$myo rabbit

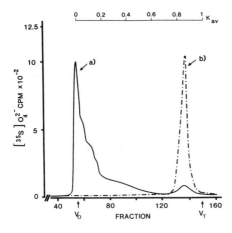

FIGURE 1. a) Medium 199 without serum incubated for 24 hours at 37°C and neutral pH with ^{35}S-labelled extracellular matrix (——); b) Free Na$_2$[^{35}S]O$_4$ (—·—·). Elution profiles after gel filtration through Sepharose 6B.

aortic smooth muscle, 8 days in primary culture, had no effect on smooth muscle phenotype after 4 days incubation. Macrophage-conditioned medium was concentrated 10-fold with an Amicon concentrator, then increasing concentrations of ammonium sulphate added together with bovine serum albumin. Precipitates were obtained in the presence of 0–25%, 25–50%, 50–75% and 75–100% ammonium sulphate. Each of the four precipitates was dissolved in 1 ml medium 199 without serum, and 100-μl aliquots added to confluent 30-mm dishes of rabbit aortic smooth muscle. After 4 days, the $V_v$myo of the smooth muscle cells in fractions which precipitated with 0–25%, 25–50% and 75–100% ammonium sulphate were not significantly different from controls ($p > 0.5$), but the $V_v$myo of smooth muscle cells in the presence of fraction 50–75% had a $V_v$myo of 42.7 ± 2.9%, which was significantly lower than that of control cells (49.2 ± 1.4%, $p < 0.15$) (FIG. 3). Each of the precipitates was also tested for matrix-degrading activity. The 0–25%, 25–50% and 75–100% ammonium sulphate-precipitated fractions all produced large peaks at V_0 and another broad peak with a K_{av} of 0.37–0.42 ($M_r = 30,000$–40,000 daltons). Fraction 50–75% had a small peak at V_0 and a distinct, considerably larger peak at K_{av} 0.65. Thus the fraction that degraded the ^{35}S-labelled proteoglycans into fragments

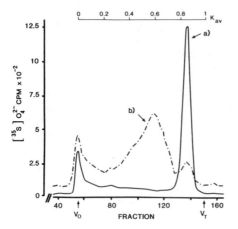

FIGURE 2. a) Living mouse peritoneal macrophages (——), and b) lysate of whole J774 macrophages (—·—·) incubated for 24 hours at 37°C and neutral pH with ^{35}S-labelled extracellular matrix. Elution profiles after gel filtration through Sepharose 6B.

of about 10,000 dalton molecular weight, was the same that induced a decrease in $V_v$myo of the rabbit aortic smooth muscle cells.

It was also clear that the matrix-degrading activity of the macrophages is stored within the cells and that only small amounts are released into the incubation medium. To identify the subcellular location of the stored enzymes that degrade the ^{35}S-labelled proteoglycans, macrophage lysosomes were prepared and 100 μl of the lysate added to confluent 30-mm dishes of rabbit aortic smooth muscle, 8 days in culture. After 4 days in the presence of the lysosomal lysate, the $V_v$myo of the cells was 38.2 ± 2.6%, which was significantly lower ($p < 0.1$) than that of control cells (48.2 ± 0.5%). Incubation of the ^{35}S-labelled matrix with 100 μl of the macrophage lysosomal lysate at neutral pH produced a degradation peak with K_{av} 0.63 that was totally inhibited when 10 μg/ml heparin was included in the incubation (FIG. 4). When the lysosomal lysate was incubated with the ^{35}S-labelled matrix at acid pH (pH 6.5 or less), the peak at K_{av} 0.63 was smaller and a second large peak at K_{av} 0.84 appeared (FIG. 4). Having established that the K_{av} 0.63 peak eluted in fractions 100 to 125, a second aliquot of the lysate was run on the same column and

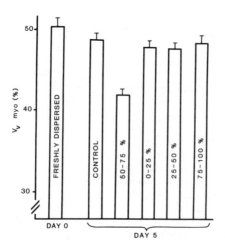

FIGURE 3. Histogram of the volume fraction of myofilaments ($V_v$myo) of smooth muscle cells from the 9–12-week-old rabbit aortic media when freshly dispersed into single cells (day 0), and after 5 days in primary culture either alone or in the presence of re-dissolved precipitates from a concentrate of macrophage-conditioned medium. The precipitates were formed by adding progressively higher concentrations of $(NH_4)_2SO_4$, and centrifuging and removing each precipitate before adding more $(NH_4)_2SO_4$. Four precipitates were prepared from 0–25%, 25–50%, 50–75%, and 75–100% $(NH_4)_2SO_4$.

fractions 100 to 125 collected (5 ml). An aliquot (0.5 ml) of these pooled fractions was treated with low pH nitrous acid which selectively results in deamination of heparan sulphate chains to fragments less than M_r 1,000. When this mixture was passed through Sepharose 6B, no peak at K_{av} 0.63 occurred, but instead a peak at K_{av} 0.84 appeared. In contrast, treatment of another 0.5 ml aliquot of pooled fractions 100–125 (peak K_{av} 0.63) with 10 units/ml chondroitin ABC lyase, which degrades chondroitin sulphate, resulted in only a very small peak at K_{av} 0.84, with most of the radioactivity continuing to elute with a K_{av} 0.63.

Addition of 10 units/ml heparinase to the extracellular matrix consistently resulted in a large peak eluting at K_{av} 0.63 (FIG. 5), identical to that obtained in the presence of macrophage lysosomal lysate at neutral pH (see FIG. 4). Again, this peak did not occur if 10 μg/ml heparin was included in the incubation, and also like the K_{av} 0.63 peak produced by lysosomal lysate, was degraded to smaller fragments and free $[^{35}S]O_4^{2-}$ (K_{av} = 0.84 to 0.87) after treatment with nitrous acid, but was unaffected by chondroitin ABC lyase. Addition of 10 units/ml heparinase to confluent aortic smooth muscle cultures induced a significantly ($p < 0.1$) lower $V_v$myo (42.8 ± 1.2%) compared with control cells (51.0 ± 3.2%) after 4 days.

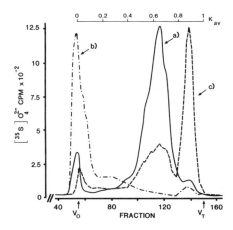

FIGURE 4. a) Lysosomal lysate (100 μl) from J774 macrophages in medium 199 without serum incubated at neutral pH for 24 hours at 37°C with ^{35}S-labelled extracellular matrix (———); b) as for a) but including 10 μg/ml sodium heparin (—·—·); c) as for a) but at pH 6.2 (- - - -). Elution profiles after gel filtration through Sepharose 6B.

These results indicate that the degradation peak which elutes at $K_{av} \approx 0.63$ consists almost exclusively of heparan sulphate fragments, and suggest that the macrophages used in the present study have in their lysosomes a heparan sulphate degrading endoglycosidase which cleaves internal glycosidic bonds, and whose action on smooth muscle cells is sufficient to induce a change in phenotypic expression. The results further suggest that macrophages also possess sulphatases and/or exoglycosidases which sequentially release inorganic sulphates and monosaccharide residues from the nonreducing ends of the heparan sulphate fragments released by the endoglycosidase. The subcellular localisation of the exoglycosidases and/or sulphatases is also lysosomal, but unlike the heparinase, they are only active at acid pH, such as occurs in intact lysosomes.

Plasma membrane preparations incubated with ^{35}S-labelled extracellular matrix produced a large, broad elution peak which began at V_0, peaked at K_{av} 0.24, then gradually tailed off (FIG. 5), indicating that they possess enzyme activity, probably proteolytic, which releases high molecular weight ^{35}S-labelled species from matrix, but little or no activity to degrade these substances further. A similar elution profile occurred when 10

μg/ml trypsin was incubated with the ^{35}S-labelled matrix (FIG. 5). One peak occurred at V_0 (undegraded proteoglycan) and another broader peak at K_{av} of about 0.20.

Cell-associated heparan sulphate proteoglycans occur as membrane-intercalated gly-coproteins where the core protein is anchored in the lipid interior of the plasma membrane, and the heparan sulphate chains bind to specific sites on collagen, laminin, and fibronectin.[11] The function of the proteoglycan-mediated interaction is to promote the organisation of actin filaments in the attaching cell which also has the effect of stabilising cell morphology; thus removal and destruction of cell-surface heparan sulphate at these sites may initiate a change in smooth muscle phenotype through disorganisation of actin filaments with subsequent influences on gene expression.[12] However, the observation that trypsin (which releases the heparan sulphate proteoglycans from the cell surface) does not by itself induce a change in smooth muscle phenotype, suggests that the heparan chains must be completely destroyed or otherwise removed from the vicinity of the cell for this to occur. The ability of free heparin to prevent a change in phenotype of those smooth muscle cells whose extracellular matrix and basal lamina have been degraded and removed during enzymatic isolation, supports this view.

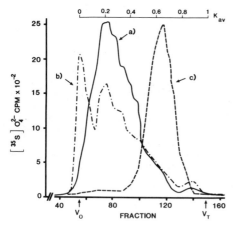

FIGURE 5. a) Plasma membrane preparation (100 μl) from J774 macrophages in medium 199 without serum (———); b) 10 μg/ml trypsin in medium 199 without serum (—·—·); c) 10 units/ml heparinase in medium 199 without serum (- - - -). Elution profiles after gel filtration through Sepharose 6B.

Heparan sulphate proteoglycans and free glycosaminoglycan chains, including heparin, bind to specific proteins at the cell surface, are internalised with a half-life of 4–6 hours, and are degraded intracellularly.[13] A small fraction of the heparan sulphate enriched in the rare 2–O-sulphate glucuronate units is transported to the cell nucleus where it has been implicated in cell growth control,[14] but whether internalised heparan sulphate/heparin affects smooth muscle phenotypic expression by the same or a similar mechanism is unknown.

Macrophages are prominent cells both in the host defense mechanism characteristic of chronic inflammatory responses and in atheroma. These mononuclear phagocytes produce a vast array of secretory products including neutral proteases which degrade the matrix macromolecules elastin, collagen, and glycoproteins, and endoglycosidic activity specific for heparan sulphate.[10] Heparan sulphate degrading enzymes have also been described in platelets,[15] T-lymphocytes,[10] neutrophils,[16] and tumor cells.[17,18] Indeed, the heparanase activity of tumours was shown to be directly related to their metastatic potential, leading to the suggestion that degradation of heparan sulphate in extracellular matrix facilitates invasion of the vessel wall by normal and malignant cells.[17,18]

Relationship to Atherogenesis

Based on the studies reported here, we suggest the following scenario in relation to the genesis of atherosclerosis: monocyte/macrophages which have entered the subendothelium release heparan sulphate proteoglycans from the surface of smooth muscle cells by the action of released proteases or those present on the plasma membrane. The proteoglycans are phagocytosed by the macrophages and the heparan sulphate chains completely degraded in the lysosomes. This temporarily removes all heparan sulphate from the surface of the smooth muscle cells, and this, by an unknown mechanism, initiates the process of phenotypic modulation.

ACKNOWLEDGMENTS

We are grateful to Ms Janet Rogers, Elpis Spanidis, and Julie Saffstrom for excellent technical assistance.

REFERENCES

1. Mosse, P. R. L., G. R. Campbell, Z-L. Wang & J. H. Campbell. 1985. Smooth muscle phenotypic expression in human carotid arteries. I. Comparison of cells from diffuse intimal thickenings adjacent to atheromatous plaques with those of the media. Lab. Invest. **53:** 555–562.
2. Campbell, G. R. & J. H. Campbell. 1990. The phenotypes of smooth muscle expressed in human atheroma. Ann. N.Y. Acad. Sci. This volume.
3. Chamley-Campbell, J. H. & G. R. Campbell. 1981. What controls smooth muscle phenotype? Atherosclerosis **40:** 347–357.
4. Herbert, J. M., D. Nuti, R. Paul & J. P. Maffrand. 1988. *In vitro* and *ex vivo* regulation of vascular smooth muscle cell growth and phenotypic modulation by sulphated polysaccharides. Artery **16:** 1–14.
5. Campbell, J. H. & G. R. Campbell. 1984. Cellular interactions in the artery wall. *In* The Peripheral Circulation. S. Hunyor, J. Ludbrook, J. Shaw & M. McGrath, Eds. 33–39. Elsevier. New York, NY.
6. Fritze, L. M., C. F. Reilly & R. D. Rosenberg. 1985. An antiproliferative heparan sulphate species produced by post-confluent smooth muscle cells. J. Cell Biol. **100:** 1041–1049.
7. Stadler, E., J. H. Campbell & G. R. Campbell. 1989. Do cultured vascular smooth muscle cells resemble those of the artery wall. If not, why not? J. Cardiovasc. Pharmacol. **14** (Suppl. 6): S1–S8.
8. Rennick, R. E., J. H. Campbell & G. R. Campbell. 1988. Vascular smooth muscle phenotype and growth behaviour can be influenced by macrophages *in vitro*. Atherosclerosis **71:** 35–43.
9. Joris, I., T. Zand, J. J. Nunnari, F. J. Krolikowski & G. Majno. 1983. Studies on the pathogenesis of atherosclerosis. I. Adhesion and emigration of mononuclear cells in the aorta of hypercholesterolemic rats. Am. J. Pathol. **113:** 341–358.
10. Savion, N., I. Vlodavsky & Z. Fuks. 1984. Interaction of T-lymphocytes and macrophages with cultured endothelial cells: attachment, invasion and subsequent degradation of the subendothelial extracellular matrix. J. Cell Physiol. **118:** 169–178.
11. Saunders, S. & M. Bernfield. 1988. Cell surface proteoglycan binds mouse mammary epithelial cells to fibronectin and behaves as a receptor for interstitial matrix. J. Cell Biol. **106:** 423–430.
12. Bissell, M. J. & M. H. Barcellos-Hoff. 1987. The influence of extracellular matrix on gene expression: is structure the message? J. Cell Sci. (Suppl. 8): 327–343.
13. Bienkowski, M. J. & H. E. Conrad. 1984. Kinetics of proteoheparan sulphate synthesis,

secretion, endocytosis, and catabolism by a hepatocyte cell line. J. Biol. Chem. **259:** 12989–12996.

14. FEDARKO, N. S. & H. E. CONRAD. 1986. A unique heparan sulfate in the nuclei of hepatocytes: structural changes with the growth state of the cells. J. Cell Biol. **102:** 587–599.

15. WASTESON, A., B. GLIMELIUS, C. BUSCH, B. WESTERMARK, C. H. HELDIN & B. NORLING. 1977. Effect of a platelet endoglycosidase on cell surface associated heparan sulphate of human cultured endothelial and glial cells. Thrombosis Res. **11:** 309–321.

16. MATZNER, Y., M. BAR-NER, J. YAHALOM, R. ISHAI-MICHAELI, Z. FUKS & I. VLODAVSKY. 1985. Degradation of heparan sulphate in the subendothelial extracellular matrix by a readily released heparanase from human neutrophils. J. Clin. Invest. **76:** 1306–1313.

17. NAKAJIMA, M., T. IRIMUA, N. DI FERRANTE & G. L. NICOLSON. 1983. Heparan sulphate degradation: relation to tumor invasive and metastatic properties of mouse B16 melanoma sublines. Science **220:** 611–613.

18. VLODAVSKY, I., Z. FUKS, M. BAR-NER, Y. ARIAV & V. SCHIRRMACHER. 1983. Lymphoma cell-mediated degradation of sulfated proteoglycans in the subendothelial extracellular matrix: relationship to tumor cell metastasis. Cancer Res. **43:** 2704–2711.

Vascular Signal Transduction and Atherosclerosis

VLADIMIR N. SMIRNOV, TATYANA A.
VOYNO-YASENETSKAYA,[a] ALEXANDER S. ANTONOV,
MATVEY E. LUKASHEV, VLADIMIR P. SHIRINSKY,
VLADIMIR V. TERTOV, AND VSEVOLOD A. TKACHUK

Institute of Experimental Cardiology
USSR Cardiology Research Center
121552 3rd Cherepkovskaya Str. 15A
Moscow, USSR

INTRODUCTION

Hormones, growth factors, neurotransmitters, and other agonists bind to specific receptors on cell plasma membrane. Receptor occupancy initiates the formation of second messenger molecules including adenosine $3',5'$-monophosphate (cAMP), guanosine $3',5'$-monophosphate (cGMP), and other recently discovered messenger molecules, diacylglycerol, and inositolphosphates formed by hydrolysis of phosphoinositides.[1,2] Second messengers control a number of cellular events including metabolism, secretion, shape change, and cellular growth.[2,3]

At present, cellular manifestations of human atherosclerosis are relatively well known. The progression of atherosclerotic plaque takes place in vascular intima; media and adventitia are not involved. It is known that in aging human vascular endothelium becomes morphologically heterogeneous; clusters of giant and small endothelial cells have been described.[4,5] Recently, using computer analysis of sudanophylic areas in human aorta, the zones with high and low probability of atherosclerosis were described.[5-7] The study of morphologic heterogeneity of endothelial lining in these regions demonstrated that in the areas of high probability of atherosclerosis (ages 30–70 years) heterogeneous clasterized endothelium is met 2.7 times more frequently than in unaffected areas, and in the age group of 20–27 years this clusterization is found exclusively in these regions.[5]

Thickening of vascular wall in the region of atherosclerotic plaque is caused by local increase in the volume of extracellular matrix[8] synthesized by modified smooth muscle cells (SMC). Statistically reliable increase in the proportion of modified SMC was demonstrated in atherosclerotic plaque leading to a drop in the number of SMC of contractile phenotype.[8]

The important cellular event in the development of atherosclerotic plaque is the appearance of macrophage- and smooth muscle cell-derived foam cells in intima.[9]

Thus, it is evident that the formation of human atherosclerotic plaque is accompanied by essential changes in morphology, functions, and cellular composition of intimal layer including endothelial cells. Therefore, it is logical to study the involvement of the second messenger systems in these events. This paper describes the results of the study of signal transduction systems and second messengers in intimal cells of human aorta in athero-

---

[a]To whom correspondence should be addressed.

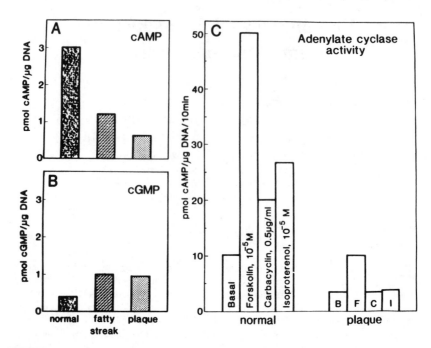

FIGURE 1. Cyclic nucleotides in atherosclerotic human intima. Aortas were collected and processed, and cyclic nucleotide concentration and adenylate cyclase activity were measured as described by Tertov *et al.*[14] (**A**) cAMP level; (**B**) cGMP level; (**C**) basal and agonist-stimulated adenylate cyclase activity.

sclerosis, including adenylate cyclase and phosphoinositide metabolism and their involvement in the control of endothelium morphology. The relationships between low density lipoproteins (LDL) and second messengers in human vascular endothelium and platelets are also discussed.

Cyclic Nucleotides in Human Intimal Cells in Atherosclerosis

Changes in the second messengers were registered in a number of pathological states, including diabetis, tumor formation, and certain infections.[10–12] Recently the data related to the changes in the system of cyclic nucleotides in animal atherosclerosis became available.[13] It was found that the progression of atherosclerotic plaque in human intima is accompanied by the changes in the metabolism of second messengers.[14] Thus, cAMP content in lipid streaks and atherosclerotic plaques decreases 3–5-fold compared to the noninvolved intimal regions, whereas the level of cGMP was elevated almost 3-fold (FIG. 1A,B). Such variations in the level of cyclic nucleotides may be explained by the changes in regulatory properties of enzymes involved in the metabolism of cAMP and cGMP. Thus, basal activity of adenylate cyclase (AC) is lowered by 3–6-fold and the hormonal activation of AC in the crude membrane preparations from atherosclerotic plaque is completely missed (FIG. 1C). The drop in forskolin-stimulated activity of AC may be explained by decline in basal enzyme activity. Whereas in normal intima basal and forskolin-stimulated activity of AC is respectively 9.4 ± 1.2 and 56.2 ± 4.2 pmol cAMP/μg DNA/10 min; these values in atherosclerotic plaque were equal to 2.2 ± 0.6 and 10.9 ± 2.8 pmol cAMP/μg DNA/10 min.[14] Thus, in normal intima forskolin stimulates adenylate cyclase by 5.9-fold, whereas in atherosclerotic plaque stimulation is 5-fold.

In our experiments the activity of cAMP phosphodiesterase in normal intima and atherosclerosis prone regions was not changed.[14] The elevation of cGMP concentration in atherosclerotic lesions may be due to the increase in the activity of guanylate cyclase and the decline in the activity of cGMP phosphodiesterase.[14] It is noteworthy that in medial layer no changes in the cyclic nucleotide levels were found.[14]

It is known that in atherosclerotic lesions of human intima lipid-laden cells are usually present.[9] If primary cultured human aortic cells are grown in the presence of 40% serum taken from patients with atherosclerosis, a 2–3-fold decrease in the level of cAMP is found in cells which accumulate lipids, while cGMP is elevated by almost 2-fold (FIG. 2) compared to cyclic nucleotide level in the control cells cultured from unaffected areas. Thus, accumulation of lipids by cells leads to the same changes in the system of cyclic nucleotides which were found in lipid streak and the atherosclerotic plaque of human aortic intima.

It is well known that cAMP controls intracellular hydrolysis of triglycerides. cAMP-dependent protein kinase phosphorylates triglyceride lipase converting this enzyme into its active form, which hydrolyzes triglycerides into free fatty acids and glycerol.[15] Proliferative activity of intimal human aortic cells is also controlled by cAMP.[16]

If intracellular level of cAMP is increased (TABLE 1), profound inhibition of cholesterol ester and triglyceride accumulation in cultured intimal cells is observed accompanied by essential inhibition of [³H]-thymidine incorporation into these cells.

Thus, the decrease of cAMP level found in human aortic intimal cells isolated from atherosclerotic plaque and in lipid-laden cultured intimal cells may accelerate lipid accumulation and proliferation of these cells. In an attempt to understand the changes in second messengers during atherosclerosis progression the effect of low density lipoproteins on this system was studied using platelets and human vascular cells.

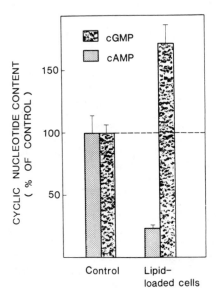

FIGURE 2. Effect of lipid accumulation of cyclic nucleotide content in human intimal cells. Cells were isolated and cultured as described by Orekhov *et al.*[16] Loading of cells with lipids was performed by 24-h incubation with 40% serum from patients having atherosclerosis. Cells were then incubated for 6 h in standard culture medium[16] and cyclic nucleotide concentration was measured as described by Tertov *et al.*[14]

TABLE 1. Effect of cAMP on Lipid Content and Proliferative Activity of Human Intimal Cells[a]

| | % of Control | | |
Agent	CE	TG	^{3}H-T
cAMP containing liposomes	69 ± 4	52 ± 6	67 ± 2
Db cAMP, 0.1 mM	53 ± 8	61 ± 5	60 ± 2
Cholera toxin, 100 ng/ml	57 ± 6	62 ± 5	63 ± 12
PGE$_2$, 10 μg/ml	69 ± 2	52 ± 4	46 ± 2
Carbacyclin, 0.5 μg/ml	52 ± 10	51 ± 8	50 ± 7
Forskolin, 0.01 mM	49 ± 11	53 ± 5	53 ± 6
Mix, 0.1 mM	47 ± 7	40 ± 6	45 ± 4

[a]Cells were isolated and cultured as described by Orekhov et al.[16] Cholesterol ester, triglyceride content, and [^{3}H]-thymidine incorporation were determined as described by Orekhov et al.[16] Agents tested were added 24 h prior to experiment. The data are presented as the per cent of control values.

"Hormone-Like" Effects of Low Density Lipoproteins

Recently some new functions of LDL have been described. Using platelets, smooth muscle cells, endothelial cells, lymphocytes, and fibroblasts it was shown that LDL activates phosphoinositide metabolism and increases cytoplasmic calcium ([Ca^{2+}]).[17] Nonspecific effects of LDL on the system of second messengers related to the changes in the viscosity of plasma membrane, the changes in the ratio of cholesterol:phospholipids or ionophore effects of LDL were discussed.[18]

In culture of human endothelial cells phosphoinositide metabolism is activated by a number of Ca^{2+}-mobilizing agonists, including histamine, platelet activation factor (PAF), and bradykinin.[19–21] Activation of phosphoinositide metabolism in endothelium by these hormones is accompanied by the synthesis of thromboxane and prostacyclin involved in the regulation of vascular tone, as well as in the function of endothelial layer in general.[19]

Comparing effects of histamine and LDL it was found that both histamine (10^{-4} M) and LDL (10 μg/ml) activate phosphoinositide metabolism in cultured human endothelial cells (FIG. 3).

It is well known that coupling of membrane receptors for vasoactive agents with phsopholipase C which hydrolyzes phosphoinositides occurs via GTP-binding proteins (G proteins).[22] α-Subunit of all G proteins is capable of binding GTP or GDP depending on the association with membrane receptors. After interaction of ligand with receptor, binding of GTP and activation of phospholipase C by corresponding G protein occurs. On the other hand, GDP binding inactivates membrane G proteins. In many cell types phosphoinositide metabolism is sensitive to guanyl nucleotides. Activation of phospholipase C and the formation of inositol phosphates in the presence of stable analogs of GTP (GTPγS) were demonstrated, in particular, in bovine pulmonary endothelium.[20]

FIGURE 3 demonstrates that GTPγS potentiates the effect of histamine, as well as of LDL. Stable analog GDPβS completely blocks the effect of the hormone and LDL. These results suggest that LDL receptors may be coupled to GTP-binding proteins, and like hormonal receptors, may stimulate the formation of second messengers.

The activation of cells by LDL may have physiological, as well as pathophysiological significance. It is noticed that EC$_{50}$ for activation of cells by LDL is close to K$_d$ of high affinity binding of LDL by cells, and similar to LDL concentrations found in interstitial fluid.[17]

Like Ca^{2+}-mobilizing hormones LDL may trigger cellular events which lead to activation of phosphoinositide metabolism, namely proliferation, endocytosis, secretion, and contraction.[23] In particular, it was found that LDL stimulates PGE_1 and prostacyclin synthesis in smooth muscle cells.[24] These syntheses are correlated with the activation of phospholipase C in the cells.[19]

At present the data are available on the physiological interaction between receptor-dependent systems of second messengers. Thus, it was found that prolonged stimulation of phosphoinositide metabolism accompanied by the activation of protein kinase C leads to desensitization of beta-adrenergic receptors and adenylate cyclase in human endothelial cells. After incubation for 1 h with protein kinase C activator, phorbol-myristate-acetate (PMA), drastic increase in the activity of adenylate cyclase in membranes isolated from these cells was found (FIG. 4A). Besides, sensitivity of enzyme to isoproterenol decreases, which is mediated by beta-adrenergic receptors (FIG. 4A). It was demonstrated that the decrease in the sensitivity of adenylate cyclase to isoproterenol is related to a decrease in the number of beta-adrenergic receptors per cell by 4–6-fold. This densensitization was observed when kinase C activation was produced directly (by PMA) or via stimulation of phosphoinositide metabolism by hormones (histamine, PAF) (FIG. 4B).

Thus, the products of phosphoinositide metabolism activating protein kinase C cause desensitization of beta-adrenergic receptors and adenylate cyclase system in endothelial cells. It is thought that the changes observed in atherosclerotic plaque of human aortic cells in the levels of cyclic nucleotides and a sharp drop in the sensitivity of adenylate cyclase to hormones (FIG. 1) may be related to desensitization of receptors involved in the activation of phosphoinositide metabolism. Thus, not only vasoactive hormones, but also LDL are capable of activating phosphoinositide metabolism in endothelium. It is well known that the level of LDL in patients with atherosclerosis is often elevated.

Besides endothelial cells "hormone-like" effects of LDL were demonstrated in human platelets. Putative receptor-operated Ca^{2+} channels in platelets, which can be activated by PAF, thrombin and other agonists, possess some common properties. The activation of receptor-gated Ca^{2+} channels is accompanied by the inward Ca^{2+} flow and by mobilization of Ca^{2+} from intracellular stores.[25] Protein kinase C and cAMP-dependent protein kinase block Ca^{2+} flow, whereas epinephrine potentiates Ca^{2+} current via receptor-activated Ca^{2+} channels.[26,27] These channels are permeable for other bivalent cations, particularly for Ba^{2+} and Mn^{2+}.[28] It was found that LDL-dependent increase in cytoplasmic $[Ca^{2+}]$ found in human platelets possesses all properties of agonist-dependent increase in Ca^{2+}.[29]

Using fluorescent probes quin-2 and fura-2 it was shown that PAF causes transient increase in intracellular $[Ca^{2+}]_i$ in human platelets. The inward flow of calcium stimulated by histamine is inhibited by protein kinase C activator, phorbol ester, and also adenylate cyclase activator prostaglandin E_1 (FIG. 5A).

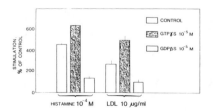

FIGURE 3. LDL stimulate phosphoinositide turnover in cultured human endothelial cells. Human umbilical vein endothelial cells were isolated and cultured as described by Resink *et al.*[19] Labeling with [^{3}H]-myoinositol was performed as described by Voyno-Yasenetskaya *et al.*[20] Cells were preincubated with 0.1 mM GTPγS or 0.1 mM GDPβS for 1 h at 37°C and subsequently incubated with 0.1 mM histamine or 10 μg/ml LDL for 10 min. Inositol phosphates were separated after cell lysis with 10% SDS.[20] Basal level of inositol monophosphate (3200 ± 238 dpm/10^6 cells) was taken as 100%.

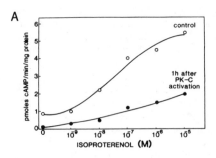

Similarly at low concentrations LDL elevates $[Ca^{2+}]_i$ in platelets and this effect is completely blocked after activation of protein kinase C and adenylate cyclase (FIG. 5B).

The similarity of LDL-dependent increase in $[Ca^{2+}]_i$ and the effect of other calcium-mobilizing agonists is confirmed by the potentiation of the effect of LDL by epinephrine. Epinephrine *per se* does not affect the level of Ca^{2+} in platelets but dramatically enhances the effects of other calcium-mobilizing agents.[27] Similarly preincubation of platelets with epinephrine leads to a profound potentiation of LDL-dependent elevation of $[Ca^{2+}]$ in the platelet cytoplasm (FIG. 5C).

It is known that LDL binding by human platelets is specific, reversible, and saturable.[17] The affinity of LDL receptors in platelets ($K_d = 5 \times 10^{-8}$ M) is not different from affinity of "classic" LDL-receptors from fibroblasts described by Goldstein and Brown.[30] At the same time, binding sites for LDL on platelets by some parameters differ from corresponding LDL binding sites on fibroblasts. Particularly, binding of LDL by platelets is blocked by HDL particles (HDL$_3$), which do not contain either E or B apoproteins and do not bind to LDL receptors on fibroblasts.[17,31]

Although there is no clear understanding of the mechanism of LDL interaction with platelets, it is possible that LDL-dependent increase of $[Ca^{2+}]_i$ in platelets occurs via the same pathways as the elevation in $[Ca^{2+}]_i$ caused by such aggregation inducers as PAF, vasopressin, histamine, thromboxane A_2, etc.

Regulatory Mechanisms Controlling Shape Changes and Orientation of Endothelial Cells in Monolayer

Two principal events in the morphology of human endothelium are noticed in aging cells: the loss of cell orientation and the appearance of morphological heterogeneity.[4,5] It was found that second messenger systems are involved in the regulation of shape changes

B

60 min incubation	Beta-adrenoceptors per cell
control	9600
histamine, 0.1 mM	2760
PMA, 0.1 nM	2460
PAF, 1 nM	1500

FIGURE 4B.

and orientation of endothelial cells in monolayer. Being in constant contact with blood, endothelium is affected by a large spectrum of hormones and other humoral mediators. *In vivo* and *in vitro* experiments demonstrated that blood vasoactive substances (serotonin, histamine) and β-TGF cause reversible changes in the permeability of endothelium and in the morphology of endothelial cells.[32–35] It was also found that in regulation of endothelial morphology cAMP and phosphoinositol metabolites may be involved, which mediate intracellular transduction of regulatory signals from humoral mediators.[36] FIGURE 6 (A–C) demonstrates the effects of forskolin which activates the synthesis of cAMP, and the activator of protein kinase C 4β-phorbol-12-myristate, 13-acetate (PMA) on the morphology of cultured endothelial human cells in confluent monolayer. It was found that forskolin at 10^{-5} M initiates evident changes in the cell shape and organization of endothelial layer (B). PMA alone had no effect on the morphology of endotheliocytes (C), but, as it

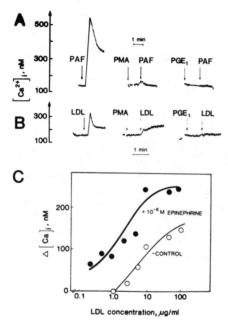

FIGURE 5. LDL-induced elevation of $[Ca^{2+}]_i$ in human platelets. Platelet isolation and loading with the fluorescent probes quin-2 and fura-2 were performed as described.[26] Quin-2 fluorescence and $[Ca^{2+}]_i$ level were measured as described by Avdonin *et al.*[26] (A) Prostaglandin E_1 PAF (10 μM) or PMA (0.1 μM) blocked PAF-induced (0.1 μM) elevation in $[Ca^{2+}]_i$; (B) prostaglandin E_1 (10 μM) or PMA (0.1 μM) blocked LDL-induced (10 μg/ml) elevation in $[Ca^{2+}]_i$; (C) dose-response for LDL-dependent $[Ca^{2+}]_i$ rise in fura-2-loaded platelets. Preincubation with epinephrine for 2–3 min potentiated LDL-dependent $[Ca^{2+}]_i$ elevation.

was shown earlier, significantly potentiated the effect of forskolin.[36] The analysis of forskolin and PMA effects demonstrated that both agents cause significant changes in the organization of actin cytoskeleton (microfilaments) of endothelial cells (FIG. 6, D–F). In confluent monolayer microfilaments form the system of bundles oriented along cellular edges (D). When forskolin increases intracellular level of cAMP these bundles disappear and F-actin becomes concentrated along the cell-cell borders (E). PMA also induces redistribution of microfilaments. In this case the number of microfilament bundles increases and many new bundles appear in the cell body (F). The stability and the organization of microfilaments are regulated by various actin-binding proteins including myosin playing an important role in the stabilization of microfilaments in nonmuscle cells.[37] Activation of cAMP synthesis by forskolin leads to a decrease in the amount of myosin content associated with cytoskeleton of endothelial cells. PMA, activating protein kinase

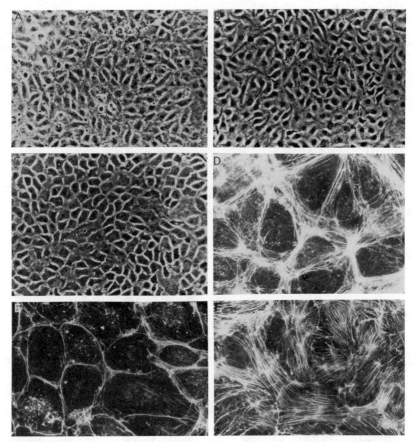

FIGURE 6. Effect of 10 μM forskolin (**B,E**) and 0.01 μM PMA (**C,F**) on cell shape (**A,C**) and microfilament organization (**D,F**) in cultured human umbilical vein endothelial cells. One-hour incubation with forskolin or PMA. A–C, phase contrast; D–F, F-actin staining with TRITC-phalloidin; A–D, controls.

C, increases the amount of myosin associated with endothelial cytoskeleton (FIG. 7A). The affinity of myosin binding for F-actin is known to be regulated by phosphorylation of myosin light chains.[38] The analysis of endothelial myosin phosphorylation using its metabolic labeling with ^{32}P and immunoprecipitation demonstrated that forskolin causes significant inhibition in the incorporation of the label in Mr 20 kD myosin light chains. In contrast to forskolin, PMA stimulated phosphorylation of Mr 20 kD myosin light chains (FIG. 7B). Phosphorylation of myosin light chains is mediated by myosin light chain kinase (MLCK). *In vitro* experiments demonstrated that MLCK is the substrate of cAMP-dependent protein kinase, and the phosphorylation of MLCK by cAMP-dependent protein kinase inhibits the activity of MLCK.[39] In our experiments it was demonstrated that forskolin causes an increase in the activity of cAMP-dependent protein kinase of endothelial cells, whereas PMA significantly decreases this activity (FIG. 7C).

The morphology of endothelial cells may also be changed as a result of periodic stretching of the substrate on which endothelial monolayer is grown.

Orientation of endothelial cells in blood vessels *in vivo* depends on blood flow and periodic stretch of the artery wall. It was shown that shear stress produced by the flow of liquid results in the elongation and orientation of cultured endothelial along flow direction.[40] As a result of shear stress *in vivo* and *in vitro* microfilament bundles in endothelium are oriented in a parallel accord to the direction of blood flow and cellular axis.[41] These findings suggest that dynamic changes in the cellular cytoskeleton and endothelial response to mechanical stimulation may be related to each other.

Periodic stretching and relaxation of endothelial monlayer, as well as the liquid flow, lead to endothelium orientation.[42] To understand the mechanism of stretch-induced orientation endothelium was grown on elastic silicone membrane, which was cyclically stretched imitating vascular wall movement.

It was shown that endothelial orientation depends on the rearrangements of actin in cellular cytoskeleton. The increase in the concentration of cAMP results in stress fiber dissasembly, redistribution of F-actin and inhibition of endothelium orientation. When cAMP and periodic stretching act simultaneously, homogeneous endothelial layer is transformed into a heterogeneous one within 3–4 h.[43]

From FIGURE 8 it is evident that periodic stretching of substrate on which endothelium is grown results in orientation of endothelial cells and in orientation of stress fiber parallel to the long axis of the cell.

Stretch-induced orientation of endothelium is inhibited after addition of forskolin. Preincubation of endothelium with 10^{-5} M forskolin for 1.5 h followed by periodic stretching of the substrate in the presence of forskolin also for 1.5 h reliably inhibits

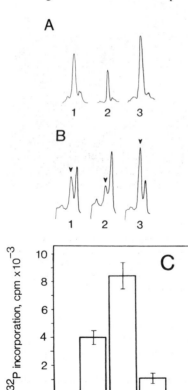

FIGURE 7. Effects of forskolin and PMA on myosin content in Triton X-100-insoluble cytoskeleton fraction (**A**), phosphorylation of 20 kD myosin light chain (**B**), and activity of cAMP-dependent protein kinase (*C*) in cultured human umbilical vein endothelial cells. A, densitogram of immunoblot of the Triton X-100-resistant fraction after immunoperoxidase detection of myosin heavy chain (antibodies were a generous gift of Drs. V. I. Gelfand and A. B. Verkhovsky, Moscow State University); B, densitogram of radioautograph obtained after metabolic labeling with ^{32}P, extraction, immunoprecipitation and SDS-PAGE of endothelial cell myosin. *Arrows* indicate the peak corresponding to 20 kD myosin light chain; C, protein kinase activity in endothelial cell lysates: ^{32}P incorporation in histone H1 inhibitable by purified termostable inhibitor of cAMP-dependent protein kinase. The lysates were incubated with [α-^{32}P]ATP and histone H1 for 10 min at 37°C. Incorporated radioactivity was measured in a liquid scintillation counter after precipitation of histone by TCA. 1, no additives; 2, 10 μM Fsk, 1 h; 3, 10 nM PMA, 1 h.

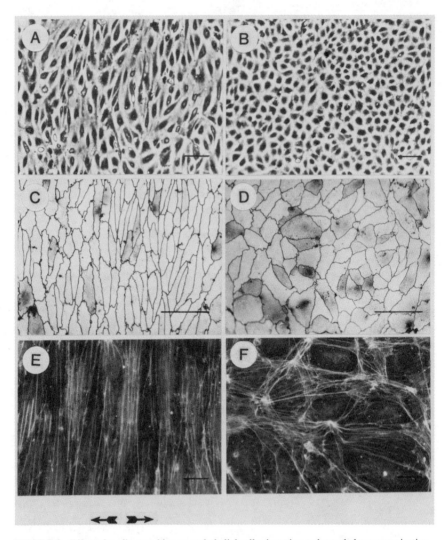

FIGURE 8. Effect of cyclic stretching on endothelial cell orientation and cytoskeleton organization. Cells were grown on silicone membranes[44] subjected to stretches and relaxations at 20% amplitude and 52 cycle/min for 48 h (**A,C,E**); cells on unstretched membranes served as a stationary control (**B,D,F**). A–B, phase contrast; C–D, silver nitrate staining; E–F, TRITC-phalloidin fluorescence.[44] *Arrows* show the direction of strain. Bars 100 μM (A–D), and 20 μM (E,F).

endothelial orientation (FIG. 9). Endothelial cells which underwent stretching in the presence of forskolin exhibit nearly random orientation (FIG. 9D), whereas the majority of cells in the absence of forskolin are oriented at 80°–120° of the direction of stretching (FIG. 9B).

Orientation of endothelial monolayer grown under conditions of periodic substrate stretching is very similar to the organization of endothelium in child aorta *in situ* (FIG.

10A,B). Periodic stretching of the confluent monolayer leads to the formation of small (3–5 cells) denuded areas. However, in the presence of forskolin these denudations are healed within 3–4 h and heterogeneous endothelial monolayer is formed which strikingly resembles adult human endothelial lining *in situ* (FIG. 10C,D). It is likely that endothelial heterogeneity and the appearance of giant endothelial cells may also be related to the spreading of endothelial cells healing monolayer defects formed after mechanical insult.[43]

Morphological heterogeneity is a typical feature of endothelium in adult human aorta and is absent in children's and animals' arteries. As was mentioned above, in the zones of high probability of atherosclerosis, the degree of endothelium heterogeneity is higher compared to the zones of low probability of atherosclerosis.[5] One of the mechanisms which explains the heterogeneity of endothelium is the accumulation of giant multinuclear cells.[44] From our data it is possible to conclude that in addition to polyploidy there exists another mechanism of the development of shape heterogeneity of endothelium *in situ*. This reaction may represent cAMP-dependent spreading of mononuclear endothelial cells in the zones of local denudation of monolayer. The possible factors which can interfere with the integrity of the endothelial layer include nonuniform stretching and turbulency in the zones of the progressing atherosclerotic plaque,[45] as well as receptor-mediated injury of endothelium caused by simultaneous stimulation of adenylate cyclase and phospho-inositide metabolism.[46]

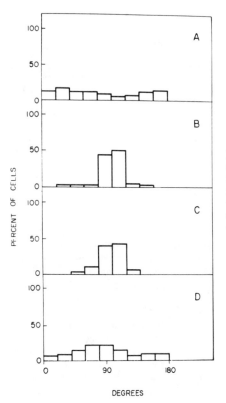

FIGURE 9. Histograms showing endothelial cell orientation in response to cyclic stretching. Percentage of endothelial cells is shown as a function of the angle between cell long axis and the stretch direction. (**A**) Stationary control; (**B**) endothelial cells after 24-h cycle stretching; endothelial cells stretched for 1.5 h in the absence (**C**) and in the presence (**D**) of 10 μM forskolin.[44]

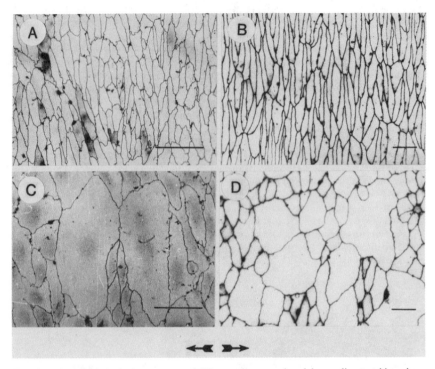

FIGURE 10. Morphological apperance of EC monolayer produced by cyclic stretching shows similarity to *in situ* organization of endothelium in human aorta. (**A**) Homogenous oriented monolayer formed after 48-h periodic stretching of preconfluent EC; (**B**) endothelial lining of infant aorta; (**C**) heterogeneous oriented monolayer is formed in response to combined action of cyclic stretching and 10 μM forskolin on confluent EC; (**D**) endothelial lining of adult aorta, A,B,D, silver nitrate staining. C, combination of silver nitrate staining and phase contrast; a single nucleus is visible in the center of each giant cell. *Arrows* show the direction of strain applied to silicone membrane and vessel wall. Bars, 40 μM.

CONCLUSION

Atherosclerotic injury of human aorta is accompanied by changes in the metabolism of second messengers in intimal cells. A dramatic drop in the level of cAMP in lipid streak and the atherosclerotic plaque of intimal layer is explained by a decrease of the basal activity of adenylate cyclase and the complete loss of its ability to be stimulated by hormones. A similar decrease in the level of cAMP is observed in the culture of human intimal cells loaded with lipids.

In endothelial cells from human vessels a prolonged activation of protein kinase C rsesults in the desensitization of beta-adrenergic receptors and the decrease in the activity of adenylate cyclase. One of the mechanisms which changes cyclic nucleotides spectrum and decreases the sensitivity of adenylate cyclase to hormones in human atherosclerotic plaque may be desensitization of receptors due to activation of protein kinase C.

"Hormone-like" effects of LDL, particularly activation of phosphoinositide metabolism in human endothelium and the activation of receptor-gated calcium channels in human platelets show that high level of LDL in blood may be one of the factors which affect the second messenger systems in atherosclerosis.

Since lipid accumulation and cell proliferation are controled by cAMP level, the decrease in [cAMP] in human aortic intima in the plaque may be one of the factors causing accelerated accumulation of lipids and the proliferation of intimal cells.

Second messengers are also involved in the regulation of morphology of vascular human endothelium. The activation of cAMP-dependent protein kinase inhibits phosphorylation of myosin light chains, thus blocking the binding of myosin to actin resulting in the changes of cytoskeleton and, consequently, of endothelial cell morphology. Morphologic changes of cells can be modulated also by protein kinase C, which inhibits the activity of cAMP-dependent protein kinase in endothelium.

Periodic stretching of the substrate on which endothelium is grown results in the orientation of cells and the rearrangment of endothelial cytoskeleton. The activation of adenylate cyclase under conditions of mechanical injury brought about by periodic stretching results in the appearance of heterogeneous shape of endothelial cells in monolayer.

All these observations suggest that the changes of the second messenger systems under certain conditions may play a pivotal role in the local changes of vascular wall observed in atherosclerosis.

REFERENCES

1. RALL, T. W. 1982. Formation and degradation of cyclic nucleotides: an overview. *In* Cyclic Nucleotides. J. A. Nathanson & J. W. Kebabian, Eds. Vol. **1**: 3–16. Springer-Verlag. Berlin, Heidelberg, New York.
2. BERRIDGE, M. J. & R. F. IRVINE. 1984. Inositol trisphosphate, a novel second messenger in cellular signal transduction. Nature **312**: 315–321.
3. EXTON, J. H. 1983. Regulation of carbohydrate metabolism by cyclic nucleotides. *In* Cyclic Nucleotides. J. A. Nathanson & J. W. Kebabian, Eds. Vol. **2**: 3–88. Springer-Verlag. Berlin, Heidelberg, New York.
4. REPIN, V. S., V. V. DOLGOV, O. E. ZAIKINA, I. D. NOVIKOV, A. S. ANTONOV, M. A. NIKOLAEVA & V. N. SMIRNOV. 1984. Heterogeneity of endothelium in human aorta. A quantitative analysis of scanning electron microscopy. Atherosclerosis **50**: 35–52.
5. ANTONOV, A. S., Y. A. ROMANOV, V. O. BROVTSEV & E. M. TARARAK. 1989. Heterogeneity of human aortic endothelium in situ: two variants of organization in atherosclerosis. International Atherosclerosis Congress, Vienna, 20–22 April.
6. CORNHILL, J. F. & M. R. ROACH. 1976. A quantitative study of the localization of atherosclerotic lesions in the rabbit aorta. Atherosclerosis **23**: 489–501.
7. CORNHILL, J. F., W. A. BARRET, E. E. HERDERICK, R. W. MAHLEY & D. L. FRY. 1985. Topographic study of sudanophylic lesions in cholesterol-fed minipigs by image analysis. Arteriosclerosis **5**: 415–426.
8. MOSSE, M. J., G. R. CAMPBELL, Z. I. WANG & J. H. CAMPBELL. 1985. Smooth muscle phenotypic expression in human carotid arteries. I. Comparison of cells from diffuse intimal thickenings adjacent to atheromatous plaques with those of the media. Lab. Invest. **53**: 556–562.
9. THOMAS, W. A. & D. N. KIM. 1983. Biology of disease. Atherosclerosis as a hyperplasic and/or neoplasic process. Lab. Invest. **348**: 245–255.
10. EXTON, J. H. 1980. Cyclic nucleotides in diabetes mellitus and obesity. Adv. Cyclic Nucl. Res. **12**: 97–123.
11. DERUBERTIS, F. R. & P. A. CRAVEN. 1980. Cyclic nucleotides in carcinogenesis: activation of guanylate cyclase and cyclic GMP by chemical carcinogens. Adv. Cyclic Nucl. Res. **8**: 85–97.
12. GILL, D. M. 1977. Mechanism of action of cholera toxin. Adv. Cyclic Nucl. Res. **8**: 85–97.
13. NUMANO, F. 1980. Cyclic nucleotides and atherosclerosis. *In* Atherosclerosis V. Proceedings

of the 5th International Symposium on Atherosclerosis. A.M. Gotto, L. C. Smith & B. Allen, Eds. 537–540. Springer-Verlag. New York.

14. TERTOV, V. V., A. N. OREKHOV, G. Y. GRIGORIAN, G. S. KURENNAYA, S. A. KUDRYASHOV, V. A. TKACHUK & V. N. SMIRNOV. 1987. Disorders in the system of cyclic nucleotides in atherosclerosis: cyclic AMP and cyclic GMP content and activity of related enzymes in human aorta. Tissue Cell **19:** 21–28.

15. FAIN, J. N. 1982. Regulation of lipid metabolism by cyclic nucleotides. *In* Cyclic Nucleotides. J. A. Nathanson & J. W. Kebabian, Eds. Vol. **1:** 89–150. Springer-Verlag. Berlin, Heidelberg, New York.

16. OREKHOV, A. N., V. V. TERTOV, S. A. KUDRYASHOV, KH. A. KHASHIMOV & V. N. SMIRNOV. 1986. Primary culture of human aortic intima cells as a model for testing antiatherosclerotic drugs. Effects of cyclic AMP, prostaglandins, calcium antagonists, antioxidants, and lipid-lowering agents. Atherosclerosis **60:** 101–110.

17. BLOCK, L. H., M. KNORR, E. VOGT, R. LOCHER, W. VETTRE, P. GROSCURTH, B. Y. QIAO, D. POMETTA, R. JAMES, M. REGENASS & A. PLETSCHER. 1988. Low density lipoprotein causes general cellular activation with increased phosphatidylinositol turnover and lipoprotein catabolism. Proc. Natl. Acad.Sci. USA **85:** 885–889.

18. KNORR, M., R. LOCHER, E. VOGT, W. VETTER, L. H. BLOCK, F. FERRACIN, H. LEFKOWITS & A. PLETSCHER. 1988. Rapid activation of human platelets by low concentrations of low-density lipoprotein via phosphatidylinositol cycle. Eur. J. Biochem. **172:** 753–759.

19. RESINK, T. J., G. Y. GRIGORIAN, A. K. MOLDABAEVA, S. M. DANILOV & F. R. BUHLER. 1987. Histamine-induced polyphosphoinositide metabolism in cultured human enodthelial cells: association with thromboxane and prostacyclin release. Biochem. Biophys. Res. Commun. **144:** 438–446.

20. VOYNO-YASENETSKAYA, T. A., V. A. TKACHUK, E. G. CHEKNYOVA, M. P. PANCHENKO, G. Y. GRIGORIAN, R. J. VAVREK, J. M. STEWART & U. S. RYAN. 1989. Guanine-nucleotide-dependent, pertussis toxin-insensitive regulation of phosphoinositide turnover by bradykinin in bovine pulmonary artery endothelial cells. FASEB J. **3:** 44–51.

21. GRIGORIAN, G. YU. & U. S. RYAN. 1987. Platelet-activating factor effects on bovine pulmonary artery endothelial cells. Circ. Res. **61:** 389–395.

22. GILMAN, A. G. 1987. G proteins: transducers of receptor-generated signals. Annu. Rev. Biochem. **56:** 615–649.

23. PHEE, S. G., P. G. SUH, S. H. RYU & S. Y. LEE. 1989. Studies of inositol phospholipid specific phospholipase C. Science **244:** 546–550.

24. POMERANTZ, K. B., A. R. TALL, S. J. FEINMARK & P. J. CANNON. 1984. Stimulation of vascular smooth muscle cell prostacyclin and prostaglandin E_2 synthesis by plasma high and low density lipoproteins. Circ. Res. **54:** 554–565.

25. BERRIDGE, M. J. 1982. Regulation of cell secretion: the integrated action of cyclic AMP and calcium. *In* Handbook of Experimental Pharmacology. J. A. Nathanson & J. W. Kebabian, Eds. Vol. **58:** 227–270. Springer-Verlag. Berlin, Heidelberg, New York.

26. AVDONIN, P. V., I. B. CHEGLAKOV, E. M. BOOGRY, I. V. SVITINA-ULITINA, A. V. MAZAEV & V. N. TKACHUK. 1987. Evidence for the receptor-operated calcium channels in human platelet plasma membrane. Thromb. Res. **46:** 29–37.

27. CROUCH, M. F. & E. G. LAPETINA. 1988. A role for G_i in control of thrombin receptor-phospholipase C coupling in human platelets. J. Biol. Chem. **263:** 3363–3371.

28. HALLAM, T. J. & T. J. RINK. 1985. Agonists stimulate divalent cation channels in the plasma membrane of human platelets. FEBS Lett. **186:** 175–179.

29. TKACHUK, V. A., V. N. BOCHKOV, T. A. VOYNO-YASENETSKAYA & P. V. AVDONIN. Mechanism of low density lipoprotein-induced rise of free cytoplasmic Ca^{2+} in human blood platelets. In preparation.

30. BROWN, M. S. & J. L. GOLDSTEIN. 1986. A receptor-mediated pathway for cholesterol homeostasis. Science **232:** 34–47.

31. BROWN, M. S., P. T. KOVANEN & J. L. GOLDSTEIN. 1981. Regulation of plasma cholesterol by lipoprotein receptors. Science **212:** 628–635.

32. MAJNO, G., S. M. SHEA & M. LEVENTAL. 1969. Endothelial contraction induced by histamine-type mediators. J. Cell Biol. **42:** 647–672.

33. WELLES, S. L., D. SHEPRO & H. B. HECHTMAN. 1985. Vasoactive amines modulate actin

cables (stress fibers) and surface area in cultured bovine endothelium. J. Cell. Physiol. **123:** 337–342.

34. BOTTARO, D., D. SHEPRO, S. PETERSON & H. B. HECHTMAN. 1986. Serotonin, norepinephrine, and histamine mediation of endothelial cell barrier function *in vitro*. J. Cell. Physiol. **128:** 189–194.

35. MADRI, J. A., B. M. PRATT & A. M. TUCKER. 1988. Phenotypic modulation of endothelial cells by transforming growth factor-beta depends upon the composition and organization of the extracellular matrix. J. Cell Biol. **106:** 1375–1384.

36. ANTONOV, A. S., M. E. LUKASHEV, Y. A. ROMANOV, V. A. TKACHUK, V. S. REPIN & V. N. SMIRNOV. 1986. Morphological alterations in endothelial cells from human aorta and umbilical vein induced by forskolin and phorbol 12-myristate 13-acetate: a synergistic action of adenylate cyclase and protein kinase C activators. Proc. Natl. Acad. Sci. USA **83:** 9704–9708.

37. LAMB, N. J., A. FERNANDEZ, M. A. CONTI, R. ADELSTEIN, D. B. GLASS, W. J. WELCH & J. R. FERAMISCO. 1988. Regulation of actin microfilament integrity in living nonmuscle cells by the cAMP-dependent protein kinase and the myosin light chain kinase. J. Cell Biol. **106:** 1955–1971.

38. WAGNER, P. P. & J. N. GEORGE. 1986. Phosphorylation of thymus myosin increases its apparent affinity for actin but not its maximum adenosine triphosphatase rate. Biochemistry **25:** 913–918.

39. CONTI, M. & R. S. ADELSTEIN. 1981. The relationship between calmodulin binding and phosphorylation of smooth muscle myosin kinase by the catalytic subunit of $3',5'$cAMP-dependent protein kinase. J. Biol. Chem. **256:** 3178–3181.

40. DEWEY, S. F., S. R. BUSSOLARI, M. A. GIMBRONE, JR. & P. F. DAVIES. 1981. The dynamic response of vascular endothelial cells to fluid shear stress. J. Biomech. Eng. **103:** 177–185.

41. WONG, A. J., T. D. POLLARD & I. M. HERMAN. 1983. Actin filament stress fibers in vascular endothelial cell *in vivo*. Science **219:** 867–869.

42. IVES, S. L., S. G. ECKIN & L. V. MCINTIRE. 1986. Mechanical effects on endothelial cell morphology: *In vivo* assessment. In Vitro Cell. Dev. Biol. **22:** 500–507.

43. SHIRINSKY, V. P., A. S. ANTONOV, K. G. BIRUKOV, A. V. SOBOLEVSKY, Y. A. ROMANOV, N. V. KABAEVA, G. N. ANTONOVA & V. N. SMIRNOV. 1989. Mechano-chemical control of human endothelium orientation and size. J. Cell Biol. **109:** 331–339.

44. ANTONOV, A. S., M. A. NIKOLAEVA, T. S. KLUEVA, Y. A. ROMANOV, V. R. BABAEV, V. B. BYSTREVSKEAYA, N. A. PEROV, V. S. REPIN & V. N. SMIRNOV. 1986. Primary culture of endothelial cells from atherosclerotic human aorta. I. Identification, morphological and ultrastructural characteristics of two endothelial subpopulations. Atherosclerosis **59:** 1–19.

45. HERMAN, I. M., A. M. BRANT, V. S. WARTY, J. BONACCORO, E. C. KLEIN, R. L. KORMOS & H. S. BOROVETZ. 1987. Hemodynamics and the vascular endothelial cytoskeleton. J. Cell Biol. **105:** 291–302.

46. VOYNO-YASENETSKAYA, T. A., I. K. KONDAKOV, V. S. REPIN, V. A. TKACHUK & V. N. SMIRNOV. 1986. Synergistic interaction of adenylate cyclase and phosphoinositide turnover stimulators. Dokl. Acad. Sci. USSR (Russian) **5:** 56–61.

The Control of Vascular Endothelial Cell Injury

SEI-ITSU MUROTA, IKUO MORITA, AND NAOTO SUDA

Section of Physiological Chemistry
Faculty of Dentistry
Tokyo Medical and Dental University
Tokyo 113, Japan

INTRODUCTION

The initiation of atherogeneis is said to be in endothelial cell injury.[1] Therefore, it is important to know what causes this endothelial cell injury, what the mechanism of this endothelial cell injury is, and how to protect endothelial cells from the injury. We established some *in vitro* assay systems for endothelial cell injury by using cultured endothelial cells,[2,3] and examined the effects of various arachidonic acid metabolites and related compounds on endothelial cell injury. Among the substances tested 15-HPETE(15-L-hydroperoxy-5,8,10,14-eicosatetraenoic acid) was found to have a potent capacity to cause severe endothelial cell injury.[2-4] Later, 12-HPETE was found to have a similar cytotoxic activity to 15-HPETE (the data will be shown elsewhere).

Arachidonic acid is known to be oxidized by various kinds of lipoxygenase to their corresponding lipoxygenase products (FIGURE 1). 5-HPETE and 15-HPETE are known to be produced by activated leukocytes, while 12-HPETE is produced by activated platelets. These HPETEs are kinds of lipid peroxides. Releasing hydroxylradicals, a kind of active oxygens, they are metabolized to the corresponding HETEs (hydroxy-5,8,10,14-eicosatetraenoic acid) by hydroperoxidase. Though the HPETEs are very cytotoxic, none of these HETEs is cytotoxic any longer.[2-4] Therefore, it is suggested that the structure of lipid peroxide itself in HPETEs or the released active oxygens must be responsible for the cytotoxicity.

During the course of search for cytoprotective drugs, we found MCI-186 having a remarkable cytoprotective effect on the endothelial cell injury due to 15-HPETE. The protective effect of MCI-186 on the endothelial cell injury was dose dependent. 3×10^{-5} M 15-HPETE caused cell death by 60%. But this cytolytic activity of 15-HPETE was almost completely abolished by the treatment of endothelial cells with 10^{-5}–10^{-4} M of MCI-186.[2,4]

Regarding the mechanism by which MCI-186 shows such a potent cytoprotective activity, we suggested in previous papers[2,4] the possibility that the activities of MCI-186 capable of enhancing prostacyclin production in endothelial cells and inhibiting 5-lipoxygenase in RBL-1 cells might bring about such remarkable cytoprotection as mentioned above. However, we found afterward that prostacyclin had nothing to do with the protection of endothelial cell injury due to 15-HPETE.[5]

In this paper, we shall present the possibility that a potent radical scavenging capacity of MCI-186 may be deeply involved in its remarkable cytoprotective activity.

EXPERIMENTAL METHODS

Chemicals

MCI-186 (FIGURE 2) was synthesized at the Research Center of Mitsubishi Chemical Industries, Ltd., Japan. [^{51}Cr] Sodium chromate (250–500 mCi/mg) was purchased from Amersham International (Amersham, UK).

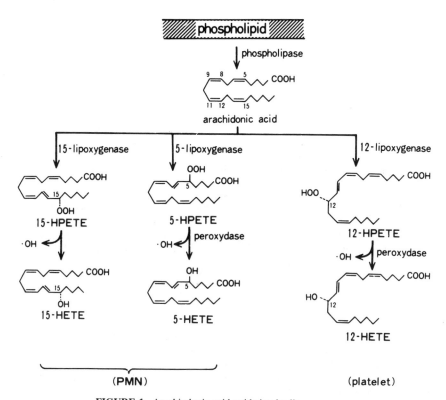

FIGURE 1. Arachindonic acid oxidation by lipoxygenases.

Endothelial Cell Culture

Endothelial cells were isolated from bovine carotid arteries and cultured with an Eagle's MEM (minimum essential medium) containing 10% fetal calf serum.[6]

Preparation of 15-HPETE

15-HPETE was enzymatically prepared as previously described.[3–5] In brief, arachidonic acid (99% pure) was incubated with soybean lipoxygenase in 0.1 M Tris-HCl buffer

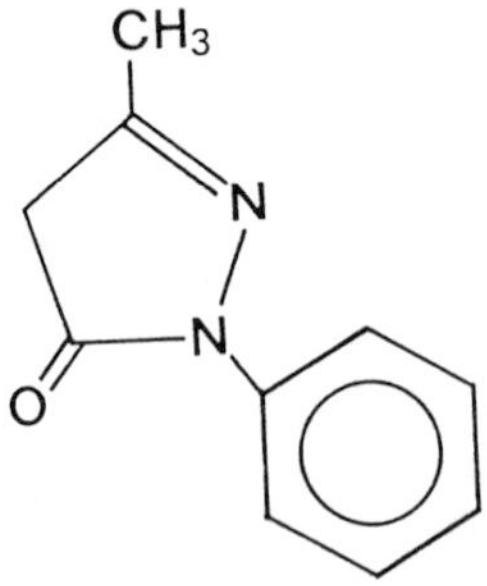

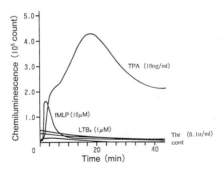

FIGURE 2. Chemical structure of MCI-186.

MCI-186
(3-Methyl-1-phenyl-2-pyrazolin-5-one)

(pH 9.5). The reaction mixture was then acidified and extracted with ethylether. The ethereal extract was evaporated and then the residue was subjected to thin-layer chromatography on Silica gel G ($60F_{254}$, E. Merk, Darmstadt, FRG) with the solvent mixture of hexane/ethylether/acetic acid (70:30:1). Silica gel corresponding to a standard of 15-HPETE under UV light was scraped off and then the prepared 15-HPETE in the silica gel was extracted with a mixture of ethylether/petroleum ether (1:3). After evaporation of the solvent, the purified 15-HPETE was dissolved in absolute ethanol and stored at $-20°C$ until use.

The purity of 15-HPETE was estimated as more than 95%. The concentration of 15-HPETE was also determined spectrophotometrically by using a molar extinction coefficient at 237 nm of 30000 M^1cm^1 (7).

Estimation of Endothelial Cell Injury

Endothelial cell injury was estimated by the release of [51]chromium as previously described.[3,5] In brief, confluent monolayers in 24 multiwell dishes (Falcone Labware) were prelabeled with 2 μCi of [^{51}Cr] sodium chromate for 18 hours in the growth medium. After labeling, the cells were washed twice with MEM and then exposed to 15-HPETE or other test compounds for 6 hours in MEM.

After the 6-hour cultivation, aliquots of the culture medium were removed and the

FIGURE 3. Chemiluminescence released from human leukocytes stimulated by various chemical mediators.

radioactivities due to ^{51}Cr released out of the injured cells were measured by gamma-scintilation spectrophotometer.

Measurement of Chemiluminescence of Activated Polymorphonuclear Leukocytes by Biolumat

Heparinized blood was withdrawn from healthy volunteers. Polymorphonuclear leukocytes were obtained using Ficoll/Hypaque gradient centrifugation and hypotonic lysis of contaminated erythrocytes. The leukocytes were washed three times in a Hank's balanced salt solution, and finally resuspended in the Hank's solution containing 10 mM HEPES (pH 7.4) at a concentration of 1×10^7 cells/ml. The final cell suspension was more than 94% in purity of neutrophils, and platelet contamination was below 1%. In experiments of chemiluminescence, 0.4 ml of the leukocyte solution and 10 µl luminol (1 mg/ml) were incubated in reaction tubes of multichannel Biolumat (LB 9505, Bertold). After 5 min incubation, one of the various kinds of chemical mediators was added into the reaction tube and the chimiluminescence was measured for 30 min. The intensity of total chemiluminescence was expressed as the summation area.

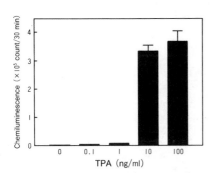

FIGURE 4. Dose response of chemiluminescence in human leukocytes stimulated by TPA.

RESULTS AND DISCUSSION

Activated Leukocytes Produce Chemiluminescence

To discover the mechanism of the cytoprotective effect of MCI-186, we did the following experiments. Human peripheral leukocytes were isolated, and fractionated by using Percoll. The purified leukotcytes were then stimulated with various kinds of chemical mediators, which caused activation and aggregation of the leukocytes, and resulted in having the leukocytes release active oxygens. The amount of the released active oxygens could be measured by luminol-dependent chemiluminescence.

As shown in FIGURE 3, TPA (12-O-tetradecanoylphorbol-13-acetate) could release the active oxygens the most of the mediators tested, and next came fMLP (formyl-methionyl-leucyl-phenylalanine) and LTB$_4$ (leukotriene B$_4$). Thrombin showed little effect at the dose used. The chemiluminescence due to TPA was dose dependent (FIGURE 4).

Activated Leukocytes Elicit Endothelial Cell Injury

Next, we put leukocytes directly on the monolayer of cultured endothelial cells, and stimulated the leukocytes with TPA. The leukocytes activated with TPA elicited endothelial cell injury, which depended on the dose of TPA (FIGURE 5). There was good correlation between the active oxygen-releasing activity and the cytolitic activity.

To confirm the fact that the cytotoxicity due to the TPA-stimulated leukocytes was actually caused by the active oxygens released, we examined it by using some special device which had been developed for culturing 2 different types of cells without having them contact each other. When leukocytes were put directly on a monolayar of endothelial cells and stimulated with TPA, a severe endothelial cell injury was observed, as shown in FIGURE 5. However, when leukocytes were placed on a filter which was set apart from a monolayer of endothelial cells, and stimulated the leukocytes with TPA, the cytotoxicity was completely abolished. Thus, the cyotoxicity must be caused by some very short-lived labile substance, presumably active oxygens.

MCI-186 is a Kind of Radical Scavenger

To find out the mechanism of the cytoprotective effect of MCI-186, we examined whether MCI-186 could quench the chemiluminescence due to active oxygens. Addition of MCI-186 to the assay system caused a remarkable quenching of the chemiluminescence due to TPA-stimulated leukocytes. The radical scavenging effect of MCI-186 appeared immediately after the addition of MCI-186 to the assay system (FIGURE 6). These results suggest that the potent cytoprotective effect of MCI-186 is likely due to its specific radical scavenging activity.

SUMMARY

The mechanism by which MCI-186 showed a potent cytoprotective effect on the *in vitro* endothelial cell injury due to 15-HPETE was studied. Stimulation of human leukocytes with various chemical mediators such as TPA, f-Met-Leu-Phe, LTB_4, etc. elicited the production of active oxygens, which could be detected by luminol-dependent chemiluminescence. Among the chemical mediators tested, TPA elicited the chemiluminescence the most, and f-Met-Leu-Phe and LTB_4 came next.

When the leukocytes were directly placed on a monolayer of cultured endothelial cells, followed by stimulating the leukocytes with TPA, severe endothelial cell injury was observed. The effect of TPA was dose dependent. There was good correlation between the active oxygen releasing activity and the cytotoxic activity. When the leukocytes were placed on a filter which was set apart from the monolayer of endothelial cell in a culture

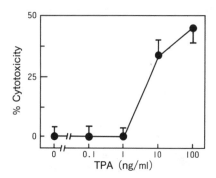

FIGURE 5. Endothelial cell injury by TPA-stimulated human leukocytes.

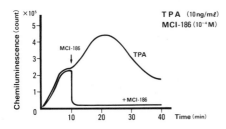

FIGURE 6. Effect of MCI-186 on the chemiluminescence due to TPA-stimulated human leukocytes.

dish, and stimulated the leukocytes with TPA, no cytotoxicity was observed. These data strongly suggest that the substance responsible for the cytotoxicity must be a very labile and short-lived substance, presumably active oxygens.

On the other hand, MCI-186 was found to have a complete quenching acitvity to the chimiluminescence due to active oxygens in the TPA-leukocyte system. Taken together, these factors indicate that the potent cytoprotective effect of MCI-186 may be due to its specific radical scavenging activity.

REFERENCES

1. Ross, R. & J. A. Glomeset. 1976. The pathogenisis of atherosclerosis. N. Engl. J. Med. **8:** 420–425.

2. Murota, S., I. Morita & K. Kato. 1988. An *in vitro* assay system for measuring both vascular permeability and endothelial cell damage. *In* Role of Blood Flow in Atherosclerosis. Y. Yoshida, Y. Yamaguchi, C. G. Caro, S. Glagov & R. M. Nerem, Eds. 223–229, Springer-Verlag. Tokyo.

3. Abe, M., I. Morita & S. Murota. 1988. A new *in vitro* method using fura-2 for the quantification of endothelial cell injury. Prostaglandins Leukotrienes Essent. Fatty Acids **34:** 69–74.

4. Watanabe, T., I. Morita, H. Nishi & S. Murota. 1988. Preventive effect of MCI-186 on 15-HPETE induced vascular endothelial cell injury *in vitro*. Prostaglandins Leukotrienes Essent. Fatty Acids 33: 81–87.

5. Ochi, H., I. Morita & S. Murota. Endothelial cell injury caused by 15-HPETE, a lipoxygenase product of arachidonic acid. Acta Med. Biol. **37.** In press.

6. Neichi, T., W. C. Chang, Y. Mitsui & S. Murota. 1982. Comparison of prostaglandin biosythetic acitvity between pocine aortic endothelial cell and smooth moscle cells in culture. Artery **11:** 47–63.

7. Bild, G. S., C. S. Ramadoss, S. Lim & B. Axelrod. 1977. Double dioxygenation of arachidoinc acid by soybean, Lipoxygenase-1. Biochem. Biophys. Res. Commun. **74:** 949–954.

The Role of Atherogenic Low Density Lipoproteins (LDL) in the Pathogenesis of Atherosclerosis[a]

TORU KITA,[b,d] MASAYUKI YOKODE,[c] KENJI ISHII,[b]
HIDENORI ARAI,[c] AND YUTAKA NAGANO[c]

[b]*Department of Geriatric Medicine*
and
[c]*Department of Internal Medicine*
Faculty of Medicine
Kyoto University
Kyoto 606, Japan

INTRODUCTION

Several epidemiologial studies reveal that more than half the people in industrialized societies have a high level of plasma cholesterol that puts them at high risk for developing atherosclerosis. The more cholesterol in the blood, the more rapidly atherosclerosis develops.[1,2] However, we do not know yet the ideal level of cholesterol in human blood. The plasma levels of cholesterol now believed ''normal'' may well be too high in view of such a prevailing high risk of atherosclerotic lesions. What determines the blood level of cholesterol? The number of LDL receptors on the surface of cells varies with the demand for cholesterol of the cells.[3] Because of the size and the high concentration of LDL receptors, it is proved that liver is the key organ in cholesterol homeostasis.[4]

Especially in patients with familial hypercholesterolemia (FH), there are elevations of plasma cholesterol level and premature coronary atherosclerosis because of decreased activity or deficiency of the LDL receptor.[3,5] In autopsy specimens of FH patients, the characteristic feature of the early stage of atherosclerosis is the migration and accumulation of macrophages in the subendothelial spaces and the conversion of macrophages into foam cells.

Studies of lipoprotein metabolism in macrophages were initiated to explain the paradoxical finding that even FH patients who have no LDL receptor can accumulate lipoprotein-bound cholesteryl esters in macrophages.

A new animal model of human FH, known as the Watanabe heritable hyperlipidemic (WHHL) rabbit, has recently become available.[3,6-8] Homozygous WHHL-rabbits resemble their human counterparts in having an accumulation of very low density lipoprotein (VLDL) and LDL on a low-fat diet, severe fulminant atherosclerosis, and a genetic defect

[a]This work was supported in part by a grant from the Japanese Foundation on Metabolism and Diseases, research grants from the Ministry of Education, Science, and Culture of Japan (No. 63870014 and 01619503), a research grant from the Ministry of Health and Welfare of Japan, a research grant from Osaka Gas Group Welfare Foundation, and a research grant from the Tokyo Biochemical Research Foundation.

[d]Address for correspondence: Toru Kita, Department of Geriatric Medicine, Faculty of Medicine, Kyoto University, 54 Kawara-cho Shogoin, Sakyo-ku, Kyoto 606, Japan.

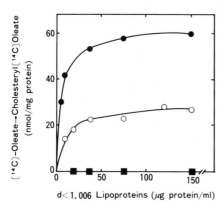

FIGURE 1. Cholesteryl ester formation in mouse peritoneal macrophages incubated with varying concentrations of d <1.006 g/ml lipoproteins from control, cholesterol-fed, and WHHL rabbits. Each monolayer received 0.6 ml of DME containing 0.2 mM [^{14}C]oleate–2.4 mg/ml albumin and the indicated concentration of d <1.006 g/ml lipoproteins obtained from one of the following animals: (■) control rabbits fed commercial rabbit chow; (●) control rabbits fed commercial chow which contained 2% cholesterol–10% corn oil; (○) WHHL-rabbits fed commercial rabbit chow. After incubation for 6 h at 37°C, the cellular contents of cholesteryl [^{14}C]oleate were determined. The content of cholesteryl [^{14}C]oleate in cells incubated without d <1.006 g/ml lipoproteins was 0.17 nmol/mg protein. (Modified from Kita *et al.*[20])

in the LDL receptor in all tissues. Due to the availability of this rabbit, we have been able to study lipoprotein metabolism and to ascertain the accumulation of VLDL and LDL.

In this report we ask the following questions:

1. What kind of lipoproteins could transform macrophages into foam cells? If there is a candidate, what kind of mechanism is involved?
2. Is it possible to prevent the progression of atherosclerosis in WHHL rabbits *in vivo?*

Lipoproteins That Could Transform Macrophages into Foam Cells

VLDL, Intermediate Density Lipoprotein (IDL), and β-VLDL

Previous studies have demonstrated that WHHL-rabbits have a pattern of endogenous atherosclerosis which is similar to that in human beings, with or without familial hypercholesterolemia, except WHHL rabbits have a high plasma level of VLDL. The concentration of apoB in each plasma fraction of density <1.063 g/ml was increased in WHHL-rabbit as compared with normal rabbit (VLDL 25 vs 10 mg/dl; LDL, 168 vs 16 mg/dl). These facts imply the LDL receptor normally participates in clearance of VLDL and LDL from plasma. How does the elevated level of VLDL and LDL promote atherosclerosis in these rabbits, especially fatty streak formation? When we examined the atheromatous lesions by electronmicroscopy, we found numerous foam cells that originated from both macrophages and smooth muscle cells.[9,10] It is generally accepted that foam cells in atherosclerotic lesions, in the early stage, are derived from monocyte-macrophages. The origin of cholesteryl ester in cholesterol-filled macrophages in these lesions is thought to be derived from plasma lipoproteins. To ascertain atherogenic lipoproteins in WHHL-rabbits, we checked the ability of VLDL, IDL, and LDL to transform macrophages into foam cells. Cells incubated with WHHL-VLDL had numerous oil red 0-positive droplets within cytoplasma. In case of control-VLDL, there is no oil red 0-positive droplets. To clarify the uptake mechanism of WHHL-VLDL, we used two methods—cholesterol reesterification, and degradation of ^{125}I-labeled lipoprotein. Experimental data shows the saturation kinetics of cholesteryl [^{14}C]oleate reesterification (FIG. 1). Maximum uptake of WHHL-VLDL is about 22.4 nmol/mg protein, which is about half of the uptake of β-VLDL (TABLE 1). Degradation of ^{125}I-VLDL from WHHL-rabbit also shows the saturation kinetics as a function of VLDL concentration. Cold express β-VLDL complete for the binding of ^{125}I-VLDL from WHHL-rabbits (data not shown). Fucoidin, poly I or acetyl-LDL could not inhibit the uptake of WHHL-VLDL. It is well known that macrophage has at least two kinds of receptors—β-VLDL receptor and acetyl-LDL receptor—, certain polypurines—polyinosinic acid and polyguanylic acid—, and fucoidins complete effectively for binding ^{125}I-acetyl-LDL.[11] Therefore we assumed our data indicated that the uptake of WHHL-VLDL in macrophages is via β-VLDL receptor.[8] In addition, we analyzed WHHL-VLDL particles and found that the properties of WHHL-VLDL were similar to those of β-VLDL, *i.e.*, richness in apoE and cholesteryl ester.[12] Moreover, as shown in TABLE 1., not only WHHL-VLDL, but also IDL from control and WHHL rabbits stimulates cholesteryl ester synthesis. Because WHHL rabbits lack the LDL re-

TABLE 1. Stimulation of Cholesteryl Ester Formation in Mouse Macrophages by Lipoproteins[a]

Sourse of Lipoproteins	Lipoprotein Fraction Added to Medium	Concentration in Medium		[14C]oleate→Cholesteryl [14C]oleate (nmol/mg Protein)
		Protein (μg/ml)	Cholesterol (μg/ml)	
	none	0	0	0.18
Control rabbit	βVLDL (d <1.006)	3	50	26.2
(2% cholesterol diet)		18	300	45.6
Control rabbit	VLDL (d <1.006)	38	50	0.13
(chow diet)		228	300	0.18
	IDL (1.006–1.019)	56	50	3.8
		337	300	9.2
	LDL (1.019–1.063)	39	50	0.51
		234	300	0.95
WHHL rabbit	VLDL (d <1.006)	9	50	10.9
(chow diet)		54	300	22.4
	IDL (1.006–1.019)	19	50	5.5
		114	300	13.8
	LDL (1.019–1.063)	45	50	0.54
		270	300	0.93

[a]Modified from Kita *et al.*[20]

ceptor, VLDL is converted to IDL at a relatively normal rate, but most IDL particles fail to enter the liver for catabolism. Therefore IDL particles remain in the circulation where it is converted to LDL.[3,4] On the other hand, in the control rabbits, the vast majority of IDL particles disappear rapidly from the blood stream because it binds to the LDL receptors on the surface of hepatic cells, due to the presence of apoprotein E, which has a higher affinity for LDL receptors than apoprotein B-100.[3,11] Even though IDL particles stimulate cholesteryl ester formation on macrophages, IDL particles are not present in the plasma for a long time in the control rabbits. Therefore, IDL particles are not dangerous in atherosclerosis in control rabbits.

Modified LDL

On the other hand, native LDL, from either the control or WHHL rabbit could not be recognized by macrophages (TABLE 1). Recently, several groups have demonstrated *in vitro* that macrophages can ingest large amounts of certain chemically modified lipopro-

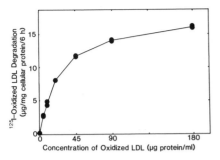

FIGURE 2. Degradation of ^{125}I-oxidized LDL by mouse peritoneal macrophages. Each monolayer received 1 ml of DME and the indicated concentration of ^{125}I-oxidized LDL. After incubation for 5 h at 37°C, the amount of ^{125}I-labeled acid-soluble material in the medium (●) was determined.

teins such as acetyl-LDL and malondialdehyde-treated LDL through the process of receptor-mediated endocytosis, becoming foam cells. However, *in vivo,* this process has not been verified. Recently, Steinbrecher,[13] Morel,[14] and ourselves[9,15] suggested that when LDL is oxidatively modified, it is taken up by macrophages, which facilitates the accumulation of lipids in macrophages *in vitro.*[15,16] Degradation study of oxidized LDL indicated that oxidized LDL is taken up by macrophages via specific receptors (FIG. 2). We performed the cross competition studies to compare the receptor-mediated incorporations of acetyl LDL and oxidized LDL. FIGURE 3 shows that cold excess oxidized LDL was effective in inhibiting the uptake and degradation of ^{125}I-oxidized LDL. In contrast, cold excess acetyl-LDL at concentrations as high as 200 μg protein/ml could only partially complete with ^{125}I-oxidized LDL for binding. Therefore, the competition study suggested that oxidized LDL was recognized partially by acetyl-LDL receptor. When we incubated ^{125}I-acetyl LDL with cold excess oxidized LDL, cold excess oxidized LDL inhibits the binding of ^{125}I-acetyl-LDL only partially (data not shown). These results suggest that macrophages have one receptor for common to both acetyl-LDL and oxidized LDL and other two receptors specific for each modified LDL.[16]

Preventing the Progression of Atherosclerosis

There is growing evidence of the exsistence of oxidized LDL *in vivo.* First, recent *in vitro* studies suggest that oxidized LDL plays an important role in atherosclerosis by

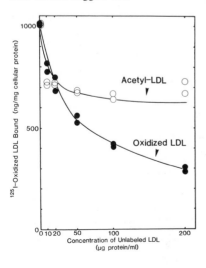

FIGURE 3. Ability of unlabeled acetyl LDL and oxidized LDL to inhibit the binding of ^{125}I-oxidized LDL by mouse peritoneal macrophages. Each monolayer received 1 ml of DME containing 10 μg protein/ml of ^{125}I-oxidized LDL and the indicated concentration of either unlabeled acetyl LDL (○) or unlabeled oxidized LDL (●). After incubation for 5 h at 37°C, the amount of ^{125}I-labeled acid-soluble material in the medium was determined.

facilitating the accumulation of lipids in macrophages. Second, probucol, an agent originally developed as an antioxidant, was shown to prevent oxidation of native LDL by copper ion *in vitro* by parthasarathy.[17] Third, Drs. Yamamoto and Matsuzawa clearly showed that probucol causes a regression of cutaneous and thendon xanthoma in homozygous FH patients.[18] In addition, the foam cell has been recognized as a characteristic feature of both xanthomas and atheromas. Therefore, given the exisiting data obtained in clinical and *in vitro* studies, we questioned whether probucol *in vivo* could prevent the progression of atherosclerosis in WHHL rabbits. At age 2 months, 4 WHHL rabbits were treated with probucol, 1 g/day for 6 months. At the end of the trial period, the animals were killed to measure the extent of aortic atheromatous plaques. The plasma concentration of probucol in WHHL rabbits was 42.9 μg/ml plasma, which is comparable with that in human probucol-treated patients.[9,17]

The mean value of plasma cholesterol in the probucol-treated group was slightly lower than that of the control group, but the difference was insignificant. The percentage of the surface area of total thoratic aorta with visible plaques was 54.2 ± 18.5% in the untreated group and only 7.0 ± 6.3% in the probucol-treated group (TABLE 2). Furthermore, the

TABLE 2. Percentages of Intimal Surface Area of Thoracic Aorta Involved with Atheromatous Plaque in WHHL Rabbits[a]

	Aortic Arch	Descending Aorta	Total Thoracic Aorta
Controls	67.8 ± 19.1	41.1 ± 20.2	54.2 ± 18.8
Probucol-fed	14.0 ± 12.4	0.2 ± 0.2	7.0 ± 6.3*

[a]Figures are percentages, mean ± SD. *$p < 0.01$. (Modified from Kita *et al.*[9])

percentage of plaque in the descending thoracic aorta in the probucol-treated rabbits was almost negligible (0.2 ± 0.2% compared with 4.1 ± 20.2% in untreated rabbits). Therefore, these data indicate that there is a strong possibility of oxidized LDL existing *in vivo*. Further study is needed for a thorough understanding of the mechanism of action of probucol in inhibiting the progression of atherosclerosis. Our preliminary data suggest that long-term treatment with probucol (start at 2 months and end at 18 months) could slow down the formation of atherosclerotic lesions. However, we could not completely prevent the formation of atherosclerotic lesions. Our data show that probucol treatment itself was not good enough for complete inhibition of lesion progression. As Nagano indicated, probucol did not affect the uptake of atherogenic lipoproteins in macrophages.[19] And also, as shown in FIGURE 1, VLDL particles in WHHL rabbits could transform macrophages into foam cells. These studies taken together, we think that VLDL particles play a role in forming the foam cell in WHHL rabbits.

REFERENCES

1. BROWN, M. S. & J. L. GOLDSTEIN. 1984. How LDL receptors influence cholesterol and atherosclerosis. Sci. Am. **251:** 58–66.
2. KANEL, W. B., W. P. CASTELLI, T. GORDON & P. M. McNAMARA. 1971. Serum cholesterol, lipoproteins, and the risk of coronary heart disease: the Framingham study. Ann. Intern. Med. **74:** 1–12.
3. GOLDSTEIN, J. L., T. KITA & M. S. BROWN. 1983. Defective lipoprotein receptors and atherosclerosis. N. Engl. J. Med. **309:** 288–296.
4. KITA, T., M. S. BROWN, D. W. BILHEIMER & J. L. GOLDSTEIN. 1982. Delayed clearance of very low density and intermediate density lipoproteins with enhanced conversion to low density lipoprotein in WHHL rabbits. Proc. Natl. Acad. Sci. USA **79:** 5693–5697.

5. GOLDSTEIN J. L. & M. S. BROWN. 1982. Insights into the pathogenesis of atherosclerosis derived from studies of familial hypercholesterolemia. *In* Metabolic Risk Factors in Ischemic Cardiovascular Disease. L. A. Carlson & B. Pernow, Eds. 17–34. Raven Press. New York, NY.

6. WATANABE, Y. 1980. Serial inbreeding of rabbits with hereditary hyperlipidemia (WHHL-rabbit): incidence and development of atherosclerosis and xanthoma. Atherosclerosis **36:** 261–268.

7. KITA, T., M. S. BROWN, Y. WATANABE & J. L. GOLDSTEIN. 1981. Deficiency of low density lipoprotein receptors in liver and adrenal gland of the WHHL rabbits, an animal model of familial hypercholesterolemia. Proc. Natl. Acad. Sci. USA 78:2268–2272.

8. KITA, T., M. YOKODE, Y. WATANABE, S. NARUMIYA & KAWAI C. 1986. Stimulation of cholesteryl ester synthesis in mouse peritoneal macrophages by cholesterol-rich very low density lipoproteins from the Watanabe heritable hyperlipidemic rabbit, an animal model of familial hypercholesterolemia. J. Clin. Invest. **77:** 1460–1465.

9. KITA, T., Y. NAGANO, M. YOKODE, K. ISHII, N. KUME, A. OOSHIMA, H. YOSHIDA & C. KAWAI. 1987. Probucol prevents the progression of atherosclerosis in WHHL rabbit, an animal model for familial hypercholesterolemia. Proc. Natl. Acad. Sci. USA **84:** 5928–5931.

10. BUJA, L. M., T. KITA, J. L. GOLDSTEIN, Y. WATANABE & M. S. BROWN. 1983. Cellular pathology of progressive atherosclerosis in the WHHL rabbit: and animal model of familial hypercholesterolemia. Arteriosclerosis **3:** 87–101.

11. BROWN, M. S. & J. L. GOLDSTEIN. 1983. Lipoprotein metabolism in the macrophage: implications for cholesterol deposition in atherosclerosis. Annu. Rev. Biochem. **52** 223–261.

12. ISHII, K., T. KITA, M. YOKODE, N. KUME, Y. NAGANO, H. OTANI, T. YAMAMURA, S. MURAYAMA, Y. MORIMOTO, Y. TERANISHI & C. KAWAI. 1989. Characterization of very low density lipoprotein from Watanabe heritable hyperlipidemic rabbits. J. Lipid Res. **30:** 1–7.

13. STEINBRECHER, U. P., S. PARTHASARATHY, D. S. LEAK, J. L. WITZTUM & D. STEINBERG. 1984. Modification of low density lipoprotein by endothelial cells involves lipid peroxidation and degradation of low density lipoprotein phospholipids. Proc. Natl. Acad. Sci. USA **81:** 3883–3887.

14. MOREL, D. W., P. E. DiCORLETO &G. M. CHISOLM. 1984. Endothelial and smooth muscle cells after low density lipoprotein in vitro by free radical oxidation. Arteriosclerosis **4:** 357–364.

15. YOKODE, M., T. KITA, Y. KIKAWA, T. OGOROCHI, S. NARUMIYA & C. KAWAI. 1988. Stimulated arachidonate metabolism during foam cell transformation of mouse peritoneal macrophages with oxidized low density lipoprotein. J. Clin. Invest. **81:** 720–729.

16. ARAI, H., T. KITA, M. YOKODE, S. NARUMIYA & C. KAWAI. 1989. Multiple receptors for modified low density lipoproteins in mouse peritoneal macrophages: different uptake mechanisms for acetylated and oxidized low density lipoproteins. Biochem. Biophys. Res. Commun. **159:** 1375–1382.

17. PARTHASARATHY, S., S. G. YOUNG, J. L. WITZTUM, R. C. PITTMAN & D. STEINBERG. 1986. Probucol inhibits oxidative modification of low density lipoprotein. J. Clin. Invest. **77:** 641–644.

18. YAMAMOTO, A., Y. MATSUZAWA, S. YOKOYAMA, T. FUNAHASHI, T. YAMAMURA & B. KISHINO. 1986. Effects of probucol on xanthomata regression in familial hypercholesterolemia. Am. J. Cardiol. **57:** 29H–35H.

19. NAGANO, Y., T. KITA, M. YOKODE, K. ISHII, N. KUME, H. OTANI, H. ARAI & C. KAWAI. 1989. Probucol does not affect lipoprotein metabolism in macrophages of Watanabe heritable hyperlipidemic rabbits. Arteriosclerosis **9:** 453–461.

20. KITA, T., M. YOKODE, Y. WATANABE, S. NARUMIYA & C. KAWAI. 1985. Foam cell and lipoprotein receptor. J. Jpn. Atheroscler. Soc. **13:** 21–31 (in Japanese).

Autocrine System for Smooth Muscle Cell Migration and Proliferation in the Arterial Wall

YASUSHI SAITO, NOBUHIRO MORISAKI,

AND NORIYUKI KOYAMA

Second Department of Internal Medicine
Chiba University
Chiba City 280, Japan

INTRODUCTION

One of the most remarkable pathological findings in atheromatous lesions is intimal thickening. The thickened intima is mainly composed of smooth muscle cells (SMC). These SMC are thought to accumulate first by active migration of SMC into the intima stimulated by migration factors such as platelet derived growth factor (PDGF) and 12-hydroxyeicosatetraenoic acid (HETE) and then by proliferation of SMC in the intima. Many growth factors for proliferation of SMC have been reported. This paper reports studies on a new factor for migration or proliferation of SMC secreted by SMC themselves.

MATERIALS AND METHODS

Preparation of Conditioned Medium Containing Smooth Muscle Derived Migration Factor (SDMF)

SMC were explanted from the thoracic aorta of Wistar rats or Japanese white rabbits essentially by the method of Fischer-Dzoga *et al.*[1] as described in detail elsewhere.[2,3] From the second passage, confluent SMC in T-75 flasks were subcultured at a 1:2 split ratio in T-75 flasks. Confluent SMC in T-75 flasks at the second to twelfth passages were washed twice with 10 ml Dulbecco's modified Eagle's medium (DME) and incubated with 10 ml of fresh DME. Every 2 days the medium was replaced by 10 ml of fresh DME, and the conditioned medium (CM) was collected three times.

Assay of Migration Activity

Migration activity was assayed in a modified Boyden's chamber using a polycarbonate filter (Nuclepore Co., USA) with pores of 5.0 μm diameter.[4] Cultured SMC were trypsinized and suspended at a concentration of 5.0×10^5 cells/ml in DME supplemented with 10% fetal bovine serum. Then 1 ml of SMC suspension was placed in the upper chamber and 0.9 ml of DME containing a migration factor was placed in the lower chamber. The chamber was incubated at 37°C and 5% CO_2 in air for 4 hours. The SMC on the upper side of the filter were then scraped off and the filter was removed. The SMC that had migrated to the lower side of the filter were fixed in ethanol, stained with hematoxylin and counted by microscopy ($\times$ 400) for the quantification of SMC migra-

194

tion. Migration activity was assayed in duplicate and expressed as the mean number of migrated cells in 10 high-power fields. Similar results were obtained in repeated experiments.

Preparation of Conditioned Medium Containing Smooth Muscle Cell Derived Growth Factor (SDGF)

SMC were cultured as described for collection of SDMF. For collection of CM, SMC at the second passage were subcultured at a 1:2 split ratio in T-75 flasks. CM without plasma was collected at the fourth to tenth passage as reported.[5] Pooled CM was used for experiments.

Culture of Endothelial Cells (EC)

EC from human umbilical cord vein were cultured as previously reported.[6] Co-culture of EC with SMC was carried out in a Millicell.[6]

DNA Synthesis

DNA synthesis was assayed as described previously.[3] Briefly, confluent SMC at the third passage in 24-well plates were synchronized to the G_0 stage by serum depletion for 24 h. Then the cells were treated with growth factor(s), and [^{3}H]thymidine incorporation into DNA during incubation for 24 h was measured. Cells were used at the third passage because at this passage they secreted little material with mitogenic activity into the medium.[4]

RESULTS AND DISCUSSION

The CM of cultured SMC from rat and rabbit aorta at passage 2 to 12 was tested for the presence of a factor that induced migration of SMC. The activity was compared with that of purified PDGF, one PDGF unit being defined as the maximum activity of PDGF. Results showed that cultured SMC secreted a factor with strong activity to induce migration of SMC. We named this factor smooth muscle derived migration factor (SDMF). The level of SDMF in the CM was independent of the passage number (data not shown).

As shown in FIGURE 1, the CM stimulated the migration of SMC dose-dependently, activity being maximal at a concentration of 50% or more. Checkerboard analysis showed that SDMF was chemotactic, but not chemokinetic (data not shown). The migration activities of 50% CMs from rabbit and rat SMC of different strains were compared with those of PDGF at 2 ng/ml and control medium (DME only). The CMs of rabbit and rat SMC had much higher activities than that of control medium: rabbit CM, 57.2 ± 46.5 (n = 26); rat CM, 81.8 ± 65.5 (n = 12) (mean ± SD, fold increase over control activity). Moreover, these activities were, respectively, 4.44 ± 1.05 and 4.60 ± 1.71 times higher than the maximal PDGF activity (= one PDGF unit).

The results of physicochemical analyses (TABLE 1) showed that SDMF is a new migration factor, distinct from various factors reported previously, such as PDGF, interleukin 1, fibronectin, leukotriene B$_4$, and 12-HETE. This conclusion was supported by immunological studies with anti-PDGF and anti-fibronectin antisera.

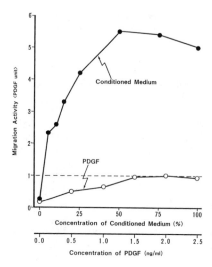

FIGURE 1. Dose-dependence of conditioned medium and platelet derived growth factor (PDGF) on the migration of rat aortic smooth muscle cells. The conditioned medium was collected from cultured rat aortic smooth muscle cells.

The migration activity of the CM of cultured intimal SMC from the thickened intima of rabbits given high cholesterol diet was about twice that of CM of medial SMC (data not shown). Thus in atheromatous lesions, SDMF may enhance the migration of the medial

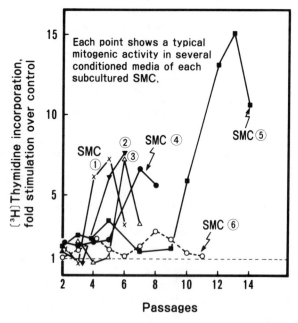

FIGURE 2. Relationship between passages of cultured smooth muscle cells and secretion of mitogenic activity. Typical mitogenic activities of several smooth muscle cells from different primary cultures are shown.

TABLE 1. Characterization of Migration Factor in CM of SMC

	Migration Activity (%)
Control (no treatment)	100
Heated at 56°C for 30 min	85
100°C for 10 min	1
Freezing and thawing	108
pH 2.5 at 22°C for 30 min	105
pH 10.0 at 22°C for 30 min	107
Dialysed (cut off MW 3500)	80
0.01% trypsin at 37°C for 30 min	21
0.1% trypsin at 37°C for 30 min	3
2 mM mercaptoethanol at 22°C for 30 min	90
Cross reactivity with	
anti-fibronectin antibody	—
anti-PDGF antibody	—

SMC to the intima, resulting in a vicious cycle of migration and proliferation of SMC. This autocrine system inducing migration of SMC may contribute to the development of atheromatous lesions.

Recently we reported that intimal SMC grew more rapidly than medial SMC.[7] In the present work we examined the reason for their rapid proliferation.

Significant mitogenic activity (defined as more than 3 times the control value) was first secreted into the CM at the fourth to tenth passage, depending on the primary culture, as shown in FIG. 2.[5] This CM stimulated the proliferation of SMC dose-dependently and its effect was synergistic with those of other growth factors.[8] TABLE 2 summarizes the characteristics of the SDGF in comparison with those of other known human growth factors. The results suggest that SDGF is a new growth factor, distinct from the factors reported previously such as PDGF, FGF, EGF, and somatomedin C. Unlike medial SMC, intimal SMC secreted a substantial amount of mitogenic activity into the CM at early

TABLE 2. Comparison between Growth Factors[a]

	PDGF	FGF	EGF	SomC	IL-1	SDGF
SMC proliferation	+	+	+	+	−	+
EC proliferation	−	+	−	−	−	−
Collabolation with SDGF	+	+	+	+		
Molecular weight (KD)	30	16	6	7.6	12–20	9.7
Heat stability (100°C)	+	−	+	+		−
Acid stability	+	−	−			+
PI	10	4.7, 9.5	4.5	8.2	5, 7–8	4.2, 5.9
Reactivity to RIA for somatomedin C				+		−
Inhibition by anti-PDGF	+					−
Receptor competition with ^{125}I-PDGF	+					−

[a]PDGF, platelet derived growth factor; FGF, fibroblast growth factor; EGF, epidermal growth factor; SomC, somatomedin C; SDGF, smooth muscle cell derived growth factor; SMC, smooth muscle cell; EC, endothelial cell.

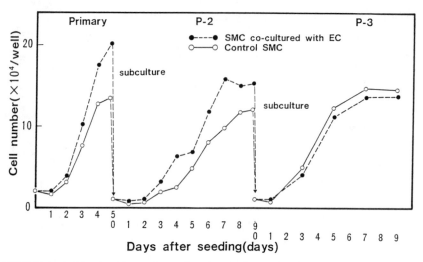

FIGURE 3. Proliferation of smooth muscle cells co-cultured with endothelial cells (EC). Medial smooth muscle cells were cultured either in the presence of or in the absence of (control) EC and then seeded into 24 plates without EC for the growth experiment (primary). Growth experiments were also carried out in the following two pasages.

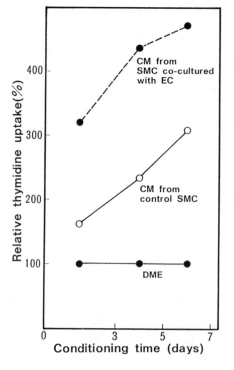

FIGURE 4. SDGF production from smooth muscle cells co-cultured with endothelial cells (EC). The conditioned media were collected from the smooth muscle cells mentioned in the legend to FIGURE 3.

passages, such as the second and third passage (data not shown). This activity was not inhibited by a polyclonal antibody to PDGF. Therefore, the high mitogenic activity of intimal SMC may be due to the autocrine secretion of SDGF.

Next, we examined the effect of endothelial cells (EC) on the mitogenic activity of SMC. As shown in FIGURE 3,[6] when medial SMC had been co-cultured with EC and then the EC were removed and the SMC were subcultured, they grew faster than control SMC. This enhanced growth persisted during two subsequent subcultures, but was not apparent during the third subculture. These results suggest that some factor(s) derived from EC changes the character of medial SMC and that the change persists for two passages.

Medial SMC not co-cultured with EC did not secrete much SDGF for the first 2 days but secreted it in the next 4 days. This is consistent with the findings on the relationship between the passage of medial SMC and their SDGF production, because the SMC used for FIGURE 3 were at passage 4 or more. Medial SMC co-cultured with EC secreted more SDGF than control SMC at the corresponding conditioning time (FIGURE 4).[6]

The above results can be summarized as follows: 1) Medial SMC are in the contractile form *in vivo,* but become in the synthetic state when cultured. However, they start to secrete SDGF only after prolonged culture. Their secretion of SDGF is probably due to their continuous stimulation with serum. 2) Intimal SMC are in a synthetic state *in vivo* and secrete SDGF. Therefore, they secrete SDGF from an early stage of culture. 3) EC enhance change of medial SMC toward intimal SMC with respect to the characters of growth and growth factor secretion. From these results we suggest that the SMC that migrate from the media to the intima are in part modulated by EC and become so-called intimal SMC. Atherosclerotic plaques must be formed by these pathological cells.

REFERENCES

1. FISCHER-DZOGA, K., R. M. JONES, D. VESSELINOVITCH & R. W. WISSLER. 1973. Exp. Mol. Pathol. **18:** 162–176.
2. MORISAKI, N., T. KANZAKI, Y. FUJIYAMA, I. OOSAWA, K. SHIRAI, N. MATSUOKA, Y. SAITO & S. YOSHIDA. 1985. J. Lipid Res. **26:** 930–939.
3. MORISAKI, N., T. KANZAKI, N. MOTOYAMA, Y. SAITO & S. YOSHIDA. 1988. Atherosclerosis **71:** 165–171.
4. OOYAMA, T., K. FUKUDA, H. ODA, H. NAKAMURA & Y. HIKITA. 1987. Arteriosclerosis **7:** 593–598.
5. MORISAKI, N., T. KANZAKI, T. KOSHIKAWA, Y. SAITO & S. YOSHIDA. 1988. FEBS Lett. **230:** 186–190.
6. SAITO, Y., T. KANZAKI, N. MORISAKI, T. KOSHIKAWA & S. YOSHIDA. 1989. Clin. Terapia Cardiovasc. **8:** 261–264.
7. SAITO, Y., H. BUJO, N. MORISAKI, K. SHIRAI & S. YOSHIDA. 1988. Atherosclerosis **69:** 161–164.
8. MORISAKI, N., N. KOYAMA, S. MORI, T. KANZAKI, T. KOSHIKAWA, Y. SAITO & S. YOSHIDA. 1989. Atherosclerosis **78:** 61–67.

Pathobiology of Vascular Cells *In Vitro* in Relation to Human Atherogenesis

Organ and Species Differences[a]

ABEL LAZZARINI ROBERTSON, JR.

Department of Pathology
University of Illinois College of Medicine
1853 West Polk Street (M/C 847)
Chicago, Illinois 60612

> *Make everything as simple as possible,*
> *but* not *simpler.* Albert Einstein

INTRODUCTION

While methodology for the cultivation of mammalian cells *in vitro* has been available for almost nine decades since the early studies of Carrel and Burrows,[1] isolation and characterization of vascular cells in cell culture was limited for a long time to the microscopic evaluation of cells outgrowing tissue explants containing mostly capillaries and venules.[2-7]

Clinical application of preserved arterial homografts in the surgical treatment of symptomatic vascular disease and the belief that graft viability was essential for their functional success, provided a strong incentive for the development of tissue and organ culture methods to evaluate human arteries before transplantation.[8,9]

These studies were followed by individual attempts to study fetal and adult human arterial cells under a variety of experimental conditions.[10-12] Irrigation of adult human thoracic aortas with elastase-free proteolytic enzymes combined with timed fraction collection[13] provided a reliable source of intimal cells as well as intercellular components for biochemical studies. However, due to the limited availability to most investigators of aseptically collected fresh human arteries, the subsequent application of enzymatic digestion for cell isolation and harvesting to readily obtainable umbilical veins[14] greatly expanded the number of investigators able to study and characterize fairly homogeneous populations of pooled fetal endothelial and/or smooth muscle cells in culture for relatively long periods.

Due to the efforts of many laboratories worldwide, major parallel advances, too long to enumerate, on the application of new or greatly improved biochemical, immunocytochemical, genetic, and/or ultrastructural research techniques to the study of vascular cells *in vitro* have exponentially expanded our knowledge of the general metabolic characteristics, growth requirements, and functional similarities or differences between endothelial[15-25] and vascular smooth muscle cells[26-34] not only from arteries, but also from veins and capillaries in man and animal models. However, for those investigators specifically interested in human atherogenesis, major questions remain regarding intimal-medial cell interactions as well as with the extracellular environment and circulating blood

[a]These studies are partially supported by Grant HL-30533 from the National Institutes of Health.

components. It is hoped that with the advent of promising new laboratory tools being rapidly developed in the field of Molecular Biology, many such questions could be addressed by *in vitro* studies on arterial cells directly involved in the development of spontaneous atheroma.

It seems therefore appropriate at this time to review available information on physiological and pathological segmental differences expressed in culture by arterial cells obtained during the initial stages of human atherogenesis as well as from atheroma-free specimens and to compare them with those obtained from major veins and fetal blood vessels. Furthermore, while keeping in mind the unavoidable limitations of organ, tissue, and cell culture methods compared with *in vivo* experiments, the former offer, due to their relative simplicity and reproducibility under laboratory conditions, an unique opportunity to compare the *in vitro* behavior of human adult arterial cells with those from animal models recognized to be less susceptible than man to the development of spontaneous atherogenesis.

MATERIALS AND METHODS

For the studies described herein, all human tissues were aseptically obtained at autopsy during collection of arteries for clinical transplantation as previously described,[35,36] except that specimens for culture were limited to those within 24 hours postmortem and less than 30 years of age or from vascular samples collected during reconstructive vascular surgery.

In all cases, specimens were transported to the laboratory in Hank's balanced salt solution at 4°C and processed for organ or tissue culture studies without delay. After careful aseptic dissection of adventitial fat (FIG. 1), organ cultures of vascular rings were prepared in culture medium containing 20% homologous serum without antibiotics. Outgrowing intimal and medial cells from the same vascular segments were harvested under an inverted microscope with micromanipulator attachments and cells aspirated with a micropipette (FIG. 2). After cell cloning on agar films, intimal and adventitial cells were separately counted and distributed in specially designed "candelabra" shaker flasks that allowed periodic refeeding, addition of labeled substrates, and predetermined oxygen-CO_2 concentrations without disturbing the cell suspensions[37] (FIG. 2).

For large blood vessels such as the aorta and vena cava, the vascular segments were opened longitudinally and cross sections from disease-free or grossly atheromatous regions further dissected under an inverted microscope in order to prepare 1–1.5 mm full thickness explants containing either intima-media or media-adventitial layers (FIG. 3) by the "double coverslip" method.[38] Outgrowing cell colonies were then harvested and processed as described above.

Human umbilical veins were processed by enzymatic digestion as originally proposed by Jaffe *et al.*[14] Intimal cells from umbilical arteries were similarly collected but following a 30 minutes incubation in a solution of 0.05% papaverine hydrochloride at 37°C, careful catheterization, and enzymatic digestion. After intimal cells were collected, a preheated enzyme mixture containing supplemental elastase was irrigated following gentle disruption of the medial layer with a glass "micropoliceman."

Endothelial, intimal, and medial cells were then individually transferred to culture flasks in medium M199, 10–20% homologous normolipemic sera without antibiotics. After reaching confluence, cells from each vascular layer were karyotyped and immunochemically characterized before use. Representative cell samples were also cryopreserved for future metabolic and functional comparisons with those undergoing multiple subcultures.

For some of the *in vitro* studies described under Results, intimal cells were also collected *in vivo* from arteries and veins of normo- and hyperlipemic laboratory animals (FIG. 4). The technique allowed repetitive sampling of different segments of the same blood vessel for biochemical, ultrastructural, and/or culture studies. The method also proved useful for the timed evaluation of vascular repair following segmental enzymatic deendothelialization.[39]

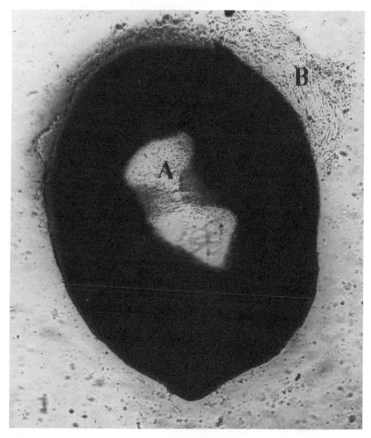

FIGURE 1. Organ culture method used to isolate arterial cells by tissue layers. Cross section of human anterior descending coronary artery after 24 days in culture. Note intimal cells growing into the arterial lumen (A) in contrast to adventitial and medial cells in the periphery of the explant (B). May Grünwald-Giemsa staining. Magnification 20 ×.

Oxygen requirements of suspension cultures of intimal cells from human blood vessels were determined by the cartesian diver method proposed by Linderstrom-Lang[40] as modified by Paul and Danes[41] and Robertson.[42]

Pooled human and animal sera were studied exclusively in homologous cell cultures. Lipoprotein fractions were prepared according to the method of Havel *et al.*[43] by repeated

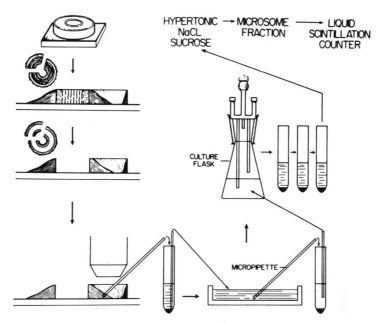

FIGURE 2. Schematic illustration of isolation of intimal, medial, and/or adventitial cells by cloning preceding biochemical-immunochemical characterization of subcellular fractions and evaluation of uptake of radiolabeled lipid fractions compared with *de novo* intracellular synthesis.

ultracentrifugation in increasing density gradients and exchanged-labeled with ^{125}I or ^{3}H markers.

De novo cholesterol synthesis was measured from ^{3}H acetate or mevalonate as previously reported.[37] Chylomicrons were collected by cannulation of the thoracic duct as proposed by Zilversmit *et al.*[44] Total cholesterol was measured by a modification of the method of Abell *et al.*[45] and total lipids as described by Swahn.[46]

Cell growth was measured by electronically counting harvested cells following repeated rinses in cold substrate. Monolayer cell cultures were gently separated and rinsed as above. ^{3}H thymidine labeled (1 μ Ci/ml) cultures were evaluated by autoradiography and results determined by computerized scanning of all monolayers to determine percentages of labeled nuclei per unit surface area.

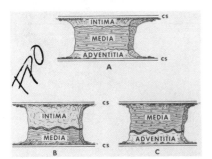

FIGURE 3. Application of the "double coverslip" method to isolate cells from each tissue layer of the vascular wall in large blood vessels such as the aorta or vena cava. When the vascular wall exceeds 2 mm in thickness, the media is carefully bisected and separated, matching cultures prepared of intima-media (B) and media-adventitia (C) cells.

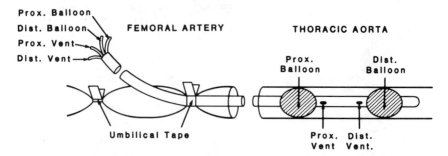

FIGURE 4. Method developed in our laboratory for *in vivo* collection of intimal cells in normo-and/or hyperlipemic animal models. A four channel catheter of appropriate size was introduced by distal arteriotomy or venous puncture and guided to the preselected branchless collection site by fluoroscopy. Both proximal and distal balloons were inflated to slightly above mean systolic or diastolic pressures and entrapped blood rinsed away with prewarmed Hank's solution. Elastase-free enzyme mixtures were then perfused at 37°C and physiological pressures and cells sequentially harvested in 10% homologous serum in balanced salt solution at 4°C with the aid of a fraction collector before isolation, gradient centrifugation, subculture, and immunocytochemical identification preceding metabolic studies on lipoprotein transport and *de novo* lipid synthesis as described under Experimental Results.

EXPERIMENTAL RESULTS

Matching suspension cultures of human intimal cells from atherosclerotic arteries showed elevation of all intracellular lipid fractions after 120 minutes incubation in pooled hypercholesterolemic homologous sera compared to those maintained in normocholesterolemic media (TABLE 1). Cholesterol esters in particular increased an average 16 fold. Furthermore, *de novo* cholesterol synthesis was not inhibited, in contrast to cells from atheroma-free arteries, and substantive elevations of cholesteryl esters were noted in spite of increased uptake from extracellular sources.[47]

The above responses were also not found when human skin fibroblasts, skeletal muscle or fetal arterial cells were similarly tested, suggesting that both receptor-mediated autoregulation of cholesterol uptake and ultracellular feedback mechanisms overseeing

TABLE 1. *In vitro* Effects of Hyperliproteinemic Human Sera on Arterial Intimal Cells Lipid Uptake and *de novo* Synthesis

Intracellular Total Lipids (μg/mg Cell Protein)[a]	in NHS*	in HHS**
Triglycerides	52	142
Free cholesterol	84	194
Cholesterol esters	32	520
FC/CE	2.6	0.37
de novo Synthesis[b]		
Free cholesterol	96/620[b]	8/28
Cholesterol esters	12/94	81/146

[a]Average results of 32 cultures incubated in M199–20% * or ** for 120° in 5% CO_2-Air.
[b]From ^{3}H mevalonate.
*Pooled normolipemic human serum—TC:220; CE:184; TG:89; PH:292 mg/dl.
**Pooled hyperlipemic human serum—TC:396; CE:294; TG:104; PH:290 mg/dl.

cholesterol esters synthesis present in other human cells, may be inoperative or severely inhibited in human atheroma.

The above response of human atheroma cells to lipoprotein cholesterol was, however, not uniform. A majority responded with rapid accumulation of abundant and increasingly larger cytoplasmic membrane-bound lipid droplets, containing a high proportion of cholesteryl esters, transforming eventually *in vitro* into typical "foam" cells. In contrast, other cells were able to resist, even after prolonged incubation in the same culture, increased uptake and *de novo* sterol synthesis (FIG. 5). The presence of these spindle

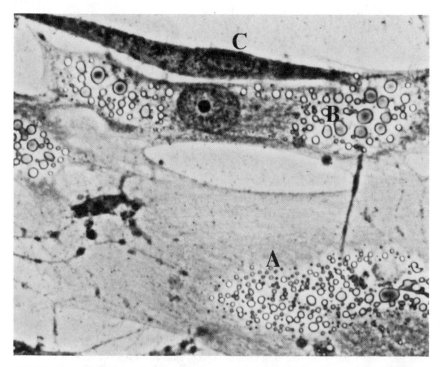

FIGURE 5. Differences in cellular response of human coronary intimal cells (isolated as shown on FIG. 2) following incubation in pooled homologous hypercholesterolemic sera under standardized conditions. Note that while cells (A) and (B) show extensive cytoplasmic accumulation of membrane-bound lipid droplets, cell (C) is not affected, suggesting a heterogenous intimal cell population. Sudan IV staining. Magnification 840 × .

shaped "fibrophils"[48] in the intima of atherosclerotic arteries has suggested to us the presence of a metabolically heterogenous cell population during the early stages of human atherogenesis.[49] Parenthetically, no evidence of similar cellular differences was found in parallel studies with arterial cells from cholesterol-fed rats, rabbits, or dogs.

When internalization and lysosomal degradation of homologous low density (LDL) and very low density lipoprotein (VLDL) fractions by human arterial intimal cells were followed by time-lapse microcinematography (FIG. 6), the first observable changes occurred within the Golgi apparatus, suggesting that at that early stage of accumulated lipid uptake, physiological subcellular mechanisms were still operational and the cell was attempting to "pack" the excess lipids for exocytosis.[47] When that response failed, transmission electronmicroscopy of cultures of aortic intima from atheroma-prone regions showed (FIG. 7) diffuse cytoplasmic lipid storage in membrane-bound vacuoles of varied electron density as well as in dilated canaliculi of endoplasmic reticulum. Fluorescence microscopy confirmed those findings (FIG. 8) by the demonstration of discrete cytoplasmic accumulation of neutral lipids.[50]

Cloned-factor VIII positive-human aortic endothelial cells in short term cultures were

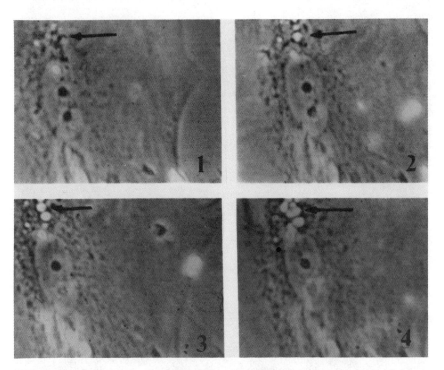

FIGURE 6. Initial stages of *in vitro* foam cells formation. Intracellular lipid accumulation in human coronary intimal cells incubated in culture medium containing homologous hypercholesterolemic sera equivalent to 280 mg/dl of total cholesterol and 150 mg/dl triglycerides. Individual frames from phase-contrast, time lapse microcinematography **(1)** after 60 minutes incubation at 37°C in air-5% CO_2 and **(2)**, **(3)**, and **(4)** every 10 minutes thereafter. Note birefrigent droplets selectively appearing in the Golgi zone (*arrows*) and their expansion and fusion into layer membrane bound vacuoles that will eventually extend to the whole cytoplasm. Original magnification 787 ×.

found to differ on their uptake of LDL-cholesterol depending on whether they originated from lesion-prone branching sites or less susceptible ventral aorta.[51]

As shown on TABLE 2, the uptake of homologous ^{125}I labeled LDL was accompanied in the above cells by increased de novo cholesterol synthesis, accelerated *in vitro* cell proliferation, and shortened generation times. Human aortic endothelial cells seem therefore to be preprogrammed, at sites prone to accelerated atherosclerosis, for rapid cell turnover and increased free and esterified cholesterol accumulation, potentiating the recognized hemodynamic effects of changes in flow patterns at branching sites.[52]

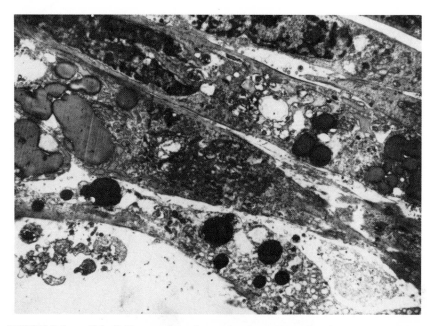

FIGURE 7. Intracellular lipid accumulation in cytoplasmic membrane-bound vacuoles as well as in dilated cisternae of endoplasmic reticulum. Culture of intimal cells from lesion-prone areas of the abdominal aorta (dorsal region) incubated for 24 hours with pooled hypercholesterolemic serum. Note significant variations on electron density related to variable content of neutral lipids in individual vacuoles. Water embedding method following osmication. Uranyl acetate-lead citrate staining. Magnification 8,600 × .

TABLE 3 summarizes differences on lipid metabolism found when human intimal arterial cells were compared with matching skeletal muscle cell cultures from the same donors, incubated in homologous hypercholesterolemic sera. Average uptake of lipids, particularly cholesterol esters, increased dramatically compared to striated muscle cells, while the average free to esterified cholesterol ratio was reduced as previously shown in TABLE 1.

To determine whether the above metabolic changes extended to other key cellular functions, oxygen consumption rates, as a measure of oxidative phosphorylation, were determined in cloned aortic intimal cell suspensions.

TABLE 2. Summary of Regional Variations on Homologous ^{125}I-LDL Uptake *in vitro* by Endothelial Cells from Dorsal Branching Sites Compared to Ventral Regions of the Human Thoracic Aorta[a]

1. Accelerated LDL uptake
2. Increased *de novo* FC/CE synthesis (from ^{3}H acetate)
3. Elevated ^{3}H thymidine incorporation
4. Shorten generation times

[a]Average results of 24 matching cultures each.

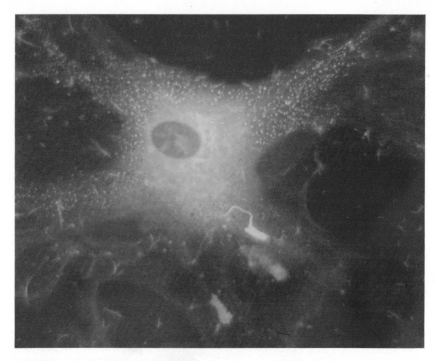

FIGURE 8. Diffuse cytoplasmic distribution of fluorescent unesterified cholesterol and other neutral lipids following incubation of HSV-1 infected human aortic intimal cells following 120 minutes incubation in culture medium containing mg/dl of LDL-cholesterol. Nile red staining.[50] Ultraviolet illumination at 450–500 nm. Yellow-gold fluorescence. Original magnification 840×.

TABLE 4 illustrated significant differences found between cells from lesion-prone compared with less susceptible aortic regions and with those from the inferior vena cava.[42] While aortic cells from the dorsal (lesion prone) region had twice as high oxygen

TABLE 3. *In vitro* Lipid Metabolism of Human Coronary Intimal Cells (CAI) Compared with Homologous Skeletal Muscle Cells (SKM)[a]

	CAI[b]	SKM[b]
Triglycerides	298.3	46.4
Free cholesterol	560.2	88.1
Cholesterol esters	1440.3	30.1
FC/CE ratios	0.389	2.927
Synthesized FC/CE[c]		
Average % total	72.5/328.2	16.2/10.4
Average dpm/μg	52.3/456.4	2.2/9.5

[a]Changes in total intracellular lipids including *de novo* sterol synthesis following 180 minutes incubation in 20% human HS (TC = 396, CE = 294, TG = 104, PH = 290 mg/dl) in medium M199 (28 cultures each).
[b]Average values in μg lipids/mg cell protein.
[c]From ^{3}H acetate.

TABLE 4. Differences in Oxygen Consumption Rates[a] of Human Aortic Intimal Cells Compared with Those from the Inferior Vena Cava

Ventral thoracic aorta	0.098 ± 0.028 μM/hour/10^7 cells
Dorsal thoracic aorta (lesion prone)	0.184 ± 0.038 μM/hour/10^7 cells
Inferior vena cava	0.018 ± 0.012 μM/hour/10^7 cells

[a]Average of 12 determinations each by the Cartesian Diver Method; M 199/20% normolipemic human serum.

consumption rates as those isolated from the ventral aortic intima, their oxygen requirements were 10 fold higher than those from the vena cava. These findings confirmed observations by other investigators studying experimental atherosclerosis in rats[53] and rabbits.[54] In our own studies, it was observed that oxygen concentrations below 5% in the gas phase of the cultures did not significantly inhibit uptake of ^{14}C acetate or ^{3}H mevalonate in spite of significant reductions of measurable *de novo* cholesterol synthesis. For that reason, quantitative measurements of intracellular squalene[55] were made. They showed that under hypoxic culture conditions, human arterial cells were unable to complete cholesterol synthesis resulting in cytotoxic intracellular levels of squalene.[42] These experimental findings agree with biochemical evidence that the cyclization of squalene into lanosterol is oxygen dependent and that low oxygen levels will block completion of cholesterol synthesis.

Since the seminal studies of Zilversmit *et al.*[44] on the transport of exogenous cholesterol by rabbit chylomicrons, the potential atherogenic role of small chylomicrons remaining in the systemic circulation for long periods postprandially, was suspected. In man, they carry up to 2% as free cholesterol (dry weight) and their attachment to arterial endothelial cells was studied following stimulation with rapidly acting vasopressor agents.[56]

TABLE 5 illustrates results obtained after such stimulation with adult human arterial endothelium compared to those of venous or fetal origin.

While no statistical differences were found between adult endothelial cells of the aortic and carotid arteries, a significant response to angiotensin II, 5-hydroxytryptamine, or prostaglandin E_1 stimulation occurred. In contrast to the endothelia of umbilical vein or vena cava, it consisted of increased surface binding of the small chylomicrons followed by rapid intracellular accumulation of free cholesterol.

To determine whether significant cellular differences on lipoprotein cholesterol uptake *in vitro* may exist between human adult arterial intimal cells and those from some of the

TABLE 5. Comparative "Stickiness" of Homologous ^{3}H Labeled Small Chylomicrons[a] to Confluent Human Endothelial Monolayer Cultures under Perfusion[b] following *in vitro* Stimulation

	Vasoactive Agents		
Vascular Origin	I	II	III
Thoracic aorta	82.4	69.3	42.8
Carotid arteries	62.1	52.6	39.7
Umbilical vein	8.9	2.3	2.8
Inferior vena cava	15.0	16.4	1.2

[a]Average %, 6×10^8 labeled cells, 20 cultures each.
[b]Perfused at 37.2°C, 240 minutes, 2.5 ml medium/hour: (I) Angiotensin II: 1×10^9 g; (II) 5-Hydroxytriptamine (SO$_4$): 1×10^8 g; (III) Prostaglandin E_1: 1×10^7 g.

most widely used animal models for experimental atherosclerosis, a comparative study, summarized on TABLE 6, was carried out. Average results of cultures from each subgroup tested showed that final intracellular cholesterol concentrations were substantially higher in cells from human arteries than in any of those obtained from arteries harvested from mature laboratory animals.

Furthermore, significant differences on lipoprotein cholesterol uptakes were found between human endothelial cells under similar laboratory conditions. Adult coronary endothelium was found to have much higher uptake rates than those from the ventral aspect of the thoracic aorta or the umbilical vein.[57]

DISCUSSION

Application of tissue and cell culture techniques in many laboratories to the study of mammalian vascular cells has shed new light on our understanding of blood vessel morphology and function. Endothelial and smooth muscle cells from human and laboratory animal sources have been successfully isolated, immunochemically characterized,

TABLE 6. Comparative Species Differences in *in vitro* Extracellular Lipoprotein Cholesterol[a] Uptake by Vascular Cells

	Incubation Time (Minutes)		
	60	120	240
Human aorta	[b]246.2/0.8	548.4/0.4	847.3/0.2
Human vena cava	9.6/2.8	42.4/2.6	84.6/2.3
Chicken aorta	0.2/4.0	0.3/3.8	0.5/3.6
Rabbit aorta	0.6/4.2	0.8/3.9	1.2/3.3
Rat aorta	0.4/3.8	0.5/3.6	0.4/3.9
Swine aorta	2.4/4.1	4.9/3.2	16.3/2.7

[a]Challenged with matching concentrations of homologous sera in the culture medium.
[b]Average μg of total cholesterol per mg cell protein/FC/CE ratios.

cloned and subcultured to establish cell strains for long-term physiological and/or pharmacological investigations. However, in applying such established techniques to the elucidation of some major unanswered questions regarding the pathogenesis of human atherosclerosis, investigators should be aware of substantial methodological limitations when cells other than those from adult human arteries are used. The arterial wall is a complex multicellular organ and intimal cells, primarily involved during the initial stages of human atherogenesis, actively interact with one another as well as with extracellular components and the circulating blood during lesion development. For that reason, extrapolation to the clinical setting of experimental data obtained by the study of isolated monolayer cultures of vascular cells after continued subcultivation is at best, limited. These concerns are reflected in the dictum: "*In vivo,* Veritas; *in vitro,* maybe. . . ." It should also be recognized that isolation by repeated enzymatic digestion of highly differentiated cells and subsequent subculture, significantly alters by growth selection or spontaneous mutations metabolic cellular differences found in primary or short-term diploid cultures. After repeated subcultivation, most cultures consist of fairly homogenous polyploidy cell populations metabolically quite distinct from those found in the tissue of origin.

Our own studies as well as those from an increasing number of other laboratories strongly suggest significant and quite variable phenotypic diversity between cells from adult and fetal human arteries, veins, and capillaries as well as with those from different organs.[58-62]

Recent cell culture studies have also shown variability on cell surface receptors, response to growth factors and/or hormones as well as cell-to-cell interactions.[19,22,31,32,63-65] For instance, *in vitro* studies of isolated vascular smooth muscle cells from human and laboratory models have shown significant differences influenced by such factors as blood pressure and age of the donor,[66] contractile proteins,[67] oxygen availability,[68] growth promoting agents,[31,69-71] and inflammatory mediators.[72-76]

A still unresolved question is whether such noted differences could also be similarly expressed when a heterogenous cell population as the one that is found in the adult arterial intima *in vivo* could be maintained in primary organ cultures.[77-81] A potentially important contribution of that type of short-term culture is the preservation of autocrine and paracrine arterial cell functions that may play key roles in the metabolic regulation of the arterial intima. Recent studies employing cocultivation of arterial and blood cells[82] could also provide valuable information on intercellular communications between the vessel wall and circulating cells. More comparative metabolic studies, like those shown on TABLE 6 between adult human arterial intimal cells and those of mature laboratory animals known to be less susceptible to spontaneous atherosclerosis, are urgently needed. Our investigations showed that such human cells have considerably greater affinity for lipoprotein cholesterol uptake than any of the laboratory models tested. Indeed, detailed *in vitro* exploration of metabolic cellular differences utilizing newly developed molecular markers should also help to explain the noted resistance of some of these models to experimental atherosclerosis and indirectly aid the search for new therapeutic approaches to human atherogenesis.

Finally, one of the currently most promising research areas in the pathogenesis of spontaneous atherosclerosis that is adaptable to study by short-term organ cultures of adult human arterial intimal cells is that of considering atherogenesis as the tissue expression of a hyperplastic or neoplastic process[83,84] resulting from altered gene expression.[85]

Characteristic intimal cellular changes inducing excessive accumulation of intracellular cholesteryl esters could thus represent the effects of cholesterol-induced mutagens,[86] inducers, oncogens,[87,88] and/or transforming agents such as common viruses[89,90] illustrated in FIGURE 8. Any one of these mechanisms of genetic injury and subsequent DNA repair[91] could then favor focal intimal cell proliferation, "foam" cell formation, and eventual development of full-fledged atheromata.

CONCLUSIONS

For the past four decades, investigators in many countries have made valuable contributions to our understanding of the structure and function of the mammalian vascular wall by applying newly developed organ, cell, and tissue culture methods. Standardized *in vitro* studies with vascular cells from man and laboratory animals have shown that:

1. There are significant metabolic differences between cultures of adult human arterial and venous cells and between them and those of fetal origin;
2. In short-term cultures, adult human arterial intimal cells from atheroma-prone regions have higher oxygen consumption requirements and metabolize extracellular lipoproteins as well as synthesize *de novo* cholesterol at faster rates than those from atheroma-free regions or from major veins; and
3. When arterial intimal cells from adult or fetal laboratory models, known to be less

susceptible to spontaneous atherogenesis were also compared *in vitro,* they failed to show similar metabolic differences.

These findings strongly suggest that further advances on the application of *in vitro* metabolic and functional studies to better define the role of vascular cells during the initial stages of human atherogenesis require the selective use of low-passage cultures of adult diploid human arterial intimal cells and appropriate controls. While this approach is undoubtedly technically more difficult and time consuming, it should prove to be significantly more meaningful and rewarding to the atherosclerosis researcher.

ACKNOWLEDGMENTS

The technical support of Rose Harper and Francis Norris and the assistance of Patricia Berg and Irene Robertson in the preparation of the manuscript are gratefully recognized.

REFERENCES

1. CARRELL, A. & M. T. BURROWS. 1910. Cultivation of adult tissues and organs outside the body. J. Am. Med. Assoc. **55:** 1379–1381.
2. MAXIMOW, A. A. 1925. Behavior of endothelium of blood vessels in tissue culture. Anat. Rec. **29:** 369 (Abstract).
3. SILBERBERG, M. 1929. Endothelium in der Geveweskultur. Arch. Exp. Zellforsch. **9:** 36–53.
4. SHIBUYA, T. 1931. On the pure cultivation of endothelial cells from aorta and their differentiation. Kitasato Arch. Exp. Med. **8:** 68–88.
5. HERZOG, G. & W. SCHOPPER. 1931. Über das verhalten der blutgefasse in der Kultur. Arch. Exp. Zellforsch. **11:** 202–218.
6. LEWIS, W. H. 1931. The outgrowth of endothelium and capillaries in tissue culture. Johns Hopkins Med. J. **48:** 243–253.
7. WHITE, J. F. & M. S. PARSHLEY. 1951. Growth *in vitro* of blood vessels from bone marrow of adult chicken. Am. J. Anat. **89:** 321–345.
8. PEIRCE, E. C., R. E. GROSS, A. H. BILL & K. MERRILL. 1949. Tissue culture evaluation of the viability of blood vessels by refrigeration. Ann. Surg. **129:** 333–348.
9. ROBERTSON, A., LAZZARINI, JR. 1952. Vascular homografts. Viability testing by tissue culture methods. (In Spanish) Prensa Med. Argentina **39:** 2637–2645.
10. KEMENSKAYA, N. L. 1956. Endothelium of the embryonal aorta of man. Dok. Akad. Nauk. SSSR. **110:** 1096.
11. INGENITO, F., J. M. CRAIG, J. LABESSE, M. GAUTIER & D. D. RUTSTEIN. 1958. Cells of human heart and aorta grown in tissue culture. AMA Arch. Pathol. **65:** 355–359.
12. ROBERTSON, A., LAZZARINI, JR. 1961. The effects of fatty acids and heparin in the absorption and metabolism of cholesterol microemulsions by organ cultures of human and animal arterial wall. *In* Drugs Affecting Lipid Metabolism. S. Garattini & R. Paoletti, Eds. 306–333. Elsevier Publishers. Amsterdam–New York.
13. ROBERTSON, A. L., JR. & W. INSULL, JR. 1967. Dissection of normal and atherosclerotic human artery with proteolytic enzymes *in vitro.* Nature **214:** 821–823.
14. JAFFE, E. A., R. L. NACHMAN, C. G. BECKER & C. R. MINICK. 1973. Culture of human endothelial cells derived from umbilical veins. J. Clin. Invest. **52:** 2745–2756.
15. ROBERTSON, A., LAZZARINI, JR. 1961. Effects of heparin on the uptake of lipids by isolated human and animal arterial endothelial type cells. Angiology **12**(10): 525–533.
16. MARUYAMA, Y. 1973. The human endothelial cell in tissue culture. Z. Zellforsch. Mikrosk. Anat. **60:** 69–79.
17. LEWIS, L. J., J. C. HOAK, R. D. MACA *et al.* 1973. Replication of human endothelial cells in culture. Science **181:** 453–454.
18. BECKER, C. G. & R. L. NACHMAN. 1973. Contractile proteins of endothelial cells, platelets and smooth muscle. Am. J. Pathol. **71:** 1–22.

19. GIMBRONE, M. A., JR., R. S. COTRAN & J. FOLKMAN. 1974. Human vascular endothelial cells in culture. Growth and DNA synthesis. J. Cell Biol. **60:** 673–684.
20. DEBONO, D. 1975. En face organ culture of vascular endothelium. Br. J. Exp. Pathol. **56:** 8–13.
21. THORGEIRSSON, G. & A. L. ROBERTSON, JR. 1978. The vascular endothelium: Pathobiologic significance. Am. J. Pathol. **93:** 803–848.
22. HENRICKSEN, T., E. M. MAHONEY & D. STEINBERG. 1982. Interaction of plasma lipoproteins with endothelial cells. Ann. N.Y. Acad. Sci. **401:** 109–116.
23. WATANABE, K. & K. TANAKA. 1983. Influence of fibrin, fibrinogen and fibrinogen degradation products in cultured endothelial cells. Atherosclerosis **48:** 57–70.
24. PEDERSON, D. C. & D. E. BOWYER. 1985. Endothelial injury and healing *in vitro*. Studies using an organ culture system. Am. J. Pathol. **119:** 264–272.
25. LANGELER, E. G., I. SNELTING-HAVINGA & V. W. VAN HINSBERG. 1989. Passage of LDL through monolayers of human arterial endothelial cells. Atherosclerosis **9:** 550–559.
26. ROSS, R. 1971. The smooth muscle cell. II. Growth of smooth muscle in culture and formation of elastic fibers. J. Cell Biol. **50:** 172–186.
27. FISCHER-DZOGA, K., R. M. JONES, D. VESSELINOVITCH & R. W. WISSLER. 1973. Ultrastructural and immunocytochemical studies of primary cultures of aortic medial cells. Exp. Mol. Pathol. **18:** 162–176.
28. GIMBRONE, M. A., JR. & R. S. COTRAN. 1975. Human vascular smooth muscle in culture: Growth and ultrastructure. Lab. Invest. **33:** 16–27.
29. BIERMAN, E. L. & J. J. ALBERS. 1976. Lipid uptake and degradation of human arterial smooth muscle cells in tissue culture. Ann. N.Y. Acad. Sci. **275:** 199–203.
30. FISCHER-DZOGA, K., R. FRASER & R. W. WISSLER. 1976. Stimulation of proliferation in stationary primary cultures of monkey and rabbit aortic smooth muscle cells. I. Effects of lipoprotein fractions of hyperlipemic serum and lymph. Exp. Mol. Pathol. **24:** 346–359.
31. LIBBY, P., S. J. C. WARNER, R. N. SALOMON & L. K. BIRINY. 1988. Production of platelet derived growth factor like mitogen by smooth muscle cells of human atheroma. N. Engl. J. Med. **318:** 1493–1498.
32. CAMPBELL, G. R., J. H. CAMPBELL, J. A. MANDERSON, S. HORRIGAN & R. E. RENNICK. 1988. Arterial smooth muscle, a multifunctional mesenchymal cell. Arch. Pathol. Lab. Med. **112:** 977–986.
33. MAJACK, R. A., C. K. CASTLE, L. V. GOODMAN, K. H. WEISGRABER, R. W. MAHLEY, E. M. SHOOTER & P. J. GEBICKE-HAERTER. 1988. Expression of apolipoprotein E by cultured vascular smooth muscle cells is controlled by growth state. Rat vascular SMC, a source for Apo E cells, contain Apo E in RNA. J. Cell Biol. **107:** 1207–1213.
34. MITSUMATA, M., K. FISCHER-DZOGA, G. S. GETZ & R. W. WISSLER. 1988. Sequential change of DNA synthesis in cultured aortic smooth muscle cells stimulated by hyperlipemic serum. Exp. Mol. Pathol. **48:** 24–36.
35. KEEFER, E. B. C., W. D. ANDRUS, F. GLENN, G. H. HYMPHREYS, J. W. LORD, JR., W. B. MURPHY & A. S. W. TOUROFF. 1951. The blood vessel bank. J. Am. Med. Assoc. **145**(12): 888–893.
36. ROBERTSON, A. LAZZARINI, JR. 1953. Blood vessel bank—its possibilities. Angiology **4:** 516–525.
37. ROBERTSON, A. LAZZARINI. 1965. Studies on the effects of local factors in the development of spontaneous and experimental atherosclerosis. *In* Cerebral Vascular Diseases. R. G. Siefert and J. P. Whisnant, Eds. 153–158. Grune & Stratton. New York, NY.
38. ROBERTSON, A. L., JR. 1975. Envelope technique for selective isolation of cells from multilayer organ cultures for metabolic studies. Tissue Culture Assoc. Manual **1:** 139–144.
39. ROBERTSON, A. L. 1980. Arterial endothelium in the initial stages of atherogenesis. *In* Atherosclerosis V. A. M. Gotto, L. C. Smith & B. Allen, Eds. 103–111. Springer-Verlag. New York–Heidelberg.
40. LINDERSTROM-LANG, K. 1937. Principle of the cartesian diver applied to gasometric techniques. Nature **140:** 108–110.
41. PAUL, J. & B. DANES. 1961. A modified cartesian diver method permitting measurement of oxygen uptake in the presence of carbon dioxide. Analyt. Biochem. **2**(5): 470–485.

42. ROBERTSON, A. L. 1968. Oxygen requirements of the human arterial intima in atherogenesis. Prog. Biochem. Pharmacol. **4:** 305–316.

43. HAVEL, R. J., H. A. EDER & J. N. BRAGDON. 1955. The distribution and chemical composition of ultracentrifugally separated lipoproteins in human serum. J. Clin. Invest. **34:** 1345–1353.

44. ZILVERSMIT, D. B., F. C. COURTICE & R. FRASER. 1968. Cholesterol transport in the thoracic lymph of the rabbit. J. Atheroscler. Res. **7:** 319–329.

45. ABELL, L. L., B. LEVY, B. B. BRADIE & F. E. KENDALL. 1952. A simplified method for the esterification of total cholesterol in serum and demonstration of its specificity. J. Biol. Chem. **195:** 357–366.

46. SWAHN, B. 1953. A method for determination of total lipids in serum. J. Clin. Invest. **5**(Suppl. IX): 7–38.

47. ROBERTSON, A. L., JR. 1974. Functional characterization of arterial cells involved in spontaneous atheroma. *In* Atherosclerosis III. G. Schettler & A. Weizel, Eds. 175–184. Springer-Verlag. Berlin–New York.

48. ROBERTSON, A. LAZZARINI, JR. 1969. Structure of the coronary arteries and hypothesis on the pathogenesis of human atherosclerosis. *In* The Ciba Collection. F. H. Netter, Ed. Vol. **5:** 212–213. New York, NY.

49. ROBERTSON, A. LAZZARINI, JR. 1977. The pathogenesis of human atherosclerosis. *In* Atherosclerosis. A. M. Gotto (cons. author). H. L. Gross, Ed. 37–54. A Scope Publication. Upjohn, MI.

50. GREENSPAN, P., E. P. MAYER & S. D. FOWLER. 1985. Nile red: A selective fluorescent stain for intracellular lipid droplets. J. Cell Biol. **100:** 965–973.

51. ROBERTSON, A. LAZZARINI, JR. 1976(a). Regional functional variations of human arterial endothelium and atherogenesis. Circulation **54**(II): 217.

52. KARINO, T., T. ASAKURA & S. MABUCHI. 1989. Vascular geometry, flow patterns and preferred sites of atherosclerosis in human coronary and cerebral arteries. *In* Atherosclerosis VIII. G. Crepaldo, A. M. Gotto, E. Manzato & G. Baggio, Eds. 417–420. Elsevier Publishers. Amsterdam–New York.

53. LOOMEIJER, F. J. & J. P. OSTENDORF. 1959. Oxygen consumption of the thoracic aorta of normal and hypercholesterolemic rats. Circulation Res. **7:** 466–467.

54. WHEREAT, A. F. 1961. Oxygen consumption of normal and atherosclerotic intima. Circ. Res. **9:** 571–575.

55. ROTHBLAT, G. H., D. S. MARTAK & D. KRITCHEVSKY. 1962. A quantitative colorimetric assay for squalene. Analyt. Biochem. **4:** 52–56.

56. ROBERTSON, A. L., JR. 1978. Role of vasoactive agents and hypertension in accelerated atherogenesis. Proc. International Symposium on State of Prevention and Therapy in Human Arteriosclerosis and in Animal Models. W. H. Hauss, R. W. Wissler & R. Lehman, Eds. 289–300. Westdeutscher Verlag. Opladen, West Germany.

57. ZIATS, N. P., E. D. MEDVEDEFF & A. L. ROBERTSON, JR. 1980. Culture techniques and growth requirements of human coronary endothelial cells compared with those of aorta or umbilical veins. (Unpublished data).

58. SAGE, H., P. PRITZL & P. BORNSTEIN. 1981. Secretory phenotypes of endothelial cells in culture. Comparison of aortic, venous, capillary and corneal endothelium. Arteriosclerosis **1:** 427–442.

59. PIETRA, G. G., A. P. FISHMAN, P. N. LANKEN, P. SAMPSON & J. HANSEN-FLASCHEN. 1982. Permeability of pulmonary endothelium to neutral and charged macromolecules. Ann. N.Y. Acad. Sci. **401:** 241–246.

60. KUMAR, S., D. C. WEST & A. AGER. 1987. Heterogeneity in endothelial cells from large vessels and microvessels. Differentiation **36:** 57–70.

61. RUPNICK, M. A., A. CAREY & S. K. WILLIAMS. 1988. Phenotypic diversity in cultured cerebral microvascular endothelial cells. In Vitro Cell Dev. Biol. **24:** 435–440.

62. FAYED, Y. M., J. C. TSIBRIS, P. W. LANGENBERG & A. L. ROBERTSON, JR. 1989. Human uterine leiomyoma cells: Binding and growth responses to epidermal growth factor, platelet-derived growth factor and insulin. Lab. Invest. **60:** 30–37.

63. KARNOVSKY, M. J. 1981. Endothelial-vascular smooth muscle cell interactions. Am. J. Pathol. **105:** 200–206.

64. SIMIONESCU, M., N. SIMIONESCU & G. E. PALADE. 1982. Biochemically differentiated microdomains of the cell surface of capillary endothelium. Ann. N.Y. Acad. Sci. **401:** 9–23.

65. FRY, G., T. PARSONS, J. HOAK, H. SAGE, R. D. GINGRICH, L. ERCOLANI, D. NGHIEM & R. CZERVIONKE. 1984. Properties of cultured endothelium from adult human vessels. Arteriosclerosis **4:** 4–13.

66. GRUNWALD, J., J. MEY, W. SCHONLEBEN, J. HAUSS & W. H. HAUSS. 1983. Cultivated human arterial smooth muscle cells. The effects of donor age, blood pressure, diabetes and smoking on *in vitro* cell growth. Pathol. Biol. **31:** 819–823.

67. FAGER, G., G.K. HANSSON, A. M. GOWN, D. M. LARSON, O. SKALLI & G. BONDJERS. 1989. Human arterial smooth muscle cells in culture. Inverse relationship between proliferation and expression of contractile proteins. In Vitro Cell Dev. Biol. **25:** 511–520.

68. TSUKITANI, M., R. OKAMOTO & H. FUKUZAKI. 1984. Effect of hypoxia on cholesterol accumulation in cultured rabbit aortic smooth muscle cells. Atherosclerosis **52:** 167–174.

69. THORGEIRSSON, G. & A. L. ROBERTSON, JR. 1978. Platelet factors and the human vascular wall: Variations in growth response between endothelial and medial smooth muscle cells. Atherosclerosis **30:** 67–68.

70. LIBBY, P., M. W. JANICKA & C. A. DIANARELLO. 1985. Interleukin-1 promotes production by human endothelial cells of activity that stimulates the growth of arterial smooth muscle cells. Fed. Proc. **44:** 737.

71. ROSS, R. 1986. The pathogenesis of atherosclerosis. An update. N. Engl. J. Med. **314:** 488–500.

72. ZIATS, N. P. & A. L. ROBERTSON, JR. 1981. Effects of peripheral blood monocytes on human vascular cell proliferation. Atherosclerosis **38:** 401–410.

73. ALBRIGHTSON, C. R., N. L. BAENZIGER & P. NEEDLEMAN. 1985. Exaggerated human vascular cell prostaglandin biosynthesis mediated by monocytes: Role of monokines and interleukin-1. J. Immunol. **135:** 1872–1877.

74. ROSSI, V., F. BREVIARIO, P. GHEZZI, E. DEJANA & A. MANTOVANI. 1985. Prostacyclin synthesis induced in vascular cells by interleukin-1. Science **229:** 174–176.

75. BEVILACQUA, M. P., R. SCHLEEF, M. A. GIMBRONE, JR. & D. J. LOSKUTOFF. 1986. Regulation of the fibrinolytic system of human vascular endothelium by interleukin-1. J. Clin. Invest. **78:** 587–591.

76. WARNER, S. J. C., K. R. AUGER & P. LIBBY. 1987. Human interleukin-1 induces interleukin-1 gene expression in human vascular endothelial cells. J. Exp. Med. **165:** 1316–1331.

77. OREKHOV, A. N., V. V. TERTOV & V. N. SMIRNOV. 1985. Lipids in cells of atherosclerotic and uninvolved human aorta. Lipid metabolism in primary culture. Exp. Mol. Pathol. **43:** 187–195.

78. MERRILEES, M. J. & L. J. SCOTT. 1985. Effects of endothelial removal and regeneration on smooth muscle glycosaminoglycan synthesis and growth in rat carotid artery in organ culture. Lab. Invest. **52:** 409–419.

79. TERTOV, V. V., A. N. OREKHOV & V. N. SMIRNOV. 1986. Cyclic AMP and cyclic GMP content in short-term organ cultures of normal and atherosclerotic human aorta. Artery **13:** 373–382.

80. JACKMAN, R. W., S. K. ANDERSON & J. D. SHERIDAN. 1988. The aortic intima in organ culture. Response to culture conditions and partial endothelial denudation. Am. J. Pathol. **133:** 241–251.

81. SCHOEFFTER, P., C. LUGNIER, C. TRAVO & J. C. STOCLET. 1989. A comparison of cyclic AMP signaling system in rat aortic myocytes in primary culture and aorta. Lab. Invest. **61:** 177–182.

82. NAVAB, M., G. P. HOUGH, L. W. STEVENSON, D. C. DRINKWATER, H. LAKS & A. M. FOGELMAN. 1988. Monocyte migration into the subendothelial space of a coculture of adult human aortic endothelial and smooth muscle cells. J. Clin. Invest. **82:** 1853–1863.

83. THOMAS, W. A. & D. N. KIM. 1983. Atherosclerosis as a hyperplastic and/or neoplastic process. Lab. Invest. **48:** 245–255.

84. MURRAY, C. D., K. T. LEE, M. KROMS & K. JANAKIVEDI. 1988. Clonal nature of atherosclerotic plaques. Exp. Mol. Pathol. **48:** 391–402.

85. BENDITT, E. P. 1988. Origin of human atherosclerotic plaques. The role of altered gene expression. Arch. Pathol. Lab. Med. **112:** 997–1001.

86. SEVANIAN, A. & A. R. PETERSON. 1988. Cholesterol epoxide as a direct-acting mutagen. Proc. Natl. Acad. Sci. USA **81:** 4198–4202.
87. BARRETT, T. B., C. M. GAJDUSEK, S. M. SCHWARTZ, J. K. McDUGALL & E. P. BENDITT. 1984. Expression of the *sis* gene by endothelial cells in culture and *in vivo*. Proc. Natl. Acad. Sci. USA **81:** 6772–6774.
88. TONG, B. D., S. E. LEVINE, M. JAYE, G. RICCA, W. DROHAN, T. MACIAG & T. F. DEVEL. 1986. Isolation and sequencing of a cDNA clone homologous to the v-*sis* oncogene from human endothelial cells. Mol. Cell. Biol. **6:** 3018–3022.
89. HAJJAR, D. P., D. J. FALCONE, C. G. FABRICANT & J. FABRICANT. 1985. Altered cholesteryl ester cycle is associated with lipid accumulation in herpes virus infected arterial smooth muscle cells. J. Biol. Chem. **260:** 6124–6128.
90. YAMASHIROYA, H. M., L. GHOSH, R. YANG & A. L. ROBERTSON, JR. 1988. Herpesviridae in the coronary arteries and aorta of young trauma victims. Am. J. Pathol. **130:** 71–79.
91. BOHR, V. A., M. K. EVANS & A. J. FORNACE. 1989. Biology of disease. DNA repair and its pathogenetic implications. Lab. Invest. **61:** 143–161.

Multinucleated Variant Endothelial Cell

Its Characterization and Relation to Atherosclerosis[a]

TERUO WATANABE AND OSAMU TOKUNAGA

Department of Pathology
Saga Medical School
Saga 840-01, Japan

INTRODUCTION

The recent rediscovery of heterogeneity in human aortic endothelium suggests an alternative relationship between the role of endothelial cells and the development of vascular disease, especially atherosclerosis. Vascular endothelial cells have long been thought to be polygonal and to comprise a homogeneous population forming an *en face* pavement arrangement. Although giant endothelial cells had been found in a Häutchen preparation in the 1940s and 1950s,[1] this topic was not reviewed until Repin *et al.*[2] reaffirmed a significant relationship between endothelial heterogeneity and the presence of atherosclerotic lesions, mainly on the basis of scanning electron microscopic observations. Since our previous report[3] on that human aortic endothelium consisted of a heterogeneous population *in vitro,* more data have been obtained from human aortic endothelial cells cultured at ages ranging from infancy to 83 years.[4] We report here on the morphologic heterogeneity of human aortic endothelial cells, their nature, and the relationship between endothelial heterogeneity and atherosclerosis.

Presence of Multinucleated Variant Endothelial Cells in Primary Culture from Human Aorta

Human endothelial cell culture has been successfully achieved with the addition of ECGF and heparin to the culture medium. Among more than 100 cases attempted, 29 cases, ranging from a 2-month-old infant to an 83-year-old, were analyzed in this study. These cases were pure enough for analysis; more than 95% of the constituent cells were pure with either the endothelial cell specific marker of von Willebrand factor (vWF) or phase contrast microscopic observation.

The cultured endothelial cells could be classified into two distinct types: the typical small type and the larger type. The typical type had round or polygon-shaped cytoplasm with a single nucleus, and cells of this type were arranged in a pavement pattern. This type was generally present in cultures of aortas from infants or children and in cultures of veins from a given specimen. Their diameter was fairly uniform, ranging from 50 to 70 μm. On the other hand, endothelial cells of the second type were more varied in size and shape. They were larger than the typical cells, ranging from 100 to 200 μm in diameter and had more than two nuclei. Giant endothelial cells of more than 250 μm in diameter were intermingled among the typical endothelial cells, and were usually multinucleated, occasionally with 10 or more nuclei, in primary cultures even from adolescent aortas (FIG. 1a).

[a]This work was supported in part by Grants-in-Aid for Scientific Research from the Ministry of Education, Science, and Culture, Japan.

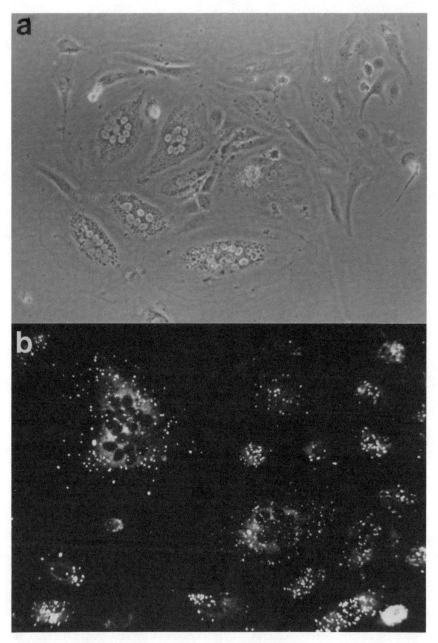

FIGURE 1. (a) Multinucleated variant endothelial cells cultured from aorta of a 24-year-old male. ×360. (b) Giant endothelial cells are vWF-positive by indirect immunofluorescence and one of them possesses 19 nuclei. 81-year-old male. ×510. ((b) from Tokunaga *et al.*[4] Reprinted by permission from J. B. Lippincott Company.)

In this study, we designated vWF-positive multinucleated cells containing more than three nuclei as *variant endothelium*. Binucleated cells were not considered to be variant cells because their possible formation as a result of dispase digestion during culture could not be ruled out.

Successful cultures of endothelial cells were reported from human aortas and arteries in which morphological heterogeneity were not mentioned except for a brief presentation by Antonov *et al.*[5] Other subtypes morphologically or functionally different from conventional typical endothelial cells have been reported by some investigators, such as ring-forming endothelial cells.[6,7] Recently, several factors including shear stress[8] and extracellular matrices[9] were shown to affect the morphological changes of endothelial cells. The presence of multinucleated endothelial cells, however, was not mentioned in any of these investigations.

Variant Cells Have Endothelial Cell Specific Markers but No Mitotic Activity

Multinucleated cells with more than three nuclei were designated as variant endothelium. More than 10 nuclei were occasionally encountered, especially in cases with severe atherosclerosis or from older persons. The multinucleated variant endothelial cells were positive for vWF by immunofluorescence technique (FIG. 1b) and contained Weibel-Palade bodies in the cytoplasm when observed with transmission electron microscopy, both of which are specific markers for endothelial cells.

No uptake of [³H]thymidine in any of these multinuclei was demonstrated by autoradiography, which ruled out the possibility of intracytoplasmic nuclear multiplication without cell division. However, the multinucleated cells survived for at least 5 passages as they were. [³H]Thymidine uptake was found only in the nuclei of mononuclear endothelial cells.

In vivo *Presence of Multinucleated Variant Endothelial Cells*

Harvested endothelial cells from the aorta with atherosclerotic lesions were centrifuged down to form cell pellets, which were not affected by culture manipulation because they were not seeded yet. The constituent cells were varied in size, were vWF-positive, and occasionally revealed more than two nuclei or lobulated nucleus, possibly nuclei. The cell pellet from the aorta of children only consisted of small and regular-sized endothelial cells.

Endothelial cells of aortas from infants and children were small, round, and regular in size, ranging from 15 to 20 μm in diameter when observed by scanning electron microscopy (FIG. 2a). In young adults in their twenties, large endothelial cells were occasionally seen. In adults, colonies of giant endothelial cells, displaying an abrupt transition from the surrounding cells were scattered throughout the aorta that showed age-related intimal thickening (FIG. 2b). The giant endothelial cells were extremely large, occasionally 10 times as large as the surrounding typical small ones. Advanced atherosclerotic lesions were almost invariably covered by large and/or giant endothelial cells. On the other hand, inferior venae cavae from cases of any age were invariably covered with small uniform cells. The *in vivo* presence of multinucleated variant endothelial cells was also confirmed by transmission electron microscopy (FIG. 2c).

The question of whether the multinucleated cells were primarily present in the aorta or secondarily formed during culture manipulation was clearly resolved, and the former theory was proved by these findings.

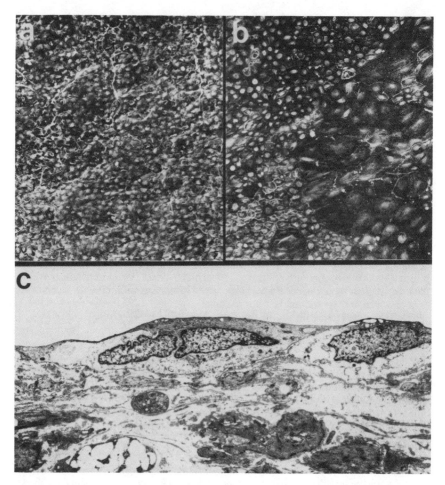

FIGURE 2. Representative picture of endothelium covering *in vivo* aorta observed by scanning and transmission electron microscopy. **(a)** Inner surface of aorta from a 5-year-old boy is thoroughly covered by typical endothelium. × 165. **(b)** Typical endothelial cells *(left half)* and colony of giant endothelial cells *(right half)* are seen in the intimal thickened aorta from a 69-year-old male. × 165. **(c)** Binucleated endothelium is observed in *in vivo* aorta by transmission electron microscopy. 59-year-old male. × 3,500. ((a) and (b) from Tokunaga *et al.*[4] Reprinted by permission from J. B. Lippincott Company.)

Multinucleated Variant Endothelial Cells Are Well Correlated with the Extent of Atherosclerosis

According to the method of Gore and Tajada,[10] atherosclerotic index (AI) of the aorta was scored after the endothelial cells had been harvested, and the ratio of variant endothelial cells per total endothelial cells was analysed in respect to AI and age. AI ranged from 0.01 in a 14-year-old boy to 21.17 in an 81-year-old man. To place a minimal AI value of 0.01 on the base line of graphic representation, conventional AI values were multiplied by 100 and converted into logarithms. The number of concomitant variant endothelial cells from the primary culture was significantly correlated with the severity of atherosclerosis (FIG. 3). The relationship between aging and the number of variant endothelial cells was not as significant as between AI and the number of these cells. This might be the result of selective cultures from older persons with less severe atherosclerotic lesions.

Antonov *et al.*[5] reported that the number of multinucleated endothelial cells at primary culture from atherosclerotic aortas was significantly higher than that from normal aortas, and similarly found no positive relationship to donor age. These authors also found no multinucleated endothelial cells in primary cultures from infant aortas. In contrast, we found that multinucleated endothelial cells were already present, to some extent, in the aorta of a 14-year-old boy.

Morphogenesis and the Role of Variant Endothelial Cells in Atherosclerosis

The presence of colonies made up of giant cells was a surprise, giving rise to questions regarding their mechanism of formation. No incorporation of [³H]thymidine was detected in nuclei of the cultured multinucleated endothelial cells, which ruled out the possibility of intracytoplasmic nuclear multiplication without cell division as mentioned above. An adhesive mechanism, probably induced by injury to the cell membrane, is therefore the most likely possibility.[11] Many factors, such as mechanical, chemical, toxic, viral, or immunologic agents and more recently cytokines[11,12] are known to cause endothelial injury. Exact morphogenesis and the role of variant endothelial cells in atherosclerosis remain unclear. Our results, however, suggest a cyclic effect of the processes. Whether they were formed primarily or secondarily by some unknown mechanism, they would

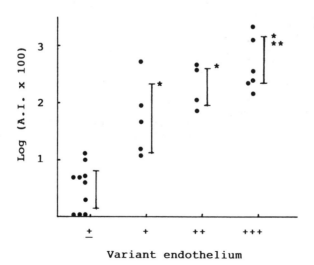

FIGURE 3. Scattergram of atherosclerotic index (A.I.) and variant endothelium. The number of concomitant variant endothelial cells is graded as follows: ±:0–5, +:5–10, + +:10–15, + + +: 15–30%. * means significance against ± grade at $p < 0.01$ and ** against + grade at $p < 0.05$ (Student t test). (From Tokunaga *et al.*[4] Reprinted by permission from J. B. Lippincott Company.)

trigger a further development of atherosclerotic lesions. The development of such lesions would then induce further formation of multinucleated variant endothelial cells.

In conclusion, the endothelial cells that cover the inner surface of the aorta are initially small, polygonal, and single-layered, but large and multinucleated giant cells emerge in correlation with atherosclerotic severity and aging. Further studies are required on the mechanism responsible for genesis of multinucleated endothelial cells and their potential role in atherosclerosis.

REFERENCES

1. McGOVERN, V. J. 1955. Reaction to injury of vascular endothelium with special reference to the problem of thrombosis. J. Pathol. Bacteriol. **69:** 283–293.
2. REPIN, V. S., V. V. DOLGOV, O. E. ZAIKINA, I. D. NAVIKOV, A. S. ANTONOV, M. A. NIKOLAEVA & V. N. SMIRNOV. 1984. Heterogeneity of endothelium in human aorta. A quantitative analysis by scanning microscopy. Atherosclerosis **50:** 35–52.
3. TOKUNAGA, O. & T. WATANABE. 1987. Atherosclerosis and endothelium. Part I. A simple method of endothelial cell culture from human atherosclerotic aorta. Acta. Pathol. Jpn. **37:** 527–536.
4. TOKUNAGA, O., J. FAN & T. WATANABE. 1989. Atherosclerosis- and age-related multinucleated variant endothelial cells in primary culture from human aorta. Am. J. Pathol. **135:** 967–976.
5. ANTONOV, A. S., M. A. NIKOLAEVA, T. S. KLUEVA, YU A. ROMANOV, V. R. BABAEV, V. B. BYSTREVSKAYA, N. A. PEROV, V. S. REPIN & V. N. SMIRNOV. 1986. Primary culture of endothelial cells from atherosclerotic human aorta. Part 1. Identification, morphological and ultrastructural characteristics of two endothelial cell subpopulations. Atherosclerosis **59:** 1–19.
6. FOLKMAN, J. & C. HAUDENSCHILD. 1980. Angiogenesis *in vitro*. Nature **288:** 551–556.
7. TOKUNAGA, O., M. MORIMATSU & T. NAKASHIMA. 1984. Ring formation by human variant endothelial cells *in vitro*. Br. J. Exp. Pathol. **65:** 165–170.
8. ZAND, T., J. NUNNARI, A. H. HOFFMAN, B. SAVILONIS, B. MacWILLIAMS, G. MAJNO & I. JORIS. 1988. Endothelial adaptation in aortic stenosis. Correlation with flow parameters. Am. J. Pathol. **133:** 407–418.
9. KUBOTA, Y., H. K. KLEINMAN, G. R. MARTIN & T. J. LAWLEY. 1988. Role of laminin and basement membrane in the morphological differentiation of human endothelial cells into capillary-like structure. J. Cell Biol. **107:** 1589–1598.
10. GORE, I., & C. TAJADA. 1957. The quantitative appraisal of atherosclerosis. Am. J. Pathol. **33:** 875–882.
11. WATANABE, T., O. TOKUNAGA, J. FAN & T. SHIMOKAMA. 1989. Atherosclerosis and macrophages. Acta Pathol. Jpn. **39:** 473–486.
12. Jørgensen, A. G., G. T. Larsen, R. L. Kinlough-Rathbone & J. F. MUSTARD. 1986. Injury to cultured endothelial cells by thrombin-stimulated platelets. Lab. Invest. **54:** 408–415.

Sustained Arterial Injury and Progression of Atherosclerosis[a]

KATSUO SUEISHI, CHIKAO YASUNAGA,
EMILIO CASTELLANOS, MASATO KUMAMOTO,
AND KENZO TANAKA[b]

Department of Pathology
Faculty of Medicine
Kyushu University
3-1-1 Maidashi, Higashi-ku
Fukuoka 812, Japan

INTRODUCTION

It is well known that various kinds of arterial injury, including those by hypercholesterolemic, immunological, viral, chemical and mechanical factors, participate in the initiation and progression of atherosclerosis. In the arterial wall, moreover, the interactions between cellular components such as endothelial cells, smooth muscle cells, and monocyte-macrophages have been considered to be essential in the atherogenic processes. The "response-to-injury hypothesis" reformulated by R. Ross[1] suggests that PDGF or PDGF-like growth factors derived from platelets, endothelial cells, and macrophages, and cellular interactions along with the increased imbibition of plasma constituents initiate the subsequent events leading to advanced atherosclerosis. The imigration of macrophages and T lymphocytes[2] and complemental deposits[3] within arterial wall have recently caused investigators to refocus on inflammatory aspects in atherogenesis.[4].

It is the purpose of the present report to review our evidence for the possible participation of immune-mediated reaction and angiogenic process as a chronic inflammation-repair process to the pathogenesis of arteriosclerotic lesions.

Immune-Mediated Response in Arteriosclerosis

A large number of studies in a variety of species have shown that the immune system possibly participates in human atherosclerosis[2,3,5-8] and in animal models.[9,10]

The development of intimal thickening and ultrastructural characteristics of aortic lesions were investigated in rats receiving a cholesterol-rich diet from 6 weeks to 30 weeks old and/or repeated injections of ovalbumin (3 mg/Kg bodyweight), subcutaneously with complete Freund's adjuvant, followed by 2.5 mg/Kg bodyweight, intraperitoneally, weekly, 5 times) from 24 weeks to 29 weeks old.

The repeated administration of ovalbumin in hypercholesterolemic rats induced an intimal thickening, which was statistically greater than that induced only by hypercho-

[a]This work was supported in part by a Grant-in-Aid from the Ministry of Education, Science and Culture of Japan (#63304045, 63637005, 01637005, 01480161).
[b]Emeritus professor, Kyushu University.

lesterolemia in the carotid artery ($p < 0.01$), thoracic aorta ($p < 0.05$) and abdominal aorta ($p < 0.01$).

The ultrastructural features observed were characterized by widespread adhesion of mononuclear cells to the endothelial surface (FIG. 1), migration of monocytes between the endothelial cells into the intima, proliferation of smooth muscle cells in the intima, minor endothelial cell damage including endothelial desquamation without denudation, duplication of the internal elastic lamina, and fragmentation of elastic fibers. These changes were more severe in the immune-challenged animals.

These findings support the evidence that the recruitment of monocyte-macrophages in the arterial intima, accompanied with minor ultrastructural endothelial damage, is involved in the initiation and progression of arteriosclerosis, and immunologic response

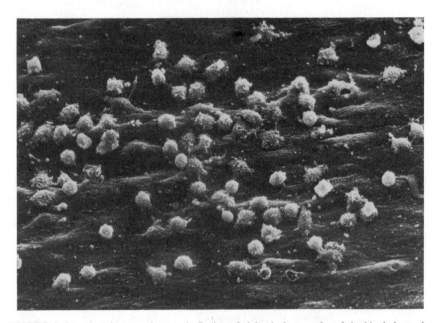

FIGURE 1. Scanning electron microscopic finding of abdominal aorta of rat fed with cholesterol-rich diet and also with repeated injections of ovalbumin. Many leukocytes adhered on the endothelial surface, which is scatteringly buldged probably due to the migration of leukocytes into the subendothelial intima. × 1,800.

plays an essential role in the atherogenesis as an inflammation-repair process. The immunological approach to the atherogenic process may explain the development of arteriosclerosis in the absence of hypercholesterolemia, hypertension, and other well-known risk factors and the earlier and greater atherosclerotic damage found in patients with immunologic disorders.

Pathophysiological Significance of Angiogenesis in Coronary Atherosclerosis

Intimal Neovascularization In Vivo

Angiogenesis is a vital response in various physiological and pathological events such as inflammation, wound repair, and solid tumor growth. In cardiovascular lesions, ne-

TABLE 1. Neovascularization in Atherosclerotic Intima of Human Coronary Arteries

	Luminal Narrowing (% Area)		
	−50 (n = 9)	50–75 (n = 17)	75– (n = 22)
Luminal stenosis (MV ± SD)	35 ± 15	62 ± 7	88 ± 7
Vascular lumen/intima (% area. MV)	0–0.10 (0.07)	0–0.42 (0.33)	0–0.90 (0.35)
No. of vessels (MV)	0–30 (5)	0–86 (14)	0–70 (19)

ovascularization occurs ubiquitously as organization and recanalization of thrombus, and aberrant vasa vasorum in atherosclerotic intima. Several reports have found that newly formed microvessels in atherosclerotic intima are relatively fragile, indicating that these vessels are related to the occurrence of intimal hemorrhage, and rupture of atheroma followed by occlusive thrombi and vascular spasm. Examination of human coronary arteries obtained at autopsy by the barium sulfate infusion method and quantitatively morphometric analysis, revealed that the extent of intimal neovascularization was correlated with the severity of atherosclerosis (TABLE 1).

Analyzing the origin of angiogenic growth from either luminal or adventitial vascular endothelial cells, using postmortem angiographs of methyl salicylate-cleared hearts with Microfil®, we segmentally documented delicate vascular plexuses or networks in close vicinity to the proper lumen of coronary arteries associated with atherosclerotic narrowing (FIG. 2). The light microscopic examination of successive sections revealed that newly

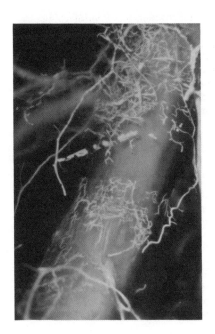

FIGURE 2. Neovascularization of coronary artery. The newly formed vascular networks are segmentally documented with Microfil® infusion, and locate in the close vicinity to the proper lumen of coronary artery with atherosclerotic narrowing.

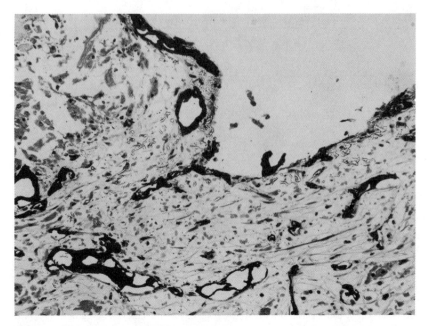

FIGURE 3. Light microscopic finding of newly formed vessels in the atherosclerotic intima. A blood vessel directly connects with the proper lumen of coronary artery, indicating that this blood vessel in the intima is derived from luminal endothelial growth. H.E. ×260.

formed blood vessels in atherosclerotic lesions were derived mainly from adventitial and partly from luminal endothelial growth (FIG. 3).

Intimal neovascularization is probably a normal response to injury and this angiogenic process may involve various factors such as platelet-, macrophage-, and smooth muscle cell-derived growth factors, and hypoxic environment. Therefore, intimal neovascularization may be essential as an inflammation-repair process in the pathogenesis of coronary atherosclerosis and the following sequelae, such as intimal hemorrhage, rupture of fibrous plaque, and formation of occlusive thrombi, possibly leading to acute myocardial infarction.

Angiogenes In Vitro

The bovine capillary endothelial cells (BCE) were isolated from the bovine adrenal cortex[11] and fifth to tenth passages of culture were used in the following studies. BCE (5 × 10^5) were seeded on type I collagen gel (2 mg/ml) in 12-well plates and cultivated in RPMI 1640 medium supplemented with 10% fetal calf serum (FCS). BCE reached confluency in 2 to 3 days and started to sprout into collagen gel, and then to organize tubular structures after about 3 days.

On Day 7 or 9 of culture, these tubular structures were randomly photographed at 9 areas in each well in triplicates under a phase-contrast microscope. The length of tubular structures in the photographs were morphometrically measured. The total length was calculated for each well. The total length of tubular structures examined with the morphometric method was well correlated with the total number of capillary-like lumina in paraffin sections.

Effects of Plasminogen, Anti-PA IgGs, and Plasmin Inhibitors on Angiogenesis

The addition of plasminogen to the gel at several concentrations up to 25 μg/ml enhanced the capillary growth in a dose-dependent manner. Although basic fibroblast growth factor (bFGF) alone at 10 ng/ml or plasminogen (25 μg/ml) alone did not enhance capillary growth, the simultaneous addition of plasminogen (25 μg/ml) and bFGF (10 ng/ml) increased the capillary growth (FIG. 4).

Therefore, the culture system of BCE on type I collagen gel containing plasminogen (5 μg/ml) and in RPMI-1640 supplemented with 10% FCS and bFGF (10 ng/ml) was used to analyze the effects of anti-PA IgGs on capillary growth of BCE. Specific anti-IgG against t-PA or u-PA (10 μg/ml)[12] was added to both culture media and gels. As shown in FIGURE 5, tube formation was significantly decreased on Day 4 in the presence of anti-IgGs to u-PA and t-PA, compared to the controls containing either nonimmunized IgG or no IgG. On Day 7, the wells treated with anti-u-PA IgG showed a significant decrease in tube formation, but not with anti-t-PA.

A plasmin inhibitor such as aprotinin (Trysylol®, 250 μ/ml), epsilon-aminocaproic acid (ε-ACA, 500 μg/ml), soybean trypsin inhibitor (100 μg/ml) or α_2 plasmin inhibitor (2.5 μg/ml) was preabsorbed into the gels containing 25 μg/ml of plasminogen, and also added to culture media containing 10% FCS and 10 ng/ml of bFGF. As shown in FIGURE 6, all plasmin inhibitors significantly reduced the capillary growth to about one-third of the control without any inhibitor.

BCE synthesize and release both t-PA and u-PA, and PA inhibitor-1 (PAI-1) under various culture conditions.[12] Culturing BCE on type 1 collagen gels, fibrin enzymographical analysis of culture media revealed that the fibrinolytic activity of t-PA with M.W. of 72,000 and 124,000 (t-PA · PAI-1 complex) and that of u-PA with M.W. of 100,000 (u-PA · PAI-1 complex) were increased, whereas the activity of free u-PA with a M.W. of 42,000 was decreased. Thus, addition of bFGF enhanced BCE to release both species

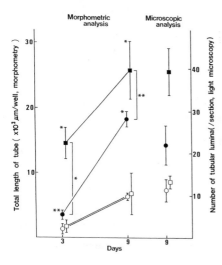

FIGURE 4. Effects of plasminogen and bFGF on tube formation of BCEs. The *right-hand points* show the number of lumina examined with light microscope of paraffin embedded collagen gels. The BCEs were cultured in the presence of plasminogen (25 μg/ml) *(solid marks)* in the gel, and in the presence *(square marks)* or absence *(circle marks)* of bFGF (10 ng/ml) in the media. Mean values (± SD) of three experiments are shown. (*p <0.01, **p <0.05.) (From Yasunaga *et al.*[22] Reprinted by permission from *Laboratory Investigation*.)

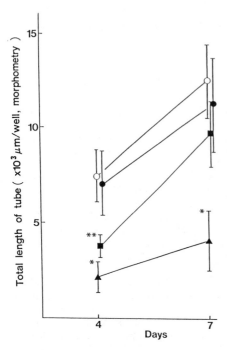

FIGURE 5. Effects of anti-plasminogen activator IgGs on tube formation of BCEs. BCEs were cultured in the media containing nonimmunized IgG (●), anti-t-PA IgG (■), anti-u-PA IgG (▲), or no IgG (○). The collagen gels were preincubated in 2.5 ml of serum-free media with or without the respective IgG for 7 days at 4°C. The final concentration of IgG added is 10 μg/ml. Plasminogen, 5 μg/ml in gel; bFGF, 10 ng/ml in medium. Mean values (± SD) of three experiments are shown. (*p <0.01, **p <0.05.) (From Yasunaga et al.[22] Reprinted by permission from *Laboratory Investigation*.)

of PA and PAI-1 into conditioned media and increased PA activity, mainly of u-PA (TABLE 2).

These findings indicate that the fibrinolysis system is involved in angiogenesis and that u-PA secreted from BCE, plays a role in the fibrinolytic activation and regulates the extracellular proteolysis in angiogenesis as well as in tumor cell migration.[13,14] Plasminogen is a zymogen found in all extracellular tissue and fluids[15] and is a specific substrate to both u-PA and t-PA. Plasmin is a broad-spectrum protease that promotes via procollagenase-plasmin-active collagenase system,[15] and the degradation of the extracellular matrices. Anti-t-PA IgG suppressed the capillary growth at the early phase. As PAI-1 participates in the regulation of fibrinolytic activation by specifically inhibiting the activity of t-PA as well as double chain u-PA at almost the same association rate constant, the effect of t-PA on angiogenesis may be associated with a t-PA-dependent decrease in

TABLE 2. PA Activity in Conditioned Media of BCEs Measured by Chromogenic Peptide (S-2251) Assay: Effects of Culturing on Collagen Gel, Plasminogen, and bFGF[a]

Culture Conditions	Control (mIU/ml)	bFGF (10 ng/ml) Treatment (mIU/ml)
Culture on plastic dish	513.4 ± 359.1	1353.3 ± 498.1[b]
Culture on collagen gel without plasminogen	160.6 ± 42.4	310.0 ± 130.0[b]
Culture on collagen gel with plasminogen (25 μg/ml)	117.3 ± 22.0	140.0 ± 70.0[b]

[a]Means ± SD for triplicated dishes.
[b]This PA activity was completely quenched by anti-uPA IgG but not by anti-tPA IgG.

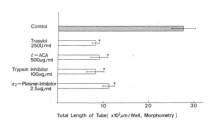

Total Length of Tube(x10³μm/Well, Morphometry)

FIGURE 6. Effects of serine-proteinase inhibitors on tube formation of BCEs on sixth day. Control medium, Trasylol®, ε-aminocaproic acid (ε-ACA), soybean trypsin inhibitor (trypsin inhibitor) and α₂-plasmin inhibitor were added in the same experimental condition as described in FIGURE 4. Plasminogen, 25 μg/ml in gel; bFGF, 10 ng/ml in medium. Mean values (± SD) of three experiments are shown. (*p <0.01.) (From Yasunaga *et al.*[22] Reprinted by permission from *Laboratory Investigation.*)

PAI-1 and the subsequent increase of u-PA activity. (From Yasunaga *et al.*[22] Reprinted by permission from *Laboratory Investigation.*)

Effects of Growth Factors and Cytokines on Angiogenesis

The effects of bFGF (10 ng/ml), transforming growth factor β, (TGFβ, 10 ng/ml), recombinant insulin-like growth factor-1 (rIGF-1, 200 ng/ml), recombinant tumor necrosis factor α (rTNFα, 100 u/ml), recombinant interleukin-1 (rIL-1 10 u/ml) and recombinant interleukin-2 (rIL-2, 10 u/ml), which were added to in condition media, on the capillary growth of BCE in type I collagen gel containing 25 μg/ml of plasminogen were morphometrically examined. As shown in FIGURES 4 and 7, bFGF and TGFβ increased the angiogenesis (p <0.05), but rTNFα and rIL-1 suppressed it (p <0.01). These growth factors and cytokines have been shown to modulate the production of PA and PAI-1 from normal and neoplastic cells. bFGF enhances the synthesis and secretion of PA and PAI-1 from endothelial cells, whereas rTNF and IL-1 suppress the fibrinolytic activity by increasing PAI-1 activity and decreasing PA activity.[16] rTNF also induces the synthesis and expression of biologically active IL-1 from endothelial cells. Thus, these cytokines alter the endothelial cell functions including angiogenesis. The effect of TGFβ, however, on the fibrinolysis system has been reported to be diverse,[17] especially concerning the secretion of u-PA, although TGFβ enhances the expression and secretion of PAI-1 in pericellular matrix.[18] TGFβ also enhances capillary tube formation *in vitro* through the modulation of extracellular matrix formation.[19] Therefore, the enhancement of angiogenesis by TGFβ may be associated with other factors besides the fibrinolytic system.

The Role of Fibrinolytic Activity In Angiogenesis

In cultured endothelial cells u-PA is primarily cell-associated with its receptors on endothelial cells.[20] The autocrine production of u-PA from endothelial cells suggests that

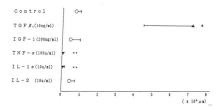

(x 10⁹ μm)

FIGURE 7. Effects of growth factors and cytokines on angiogenesis in *in vitro* assay system. Bovine capillary endothelial cells (BCEs) were cultured on the collagen gel containing 2.0 mg/ml of type I collagen and 25 μg/ml of plasminogen. TGFβ₂ increased the angiogenesis *in vitro* (*p <0.05). TNF-α and IL-1α decreased the angiogenesis *in vitro*, respectively (**p <0.01). Mean values ± SD. n = 4.

the pericellular proteolysis of matrix by plasmin itself or plasmin activated collagenase is of importance in localized precesses. u-PA has been shown to enhance the endothelial migration in the presence of plasminogen.[21] These *in vitro* findings support the hypothesis that the activation of the fibrinolysis system is closely related to antiogenesis (FIG. 8).[22] Thus, neovascularization in atherosclerotic intima can be modulated not only by hypoxic environment but also by several growth factors and cytokines, which may themselves modulate their receptor expression of vascular cells, leading to the particular perspective that the monocyte-macrophages and lymphocytes play an essential role in atherosclerosis as the inflammation-repair process.

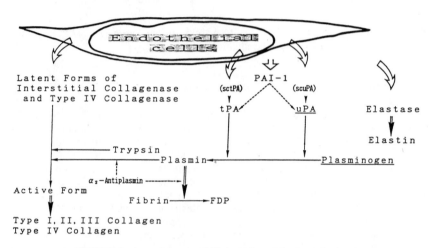

FIGURE 8. A possible role of fibrinolytic activity in angiogenesis.

SUMMARY

In this paper the following findings were described: 1) Murine arteriosclerosis induced by immune challenge was ultrastructurally characterized by intimal monocyte-macrophage recruitment and minor endothelial alterations; 2) Atherosclerotic lesions of human coronary arteries exhibited frequently segmental or patchy neovascularization, probably representing a response to intimal injury as an example of repair process. Newly formed blood vessels in the intima were derived from both adventitial and luminal endothelial growth; 3) Angiogenesis *in vitro* was related to the activation of fibrinolytic system especially via the autocrine production of u-PA from endothelial cells, and this process was modulated by cytokines and TGFβ.

These findings add more evidence for the hypothesis that the chronic inflammation-repair process plays an essential role in the initiation and progression of atherosclerosis.

REFERENCES

1. Ross, R. 1986. The pathogenesis of atherosclerosis—An update. N. Engl. J. Med. **314:** 488–500.
2. WAL, A.C., P. K. VAN DER DAS, D. B. VAN DE BERG, C. M. VAN DER LOOS & A. E. BECKER.

1989. Atherosclerotic lesions in humans. In situ immunophenotypic analysis suggesting an immune mediated response. Lab. Invest. **61:** 166–170.

3. RUS, H. G., F. NICULESCU & R. VLAICU. 1988. The relationship between macrophages and C5b-9 component complexes in human atherosclerosis. Clin. Immunol. Immunopathol. **48:** 307–316.

4. WATANABE, T., O. TOKUNAGA, J. FAN & T. SHIMOKAMA. 1989. Atherosclerosis and macrophages. Acta Pathol. Jpn. **39:** 473–486.

5. ROMANO, E. L., M. SOTOLONGO-PONS, G. CAMEJO & A. SOYANO. 1984. Circulating immune complexes, immunoglobulins, complement, antibodies to dietary antigens, cholesterol and lipoproteins levels in patients with occlusive coronary lesions. Atherosclerosis **53:** 119–128.

6. CAPLAN, M., A. HASTILLO, T. MOHANAKUMAR & M. HESS. 1984. Immunologic mechanisms in the atherosclerotic process. Cardiovasc. Rev. Rep. **7:** 713–721.

7. FUKUMOTO, S., T. TSUMAGARI, M. KINJO & K. TANAKA. 1987. Coronary atherosclerosis in patients with systemic lupus erythematosus at autopsy. Acta Pathol. Jpn. **37:** 1–9.

8. TANAKA, K., J. MASUDA, T. IMAMURA, K. SUEISHI, T. NAKASHIMA, I. SAKURAI, T. SHOZAWA, Y. HOSODA, Y. YOSHIDA, Y. NISHIYAMA, C. YUTANI & S. HATANO. 1988. A nation-wide study of atherosclerosis in infants, children and young adults in Japan. Atherosclerosis **72:** 143–156.

9. MINICK, C. R. & G. E. MURPHY. 1973. Experimental induction of athero-arteriosclerosis by the synergy of allergic injury to arteries and lipid-rich diet. II. Effect of repeatedly injected foreign protein in rabbits fed a lipid-rich, cholesterol-poor diet. Am. J. Pathol. **73:** 265–300.

10. MAJNO, G., I. JORIS & T. ZAND. 1985. Atherosclerosis: New horizons. Hum. Pathol. **16:** 3–5.

11. FOLKMAN, J., C. C. HAUDENSCHILD & B. R. ZETTER. 1979. Long-term culture of capillary endothelial cells. Proc. Natl. Acad. Sci. USA **76:** 5217–5221.

12. NAKASHIMA, Y., K. SUEISHI & K. TANAKA. 1988. Thrombin enhances production and release of tissue plasminogen activator from bovine venous endothelial cells. Fibrinolysis **2:** 227–234.

13. MIGNATTI, P., E. ROBBINS & D. B. RIFKIN. 1986. Tumor invasion through the human amniotic membrane. Cell **47:** 487–498.

14. REICH, R., E. W. THOMPSON, Y. IWAMOTO, G. R. MARTIN, J. R. DEASON, G. C. FULLER & R. MISKIN. 1988. Effects of inhibitors of plasminogen activator, serine proteinases, and collagenases IV on the invasion of basement membranes by metastatic cells. Cancer Res. **48:** 3307–3312.

15. BLASI, F. 1988. Surface receptors for urokinase plasminogen activator. Fibrinolysis **2:** 73–84.

16. SCHLEEF, R. R., M. P. BEVILACQUA, M. SAWDEY, M. A. GIMBRONE & D. J. LOSKUTOFF. 1988. Cytokine activation of vascular endothelium. Effects on tissue-type plasminogen activator and type 1 plasminogen activator inhibitor. J. Biol. Chem. **263:** 5797–5803.

17. SAKSELA, O., D. MOSCATELLI & D. B. RIFKIN. 1987. The opposing effects of basic fibroblast growth factor and transforming growth factor beta on the regulation of plasminogen activator activity in capillary endothelial cells. J. Cell Biol. **105:** 957–963.

18. LAIHO, M. 1988. Modulation of extracellular proteolytic activity and anchorage-independent growth of cultured cells by sarcoma cell-derived factors: Relationships to transforming growth factor-β. Exp. Cell Res. **176:** 297–308.

19. ROBERTS, A. B., M. B. SPORN, R. A. ASSOIAN, N. S. ROCHE, L. M. WAKEFIELD, U. I. HEINE, L. A. LIOTTA, V. FALANGA, J. H. KEHRL & A. S. FAUCI. 1986. Transforming growth factor type: Rapid induction of fibrosis and angiogenesis *in vivo* and stimulation of collagen formation *in vitro*. Proc. Natl. Acad. Sci. USA **83:** 4167–4171.

20. MOSCATELLI, D. 1986. Urokinase-type and tissue-type plasminogen activators have different distributions in cultured bovine capillary endothelial cells. J. Cell. Biochem. **30:** 19–29.

21. PEPPER, M. S., J. D. VASSALLI, R. MONTESANO & L. ORCI. 1987. Urokinase-type plasminogen activator is induced in migrating capillary endothelial cells. J. Cell Biol. **105:** 2535–2541.

22. YASUNAGA, C., Y. NAKASHIMA & K. SUEISHI. 1989. A role of fibrinolytic activity in angiogenesis. Quantitative assay using *in vitro* method. Lab. Invest. **61:** 698–704.

Competence Growth Factors Evoke the Phenotypic Transition of Arterial Smooth Muscle Cells[a]

MITSUYASU KATO AND MASAHISA KYOGOKU

Department of Pathology
Tohoku University School of Medicine
Sendai 980, Japan

INTRODUCTION

Arteriosclerosis is one of the most important diseases to be overcome. It is thought to be the result of response to an injury[1] on the arterial wall which could have several causes, such as atheromatous change, hypertension, arteritis, and drug-induced injury. Common histopathological appearance in these circumstances is the accumulation of extracellular matrices such as collagens, elastin, and proteoglycans on the wall. It occurs mostly in the intima and is a consequence of cellular intimal thickening.

One of the most important discoveries about the pathogenesis of arteriosclerosis has been that the smooth muscle cells can secrete fibrous matrices to make fibrous intimal thickening.[2-5] Smooth muscle cells that migrate to the intima and accomplish phenotypical transformation are called, "modified smooth muscle cells" or "synthetic form."[5-7] In their normal condition, vascular smooth muscle cells are confined to the arterial media and have numerous contractile filaments in their cytoplasm to give tension to the arterial wall. In response to injury, the same cells produce extracellular matrices and resemble fibroblasts. Such matrix syntheses repair the injured arterial wall on the one hand, but on the other hand bring an irreversible structural change to the arterial wall. This is the arteriosclerosis itself. In this paper, we are going to present *in vitro* studies to examine how isolated vascular smooth muscle cells (V-SMC) from human aorta accomplish phenotypic change in relation to its growth. V-SMC are suspected of losing contractile components and getting synthetic traits during the cell division cycle, and reconstructing contractile equipment after they stop growing, under the influence of competence factors.

EXPERIMENTAL PROCEDURE

Materials

Human arterial tissues were obtained from autopsy cases in our laboratory. Collagenase (type I), insulin, and ribonuclease A were purchased from Sigma Chemical Company (St. Louis, MO). Daigo's T nutrient medium was from Nippon Pharmaceutical Corporation (Tokyo, Japan). Minimum essential medium (MEM) and phosphate-buffered saline

[a]Financial support was obtained in part from Grants-in-Aid for Scientific Research from the Ministry of Education, Science, and Culture of Japan, Research Grants for Intractable Diseases from the Ministry of Health and Welfare of Japan, and Research Grants from the Uehara Memorial Foundation.

232

(PBS) were from Nissui (Tokyo, Japan). PDGF was from Bioprocessing (Durham, England). Epidermal growth factor (EGF) and collagen (type I) were from Collaborative Research (Bedford, MA). Monoclonal antibody to α-smooth muscle actin and propidium iodide (PI) were from Sigma (St. Louis, MO). Anti-prolyl 4-hydroxylase was from Fuji Chemical Corporation (Takaoka, Japan). Biotinized anti-mouse IgG and fluorescein isothiocyanate (FITC)-labeled avidin were from Vector Laboratories (Burlingame, California).

Isolation and Culture of Smooth Muscle Cells from Human Vascular Tissue

Human thoracic aortae were obtained one to 5 hr postmortem, placed in MEM containing gentamycin (5 μg/ml), penicillin G (100 μg/ml), and amphotericin B (5 μg/ml), and maintained at 4°C until processing. Adventitial tissues were totally removed and after extensive washing with PBS, aortic tissues were incubated with 0.1% collagenase in MEM at 37°C for 1 hr. Its intima was scraped with a scalpel blade and extensively washed to obtain the medial plates composed of only smooth muscle cells. This medial plate was minced and digested to single cells with 0.1% collagenase in MEM containing bovine serum albumin (BSA) and antibiotic drugs at 20°C for 15 to 24 hr. Cells were passed through mesh and harvested by centrifugation at $100 \times$ g for 5 min, then suspended in Daigo's T medium and plated in T-25 culture flasks coated with collagen. Growth medium for primary and serial stock cultures of V-SMC consisted of Daigo's T medium containing EGF (10 ng/ml), insulin (1 μg/ml), and 5% FBS. Cells that started to grow were subcultured once weekly at 1:3 dilution, and the second passage cells were used for following experiments.

Immunocytochemical Staining and Flowcytometry

Freshly isolated cells and cells harvested from each culture condition were fixed with 80% acetone and washed three times with PBS containing 0.1% BSA (PBS/BSA). The cells were then exposed to unlabeled primary antibodies for 2 hr. Secondary exposure to biotinized anti-mouse IgG was followed by the exposure to FITC-avidin for 1 hr. For DNA staining, digestion with ribonuclease (37°C, 30 min) was followed by exposure to PI (50 μg/ml in PBS) for 10 min. Then, the cells were offered to FACScan analysis (Becton Dickinson). All antibodies and FITC-avidin were diluted in PBS, containing 10% normal horse serum. Staining reaction were performed at 4°C. Between each step from fixation to flowcytometry, the cells were washed three times with PBS/BSA.

Immunofluorescence Microscopy

Cells were cultured on glass coverslips coated with collagen. Fixation and staining method were the same as those mentioned above. After extensive rinsing in PBS, the coverslips were mounted in glycerol. The specimens were examined and photographed using a Zeiss Axiomat fluorescence microscope.

RESULTS

Phenotypic Change of V-SMC Could Be Detected by Flowcytometry

Immunofluorescent staining and flowcytometry were used to detect the α-smooth muscle specific (SM) actin and prolyl-4-hydroxylase (ProHy) expressed in V-SMC. Hu-

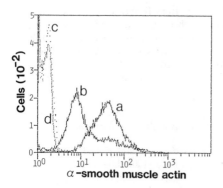

FIGURE 1. Human aortic smooth muscle cells exhibit the transitional expression of α-smooth muscle actin. X-axis, relative intensity of fluorescence reflecting the quantity of α-smooth muscle actin; Y-axis, cell number ($\times$ 10^{-2}). Cells: a & c, freshly isolated cells from human aortic media; b & d, exponentially growing cells, second passage in serum-containing medium. Staining: a & b were stained as described in Experimental Procedure using anti-α-smooth muscle actin antibody for the first antibody, and c & d were the same as a & b except for the use of dilution buffer in place of the first antibody (negative control for nonspecific fluorescence). For each condition 10^4 cells were counted.

man adult V-SMC were obtained from the aortae of autopsy cases with collagenase digestion to single cells. Some of the cells were fixed directly after digestion and stained immunocytochemically as described in Experimental Procedure and offered to flowcytometry. The others were used to establish the primary cultures and serial stock cultures.

V-SMC immediately after isolation from aortic media exhibited a single peak of strong reactivity for anti-α-SM actin antibody (FIG. 1) but no detectable specific fluorescence to indicate the reaction of anti-ProHy antibody (FIG. 2). On the other hand, cultured cells of the same origin growing exponentially in the serum-containing medium appeared to have a decreased amount of α-SM actin (FIG. 1) and increased ProHy (FIG. 2). These results told us that two different conditions of V-SMC, one just isolated from aortic media and other harvested at their growing state in culture, had different traits with regard to their functions of contraction and matrix synthesis.

They changed their phenotypic expression, which apparently associated with their growth. But we have to rule out the influence of low blood pressure, three dimensional composition, and neuronal stimuli. Therefore, we tried to confirm the reversibility of α-SM actin expression after inhibition of growth.

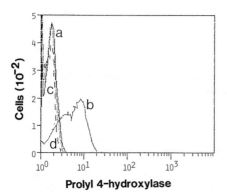

FIGURE 2. Human aortic smooth muscle cells exhibit the transitional expression of prolyl 4-hydroxylase. X-axis, relative intensity of fluorescence reflecting the quantity of prolyl 4-hydroxylase; Y-axis, cell number (10^{-2}). Cells: a & c, freshly isolated cells from human aortic media; b & d, exponentially growing cells in serum-containing medium. Staining: a & b were stained as described in Experimental Procedure using anti-prolyl-4-hydroxylase antibody for the first antibody, and c & d were the same as a & b except for the use of dilution buffer in place of the first antibody (negative control of nonspecific fluorescence). For each condition 10^4 cells were counted.

α-SM Actin Came Back Again After Growth Inhibition

Cultured V-SMC without serum stopped growing without degenerating or dying. We could continue the culture of V-SMC in such serum-free condition at least 100 days leaving an ability to regrow.

Growth-arrested cells expressed more but rearranged α-SM actin filaments (FIG. 3A and 4A). Moreover, two-dimensional analysis of α-SM actin and DNA contents revealed that the α-SM actin induction occurred only in the increased cell populations which have a low amount (2n) of DNA (FIG. 3B). The α-SM actin contents of evidently still growing

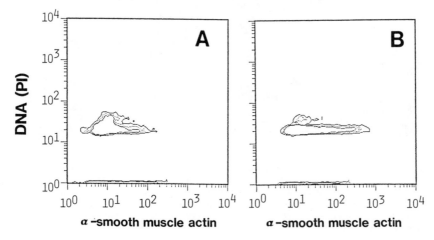

FIGURE 3. α-smooth muscle actin came back after serum starvation which was limited to the cells of low DNA quantity. X-axis, relative intensity of fluorescence (wave length = 515–545 nm) reflecting the quantity of α-smooth muscle actin; Y-axis, relative intensity of fluorescence (wave length = 563–607 nm) reflecting the quantity of DNA (2×10^1 equivalent to the DNA quantity of diploid cells). Cells: **(A)** exponentially growing cells in serum containing medium; **(B)** the cells in (A) were placed in serum-free and growth-factor-free medium for 2 days and reseeded on new dishes coated with collagen to culture without growth factors for another 2 days. Staining: (A) & (B) were stained as described in Experimental Procedure using anti-α-smooth muscle actin antibody for the first antibody. For each assay 10^4 cells were counted.

cells despite serum starvation showed no difference from that of exponentially growing cells in serum-containing media. This suggests that serum starvation worked not directly but with intervention of growth arrest.

Rearrangement of α-SM Actin Filaments Blocked by Competence Factors

The hypothesis that phenotype modulation (at least the expression of α-SM actin) depends on growth states was confirmed by the effects of growth factors.

The rearrangement of α-SM actin induced by serum starvation was completely blocked by the addition of PDGF which was a well-known competence factor for V-SMC in the well (FIG. 4B). Furthermore, PDGF broke down the α-SM actin filaments which had already induced under the serum-free condition. Another competence factor such as

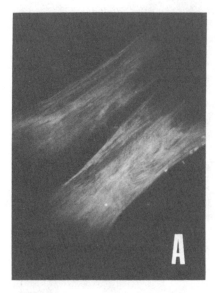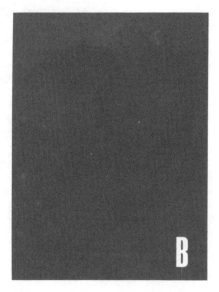

FIGURE 4. Immunocytochemical demonstration of rearrangement of α-smooth muscle actin and its inhibition by PDGF. Cells: **(A)** exponentially growing cells in serum-containing medium were placed in serum-free and growth-factor-free medium for 2 days and reseeded on glass coverslips coated with collagen to culture without growth factors another 2 days; **(B)** the same as (A) except for the addition of PDGF (2.5 U/ml) after reseeding. Staining: (A) & (B) were stained as described in Experimental Procedure using anti-α-smooth muscle actin for the first antibody. Fixation, staining, and photographing were all performed under the same conditions for (A) & (B).

basic FGF also brought the same effect. These results told us α-SM actin expression was dependent on whether the cells are in the competent state or not.

DISCUSSION

Phenotypic modulation of V-SMC had been studied previously by the aid of electron microscopy, and of chemical[8,9] and cytochemical[6,10] analysis. In this report, flowcytometry was introduced to examine the cells of transitional phenotype expression. These differences could not come from the differences of cellular subtype. It must be the altered expression of some traits in the same cells. Because, the cells belonging to the minor subtype must be, if anything, less than 0.01 percent of the population estimated from the unicellularity of obtained cells and ensured by flowcytometry (FIG. 1). Such cells must be passed more than 13 generation times to overcome the major cell group. This would not be possible.

We could introduce not only unidirectional transition from contractile to synthetic phenotype in primary culture but also bidirectional phenotypic change in cultured V-SMC by chemically defined single factors. This process is interesting biologically in itself, but is also worthy of attention clinicopathologically because of its resemblance to the modification of smooth muscle structure and function that occurs during the formation of arteriosclerotic lesion.

Arterial injuries have two ultimate forms that cause arterial dysfunction, which is fatal. They are "obstruction" and "rupture." These two very different forms could be regarded as an accumulated cicatrix of repair reaction and a "behind time" repair. The success of antiinflammatory and antithrombotic therapies for arteritis syndrome reduced the high death rate from rupture or thrombosis, but it left arteriosclerosis in their place. Our system is useful for detailed studies on the cellular and molecular mechanism of arterial smooth muscle phenotypic change and subsequently for finding a clue to prevention or effective treatment of arteriosclerosis.

SUMMARY

Vascular smooth muscle cells (V-SMC) alter their functions from contraction to production of extracellular matrices during the response to injury of the arterial wall. Accumulation of these matrices characterize the chronic structural change of arteriosclerosis. In this paper, we reported as follows. (1) V-SMC freshly isolated from human aortic media had strong reactivity with anti-smooth muscle specific α-actin (α-SM actin) antibody but not with anti-prolyl 4-hydroxylase (ProHy) antibody. (2) The exponentially growing cells in serum-containing culture media reduced α-SM actin and induced ProHy distinctly. (3) Growth-arrested cells with serum starvation rearranged numerous α-SM actin fibers in their cytoplasm. And the rearrangement of contractile filaments inhibited by the addition of single competence growth factor, such as platelet derived growth factor (PDGF) or basic fibroblast growth factor (bFGF). These results suggest that V-SMC change their phenotype in a competence-factor-dependent manner.

ACKNOWLEDGMENTS

We are extremely grateful to Ryo Ichinohasama, M.D., Ph.D. (Department of Pathology, Tohoku University Hospital) and to Fujisawa Pharmaceutical Co., Ltd. for generously allowing us to use the FACScan analyzer.

REFERENCES

1. Ross, R. 1986. N. Engl. J. Med. **314:** 488–500.
2. Altschul, R. 1950. Selected Studies on Atherosclerosis. 182. Charles Thomas. Springfield, IL.
3. Parker, F. 1960. Am. J. Pathol. **36:** 19–53.
4. Webster, W. S., S. P. Bishop & J. C. Geer. 1974. Am. J. Pathol. **76:** 245–264.
5. Campbell, J. C. H. & G. R. Campbell. 1981. Atherosclerosis **40:** 347–357.
6. Sjölund, M., K. Madsen, K. von der Mark & J. Thyberg. 1986. Differentiation **32:** 173–180.
7. Sjölund, M., U. Hedin, T. Sejersen, C. H. Heldin & J. Thyberg. 1988. J. Cell Biol. **106:** 403–413.
8. Burke, J. M., G. Balian, R. Ross & P. Bornstein. 1977. Biochemistry **16:** 3243–3249.
9. Goodman, L. V. & R. A. Majack. 1989. J. Biol. Chem. **264**(9): 5241–5244.
10. Kato, M., T. Sawai & M. Kyogoku. 1989. Proceedings of 3rd International Conference on Kawasaki Disease. 156–158. Japan Heart Foundation. Tokyo, Japan.

The Fibrinolytic System of the Vessel Wall and Its Role in the Control of Thrombosis

DAVID J. LOSKUTOFF AND SCOTT A. CURRIDEN

Research Institute of Scripps Clinic
10666 North Torrey Pines Road
La Jolla, California 92037

INTRODUCTION

It is generally assumed that homeostasis in the circulatory system results from the regulated interaction of the coagulation and fibrinolytic systems. These systems appear to be in dynamic equilibrium, and any imbalance in them leads to an increased risk of thrombosis or a tendency to develop a bleeding diathesis.[1] This balance may be disturbed in the atherosclerotic vessel wall since, "Commonly, the critical event that converts an asymptomatic atherosclerotic plaque into a symptomatic one is thrombosis, whereas non-diseased arteries rarely become thrombotic."[2] In this case, thrombosis is most likely initiated upon plaque rupture, a process which undoubtedly exposes the flowing blood to procoagulant activities present in the necrotic core and/or extracellular matrix of the vessel wall.[2] While such thrombi are normally removed quite efficiently by the fibrinolytic systems of the blood and vessel wall, the presence of type 1 plasminogen activator inhibitor (PAI-1) in plaque[3] may prevent these systems from being activated. These considerations emphasize that the fibrinolytic system of the vessel wall plays an integral part in controlling normal and pathological thrombi. In this discussion, we shall review this system as it is currently understood, primarily relying on our own studies using cultured bovine aortic and human umbilical vein endothelial cells (ECs) as models.

The Fibrinolytic System

In its simplest form, the fibrinolytic system consists of plasminogen and those molecules that convert this inactive proenzyme into the active, trypsin-like enzyme, plasmin.[4,5] Because plasminogen is present in most body fluids, changes in the availability and activity of plasminogen activators (PAs) appear to contribute very significantly to the dynamic regulation of this enzyme system. Two immunologically distinct PA families are known, including the urokinase (UK) or UK-like PAs (u-PAs) and the tissue-type PAs (t-PAs).[4,6] Although these PAs activate plasminogen through cleavage of the same peptide bond (Arg_{560}-Val_{561}), their mechanism of action differs in that t-PA binds to and requires fibrin for its activity while u-PA does not.[7,8]

Precise regulation of the fibrinolytic system constitutes a critical feature not only of vascular hemostasis, but also of ovulation, invasion, and many other biologic processes in which these PAs appear to be involved.[9,10] This control is achieved through several mechanisms, including the presence of both plasmin and PA inhibitors (PAIs), the formation and resolution of fibrin, and the controlled synthesis and secretion of both of the PAs, and their inhibitors.

The Endothelium and Vascular Fibrinolysis

The endothelium lies at the inner or luminal surface of blood vessels and is thus in a unique position to contribute to the regulation of the fibrinolytic system. In fact, not only do endothelial cells synthesize and secrete fibrinolytic proteins,[1,11-15] but the cell surfaces and subcellular matrices associated with these cells are emerging as very important elements of vascular hemostasis.[11,12,16-18]

Plasminogen Activators

In order to more clearly define the fibrinolytic components produced by the endothelium, endothelial cells (ECs) are generally isolated and cultured *in vitro* in the absence of plasma and other contaminating cell types. Using this model system, it was demonstrated that ECs from several species are fibrinolytically active.[1,14,19-23] Subsequent work with bovine aortic ECs revealed that these cells secrete two classes of PA, one that migrates by sodium dodecyl sulfate-polyacrylamide gel electrophoresis (SDS-PAGE) with an apparent M_r of 52,000 and does not bind to fibrin, and two others that migrate with apparent M_rs of 74,000 and 116,000 and do bind to fibrin.[14,24] Immunologic studies demonstrated that the low molecular weight PA was recognized by antibodies to u-PA, whereas both the high molecular weight forms were recognized by antibodies to t-PA.[1,24] Thus, it seems clear that bovine ECs synthesize and secrete both u-PA and t-PA.

PA Inhibitors

Despite the above results, several investigators were unable to detect PA activity associated with these cells.[25-28] This apparent discrepancy was resolved when it was discovered that ECs, in addition to synthesizing both u-PA and t-PA, also synthesize and secrete PAI-1 and PAI-2.[26,29-32] PAI-1 is a major biosynthetic product of these cells, representing between 2.5 and 12% of total ^{3}H-leucine-labeled protein secreted by the cells in 24 hours.[32] The M_r 116,000 form of t-PA secreted by both human and bovine ECs was later determined to be an inactive, high molecular weight complex between t-PA and PAI-1.[1,30] The physiologic relevance of this observation remains to be determined. However, it is apparent that t-PA/PAI-1 complexes are not unique to cultured cells, since much of the t-PA in plasma is also in complex with PAI-1.[33-37]

PAI-1 appears to be the primary regulator of t-PA activity. This conclusion is based on the observation that naturally occurring complexes between single-chain t-PA and PAI-1, but not between t-PA and other inhibitors,[38] can be detected in the blood. In addition, the second order rate constant for the interaction of single-chain t-PA with PAI-1 is approximately 20,000 times higher than the constant derived for the interaction of t-PA with PAI-2 and protease nexin,[39,40] two other molecules with PAI activity. Finally, a number of recent clinical observations relate alterations in plasma levels of PAI-1 with the pathogenesis of vascular disease. Thus, it is now clear that patients with an elevated level of PAI-1 in their plasma have, or are at risk to develop thrombotic disease. For example, the levels of PAI-1 increase 10 to 20-fold during gram negative infections,[41] and disseminated intravascular coagulation is one of the major clinical manifestations of this condition. Elevated PAI activity also appears to be associated with deep vein thrombosis,[42] myocardial infarction,[43] and pregnancy,[44] and has been detected in critically ill patients with unrelated diseases such as pancreatitis, malignancy, and liver disease.[45] Diseases of the liver may be expected to lead to altered levels of plasma PAI-1 since PAI-1 is cleared from the circulation by the liver[46] and may be produced by hepatocytes.[47,48] High PAI activity was also detected in the blood of obese[49] and elderly[50,51] individuals. PAI-1 activity in plasma frequently increases after major surgery and in response to acute trauma,[52] suggesting that PAI-1 is an acute-phase reactant. The importance of PAI-1 regulation is further emphasized by the finding that patients with decreased PAI-1 have bleeding disorders.[53,54] Finally, activated protein C stimulates the fibrinolytic activity of endothelial cells and plasma quite dramatically, and does so not by increasing t-PA or u-PA production, or by dissociating preexisting t-PA/PAI-1 complexes, but rather by decreasing PAI-1 itself (reviewed in REFS. 55,56).

These observations thus suggest that the net fibrinolytic activity of blood or cells is actually a reflection of the balance between PAs and PAI-1, and that changes in any of these molecules may lead to thrombotic problems or to a bleeding diathesis. It follows from this that understanding the nature of the signals that regulate PAI-1 itself, and delineating their mechanism of action, will provide new insights into the fibrinolytic system and its regulation in health and disease. Moreover, this information may lead to the development of new thrombolytic therapies based entirely on PAI-1 (*i.e.*, on the identification of drugs that chronically lower PAI-1 and thus effectively elevate t-PA). For these reasons, we have made a major effort to understand PAI-1 biosynthesis, both at the cellular and molecular level, and much of this review will be devoted to summarizing our results using cultured bovine ECs as a model. However, before this discussion on regulation begins, we would like to briefly summarize some of the more relevant and interesting properties of PAI-1 itself.

TABLE 1. PAI-1 Concentration in Various Biological Samples

Sample	PAI-1 Concentration (ng/ml)	Protein Concentration (mg/ml)
Plasma (normal)	5–20	70
Plasma (sepsis)	50–200	
Platelets (10^9)	100–300	
Endothelial cells[a]	1000–5000	0.05

[a] Also human fibrosarcoma (HT-1080) and melanoma (MJZJ) cells.

Properties of PAI-1

The explosive growth of information on the biochemistry and the cell and molecular biology of PAI-1 can be traced back directly to the decision by a number of the early workers to study PAI-1 production by cultured cells, including ECs. This was a critical decision because while PAI-1 is a trace protein in plasma (TABLE 1), it is a major biosynthetic product of ECs, and may represent 10–15% of the protein secreted by these cells into the serum-free conditioned medium. The high rate of production of PAI-1 by these cells, together with the relative simplicity of conditioned medium compared to plasma, made the purification[32,57,58] and cloning[59-61] of PAI-1 relatively straightforward, and led to the development of monoclonal and polyclonal antibodies that could be used in assays to quantitate PAI-1 not only in cells, but also in plasma.

The structure of PAI-1 has been investigated using both the purified protein and its cDNA (reviewed in REF. 56). These studies indicate that PAI-1 is a single-chain glycoprotein with an approximate molecular weight of 50,000 and an isoelectric point of 4.5–5.0. More precisely, the cDNA revealed that the mature human protein consists of 379 amino acids, three of which represent potential sites for the attachment of n-linked carbohydrate side chains. Carbohydrates constitute approximately 13% of the mass of the molecule. Comparison of the sequence of the PAI-1 cDNA with that of α_1-antitrypsin indicates that its reactive center is located at the carboxyterminal end of the molecule, at Arg_{346}-Met_{347},[62] and that it is a member of the serine proteinase inhibitor (Serpin) gene family. It is noteworthy that PAI-1 lacks cysteine residues, a property that may account for its stability under reducing conditions.

Even at the early times during the initial characterization of PAI-1, it was obvious that this was an unusual protease inhibitor. For example, it appeared to migrate with β-mobility when analyzed by agarose zone electrophoresis,[63] while most plasma protease inhibitors displayed α-mobility when analyzed in this way. Moreover, its activity was still apparent after SDS-PAGE and reduction,[32] treatments that irreversibly inactivate most other inhibitors. In spite of this unusual stability, the molecule was rapidly and efficiently inactivated by oxidants.[64] This sensitivity to oxidants may represent a means by which activated neutrophils locally inactivate PAI-1 during inflammatory processes when large amounts of oxidants are liberated. Finally, an unexpected but rather consistent finding is that a latent form of PAI-1 exists in the conditioned medium of a large variety of cells, and also may be present in platelets.[65] The basis for this conclusion is that while PAI-1 antigen is readily detected in these samples, it frequently has less than 1% of its theoretical activity. However, the inactive form can be converted into the active inhibitor by treatment with denaturants,[66] heat,[67] negatively charged phospholipids,[68] and vitronectin.[69] These observations have led to the hypothesis that PAI-1 may be produced and stored in this latent (pro-inhibitor) form, and as such, may represent a large potential reservoir of inhibitory activity. This hypothesis lacks experimental support since biologically relevant activators of latent PAI-1 in plasma and cells have not yet been identified. For example, the activation time required for vitronectin to convert latent PAI-1 into its active form is many days,[69] but the clearance time for PAI-1 *in vivo* is only minutes.[46] In fact, the available data argues against this hypothesis of a pro-inhibitor. Thus, all detectable intracellular PAI-1 appears to be active,[70,71] suggesting that it is synthesized in the active, not latent form. Moreover, intracellular PAI-1 is quite labile, decaying into the latent form with a half-life of 2–3 hours after it is secreted.[72] These observations are most consistent with the simple idea[56] that PAI-1 is produced in an active form but is inherently unstable and rapidly decays into the inactive form once secreted, perhaps because of conformational changes in the molecule. It is likely that denaturants also alter the 3-dimensional structure of the molecule, perhaps re-exposing its reactive center. Interestingly, PAI-1 is present in the extracellular matrix (ECM) of a variety of cells,[18,73,74] where it appears to be distributed as a rather homogeneous carpet under the cells.[75] In contrast to the situation in conditioned medium, the majority of PAI-1 in extracellular matrix[76] and plasma[77] is active, not latent. These samples contain molecules that specifically bind to PAI-1 and protect it from this spontaneous loss of activity, presumably by stabilizing it in the active configuration.

These results indicate that the PAI-1 binding protein is an important regulator of PAI-1 activity, and we thus set out to purify it. We used bovine plasma as our starting material both because it was difficult to obtain enough protein from matrix and because PAI-1 in plasma is also bound to a high molecular weight protein.[78,79] We employed affinity chromatography using PAI-1 immobilized on Sepharose to isolate a polypeptide greatly enriched in PAI-1 binding protein activity[80] and showed that it was vitronectin, an adhesive glycoprotein also known as serum-spreading factor[81] and the S-protein of the complement system.[82] A PAI-1 binding protein was purified recently from human plasma and also shown to be vitronectin.[79] The biological significance of the interaction between PAI-1 and vitronectin in plasma remains unclear. For example, it was reported that plasma vitronectin stabilizes PAI-1 in solution,[79] increasing its half-life from 2 hours to

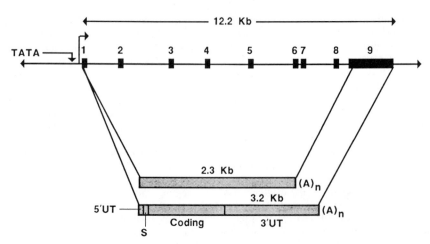

FIGURE 1. Structure of the human PAI-1 gene.

4 hours, a significant prolongation. However, since the clearance time for PAI-1 *in vivo* is only 5–10 minutes[46] the increase does not appear to be biologically relevant.

The human PAI-1 gene is located on chromosome number 7,[61] close to the locus for cystic fibrosis.[83] The entire PAI-1 gene was isolated and shown to be 12.2 Kb in length and to be organized into 8 introns and 9 exons (84,85; FIG. 1). It specifies two distinct transcripts of 3.2 and 2.3 Kb which are co-linear from their 5'-end and appear to be formed by alternative polyadenylation. The 3.2 Kb cDNA contains a small 5' nontranslated region, a region that codes for a 23 amino acid signal peptide, the coding region, and a rather large, 3' nontranslated region which accounts for over 50% of the cDNA.[59–61]

Regulation of PAI-1 Biosynthesis

PAI-1 is interesting not only because it is the primary inhibitor of t-PA in the blood, but also because it is a major biosynthetic product of ECs and its synthesis is highly regulated.[56] For these reasons we have been trying to define some of the signals that modulate PAI-1 production by these cells, and to understand their mechanisms of action. We have focused on molecules likely to be released by activated leukocytes and platelets. In initial experiments, we compared the effects of the immune monokines interleukin 1 (IL-1) and tumor necrosis factor (TNF) on PAI-1 synthesis in human umbilical vein ECs.[86] Both molecules increased PAI-1 antigen levels by 5 to 6-fold as compared to untreated controls, and both also appeared to suppress t-PA production by these cells. Northern blot analysis showed that these increases in PAI-1 antigen occur as a result of similar increases in the steady state level of PAI-1 mRNA. As already mentioned, these cells produce 2 transcripts for PAI-1, and both are increased 6 to 9-fold.

Now, the endothelium *in vivo* is a nongrowing, quiescent tissue. However it can be induced to undergo explosive growth at sites of vascular injury, presumably in response to growth factors elaborated from platelets and leukocytes. Thus, growth factors represent another group of molecules that may modulate PAI-1 biosynthesis. We examined the effect of a variety of growth factors on PAI-1 synthesis and secretion using cultured bovine ECs as a model.[87] Of those tested, only transforming growth factor beta (TGFβ), a growth modulator from platelets, induced PAI-1. Platelet-derived growth factor (PDGF) and epidermal growth factor were without effect in this system. The TGFβ effect was dose-dependent with a half-maximal response at 0.5–1.0 ng/ml, and increased secreted PAI-1 by over 100-fold. These results with TGFβ thus raised the possibility that activated platelets may be able to suppress the fibrinolytic system of the vessel wall by releasing TGFβ which in turn stimulates PAI-1 biosynthesis in ECs. To test this possibility, we added thrombin-induced platelet releasates to ECs in the presence of ^{35}S-methionine, and looked for changes in PAI-1 biosynthesis.[88] We found that the platelets increased the rate of PAI-1 biosynthesis and did so in a dose- and time-dependent manner. This increase could be blocked by pre-treating the platelet releasates with antisera to TGFβ but not with pre-immune sera. Thus, platelets can communicate with ECs to modulate their fibrinolytic system. This result suggests that platelet-rich thrombi may have high local concentrations of PAI-1, both as a direct consequence of its release from platelet α-granules, and because its production by surrounding ECs is stimulated by platelet-derived TGFβ. Again, the induction of PAI-1 antigen by TGFβ is preceded by an increase in the steady state level of PAI-1 mRNA,[89] and the kinetics of induction are similar to those obtained with TNF and endotoxin (or LPS), a molecule shown previously[41] to stimulate PAI-1 synthesis by ECs.

The intracellular mechanism of PAI-1 induction by these various agents is largely unknown. The existence of specific and distinct cellular receptors for TGFβ,[90] TNFα,[91] IL-1,[92] and glucocorticoids[93] has been reported. However, with the exception of the glucocorticoid receptor (glucocorticoid induction of PAI-1 is discussed below), the method of signal transduction by these agents has not been elucidated. Since the protein kinase C pathway is activated by phorbol esters, and phorbol esters have been shown to stimulate PAI-1 production by some cells,[94] this pathway seemed a likely candidate. However, our preliminary results[95] indicate that signal transduction for the above agents does not involve activation of the protein kinase C pathway.

As already mentioned, these agents all increase the steady-state level of PAI-1 mRNA. This induction of PAI-1 mRNA does not appear to require new protein synthesis since each agent induces PAI-1 mRNA in the presence of cycloheximide,[89] an inhibitor of protein synthesis. Although the half-life of PAI-1 mRNA in bovine ECs was short (2 1/2 hours), it was not altered by any of these agents, suggesting that they do not act by increasing the half-life of PAI-1 mRNA. And finally, nuclear run-on experiments[89] indicate that the increases in PAI-1 mRNA caused by these agents result primarily from an increase in the rate of transcription of the PAI-1 gene. Based on these observations, our working hypothesis is that these agents act directly on the gene to increase the rate of transcription of PAI-1 mRNA.

The large diversity of molecules that alter PAI-1 biosynthesis[56] implies that the regulatory region of the PAI-1 gene must be unusually complex containing DNA elements responsive to all of these molecules. Thus, in order to study PAI-1 gene expression in detail, we have begun to characterize the 5'-flanking region,[96] since it is likely to contain regulatory information. Initially, we focused on the 874 bp EcoRI-Hind III fragment shown in FIGURE 2. Nuclease protection experiments established the transcription initiation site at the "A" nucleotide *(arrow)* located 145 bp upstream of the methionine initiation codon, and a perfect TATA box was located at −23 to −28, the consensus

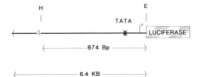

FIGURE 2. Analysis of the 5'-flanking region of the PAI-1 gene.

distance from the cap site. These results suggest that this region contains the PAI-1 promoter.[97] Transfection experiments were performed to verify this conclusion experimentally, and at the same time, to begin to identify those DNA elements in the region that might be important in regulation by some of the above agents. In these experiments, we used restriction fragments from this region that were fused to the promoterless firefly luciferase gene (FIG. 2) as a reporter gene. We asked whether the cloned fragments provide the necessary information to activate the reporter gene as indicated by the generation of luciferase activity and light. We found[96] that fragments 187 bp and 1500 bp in length exhibited high promoter activity in mouse fibroblasts and in bovine ECs, consistent with the observations that these cells also express PAI-1 in culture. HeLa cells do not express significant amounts of PAI-1 under normal conditions, and very little promoter activity was detected in transfection experiments using these cells. On the other hand, rat hepatoma cells, which normally do not make PAI-1, can be induced to synthesize high amounts of PAI-1 by the synthetic glucocorticoid, dexamethasone, and dexamethasone induced the PAI-1 promoter activity of both fragments transfected into the rat hepatoma cell line, FT02B. Taken together, these results indicate the presence of a strong, and relatively tissue-specific promoter within the first 187 bp of the 5' flanking region of the PAI-1 gene. This promoter is inducible by dexamethasone in rat FT02B hepatoma cells.

There appear to be two regions in the promoter that mediate a dexamethasone-dependent rise in promoter efficiency.[96] The first, located in the region between nucleotides −90 and +75 raises promoter activity about 10-fold. The second is located in the sequence −800 to −549 and mediates an additional 4-fold increase in promoter efficiency. We have been able to establish that the proximal element functions in both the normal and reversed orientation suggesting that it is an authentic glucocorticoid responsive enhancer. Finally, we have made a series of overlapping substitution mutants through the proximal region and shall employ them to perform transfection experiments as well as DNA "footprinting" and gel shift analysis to more precisely define the relevant sequences. We are taking similar approaches to localize the CIS-acting elements responsible for the TGFβ and TNF effects. Such experiments should provide important clues concerning the mechanism of PAI-1 regulation in the normal and atherosclerotic vessel wall.

REFERENCES

1. LOSKUTOFF, D. J. 1986. In Vascular Endothelium in Hemostasis and Thrombosis. M. A. Gimbrone, Jr., Ed. 120–141. Churchill Livingston. London.
2. WILCOX, J. N., K. M. SMITH, S. M. SCHWARTZ & D. GORDON. 1989. Proc. Natl. Acad. Sci. USA **86:** 2839–2843.
3. GORDON, D., A. J. AUGUSTINE, K. M. SMITH, S. M. SCHWARTZ & J. N. WILCOX. 1989. Thromb. Haemostasis **62:** 131.
4. COLLEN, D. 1980. Thromb. Haemostasis **43:** 77–89.
5. ERICKSON, L. A., R. R. SCHLEEF, T. NY & D. J. LOSKUTOFF. 1985. Clin. Haematol. **14:** 513–530.
6. BACHMANN, F. & E. K. O. KRUITHOF. 1984. Semin. Thromb. Hemost. **10:** 6–17.
7. THORSEN, S., P. GLAS-GREENWALT & T. ASTRUP. 1972. Thromb. Diath. Haemorrh. **28:** 65–74.
8. HOYLAERTS, M., D. C. RIJKEN, H. R. LIJNEN & D. COLLEN. 1982. J. Biol. Chem. **257:** 2912–2919.
9. REICH, E. 1978. In Molecular Basis of Biological Degradative Proteases. R. D. Berlin, H. Herrmann, I. H. Lepou & J. M. Tanzer, Eds. 155–169. Academic Press. Orlando, FL.
10. DANO, K., P. A. ANDREASEN, J. GRONDAHL-HANSEN, P. KRISTENSEN, L. S. NIELSEN & L. SKRIVER. 1985. Adv. Cancer Res. **44:** 139–266.
11. PODOR, T. J., S. A. CURRIDEN & D. J. LOSKUTOFF. 1988. In Endothelial Cells. U. S. Ryan, Ed. Vol. 1: 127–148. CRC Press. Boca Raton, FL.

12. NAWROTH, P. P. & D. M. STERN. 1985. J. Cell. Biochem. **28:** 253–264.
13. CERVENY, T., D. FASS & K. G. MANN. 1984. Blood **63:** 1467–1474.
14. LEVIN, E. G. & D. J. LOSKUTOFF. 1982. J. Cell Biol. **94:** 631–636.
15. BEVILACQUA, M. P., J. S. POBER, G. R. MAJEAU, R. A. COTRAN & M. A. GIMBRONE. 1984. J. Exp. Med. **160:** 618–623.
16. HAJJAR, K., P. HARPEL, E. JAFFE & R. NACHMAN. 1986. J. Biol. Chem. **261:** 11656–11662.
17. MILES, L., E. LEVIN & E. PLOW. 1986. Circulation **74** (Suppl. II): 246.
18. LAIHO, M., O. SAKSELA, D. A. ANDREASEN & J. KESKI-OJA. 1986. J. Cell Biol. **103:** 2403–2410.
19. BUONASSISI, V. & J. C. VENTER. 1976. Proc. Natl. Acad. Sci. USA **73:** 1612–1616.
20. SHEPRO, D., R. SCHLEEF & H. B. HECHTMAN. 1980. Life Sci. **26:** 415–422.
21. BOOYSE, F. M., J. SCHEINBUKS, J. RADEK, G. OSIKOWICZ, S. FEDOR & A. QUARFOOT. 1981. Thromb. Res. **24:** 495–504.
22. LAUG, W. 1981. Thromb. Haemost. **45:** 219–224.
23. GROSS, J. L., D. MOSCATELLI & D. B. RIFKIN. 1983. Proc. Natl. Acad. Sci. USA **80:** 2623–2627.
24. LOSKUTOFF, D. J. & L. M. MUSSONI. 1983. Blood **62:** 62–68.
25. LOSKUTOFF, D. J. & T. S. EDGINGTON. 1977. Proc. Natl. Acad. Sci. USA **74:** 3903–3907.
26. DOSNE, A. M., E. DUPUY & E. BODEVIN. 1978. Thromb. Res. **12:** 377–378.
27. MOSCATELLI, D., E. JAFFE & D. B. RIFKIN. 1980. Cell **20:** 343–351.
28. GOLDSMITH, G. M., N. P. ZIATS & A. L. ROBERTSON. 1981. Exp. Mol. Pathol. **35:** 257–264.
29. EMEIS, J. J., V. W. M. VAN HINSBERGH, J. H. VERHEIJEN & G. WIJNGAARDS. 1983. Biochem. Biophys. Res. Commun. **110:** 392–398.
30. LEVIN, E. G. 1983. Proc. Natl. Acad. Sci. USA **80:** 6804–6808.
31. LOSKUTOFF, D. J., J. A. VAN MOURIK, L. A. ERICKSON & D. LAWRENCE. 1983. Proc. Natl. Acad. Sci. USA **80:** 2956–2960.
32. VAN MOURIK, J. A., D. A. LAWRENCE & D. J. LOSKUTOFF. 1984. J. Biol. Chem. **259:** 14914–14921.
33. THORSEN, S. & M. PHILIPS. 1984. Biochim. Biophys. Acta **802:** 111–118.
34. RIJKEN, D. C., I. JUHAN-VAGUE, F. DE COCK & D. COLLEN. 1983. J. Lab. Clin. Med. **101:** 274–284.
35. MACGREGOR, I. R. & C. V. PROWSE. 1983. Thromb. Res. **31:** 461–474.
36. BERGSDORF, N., T. NILSSON & P. WALLEN. 1983. Thromb. Haemost. **50:** 740–744.
37. MATSUO, O., K. KATO, C. MATSUO & T. MATSUO. 1983. Anal. Biochem. **135:** 58–63.
38. HANSS, M. & D. COLLEN. 1987. J. Lab. Clin. Med. **109:** 97–104.
39. COLUCCI, M., J. A. PARAMO & D. COLLEN. 1986. J. Lab. Clin. Med. **108:** 53–59.
40. HEKMAN, C. M. & D. J. LOSKUTOFF. 1988. Arch. Biochem. Biophys. **262:** 199–210.
41. COLUCCI, M., J. A. PARAMO & D. COLLEN. 1985. J. Clin. Invest. **75:** 818–824.
42. PARAMO, J. A., A. DEBOER, M. COLUCCI & J. J. C. JONKER. 1985. Thromb. Haemost. **54:** 725.
43. ALMER, L. & H. OHLIN. 1987. Thromb. Res. **47:** 335–339.
44. KRUITHOF, E. K. O., C. TRAN-THANG, A. GUDINCHET, J. HAUERT, G. NICOLOSO, C. GENTON, H. WELTI & F. BACHMANN. 1987. Blood **69:** 460–466.
45. JUHAN-VAGUE, I., B. MOERMAN, F. DE COCK, M. F. AILLAUD & D. COLLEN. 1984. Thromb. Res. **33:** 523–530.
46. EMEIS, J. J. 1985. Thromb. Haemost. **54:** 230.
47. SPRENGERS, E. D., H. M. B. PRINCEN, T. KOOISTRA & V. W. N. VAN HINSBERGH. 1985. J. Lab. Clin. Med. **105:** 751–758.
48. RISBERG, B., G. K. HANSSON, E. ERIKSSON & B. WIMAN. 1987. Thromb. Haemost. **58:** 446.
49. VAGUE, P. H., I. JUHAN-VAGUE, M. C. ALESSI, C. BADIER & J. VALADIER. 1987. Thromb. Haemost. **58:** 326–328.
50. KRUITHOF, E. K. O., G. NICOLOSA & F. BACHMANN. 1987. Blood **70:** 1645–1653.
51. AILLAUD, M. F., F. PIGNOL, M. C. ALESSI, J. R. HARLE, M. ESCANDE, M. MONGIN & I. JUHAN-VAGUE. 1986. Thromb. Haemost. **55:** 330–332.
52. KLUFT, C., J. H. VERHEIJEN, A. F. H. JIE, D. C. RIJKEN, F. E. PRESTON, H. M. SUE-LING, J. JESPERSEN & A. D. AASEN. 1985. Scand. J. Clin. Lab. Invest. **45:** 605–610.

53. SCHLEEF, R. R., D. L. HIGGINS, E. PILLEMER & L. J. LEVITT. 1989. J. Clin. Invest. **83:** 1747–1752.
54. FRANCIS, R. B., JR., H. LIEBMAN, S. KOEHLER & D. I. FEINSTEIN. 1986. Blood **68:** 333a.
55. SPRENGERS, E. D. & C. KLUFT. 1987. Blood. **69:** 381–387.
56. LOSKUTOFF, D. J., M. SAWDEY & J. MIMURO. 1988. *In* Progress in Hemostas. Thromb. B. S. Coller, Ed. Vol. **9:** 87–115. WB Saunders Company. Philadelphia, PA.
57. WAGNER, O. F. & B. BINDER. 1986. J. Biol. Chem. **261:** 14474–14481.
58. ANDREASEN, P. A., L. S. NIELSEN, P. KRISTENSEN, J. GRONDAHL-HANSEN, L. SKRIVER & K. DANO. 1986. J. Biol. Chem. **261:** 7644–7651.
59. NY, T., M. SAWDEY, D. A. LAWRENCE, J. L. MILLAN & D. J. LOSKUTOFF. 1986. Proc. Natl. Acad. Sci. USA **83:** 6776–6780.
60. PANNEKOEK, H., H. VEERMAN, H. LAMBERS, P. DIERGAARDE, C. L. VERWEIJ, A. J. VAN ZONNEVELD & J. A. VAN MOURIK. 1986. EMBO J. **5:** 2539–2544.
61. GINSBURG, D., R. ZEHEB, A. Y. YANG, U. M. RAFFERTY, P. A. ANDREASEN, L. NIELSEN, K. DANO, R. V. LEBO & T. D. GELEHRTER. 1986. J. Clin. Invest. **78:** 1673–1680.
62. ANDREASEN, P. A., A. RICCIO, K. G. WELINDER, R. SARTORIO, L. S. NIELSEN, C. OPPEN-HEIMER, F. BLASI & K. DANO. 1986. FEBS Lett. **209:** 213–218.
63. ERICKSON, L. A., C. M. HEKMAN & D. J. LOSKUTOFF. 1986. Blood **68:** 1298–1305.
64. LAWRENCE, D. A. & D. J. LOSKUTOFF. 1986. Biochem. **25:** 6351–6355.
65. BOOTH, N. A., A. J. SIMPSON, A. CROLL, B. BENNETT & I. R. MACGREGOR. 1988. Br. J. Haematol. **70:** 327–333.
66. HEKMAN, C. M. & D. J. LOSKUTOFF. 1985. J. Biol. Chem. **260:** 11581–11587.
67. KATAGIRI, K., K. OKADA, H. HATTORI & M. YANO. 1988. Eur. J. Biochem. **176:** 81–87.
68. LAMBERS, J. W. J., M. CAMMENGA, B. KONIG, H. PANNEKOEK & J. A. VAN MOURIK. 1987. J. Biol. Chem. **262:** 17492–17496.
69. WUN, T. C., M. O. PALMIER, N. R. SIEGEL & C. E. SMITH. 1989. J. Biol. Chem. **264:** 7862–7868.
70. LEVIN, E. G. & L. SANTELL. 1987. Blood **70:** 1090–1098.
71. KOOISTRA, T., E. D. SPRENGERS & V. W. M. VAN HINSBERGH. 1986. Biochem. J. **239:** 497–503.
72. HEKMAN, C. M. & D. J. LOSKUTOFF. 1988. Biochem. **27:** 2911–2918.
73. KNUDSEN, B. S., P. C. HARPEL & R. L. NACHMAN. 1987. J. Clin. Invest. **80:** 1082–1089.
74. LEVIN, E. G. & L. SANTELL. 1987. J. Cell Biol. **105:** 2543–2549.
75. POLLANEN, J., O. SAKSELA, E. M. SALONEN, P. ANDREASEN, L. NIELSEN, K. DANO & A. VAHERI. 1987. J. Cell Biol. **104:** 1085–1096.
76. MIMURO, J., R. R. SCHLEEF & D. J. LOSKUTOFF. 1987. Blood **70:** 721–728.
77. CHMIELEWSKA, J., T. CARLSSON, G. URDEN & B. WIMAN. 1987. Fibrinolysis **1:** 67–73.
78. WIMAN, B., T. LINDAHL & A. ALMQVIST. 1988. Thromb. Haemostas. **59:** 392–395.
79. DECLERCK, P. J., M. DE MOL, M. C. ALESSI, S. BAUDNER, E. P. PAQUES, K. T. PREISSNER, G. MULLER-BERGHAUS & D. COLLEN. 1988. J. Biol. Chem. **263:** 15454–15461.
80. MIMURO, J. & D. J. LOSKUTOFF. 1989. J. Biol. Chem. **264:** 936–939.
81. HAYMAN, E. G., M. D. PIERSCHBACHER, Y. OHGREN & E. RUOSLAHTI. 1983. Proc. Natl. Acad. Sci. USA **80:** 4003–4007.
82. DAHLBACK, B. & E. R. PODACK. 1985. Biochem. **24:** 2368–2374.
83. KLINGER, K. W., R. WINQVIST, A. RICCIO, P. A. ANDREASEN, R. SARTORIO, L. S. NIELSEN, N. STUART, P. STANISLOVITIS, P. WATKINS, R. DOUGLAS, K. H. GRZESCHIK, K. ALITALO, F. BLASI & K. DANO. 1987. Proc. Natl. Acad. Sci. USA **84:** 8548–8552.
84. LOSKUTOFF, D. J., M. LINDERS, J. KEIJER, H. VEERMAN, H. VAN HEERIKHUIZEN & H. PANNEKOEK. 1987. Biochemistry **26:** 3763–3768.
85. BOSMA, P. J., E. V. VAN DEN BERG & T. KOOISTRA. 1988. J. Biol. Chem. **263:** 9129–9141.
86. SCHLEEF, R. R., M. P. BEVILACQUA, M. SAWDEY, M. A. GIMBRONE, JR. & D. J. LOSKUTOFF. 1988. J. Biol. Chem. **263:** 5797–5803.
87. MIMURO, J. & D. J. LOSKUTOFF. 1987. Thromb. Haemost. **58:** 1647.
88. SLIVKA, S. & D. J. LOSKUTOFF. Manuscript in preparation.
89. SAWDEY, M., T. J. PODOR & D. J. LOSKUTOFF. 1989. J. Biol. Chem. **264:** 10396–10401.
90. FANGER, B. O., L. M. WAKEFIELD & M. B. SPORN. 1986. Biochem. **25:** 3083–3091.

91. KULL, F. C., JR., S. JACOBS & P. CUATRECASAS. 1985. Proc. Natl. Acad. Sci. USA **82:** 5756–5760.
92. DOWER, S. K., S. R. KRONHEIM, C. J. MARCH, P. J. CONLON, T. P. HOPP, S. GILLIS & D. L. URDAL. 1985. J. Exp. Med. **162:** 501–515.
93. GUSTAFSSON, J. A., J. CARLSTEDT-DUKE, L. POELLINGER, S. OKRET, A. C. WIKSTROM, M. BRONNEGARD, M. GILLNER, Y. DONG, K. FUXE, A. CINTRA, A. HÄRFSTRAND & L. AGNATI. 1987. Endocr. Rev. **8:** 185–234.
94. THALACKER, F. W. & M. NILSEN-HAMILTON. 1987. J. Biol. Chem. **262:** 2283–2290.
95. SLIVKA, S. & D. J. LOSKUTOFF. Manuscript in preparation.
96. VAN ZONNEVELD, A. J., S. A. CURRIDEN & D. J. LOSKUTOFF. 1988. Proc. Natl. Acad. Sci. USA **85:** 5525–5529.
97. PTASHNE, M. 1988. Nature **335:** 683–689.

Vascular Injuries Induced by Materials Released from White Mural Thrombus and Hypercholesterolemia *In Vivo*[a]

AKINOBU SUMIYOSHI AND YUJIRO ASADA

First Department of Pathology
Miyazaki Medical College
Miyazaki, Japan

INTRODUCTION

Endothelial cell injury has been considered to be an essential event for the development of atherosclerosis, and many factors, such as immunological damage, hemodynamic stress, endotoxin, anoxia, hypercholesterolemia,[1] and platelet-releasing materials[2] have been postulated to cause endothelial injuries. One of the most difficult things in this consideration is a determination of what is meant by "endothelial injury." In addition, whether any of these factors is important for endothelial injury *in vivo* is unclear. A role for platelets in the initiation and development of atherosclerotic lesions has been widely discussed. Jørgensen and co-workers[3] reported that within 10 min of the infusion of a large dose of adenosine diphosphate into the artery, a focal endothelial cell damage was seen in the microcirculation. Lough and Moore[4] observed that thrombin-stimulated platelets and thrombin alone were unable to induce endothelial injury in the isolated rabbit aorta. On the other hand, Joris and Braunstein[5] reported that platelet aggregates caused by infusion of collagen into the pulmonary circulation of experimental animals did not damage the endothelium. However, most of these studies have been carried out in the microcirculation or in an *ex vivo* system.

The effect of hypercholesterolemia on vascular endothelium has been widely discussed. Ross and Harker[6] described large areas of endothelial sloughing in the arteries of monkeys fed a diet rich in cholesterol. Stefanovich and Gore[7] showed increased permeation of material into the vessel wall in animals with elevated levels of serum cholesterol. Stemerman[8] reported that hypercholesterolemia did not cause endothelial sloughing, but did cause increased endothelial permeability in localized area of endothelium, whether regenerated or intact. On the other hand, Lin and co-workers[9] reported that hypercholesterolemia increased mitoses of aortic endothelial cells, and Pesonen and co-workers[10] showed that a mild hypercholesterolemia induced endothelial cell damage parallel to serum cholesterol levels.

In this experiment, we studied whether or not products released from activated platelets and/or thrombi *in situ* could cause endothelial damage and proliferation of smooth muscle cells in large vessels *in vivo*. And also, we attempted to determine whether or not hypercholesterolemia could cause endothelial damage and proliferation of smooth muscle cells in large arteries *in vivo* and in addition, what kind of effects on the vascular wall could be induced by a combination of these two factors.

[a]This work was supported by a Grant-in-Aid for Thrombosis Research from Takeda Medical Research Foundation, and a Grant-in-Aid for Special Project (No. 63113007) from the Ministry of Education, Science and Culture, Japan.

MATERIALS AND METHODS

Twenty-four male New Zealand white rabbits weighing between 2.0 and 2.7 kg were randomly divided into four groups. Group I (n = 6) was a control group being fed a standard rabbit chow. Group II (n = 6) was a tubing group, in which radiopaque polyethylene tubing (3.0 F, Cook Group Company, Bloomington, Indiana) was inserted into the ascending aorta via the right common carotid artery under fluoroscopy at the 7th day and placed for 7 days continuously to induce vessel wall injury and fresh mural thrombi. Group III (n = 6) was fed a diet containing 0.5% cholesterol for 7 days and 0.2% cholesterol for the following 7 days to maintain about the same serum cholesterol level. Group IV (n = 6) was fed the same diet as Group III, and polyethylene tubing was inserted at the 7th day and placed for 7 days as in Group II.

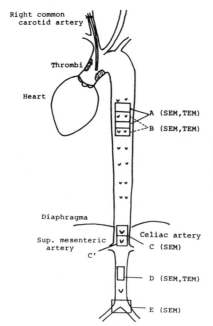

FIGURE 1. Schematic representation of tissue sampling from rabbit aorta. The *framed areas* indicate the segments examined. (From Asada *et al.*[11] Reprinted by permission from *Atherosclerosis.*)

Each animal was injected intravenously with [³H]thymidine (0.5 mCi/kg of body weight) 2, 16, and 24 h before killing. Each animal was perfusion-fixed as previously described.[11]

Total serum cholesterol level was determined using Determiner TC 555 (Kyowa Medex Co., Ltd., Tokyo, Japan).

For morphological studies, tissue blocks from direct noninjured segments from the descending thoracic and abdominal aorta and bifuraction of the common iliac arteries, which were downstream from mural thrombi, were obtained equally from each animal as shown in FIGURE 1. Pieces of each segment were examined with a scanning electron microscopy (SEM) (Hitachi S-800, Tokyo, Japan) and a transmission electron microscopy (TEM) (JEM-100S, Tokyo, Japan).[11]

To determine the number of replicating endothelial cells indicating a repair process of endothelial cell injuries, we autoradiographically examined "*en face*" preparations from four different segments of the thoracic and abdominal aorta from each animal, as previously described.[11] The number of endothelial nuclei and the labeled endothelial ones were counted.

For [³H]thymidine incorporation into the intima and media, each aortic specimen, after completely removing the adventitia, was completely dissolved in 2 ml of 1 N NaOH and then 0.4 ml of each dissolved sample added to 5 ml liquid scintillator (ACS II) was counted by a liquid scintillation system (LSC-700, Aloka, Tokyo, Japan). DNA concentration of each sample was also measured. [³H]Thymidine incorporation was then calculated and expressed as dpm/μg of DNA as described previously.[11]

All data were expressed as the mean ± SE. Statistical analysis was performed by unpaired Student t test. A p value less than 0.05 was taken as the level of statistical significance.

RESULTS

The weight gain of animals was similar in all groups. The mean serum cholesterol concentrations of each group at the time of killing were 32.3 ± 2.0 in Group I, 34.5 ± 2.5 in Group II, 704 ± 38.9 in Group III, and 736 ± 31.0 mg/dl in Group IV.

Platelet-rich mural thrombi with a few white and red blood cells were induced in the ascending aorta in Groups II and IV. Prominent degranulation and degeneration of platelets associated with fibrin threads were observed by TEM (FIG. 2). By SEM, the descending aorta in Group II showed various degrees of scattered endothelial damage such as cytoplasmic shrinkage and lifting-up and sloughing-off of the endothelial cells (FIGS. 3 and 4) as previously described.[11] Moreover, in Groups III and IV there were many monocytes which were adherent on the endothelium and penetrating into the subendothelium. Damaged endothelial cells as well as in Group II were also found in these groups, more prominently in Group IV. However, there was no endothelial denudation nor platelet adhesion on the surface in any group. By TEM, adherent and trapped monocytes containing lipid droplets were observed between and beneath endothelial cells. Modified smooth muscle cell migration into the intima was also found in Groups III and IV as well as Group II. These findings were observed more frequently in Group IV than in Group III.

On the autoradiographs of the "*en face*" preparation of the endothelial layer, there was a significant increase in the [³H]thymidine-labeled index in Groups II, III, and IV compared with Group I, and the most prominent increase was noted in Group IV at both thoracic and abdominal aortas (FIG. 5).

[³H]Thymidine uptake in the intima and media significantly increased in Groups II, III, and IV, and the most significant increase was noted in Group IV (FIG. 6). Similar results were obtained in the subendothelium and media after removal of endothelial cells (FIG. 7).

DISCUSSION

The results of this study indicate that materials released from activated platelets and/or platelet-rich thrombi into the arterial circulation can cause endothelial injury and regeneration and may also cause smooth muscle cell migration and proliferation at downstream and remote vascular segments. Hypercholesterolemia is one of the most important risk factors (hypercholesterolemia, hypertension and smoking) in atherogenesis. A number of mechanisms such as increase of permeability,[12] increase of endothelial cell replication,[13] alternation of anionic sites of endothelial cells,[14] and increase of monocyte adhesion[15,16] have been postulated to account for the role of lipids in lesion formation. LDL and oxidized LDL have cytotoxic effect in cultured endothelial cells.[17] However, there have been a few reports of quantitative *in vivo* studies on the significance of hypercholesterolemia to induce endothelial injury. The results of this study clearly indicate that dietary hypercholesterolemia can cause endothelial injury, though its true mechanism is unclear.

Monocyte adhesion itself is associated with foci of increased permeability *in vivo,* and it has been shown that monocyte migration leads to increased LDL transport across aortic endothelial cell layer *in vivo.*[18] A monocyte can produce toxic substances to endothelial

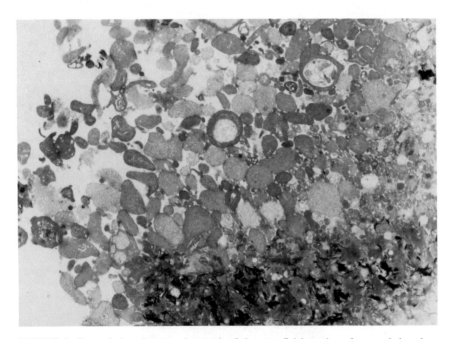

FIGURE 2. Transmission electron micrograph of the superficial portion of a mural thrombus. Degranulated platelets are present, and fibrin threads are noted beneath them. × 4000. (From Asada *et al.*[11] Reprinted by permission from *Atherosclerosis.*)

cells, the production of which is enhanced by modified LDL.[19] Monocytes could thus injure the overlying and neighboring endothelial cells and set the state for events culminating in the proliferative lesions of atherosclerosis. Platelet-derived growth factor (PDGF) is considered to be chemotactic for monocytes.[20] In Groups II and IV, it is considered that a large amount of PDGF was secreted into the arterial circulation. However, no monocyte adhesion on the endothelium could be detected in Group II. And also endothelial cell replication tended to be more prominent in Group III than Group II. Therefore, hypercholesterolemia itself is considered to be more toxic to endothelial cells and to be capable of activating macrophages.

[3H]Thymidine incorporation in the aortic wall was high in Groups II, III, and IV in

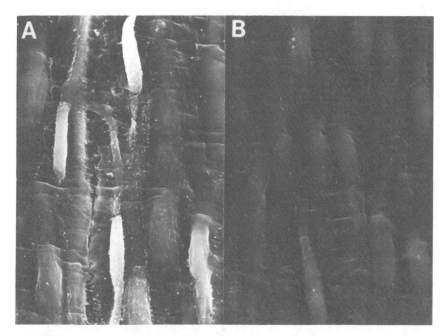

FIGURE 3. Scanning electron micrographs of the descending thoracic aorta. **(A)** Group II: cytoplasmic shrinkage and lifting-up of damaged endothelial cells are noted. ×2800. **(B)** Group I (control): there is no damaged endothelial cell. ×2200. (From Asada *et al.*[11] Reprinted by permission from *Atherosclerosis.*)

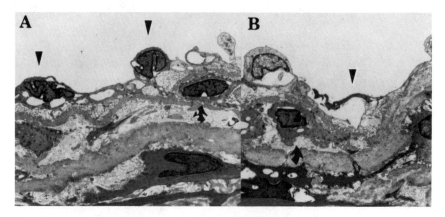

FIGURE 4. Transmission electron micrographs of the descending thoracic aorta in Group II. There are 2 damaged endothelial cells *(arrowheads)* having pyknotic cleaved nucleus, and vacuolated and osmiophilic cytoplasm **(A).** A necrotic endothelial cell with increased cytoplasmic density and marked shrinkage of cytoplasm *(arrowhead)* is noted **(B).** Modified smooth muscle cells *(arrows)* are noted. ×3300. (From Asada *et al.*[11] Reprinted by permission from *Atherosclerosis.*)

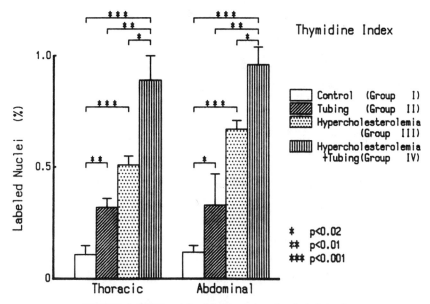

FIGURE 5. [³H]Thymidine labelling index of endothelial cells.

general and especially in segments including branching sites, indicating a synergistic effect of hemodynamic factor. An increase of [³H]thymidine uptake in the aortic cell after removal of endothelial layer is considered to represent smooth muscle cell proliferation in

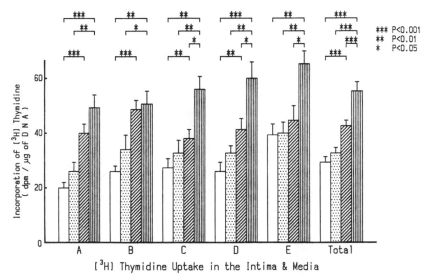

FIGURE 6. [³H]Thymidine uptake in the intima and media of the aorta.

the wall. [³H]Thymidine incorporation in the subendothelium and media was the highest in Group IV. This experiment has implicated many factors in migration and proliferation of smooth muscle cells.[21,22]

The endothelial injuries that occurred in this experiment may be minute ones, but repetition or continuation of these injuries may contribute to the development of atherosclerosis.

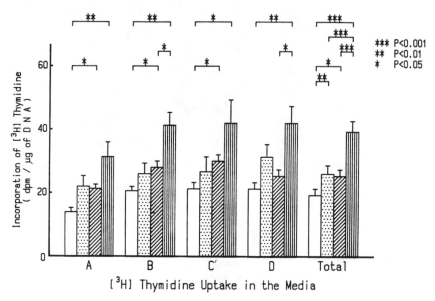

FIGURE 7. [³H]Thymidine uptake in the subendothelium and media after removal of endothelial cells. There are no data on "E" segments because all the "E" segments were used for obtaining the data in the intima and media in FIGURE 6.

SUMMARY

Materials released from platelet-rich white mural thrombi into the arterial circulation and dietary hypercholesterolemia could cause endothelial injury and regeneration, and also smooth muscle cell migration and proliferation *in vivo* in the intima. In addition, a combination of these two factors showed an additive effect on the endothelial injury *in vivo*. Further experiments are in progress to clarify how high a level of serum cholesterol and/or oxidized LDL may be sufficient for endothelial injury using this *in vivo* model for the better understanding of detailed pathogenesis of atherosclerosis.

ACKNOWLEDGMENTS

The authors wish to thank Mr. Takashi Miyamoto and Miss Ritsuko Sotomura for their excellent technical assistance.

REFERENCES

1. SILKWORTH, J. B., B. MCLEAN & W. E. STEHBENS. 1975. Atherosclerosis 22: 335–348.
2. PACKHAM, M. A. & J. F. MUSTARD. 1986. Semin. Hematol. 23: 8–6.
3. JØRGENSEN, L., T. HOVIG, H. C. ROSWELL & J. F. MUSTARD. 1970. Am. J. Pathol. 61: 161–170.
4. LOUGH, J. & S. MOORE. 1975. Lab. Invest. 33: 130–135.
5. JORIS, I. & P. W. BRAUNSTEIN. 1982. Exp. Mol. Pathol. 37: 393–405.
6. ROSS, R. & L. HARKER. 1976. Science 193: 1094–1100.
7. STEFANOVICH, V. & I. GORE. 1971. Exp. Mol. Pathol. 14: 20–29.
8. STEMERMAN, M. B. 1981. Arteriosclerosis 1: 25–32.
9. LIN, S-J., K-M. JAN, S. WEINBAUM & S. CHIEN. 1989. Arteriosclerosis 9: 230–236.
10. PESONEN, E., E. KAPRIO, J. RAPOLA, T. SOVERI, J. VIIKARI, E. SAVILAHTI, S. YLÄ-HERTTUALA & H. OKSANEN. 1987. Atherosclerosis 65: 89–98.
11. ASADA, Y., T. HAYASHI & A. SUMIYOSHI. 1988. Atherosclerosis 70: 1–6.
12. GERRITY, R. G., H. K. NAITO, M. RICHARDSON & C. J. SCHWARTZ. 1979. Am. J. Pathol. 95: 775–792.
13. FLORENTIN, R. A., S. C. NAM, A. S. DAOUD, R. JONES, R. F. SCOTT, E. S. MORRISON, D. N. KIM, K. T. LEE, W. A. THOMAS, W. J. DODDS & K. D. MILLER. 1968. Exp. Mol. Pathol. 8: 263–301.
14. LEWIS, J. C., R. G. TAYLOR, N. D. JONES, R. W. ST. CLAIR & J. F. CORNHILL. 1982. Lab. Invest. 46: 123–138.
15. ALDERSON, L. M., G. ENDEMANN, S. LINDSEY, A. PRONCZUK, R. L. HOOVER & K. C. HAYES. 1986. Am. J. Pathol. 123: 334–342.
16. ROGERS, K. A., R. L. HOOVER, J. J. CASTELLOT, JR., J. M. ROBINSON & M. J. KARNOVSKY. 1986. Am. J. Pathol. 125: 284–291.
17. HESSLER, J. R., A. L. ROBERTSON, JR. & G. M. CHISOLM, III. 1979. Atherosclerosis 32: 213–229.
18. TERRITO, M., J. A. BERLINER & A. M. FOGELMAN. 1984. J. Clin. Invest. 74: 2279–2284.
19. HARTUNG, H-P., R. G. KLADETZKY & M. HENNERICI, 1985. FEBS. Lett. 186: 211–214.
20. DEUEL, T. F., R. M. SENIOR, J. S. HUANG & G. L. GRIFFIN. 1982. J. Clin. Invest. 69: 1046–1049.
21. ROSS, R., J. GLOMSET, B. KARIYA & L. A. HARKER. 1974. Proc. Natl. Acad. Sci. USA 71: 1207–1210.
22. ROSS, R. 1989. Atherosclerosis. G. Crepaldi, A. M. Gotto, E. Manzato & G. Baggio, Eds. Vol. 8: 21–24. Excerpta Medica. Amsterdam.

The Effects of Augmented Hemodynamic Forces on the Progression and Topography of Atherosclerotic Plaques

YOJI YOSHIDA, WANG SUE, MITSUJI OKANO,
TOSHIO OYAMA, TETSU YAMANE, AND
MASAKO MITSUMATA

Department of Pathology
Yamanashi Medical College
1110 Shimokato, Tamaho
Nakakoma, Yamanashi 409–38, Japan

Some parts of the artery frequently involved with atherosclerotic lesions are easily identified, but others are not. In other words, some areas are preferential for atherogenesis but others are quite unfavorable. This suggests that blood constituents are not the sole pathognomonic factor, but hemodynamic forces are major contributing factors to initiate and develop the disease.

Careful topographical investigation of early human atherosclerosis has revealed that lesions develop preferentially in the outer lateral wall of bifurcations, the inlet to branches, and the inner distal wall of curvatures of the arteries.[1–3] Some investigated flow profiles on transparent and fixed human arteries[2,4] or on the open channel flow model[5] showed that these regions were exposed to either low but turbulent shear stress, or separation and stagnation of blood flow.

On the other hand, research on experimental animals, such as rabbits, swine, and dogs, showed topographical localization of atherosclerotic lesions different from that of human beings. For example, rabbits in acute dietary-induced hyperlipidemia had preferential lipid deposition on flow dividers at branching sites, which were expected to be laminar and high shear stress regions. The reason for the apparent difference in geographical localization of the disease between human beings and rabbits has not yet been clarified.

In this paper, we shall discuss two topics: first, ultrastructural differences of arterial walls, particularly in the intima, which are either resistant or vulnerable to atherosclerosis in the human aorta; and second, endothelial morphology and permeability at flow dividers of bifurcations in rabbit aorta which have areas either resistant or vulnerable to lipid deposition.

MATERIALS AND METHODS

Studies on Ultrastructural Differences between Apical and Outer Lateral Intimas of Bifurcations of the Human Aorta

Human aortas were obtained from 23 autopsy cases where deaths in hospitals were caused by various diseases and whose ages ranged from infancy to 51 years. Both the apex of the flow divider and the proximal lateral wall (inlet) of the inferior mesenteric artery (IMA), branching from the abdominal aorta, were investigated electron microscopically on surfaces cut longitudinally along the axis through the center of the vessel lumen.

The IMA bifurcations were fixed perfusively with a fixative (2.5% glutaraldehyde in

256

0.1 M phosphate buffer (pH 7.2) at 4°C) at 100 mm Hg within 2 hours after death. Small tissue blocks from both the apex and the outer lateral wall of the IMA were postfixed in 1% OsO_4 for 2 hours, dehydrated with alcohol, and embedded in Epon 812. Ultrathin sections were stained with uranium-lead stain. Some sections were stained additionally with tannic acid, periodic acid methenamine silver (PAM), or Ruthenium red stains.

Studies on Morphological and Functional Differences between Endothelial Cells in Areas of the Flow Divider of Bifurcations of Rabbit Aorta

Adult male rabbits, which weighed approximately 2 kg and had been placed on either a normal stock or an atherogenic diet for up to 2 weeks, were sacrificed to obtain specimens for scanning (SEM) and transmission electron microscopy (TEM) at branching sites of the brachiocephalic trunk and the left subclavian artery from the aortic arch.

Preparatory Procedures for SEM Specimens

Prior to sacrifice, rabbits were injected intravenously with 1 ml of a saline solution supplemented with 500 units of heparin and 6 mg of isosorbide dinitrate per kg of body weight to avoid clotting of the blood on the endothelial surface and undesirable contraction of the aorta. Perfusion fixation with 2.5% glutaraldehyde in 0.18 M phosphate buffer (pH 7.4) was performed after rinsing thoroughly with the same heparin-supplemented buffer in the lumen. The fixed aortas were stained with Sudan IV for 30 minutes. Borders of sudanophilic areas were marked by a 27-gauge needle under a dissecting microscope. Small specimens from the aforementioned two branchings were processed by the ordinary method, and six respective areas on the flow dividers were observed under SEM (FIG. 1).

Cell shape indices, given by an A/B ratio (A: width, B: length) and the maximum diameter of each endothelial cell, and the angle of displacement of the individual cell to the mean cell longitudinal direction were measured by an image analyzer (IBAS 2000, Zeiss).

Permeability Studies of Endothelial Cells

Horseradish peroxidase (type II, Sigma, HRP), ferritin (type I, from horse spleen, Sigma), and autologous immunoglobulin against HRP were used as tracers to investigate permeability of endothelial cells. Horseradish peroxidase (250 mg/kg) was injected intravenously 4 or 15 minutes prior to sacrifice. Ferritin (1 g/kg) was injected intravenously 30 minutes before sacrifice. Autologous immunoglobulin against HRP had been produced by immunization with HRP before the experiments. Permeability of apoprotein E was studied with an immunocolloidal gold method.

RESULTS

Studies on Morphological Changes of the Intima at the IMA Bifurcation of the Human Abdominal Aorta

Autopsy cases of newborns had thick apical intimas at the bifurcation, consisting of 3–4 layers of smooth muscle cells (SMC) as compared with outer wall intimas, which had

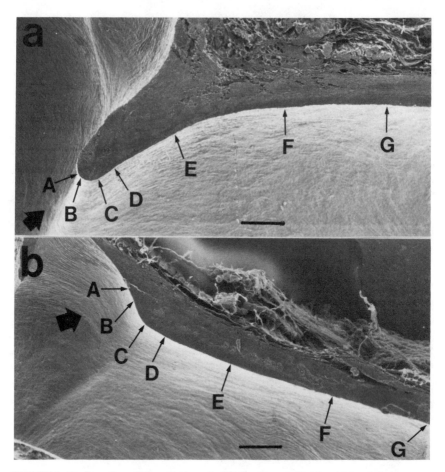

FIGURE 1. Configurations of flow dividers of rabbit brachiocephalic **(a)** and left subclavian artery **(b)** branches. Letters A–G designate the areas investigated under SEM. *Thick arrows* indicate the direction of the axial blood flow. Bars indicate 200 μm.

no or only 1 layer of SMC. Subendothelial edema, observed as electron translucent space in the subendothelium, appeared, not in the proximal outer lateral intima, but in the apical intima of newborn cases (FIG. 2).

In cases of those younger than one year old, particularly in newborns less than one month old, the apical intima (A) was thicker than the proximal lateral intima (P) of the IMA bifurcation. Consequently, the ratio of intimal thickness in the apical wall to that in the proximal lateral wall (A/P) was greater than 1, and in the most extraordinary case, infinity (FIG. 3). In that case, the apical intima was 15 μm thick while the lateral wall intima had no thickness, which means the endothelial cells lay directly on the internal elastic lamina. SMC in either apical or lateral intimas of newborns had moderate amounts of rough surfaced endoplasmic reticuli (RER) occupying a large portion of the cytoplasm, and were regarded as the synthetic type.[6,7] After one month, intimal thickness in the lateral wall developed faster than that in the apex of branchings, consequently lowering

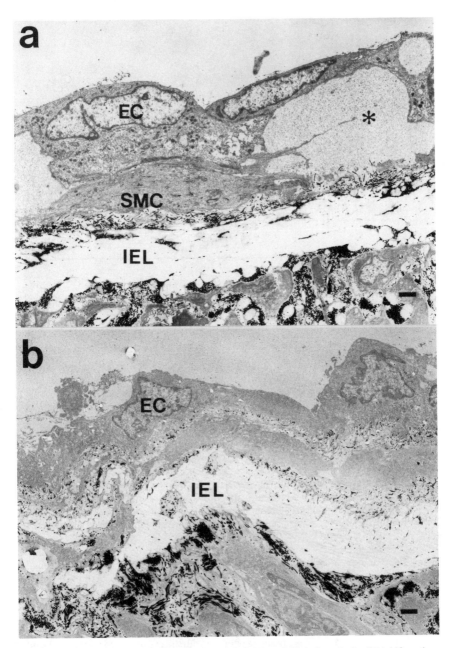

FIGURE 2. Electron micrographs of the apical **(a)** and lateral **(b)** intimas in the IMA bifurcation. Subendothelial edema is seen remarkably in the apex, but not in the lateral wall. *: edematous fluid. EC: endothelial cells. IEL: internal elastic lamina. SMC: smooth muscle cells. PAM stain. 1-month-old male. Bars indicate 2 μm.

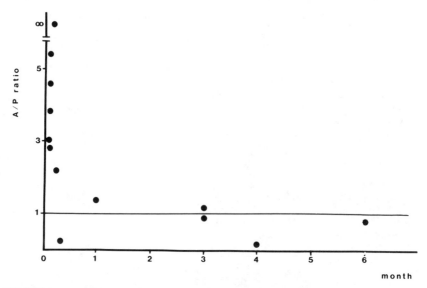

FIGURE 3. Ratio of intimal thickness in apical to proximal lateral wall (A/P) at the IMA bifurcation in cases of younger than 6 months of age. (From Yoshida *et al.*[3] Reprinted by permission from Springer-Verlag.)

the A/P ratio (FIG. 3). In all ages after the second decade, the mean maximal intimal thickness of the lateral wall surpassed that of the apex with a statistically significant difference, although both intimas thickened gradually as age increased.[3]

Stress fibers in endothelial cells (FIG. 4) and subendothelial basement membranes being more developed in the apex than in the lateral wall were apparent already in infants under one year of age. SMC in both apical and lateral intimas still had figures characteristic of the synthetic phenotype and sometimes contained lipid droplets in their cytoplasms. Within the first decade, there were no substantial differences in figures of intimal SMC of the two regions. However, when fatty streaks were observed in the outer lateral wall of the bifurcation, and not in the apical intima, many lipid-laden SMC were found among foam cells. There was a tendency for fibrous structures to be more developed and arrayed parallel to the endothelial lining in the apical intima as contrasted with those in the lateral intima, in which collagen and elastic fibers were shorter, fewer, and irregularly arranged (FIG. 4).

In the second decade, collagen, elastic fibers, and subendothelial basement membranes increased apparently in the apical intima, but intimal SMC still kept synthetic figures in the apex. Monocytes and lipid-laden macrophage invasion beneath the endothelium were not infrequent in the lateral wall.

In the 3rd and 4th decades, the apical intima, which was covered with flat endothelial cells, had a remarkable increase of collagen fibers, giving a dense appearance. Intimal SMC embedded among collagen fibers were elongated and showed contractile phenotype (FIG. 5), being rich in microfilaments and poor in synthetic organelles in their cytoplasms, which were surrounded by distinct thick basement membranes. Contrary to the apical intima, the intima of the lateral wall had a loose appearance due to the accumulation of either a matrix abundant in proteoglycans, which was proven with Ruthenium red staining, or flocculent materials and sparse collagen and elastic fibers. Intimal SMC of the lateral wall had wide cytoplasms filled with RER, so they were regarded as synthetic phenotype (FIG. 5). Basement membranes surrounded SMC incompletely. Endothelial cells covering the mucinous intima of the lateral wall were sometimes cuboidal and had many mitochondria and RER. Subendothelial basement membranes were thin and frag-

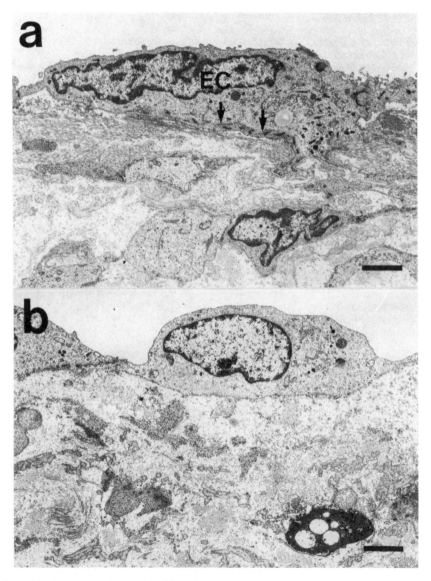

FIGURE 4. Electron micrographs of the apical **(a)** and lateral **(b)** intimas in the IMA bifurcation. Stress fibers (*arrows*) in and the basement membranes beneath the endothelial cell were more prominent in (a) than in (b). 3-month-old male. Bars indicates 2 μm.

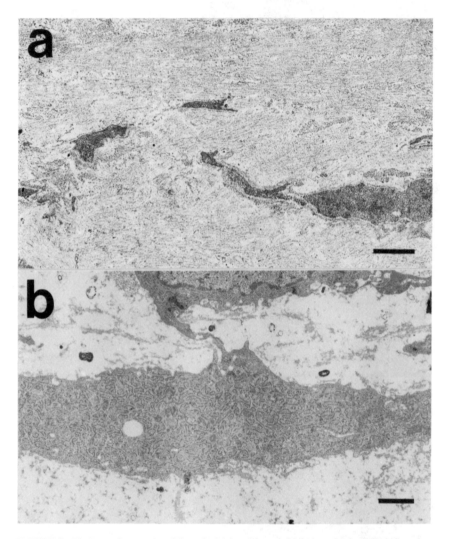

FIGURE 5. Electron micrographs of the apical **(a)** and lateral **(b)** intimas in the IMA bifurcation. Collagen fibers increased remarkably in the apex embedding SMC which show the contractile type. Contrary to the apex, SMC which are in a matrix abundant in proteoglycans continue in the synthetic type in the lateral intima. 25-year-old female. Bars indicate 2 μm.

mented. Attachment of endothelial cells to the subendothelial basement membrane appeared to be uncertain, as if floating on the mucinous intima (FIG. 6). In the subendothelial region, erythrocytes and/or lymphocytes were frequently found.

After the 4th decade, the lateral wall intima exhibited frequent denudation of endothelial cells, leading to platelet adhesion (FIG. 6) and enhancement of the insudation and accumulation of blood constituents in the inner layer of the intima. There was infiltration of lymphocytes and macrophages, as well as deposition of fibrin threads. Subsequently, cellular and fibrous components of the inner layer of the intima appeared to have been dispersed by the accumulation of edema fluid. Lipid droplets appeared in synthetic SMC in the intima, forming foam cells (FIG. 6). In the depth of the intima, the elastic muscular layer, consisting of SMC and collagen and elastic fibers, was usually unaffected by intimal edema.

Studies on the Differences of Morphology and Permeability of Endothelial Cells in Areas Which Are Either Resistant or Preferential to Lipid Deposition of the Flow Divider at Bifurcations of Rabbit Aorta

Rabbits placed on an atherogenic diet for 2 weeks showed a special geographical pattern of lipid deposition around bifurcations of the aortic arch.

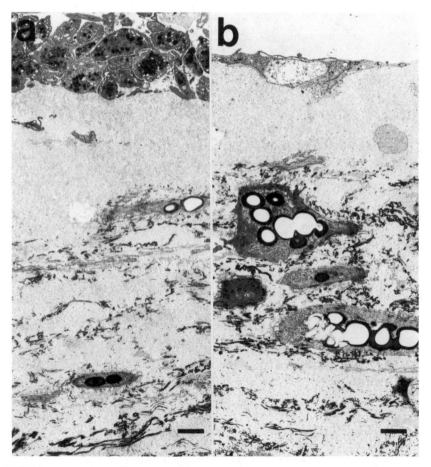

FIGURE 6. Endothelial denudation resulting in platelet adhesion and aggregation **(a)** and synthetic SMC contain lipid droplets in their cytoplasms **(b)** are observed in the lateral wall. Subendothelial basement membranes are indistinct. Tannic acid stain. 51-year-old male. Bars indicate 2 μm.

Branchings of the Brachiocephalic Trunk

Lipid depositions were band-like shaped along the full arc of the flow divider, but spared the leading edge (FIG. 7). In cases on the 2-week cholesterol feeding, the area of the flow divider of the bifurcation which was spared lipid deposition, covered 170 ± 129 μm from the apex downstream.

The form of endothelial cells observed under a scanning electron microscope varied in relation to distance from the edge (FIG. 8). Namely, just the apex of the divider was covered by round endothelial cells; the leading edge except the apex was covered by elongated cells. Beyond the leading edge, the wall was covered by ellipsoidal cells. The border between elongated and ellipsoidal cells was very clear in the bifurcation of the brachiocephalic artery. The flow divider of the bifurcation was sharper in the brachiocephalic artery than that in the subclavian artery (FIG. 1).

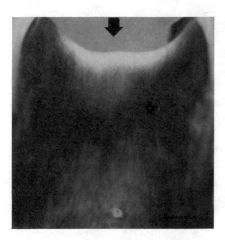

FIGURE 7. The apex and leading edge of the flow divider of the brachiocephalic trunk are spared lipid deposition in a cholesterol-fed rabbit for 2 weeks. Dark areas and spots are sudanophilic. An *arrow* indicates the direction of the blood flow. Sudan IV stain. A bar indicates 500 μm.

Branchings of the Left Subclavian Artery

Because of the wide branching angle (FIG. 1), the leading edge of this flow divider was wider and transition of the leading edge to the remaining wall of the flow divider was more gradual than in the brachiocephalic trunk. There was no sharp change in the direction of the luminal surface of the flow divider at points tangent to the leading edge. In this case, the shape of endothelial cells showed gradual change depending upon geographical distance from the impact point (stagnation point) of the flow (FIG. 9). At the bifurcation of this artery, the impact point sometimes did not correspond to the apex of the flow divider (FIG. 1).

At the point of impact from the axial blood stream, the endothelial cells were round, and in areas slightly downstream they were elongated. In regions measuring 123.5 ± 32.4 μm downstream from the impact point, elongated endothelial cells became gradually ellipsoidal.

Lipid deposition occurred consistently in areas where endothelial cells were ellipsoidal and arranged in a cobblestone-like fashion in both bifurcations.

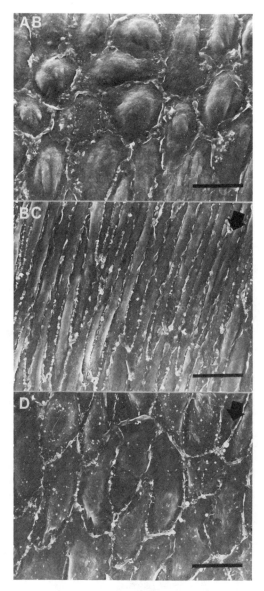

FIGURE 8. Scanning electron micrographs of endothelial cells locating on areas AB, BC, and D designated in FIGURE 1a. Cell shape varies significantly in respective areas. No cellular damage such as denudation or opening junctions of the endothelial cells is found in a cholesterol-fed rabbit for 2 weeks. Lipid deposition occurs in areas covered by ellipsoidal cells like those in D. *Arrows* show flow directions. Bars indicate 10 μm.

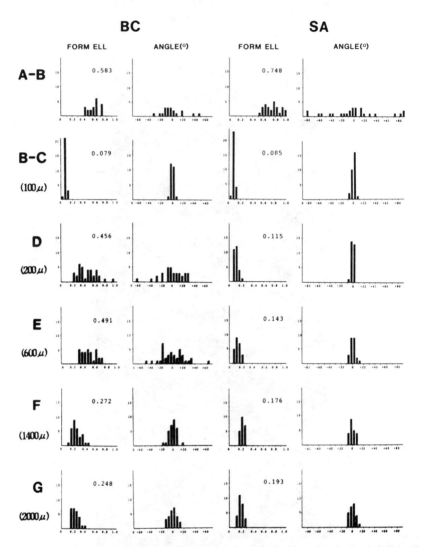

FIGURE 9. Histograms show cell shape indices given by ratio of width to length of endothelial cells (Form ELL) and angles of displacement to mean longitudinal cell direction. *Alphabetical letters* which designate areas investigated correspond to those in FIGURE 1. Each column shows the number of cells having to respective values on abscissas. BC and SA indicate brachiocephalic trunk and left subclavian bifurcation respectively.

Intact rabbits which had not received the cholesterol diet showed similar forms of endothelial cells on flow dividers in either bifurcation to those of rabbits placed on the atherogenic diet for 2 weeks. Cell shape was dependent on geographic localization, but independent of levels of hyperlipidemia.

Investigation with a transmission electron microscope on intact rabbits revealed that elongated endothelial cells, which were covering the leading edge, were most frequently equipped with thick bundles of stress fibers in their cytoplasms, fewer vacuoles, and thick subendothelial basement membranes. On the contrary, ellipsoidal endothelial cells, covering regions expected to be involved in lipid deposition after switching to the atherogenic diet, had thicker cytoplasms with many vacuoles, synthetic organelles, and mitochondria, but fewer stress fibers.

When intact animals were injected intravenously with horseradish peroxidase 4 minutes prior to sacrifice, larger numbers of pinocytotic vesicles and intracellular junctions of ellipsoidal endothelial cells contained HRP more frequently and densely than did elongated cells (FIG. 10). Subendothelial deposition of HRP was distinctly greater in the former area than in the latter. The difference between the number of vesicles and junctions of endothelial cells of the two regions remained after 15 minutes, although the number of vesicles and junctions which intensified staining increased in both areas.

After switching rabbits from stock to atherogenic diets, the number of vesicles and intercellular junctions containing HRP increased in both areas. Subendothelial connective tissue was also stained more strongly after the change of diet, but ellipsoidal cells were still dominant in permeation of HRP, rather than elongated cells at the flow divider.

When ferritin particles were injected intravenously 30 minutes prior to sacrifice, it was found that ellipsoidal endothelial cells in both normal and cholesterol-fed rabbits had more vesicles containing ferritin particles than did elongated cells covering the leading edge of the flow divider.

When rabbits which had been immunized with HRP, in order to use the endogenous antibodies against HRP in the blood as an autologous tracer, were placed on an atherogenic diet for 2 weeks, immunoglobulins were detected more frequently in ellipsoidal endothelial cells of the region with lipid deposition than in the leading edge of the flow divider. Antibody endocytosis into endothelial cells of either area was hard to find in intact animals.

DISCUSSION

Many researchers agree that areas expected to be exposed to low and turbulent shear stress, produced by local flow patterns, have been adopted as preferential sites for human atherosclerosis.[1-5,8] High and unilateral laminar shear stress regions in human beings have been recognized as areas resistant to the disease.[2,3]

In our investigation, rabbits had a geographical pattern of lipid deposition in the aorta absolutely different from that of humans. Lipid deposition in rabbits occurred in the flow divider of the bifurcation, which in the human artery was usually spared from atherosclerotic lesions. The human artery shows high probability of atherosclerotic lesions in proximal lateral walls of bifurcations or in inlets of branches, where no rabbit shows lipid deposition. As of yet, there has been no satisfactory explanation for this specific difference in localization of atherosclerotic lesions.

First, we shall discuss the preferential sites for human atherosclerosis. We selected IMA for our investigation for a number of reasons: 1) The order of magnitude of the Reynold's number at the branching site has been estimated around a few hundred.[9] Due to the low Reynold's number, the blood flow around this branching will be laminar unless there is marked irregularity of the luminar surface of the wall. 2) The IMA ostium is located in an area which has an aortic segment of sufficient length and is without major branches upward. The ostium is usually downstream from the ostia of renal arteries by 2 or 3 aortic diameters, with no other major branches between them. The length of this segment allows consistency in the blood flow at the branch of the IMA. 3) The inlet of the IMA branch has one of the highest probabilities of sudanophilia.

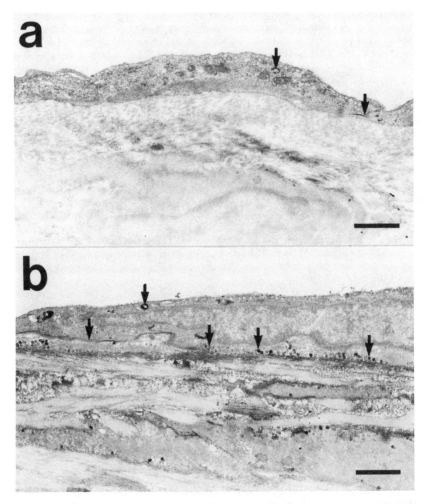

FIGURE 10. HRP permeability through junctions and pinocytotic vesicles of endothelial cells obtained from the leading edge (**a**) and the area D (**b**) of the flow divider of the brachiocephalic trunk in an intact rabbit received HRP intravenously at 4 min prior to sacrifice. Endothelial cells in the leading edge are less permeable than those in the area D. *Arrows* show the vesicles and junctions of endothelial cells containing HRP. Bars indicate 1 μm.

It was confirmed in this study that intimal thickness at the IMA bifurcation was greater in the apex than in the lateral wall in newborns under a month old. Humans over 10 years old, on the other hand, showed a thicker intima in the lateral wall. M. H. Friedman[10] stated that dependence of intimal thickening rate on mural shear was complex and changed over time; in particular, intimal thickness at sites exposed to high or more unidirectional shear stress increased more quickly to a modest value, growing slowly thereafter, while thickness at sites exposed to low or more oscillatory shear increased more slowly, but after time, reached a higher value.

Smooth muscle proliferation of the apical intima succeeded the intimal edema, which has been generally accepted as evidence of vascular injury. Four hundred dynes/cm^2 has been regarded as a critical magnitude of shear stress resulting in endothelial damage.

Shear stress on the endothelial surface of relatively uniform aortic segments were measured under basal anesthetic conditions in dogs and found to reach 100 dynes/cm^2.[11] It would be conceivable that the peak shear stress, particularly in the apex of the flow divider, could exceed the critical value.[12] Although it remains uncertain whether endothelial cells of the apex of the IMA branching of newborns were injured, it is possible that regenerating or activated endothelial cells induced by hemodynamic stimulation not only allowed an increase of their permeability, but also released growth factors to stimulate SMC proliferation.

Long-standing unidirectional shear stress may produce adaptational structures, such as bundles of cytoskeleton in and thick basement membrane beneath endothelial cells, to increase adhesion of endothelial cells to the subendothelial tissue. Development of cytoskeleton in endothelial cells seemed to decrease transcytotic activity of the cells. In rabbits, elongated endothelial cells, which were expected to be exposed to unidirectional high shear stress, showed higher volumes of cytoskeletal structures and less pinocytotic vesicles containing blood-borne tracers.

Smooth muscle cells in the intima of newborns and youths under the 2nd decade of age showed synthetic phenotype in both the apical and the outer lateral walls. Arterial SMC have two phenotypes, contractile and synthetic, in either *in vivo* or *in vitro* conditions.[6,7] Synthetic SMC are regarded as the essential form for cell division, that is, a form sensitive to growth factors which stimulate DNA synthesis in their own or other cells. Therefore, if suppressive regulation of production is not applied on the apical intima, atherosclerosis will develop in the apex equally as fast as, or faster than in the lateral wall.

We focused our attention on regulatory mechanisms which must exist in the apical intima of human bifurcations for proliferation of SMC. After the 3rd decade, collagen fibers accumulated predominantly among smooth muscle cells in the apical intima. There was no evidence that unidirectional shear stress could affect collagen synthesis of intimal SMC. It is conceivable that endothelial cells can transmit some stimuli to SMC to increase collagen synthesis, because, between endothelial and intimal SMC, there are gap junctions through which soluble mediators can pass uni- or bidirectionally to modulate cell functions. Another mechanism to stimulate SMC for production of collagen fibers in the apical intima may be oscillatory pressure generated by the blood stream running against the apex.

We assumed the effects of collagen fibers on the suppression of SMC proliferation. To clarify the effects of collagen fibers on SMC proliferation and morphology, we cultivated SMC on collagen gel consisting of approximately 90% type I and 10% type III. Our results showed that collagen gel was a potential substance for simultaneously modulating cell morphology from the synthetic to the contractile type and for suppressing DNA synthesis.[13] From these results, it is assumed that collagen may be a contributing factor to suppression of SMC proliferation.

The lateral wall intima had thinner and discontinuous basement membrane beneath the endothelium, and endothelial cells covering the lateral intima were equipped with fewer stress fibers, particularly after 3rd decade. Due to the poor appearance of the structure which consists of endothelial stress fibers and subendothelial basement membranes and anchors the endothelium to the subendothelium, it may be assumed that the endothelium of the lateral wall was likely to peel off.

Synthetic SMC existed in the lateral wall intima, which was rich in proteoglycans. It must be noted that some proteoglycans, especially dermatan sulfate, which is dominant along with chondroitin sulfate in the intima, form insoluble precipitates with LDL in the presence of calcium ions.[14] This biochemical reaction is considered responsible for extracellular deposition of lipid.

Lipid droplets appeared in only synthetic SMC, which, compared with the contractile phenotype, enhance degradation of β-VLDL and VLDL, and decrease specific activity of acid cholesteryl esterase as well as degradation of LDL.[7] As a result of disordered lipid metabolism, lipid droplets presumably appear in synthetic cells.

Accumulation of proteoglycans in the intima appears to play a very important role in characterizing vulnerability to atherogenesis in the arterial wall.

Although it is clear that proteoglycans accumulate within the lateral intima of human bifurcations, mechanisms for this accumulation are not clear. Some change of environment, induced by flow conditions in the arterial wall, is assuredly responsible for the accumulation of proteoglycans, but many factors can be nominated as additional candidates to modulate proteoglycan metabolism during the development of atherosclerosis. Cell culture studies have revealed that proteoglycan synthesis is increased when arterial smooth muscle cells are stimulated to proliferate while endothelial cells are simultaneously stimulated to migrate.[15] Other possible factors of influence of arterial cells on proteoglycan synthesis include cyclic stretching,[16] hypoxia,[17] prostaglandins,[18] interleukins,[19] lipids, lipoproteins,[20] and cell age.

In contrast to human cases, sudanophilic lesions in atherosclerotic rabbits occurred most commonly in the flow divider, which is an area expected to be exposed to high shear stress. The intensity of shear stress on the endothelial surface tends to vary from point to point, depending on local flow patterns and shapes of flow dividers. Unfortunately, there has not yet been developed an acceptable device to measure actual shear stress at each point at very short intervals in orders of hundred microns, along the vessel wall. Flow profiles and shear stress affecting the vessel wall may be estimated from both the shape and alignment of endothelial cells and the configuration of the flow divider *in vivo*. Shear stress at the apex of the flow divider of the brachiocephalic trunk has been assumed to be 0, becoming greatest a short distance from the apex because of the dividing of central blood flow with the highest velocity. At the end of the leading edge, the blood stream near the wall must separate forming turbulent and reversed flow around the flow divider, having relatively sharp curvatures (FIG. 11). As a result of flow profiles, mean shear stress, produced by turbulent and multidirectional flow, is thought to rapidly decrease downstream toward a point of flow reattachment to the vessel wall. According to the shape of the flow divider of the left subclavian artery, there was no strong curvature along the aortic side of the flow divider. Consequently, shear stress which became greatest a short distance from the impact point of the flow, decreased rapidly with distance downstream. In this case, the blood flow near the flow divider appeared to be laminar (FIG. 11).

Intimal lipid deposition occurred in areas covered by ellipsoidal endothelial cells, which were expected to be mean low shear stress areas. Areas covered by round and elongated cells were spared from lipid deposition. From the connection of cell shapes and distributions of assumed magnitudes of shear stress, we can conclude that lipid deposition in dietary-induced atherosclerotic rabbits occurred in areas with a relatively low magnitude of shear stress. Since the peak shear stress on the flow divider could approach the critical value,[12] some believe that high shear stress may trigger endothelial damage which induces lipid deposition in hyperlipidemic rabbits. However, it is difficult to observe with transmission and scanning electron microscopy endothelial injuries, such as denudation or opening of cellular junctions, in early stages of atherosclerosis in rabbits. In this study, scanning electron microscopic investigation of cell shape revealed that lipid deposition occurred in areas covered by ellipsoidal endothelial cells, but not in areas covered by round or elongated cells. *In vitro* studies applicative to shear stress on endothelial cells have shown that cells exposed to higher stress become longer and arranged parallel to the flow.[8] Cytoskeleton in the aforementioned elongated cells also become developed and aligned parallel to the long axis of the cell. Results of *in vitro* studies could be applied to *in vivo* phenomena: it could be that lipid deposition in rabbits occurs in areas exposed to relatively low mean shear stress rather than in the area exposed to the highest shear stress.

Ellipsoidal endothelial cells at the flow divider permeated, through both endothelial junctions and pinocytotic vesicles, more HRP, which had been injected into the bloodstream, than did either round or elongated cells. Ferritin was also endocytosed more often in ellipsoidal cells than in others. An increase of trans- and endocytosis of endothelial cells had already been observed in normal rabbits in a geographical distribution similar to that of hyperlipidemic rabbits. Endogenous immunoglobulin was hardly endocytosed into endothelial cells in intact rabbits. In the hyperlipidemic state, those excretory endothelial

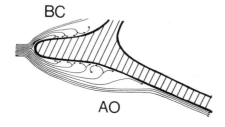

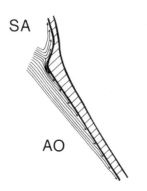

FIGURE 11. Expected flow profiles at flow dividers of brachiocephalic (BC) and left subclavian (SA) arteries. They were drown from data of the cell shape, displacement of angle, and form of flow dividers.

cells could permeate immunoglobulin and apoprotein E through pinocytotic vesicles, but not through endothelial junctions.

Ellipsoidal endothelial cells had more tracer-laden vesicles, RER, and mitochondria than did elongated cells. Endothelial cells which show fine cell structure similar to ellipsoidal cells are regarded as activated endothelial cells. Morphology and functional characteristics of activated endothelial cells have been studied *in vitro*, particularly in conditions stimulated with interleukin 1.[21] Activated endothelial cells secrete growth factors which may stimulate and enhance proliferation of SMC. Intact rabbits also have "activated endothelial cells" distributed similarly to those of atherogenic rabbits. Therefore, activation of endothelial cells might be induced by blood flow.

Endothelial activation might be the initial stage of the development of atherosclerosis.

Low and turbulent shear stress rates are very effective in stimulating the replicability of endothelial cells without rearrangement of cell alignment.[22]

SUMMARY

In order to clarify mechanisms determining different degrees of vulnerability of atherogenesis between the apical and the proximal lateral walls at branchings, both regions of the inferior mesenteric artery in human autopsy cases were investigated electron microscopically.

The lateral wall and the apex have been accepted by many researchers as the most preferential and the most resistant sites, respectively, for the disease. In regard to blood flow, the apex is exposed to laminar high shear stress, but the outer lateral wall to turbulent low shear stress. In newborns, intimal thickness in the apex was greater than that in the lateral wall, due mainly to the proliferation of SMC. After the 3rd decade, collagen fibers drastically increased in the apical intima, and SMC embedded between the collagen fibers, modulating their phenotypes from synthetic to contractile. In the lateral intima, SMC remained as the synthetic type. Synthetic SMC are considered capable of proliferation in the arterial wall.

The lateral intima was generally abundant in proteoglycans and lacked collagen (including subendothelial basement membranes) as well as elastic fibers, particularly in the upper part of the intima. Such a structural difference may cause favorable conditions for atherosclerosis.

Results of *in vitro* studies revealed that collagen gel suppressed proliferation of SMC and changed their phenotype from synthetic to contractile. Therefore, laminar high shear stress gives the arterial wall resistancy to atherogenesis through this phenotypic change.

Rabbits showed preferential regions in certain areas of the flow divider for lipid deposition which were different from those of human beings. These regions were covered by ellipsoidal endothelial cells, which should be exposed to relatively low mean shear stress. Ellipsoidal endothelial cells had already been observed in intact rabbits. Therefore, we can conclude that atherogenic processes could be initiated by relatively low mean shear stress in either humans or rabbits.

REFERENCES

1. SAKATA, N., T. JOSHITA & G. OONEDA. 1985. Heart Vessels 1: 70–73.
2. GLAGOV, S., C. ZARINS, D. P. GIDDENS & D. N. KU. 1988. Arch. Pathol. Lab. Med. 112: 1018–1031.
3. YOSHIDA, Y., T. OYAMA, S. WANG, T. YAMANE, M. MITSUMATA, T. YAMAGUCHI & G. OONEDA. 1988. Underlying morphological changes in the arterial wall at bifurcations for atherogenesis. In Role of Blood Flow in Atherogenesis. Y. Yoshida, Y. Yamaguchi, C. G. Caro, S. Glagov & R. M. Nerem, Eds. 33–40. Springer-Verlag. Tokyo.
4. KARINO, T., T. ASAKURA & S. MABUCHI. 1988. Flow patterns and preferred sites of atherosclerosis in human coronary and cerebral arteries. Ibid. REF. 3. 67–72.
5. RODKIEWICZ, C. M. 1975. J. Biochem. 8: 149–156.
6. CHAMLEY-CAMPBELL, J., G. R. CAMPBELL & R. ROSS. 1979. Physiol. Rev. 59: 1–61.
7. CAMPBELL, G. R., J. H. CAMPBELL, J. A. MANDERSON, S. HORRIGAN & R. E. RENNICK. 1988. Arch. Pathol. Lab. Med. 112: 977–986.
8. NEREM, R. M. & M. J. LEVESQUE. 1986. Endothelial cell responses to a fluid-imposed shear stress. In Atherosclerosis. N. H. Fidge & P. J. Nestel, Eds. Vol. 7: 403–409. Elsevier Science. Amsterdam.

9. CARO, C. G., T. J. PEDLEY, R. C. SCHROTER & W. A. SEED. 1978. The Mechanics of Circulation. Oxford University Press. Oxford.
10. FRIEDMAN, M. H. 1988. The relationship between intimal thickening and the hemodynamic environment of the arterial wall. Ibid. REF. 3. 41–46.
11. LING, S. C., H. B. ATABEK, D. L. FRY, D. J. PATEL & J. S. JANICKI. 1968. Circ. Res. **23:** 789–801.
12. FLAHERTY, J. T., V. J. FERRANS, J. E. PIERCE, T. E. CAREW & D. L. FRY. 1972. Localizing factors in experimental atherosclerosis. *In* Atherosclerosis and Coronary Heart Disease. W. Likoff, B. L. Segal & W. Insull, Jr., Eds. 40–83. Grune Stratton. New York, NY.
13. YOSHIDA, Y., M. MITSUMATA, M. TOMIKAWA & K. NISHIDA. 1988. Arch. Pathol. Lab. Med. **112:** 987–996.
14. WIGHT, T. N. 1989. Atherosclerosis **9:** 1–20.
15. ROBERT, L. & P. BIREMBAUT. 1989. Extracellular matrix of the arterial vessel wall. *In* Diseases of the Arterial Wall. J-P. Camilleri, C. L. Berry, J-N. Fiessinger & J. Bariety, Eds. 43–54. Springer-Verlag. London.
16. LEUNG, D. Y., S. GLAGOV & M. B. MATHEWS. 1976. Science **191:** 475–477.
17. PIETILÄ, K. & O. JAAKKOLA. 1984. Atherosclerosis **50:** 183–190.
18. PIETILÄ, K., T. MOILANEN & T. NIKKARI. 1980. Artery **7:** 509–518.
19. MONTESANO, R., L. ORCI & P. VASSALI. 1985. J. Cell Physiol. **122:** 424–433.
20. WOSU, L., R. PARISELLA & N. KALANT. 1983. Atherosclerosis **48:** 205–220.
21. POBER, J. S. 1988. Am. J. Pathol. **133:** 426–433.
22. DAVIES, P. F., A. REMUZZI, E. J. GORDON & C. F. DEWEY, JR. 1986. Proc. Natl. Acad. Sci. USA **83:** 2114–2117.

Physiological Roles of Vasa Vasorum on Micro- and Macromolecular Transport through Aortic Walls with Special Reference to the Topography of Atherosclerotic Plaques

TOSHIO OHHASHI AND YASUNOBU YOSHINAKA

First Department of Physiology
Shinshu University School of Medicine
3-1-1 Asahi
Matsumoto 390, Japan

INTRODUCTION

The nourishment of arteries is accomplished by diffusion from the lumen of arteries and from vasa vasorum.[1,2] Most arteries have a rather extensive network of adventitial, but not medial, vasa.[1,2] In the thoracic aorta of large species, branches of adventitial vasa penetrate into the media and provide an important source of nourishment.[3] One major determinant of the role of medial vasa is the thickness and lamellar unit of the vascular media.[2] When aortic media is thinner than 0.5 mm or 29 lamellar units, histological studies indicate that there are virtually no vasa vasorum in the media. In rabbit thoracic aorta, the media has about 20 lamellar units and there are few medial vasa.[4] Thus, there is a marked heterogeneity in the distribution and density of vasa vasorum in the media of large arteries.

Vasa vasorum are seen only rarely in media of normal coronary arteries in dogs and humans,[5] but they are seen much more commonly in atherosclerotic coronary arteries. Proliferation of vasa in the intima and media, with an increased propensity to intramural hemorrhage, has been proposed as one mechanism of coronary occlusion in atherosclerosis.[6] Blood flow and conductance of vasa vasorum to intima-media of coronary arteries were markedly increased in atherosclerotic monkeys.[7] They decreased significantly after regression of atherosclerosis.[7] These results may suggest that blood flow and proliferation of vasa vasorum play an important role in the development and regression of atherosclerotic lesions.

We have developed a new method that provides the continuous measurements of flow changes through vasa vasorum to intima-media of isolated dog thoracic aorta.[8] Thus, the present study was attempted to evaluate the physiological roles of vasa vasorum on the transport of substances through the aortic walls with special reference to the topography of atherosclerotic plaques.

MATERIALS AND METHODS

Mongrel dogs of both sexes, weighing 7 to 17 Kg, were anesthetized with intravenous administration of sodium pentobarbital (30 mg/kg) and killed by bleeding. FIGURE 1 shows a schematic diagram of the experimental layout. We studied the transport process

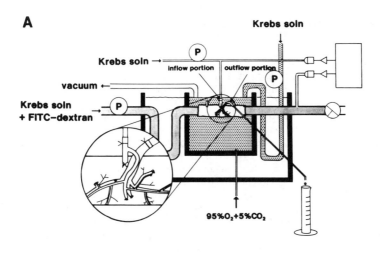

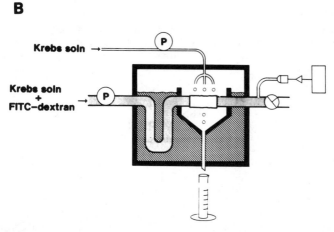

FIGURE 1. Schema of the experimental layout. **(A)** An aortic preparation with perfusion through the medial vasa vasorum. **(B)** An aortic preparation without perfusion through the medial vasa vasorum.

of FITC-labeled dextrans (FD) in isolated dog thoracic aorta with and without perfusion through the medial vasa, assessing the concentration of FD in the perfusate across the wall by means of a fluorescent spectrophotometer (Hitachi F-3000). Recently, we designed and constructed a new method to measure continuously flow changes through vasa vasorum to the intima-media of isolated dog thoracic aorta. The detail of the method was previously described.[8] Cylindrical aortic segments with intercostal arteries were carefully excised and briefly rinsed in Krebs solution. The composition of the solution was as follows (mM); NaCl 120.0, KCl 5.9, NaHCO$_3$ 25.0, NaH$_2$PO$_4$ 1.2, CaCl$_2$ 2.5, MgCl$_2$ 1.2, glucose 5.5. The solution was continuously aerated with 95% O$_2$ + 5% CO$_2$ gas mixture to give a pH of 7.4 and kept at a constant temperature of 37°C by the use of a heat exchanger. A catheter was inserted into an intercostal artery with side branches of vasa vasorum in the opposite direction of normal blood flow and then the artery was ligated completely at the adventitial portion of the aorta after the network of adventitial vasa was visualized by Evans Blue dye. The dye was clearly demonstrated in the outer layer of the media. Thus, the new preparation was morphologically confirmed to be suitable for determining flow changes through vasa vasorum in the media. The other arteries were ligated completely at the orifices of the intercostal arteries. Several branches of adventitial vasa were also ligated. Another catheter was inserted into the corresponding vein, the outflow portion of which was confirmed clearly by explosion of the injected dye, and then the perfusate through medial vasa was easily gathered in the isolated aortic preparation (FIG. 1A). The recovery of the injected dye in the corresponding vein was about 66%. The perfusion area of medial vasa was about 50% of the aortic segments, which were calculated morphologically by the injection of the dye in each preparation. The intraluminal pressure of the aortic segments was maintained at 50 mm Hg with the Krebs solution containing 300 μg/ml FD. The concentration of FD in the perfusate through the vasa vasorum was determined every 15–30 min by the spectrophotometer.

In control experiments (FIG. 1B), aortic segments of the same size without the intercostal arteries, and in which the intraluminal space was occupied by Krebs solution containing the same concentration of FD, were superfused with Krebs solution on the adventitial side. The concentration of FD in the superfusate was determined every 15–30 min after starting the superfusion.

Experimental values in the text are means ± standard error of the mean. Statistical analyses were made using Mann-Whitney's U-test for unpaired data or one way analysis of variance for multiple comparisons. The differences in means were considered significant when $p < 0.05$.

RESULTS

FIGURE 2 shows summarised data in control experiments. Each curve is depicted by 4–5 experimental results. The ordinate is the relative leakage of FD expressed as the percentage of the content of FD in the superfusate to that in the intraluminal space of aortic segment. The abscissa is the time course after an injection of FD in the intraluminal space. FD of 4 K dalton molecular weight (FD 4) appeared in the superfusate about 45 min after the injection of FD. The leakage of FD 4 increased gradually and arrived at a steady-state level, 0.2%, about 4 hr after the injection. The time course of the leakage of FD 20 was quite similar to that of FD 4. The steady-state level of FD 20, however, was smaller than that of FD 4. Leakage of FD 40 and 150 was hardly observed in the superfusate by about 6 hr after the injection.

FIGURE 3 demonstrates summarized data in the new preparations with continuous perfusion through vasa vasorum in the media by Krebs solution. The perfusion pressure of vasa vasorum was kept at 75 mm Hg throughout the experiment. Each curve is depicted by 4–5 experimental results. The ordinate is the relative leakage of FD through the aortic wall normalized by the perfusion area of medial vasa measured morphologically by the injection of Evans Blue dye. Compared with the control, the leakage of FD 4 and FD 20 in the perfusate through vasa vasorum appeared quickly, about 30 min after the injection and demonstrated higher steady-state levels, about 0.3–0.5% in the aortic preparations.

FD 40 and 150 were hardly leaked into the perfusate, which were quite similar findings to those in the control.

FIGURE 4 shows total leakage of FD expressed as the percentage of the total content of FD in the perfusate during 6 hr to that in the intraluminal space. The open and hatched columns represent control and experimental results (n = 4–5), respectively. The total leakage of FD of less than 20 k dalton molecular weight in both aortic preparations increased significantly, compared with that of FD of more than 40 k dalton. Thus, the transport of FD through the aortic wall depends upon the molecular weight of the substances in both preparations.

In the case of the transport of FD 4 and 20, adventitial and medial vasa vasorum played a facilitatory role in the transport process of substances through the aortic wall.

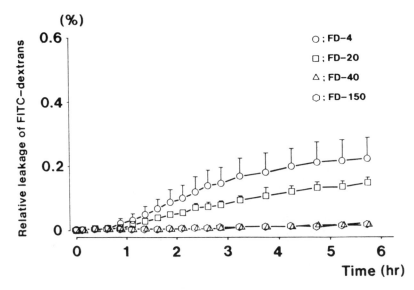

FIGURE 2. Superfusion: relationships between the relative leakage of FD and the time course after an injection of FD in isolated dog thoracic aortae superfused by Krebs solution. FD 4, 20, 40, and 150 denote FITC-labelled dextran molecular weight 4, 20, 40, and 150 K dalton, respectively.

DISCUSSION

The present results suggest that there is a net transport of macromolecules across the aortic wall and that vasa vasorum influence the transport of substances with low molecular weight within the aortic wall. Thus, heterogeneity in the network of vasa vasorum in aortic walls may be, in part, related to the topography of atherosclerotic plaques.

Nourishment of blood vessels is accomplished by diffusion from the lumen of the vessel, diffusion from adventitial vasa vasorum, and in some vessels by blood flow through medial vasa vasorum. Disruption of the medial vasa impairs diffusional support of the thoracic aorta of dogs[4] and produces medial necrosis.[4] These findings indicate that medial vasa are an essential source of nutrition to thoracic aorta. A determinant of the role of vasa vasorum in nourishment of vessels may be Po_2 in luminal blood.[9] Another determinant may be the thickness and lamellar unit of the vascular media.[2,4]

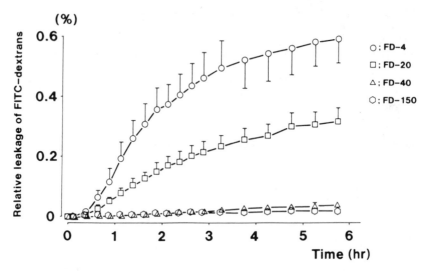

FIGURE 3. Perfusion of vasa vasorum: relationships between the relative leakage of FD in the perfusate and the time course after an injection of FD in isolated thoracic aortae with perfusion through the medial vasa. FD 4, 20, 40, and 150 show the same items as shown in FIGURE 2.

In normal humans and dogs, vasa vasorum in thoracic aortic media arose almost exclusively from adventitial vessels. In the atherosclerotic aorta, intimal proliferation extends the diffusion distance in the aorta. Thus, intimal proliferation might be expected to increase dependence on nourishment by vasa vasorum. Morphological studies suggest that vasa are more prominent in atherosclerotic than in normal aorta. Vasa have been found to penetrate the intima from the lumen to supply the media of the atherosclerotic aorta. It has not been possible, however, to quantify the extent of proliferation of vasa,

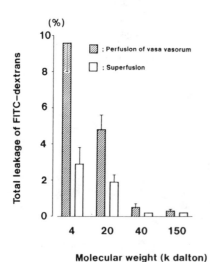

FIGURE 4. Relationships between the total leakage of FD during 6 hr and molecular weight of FD in isolated dog thoracic aortae with *(open columns)* and without *(hatched columns)* perfusion through the medial vasa.

and it has not been clear whether there is enough proliferation of vasa to produce a detectable increase in perfusion of the aortic wall in atherosclerosis.[7]

The present findings may suggest another physiological role of medial and adventitial vasa vasorum in aortic walls; vasa vasorum work as important excretory channels of waste products and metabolites in aortic walls. Thus, vasa vasorum influence the transport process of the substances through the aortic walls. The diffusion rate of waste products and metabolites in aortic walls may also depend upon the network and density of medial vasa. This hypothesis may be compatible with the following experimental findings; morphological studies and postmortem arteriograms provide qualitative evidence that atherosclerosis induces neovascularization in coronary arteries.[10] The hypothesis may also be in agreement with the well-known evidence that rabbits with few medial vasa are a suitable experimental model to develop atherosclerosis easily with feeding of high cholesterol diets. Thus, according to the hypothesis, we have suggested that the heterogeneity in the network of medial vasa in aortic walls may be, in part, related to the topography of atherosclerotic plaques.

The present study also suggests that there is a marked transport of macromolecules (FD 20) across the aortic walls. The transport process is seemingly dominantly diffusional. The findings are compatible with the experimental results obtained by Caro et al.[11] They have studied the transport of radioactively labelled albumin in the rabbit common carotid artery perfused in situ at 100 cm H_2O luminal pressure in the anesthetized living animal, assessing the distribution of concentration across the wall by means of sequential frozen sectioning. They show that there is a net transport of macromolecular (molecular weight 50,000) across the arterial wall and that the wall is inhomogenous. The distribution volume for label is greater in the adventitia than the media, which appears to offer a larger resistance. It seems warranted to speculate briefly concerning the relevance of these findings to atherogenesis. If there is net transport of lipoprotein across the aortic wall it could accumulate as the result of factors including increased intimal entry and diminished adventitial outflow. Most previous work has concentrated on the former, but there has been relevant earlier work on impairment of transmedial outflow and on the role of the adventitial circulation and lymphatics.[12] Caro et al.[11] suggest that the resistance of the media exceeds that of the adventitia, and they show the possibility that the media present a barrier to the drainage of material towards the adventitia. Thus, our present findings may suggest that the drainage barrier towards the adventitia can be weakened by the network of medial vasa in the aortic wall and that hemodynamic changes of the medial vasa can modify the concentration of macromolecules, i.e., lipoprotein in the aortic walls. Further investigations will be needed to evaluate the role of media vasa by the use of atherosclerotic preparations.

REFERENCES

1. GEIRINGER, E. 1951. Intimal vascularization and atherosclerosis. J. Pathol. Bacteriol. **63:** 201–211.
2. WOLINSKY, H. & S. GLAGOV. 1967. Nature of species differences in the medial distribution of aortic vasa vasorum in mammals. Circ. Res. **20:** 409–421.
3. WERBER, A. & D. D. HEISTAD. 1985. Diffusional support of arteries. Am. J. Physiol. (Heart Circ. Physiol.) **17:** H901–H906.
4. HEISTAD, D. D. & M. L. MARCUS. 1979. Role of vasa vasorum in nourishment of the aorta. Blood Vessels **16:** 225–238.
5. WOERNER, C. A. 1959. Vasa vasorum in arteries, their demonstration and distribution. In The Arterial Wall. A. I. Lansing, Ed. 1–14. Williams & Wilkins. Baltimore, MD.
6. SINGH, R. N., J. A. SOSA & G. E. GREEN. 1983. Internal mammary artery versus saphenous vein graft. Br. Heart J. **50:** 48–58.

7. HEISTAD, D. D., M. L. ARMSTRONG & M. L. MARCUS. 1981. Hyperemia of the aortic wall in atherosclerotic monkeys. Circ. Res. **48:** 669–675.
8. OHHIRA, A. & T. OHHASHI. 1987. A new preparation capable of the measurement of flow resistance through vasa vasorum in isolated canine thoracic aorta. *In* Microcirculation Annual 1987. M. Tsuchiya, M. Asano & Y. Mishima, Eds. 123–124. Nihon Igakukan. Tokyo.
9. OHHASHI, T., S. FUKUSHIMA & T. AZUMA. 1977. Vasa vasorum within the media of bovine mesenteric lymphatics. Proc. Soc. Exp. Biol. Med. (NY) **154:** 582–586.
10. HEISTAD, D. D. & M. L. ARMSTRONG. 1986. Blood flow through vasa vasorum of coronary arteries in atherosclerotic monkeys. Arteriosclerosis **6:** 326–331.
11. CARO, C. G., M. J. LEVER, Z. LAVER-RUDICH, F. MEYER, N. LIRON, W. EBEL, K. H. PARKER & C. P. WINLOVE. 1980. Net albumin transport across the wall of the rabbit common carotid artery perfused *in situ*. Atherosclerosis **37:** 497–511.
12. JELLINEK, H., B. VERESS, A. BALINT & Z. NAGY. 1970. Lymph vessels of rat aorta and their changes in experimental atherosclerosis. Exp. Mol. Pathol. **13:** 370–379.

A New Approach to Prevention and Treatment of Atherosclerosis by Dyslipoproteinemia

TAKEMICHI KANAZAWA, TSUGUMICHI UEMURA,
YOSHIYUKI KONTA, MAKOTO TANAKA, YUKO FUKUSHI,
KOGO ONODERA, HIROBUMI METOKI,[a]
AND YASABURO OIKE[a]

Second Department of Internal Medicine
Hirosaki University School of Medicine
and
[a]Reimeikyo Rehabilitation Hospital
5 Zaifu-Cho
Hirosaki City 036, Japan

A number of papers[1,2] have been published on the treatment and prevention of atherosclerosis. The main points of those papers were to reduce the concentrations of low density lipoprotein cholesterol (LDL-CH), apoprotein B (apo B), and lipid peroxide (LPO) or to increase that of high density lipoprotein cholesterol (HDL-CH). Furthermore, in several human and nonhuman primate experiments[3,4] it was shown that atherosclerotic lesions regressed by reducing the concentration of LDL-CH for an extended period of time.

Recently, Steinberg[5] and Kita[6] reported that the foramtion of atheroma was suppressed in WHHL rabbits by probucol treatment. They pointed out that the suppression of LPO was more important for the treatment and prevention of atherosclerosis than the reduction of LDL-CH.

In this paper, new aspects for the treatment and prevention of atherosclerosis will be discussed from the viewpoint of the composition and physical character of LDL.

EXPERIMENT I

Materials and Methods

1) In order to observe the relationships between the development of atherosclerotic lesions and the changes of LDL-CH and LDL-apo B, 24 male New Zealand white rabbits of 3 months of age were divided into 3 groups of 8 rabbits each. Group 1 rabbits were fed a commercial standard rabbit diet, group 2 rabbits were fed a standard rabbit diet plus 1% cholesterol (CH), and group 3 a standard rabbit diet, 1% CH plus 10% soycream (obtained from soybean, provided by Prof. Ohkubo of the Agricultural Department of Tohoku University, Japan).

2) To compare the regression coefficients of LDL-apo B and LDL-CH between the rabbits and humans, the blood from 16 healthy persons and 17 patients with ischemic heart diseases was drawn, and LDL-CH and LDL-apo B were measured.

3) In order to observe the changes of lipids in LDL in rabbits which were fed a

TABLE 1. A Method for Formation of Endothelial Cell Injuries on Vessel Wall by LDL Infusion in Rabbit *In Vivo*

1. Separation of LDL
a. normal rabbit
b. 1% cholesterol feeding rabbit for 10 weeks
2. Dialysis into saline solution for 48 hours
3. Dilution of LDL to the conentration of normal rabbit cholesterol
4. Infusion of 400 ml of the diluted LDL for 3 hours into
a. left external carotid artery (with 120 mm Hg)
b. auricular vein
5. Scanning electron microscope (SEM); transitional electron microscope (TEM)

standard diet plus 1% CH for 10 weeks, 8 rabbits were used, and CH, LPO, triglyceride (TG) and phospholipid (PL) in LDL were measured every two weeks for 10 weeks.

4) To produce endothelial cell injuries *in vivo*, two kinds of native LDLs, LDL from normal rabbits and LDL from rabbits fed 1% CH were diluted to the concentration of normal rabbit plasma CH (TABLE 1). These diluted LDL solutions were infused into the left external carotid artery or the auricular vein. Sixty-two male rabbits were used to separate normal LDL (1.019–1.053). The experiments were repeated 6 times.

5) The blood was drawn into the syringes containing 0,05 M EDTA after 16 hours of fasting.

6) LDL (1.019–1.063) was separated by Havel's method.[7] Cholesterol was measured by an enzymatic method and apo B was estimated by a single radial immunodiffusion method.

7) Scanning electron microscopy (SEM) and transmission electron microscopy (TEM) were carried out.[8] A negative staining method[9] was used to observe the molecular size of the LDL.

Results

1) LDL-CH and LDL-apo B in rabbits:

LDL-CH was increased markedly after feeding of 1% CH but it was significantly suppressed by adding 10% soycream in the diet with 1% CH as shown in FIGURE 1.

Although apo B also increased markedly one week after 1% CH feeding, there was no difference in LDL-CH between one and two weeks. LDL-apo B was decreased significantly by 10% soycream but the difference was not as much as that in LDL-CH.

The regression coefficients were calculated between LDL-apo B and LDL-CH in rabbits fed 1% CH and 10% soycream. As shown in FIGURE 2, the gradients of the line were reduced markedly by 1% CH feeding after one and two weeks. However, when the soycream was added to the 1% CH feed, the line moved in the direction of the gradient of the standard feeding.

2) LDL-CH and LDL-apo B in humans:

The regression coefficients between LDL-apo B and LDL-CH were calculated in the healthy persons and in the patients with ischemic heart diseases. As shown in FIGURE 2, the gradient of the line in the patients with ischemic heart diseases was smaller than that in the healthy persons.

3) A model of endothelial cell injuries in arteries *in vivo*:

Total cholesterol (TC), LPO, PL, and TG in LDL were measured periodically up to 10 weeks after 1% CH feeding. As shown in FIGURE 3, the rate of increase in TC and LPO in LDL was similar throughout the experimental period of 10 weeks.

The following results were obtained after the infusion of diluted LDLs or saline of 400 ml each with the left external carotid artery under the pressure of 120 mm Hg.

a) The surfaces of the left and right internal carotid arteries after the saline infusion were smooth, and red cells and platelets had not adhered to the surface by SEM. Furthermore, fine folds were found along the direction of the blood flow (FIG. 4).

b) When the normal LDL was infused, the surfaces of both carotid arteries were similar to those in saline-infused rabbits.

c) However, the infusion of 400 ml of diluted LDL from 1% CH rabbits made the surface of arterial endothelial cells change markedly, even when the same amount and same concentration of LDL-CH as in the diluted normal LDL was infused (FIG. 4). Many red cells, platelets, and white cells adhered to the surface, and the changes in the endothelial surface were recognized.

In order to find out whether those changes are a systemic reaction of a local phenomenon the infusion was carried out in the auricular vein, and the endothelial surface of the aorta was examined by SEM. The changes of the aortic surface were similar to those seen in the carotid arteries. Accordingly, we considered that these changes are a systemic reaction and not a direct local reaction. In addition, these changes were observed by TEM, as shown in FIGURE 5.

Numerous endocytotic vesicles were seen in the endothelial cells after the infusion of 1% CH LDL but those were not prominent after saline or normal LDL infusion.

5) To estimate the molecular ratio of CH to apo B in LDL, average molecular weight of LDL-CH was calculated and found to be 611, as shown in FIGURE 6. This was calculated on the basis of the ratio of free CH to ester CH in LDL to be approximately 1:4. The molecular weight of apo B has been reported as 30×10^4–60×10^4. Thus, the

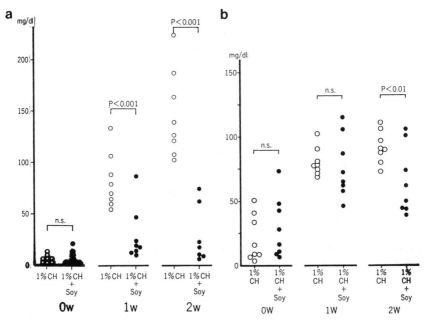

FIGURE 1. (a) LDL-cholesterol and (b) LDL-apo B after feeding standard feed plus 1% cholesterol (1% CH) and that plus 10% soycream (1% CH + Soy) for 2 weeks in rabbits. W, week.

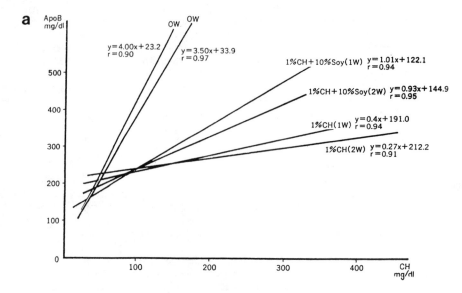

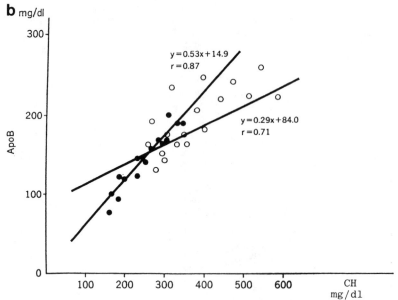

FIGURE 2. Regression coefficient between LDL-apo B and LDL-CH in each feeding in **(a)** rabbits and **(b)** humans. Rabbits: n = 8 in each group. Humans: ● healthy young person; ○ ischemic heart disease.

molecular ratio of the CH molecule to one molecule of apo B in LDL was calculated three times after 1% CH feeding. As shown in FIGURE 6, in 0 week Apo B: CH = 1:120–240, in 2 weeks 1:600–1200, and in 5 weeks 1:700–1400 were obtained.

TEM findings of normal LDL and 1% CH LDL after 5 weeks by negative staining are shown in FIGURE 6. After 5 weeks 1% CH LDL was clearly larger in molecular size than in normal LDL.

EXPERIMENT II

Materials and Methods

1) Modified LDL (ultra-water-soluble LDL [UWS-LDL]) after dialysis into filtered tap water was separated by Kanazawa's method.[10]

2) Thiobarbituric acid reactive substances (TBARS) were estimated by Yagi's method.[11]

3) Macrophages were separated by Adams' method[12] and harvested by 0.02 N NaOH. Protein was measured by Lowry's method[13] and lipids were measured by the charring method[14] after thin layer chromatography (TLC). The extraction of lipids was carried out by Bligh-Dyer's method.[15]

4) Platelet aggregability was measured by Born's method.[16] Two moles of adenosine diphosphate (ADP) were used as the concentration of the aggregants.

5) Bio-Gel A 150 was purchased from Bio-Red Laboratories. Agarose gel electrophoresis was carried out for IDL (1.006–1.019) and LDL (1.019–1.063).

6) Two kinds of solvent were used for TLC:
    a) petroleum ether 75; ethyl ether 25; acetic acid 1; and
    b) hexane 80; ethyl ether 20.

7) Lipoproteins and lipids were oxidized with 10 M Cu^{++}.

8) Cholesterol-linolate, -stearate, -linolenate, -oleate, -arachidonate, trioleate and methyl stearate were purchased from Sigma Chemical Company.

9) To prove whether modified LDL with peroxidized cholesteryl linolate can be recognized *in vivo*, native LDLs (1.019–1.063) were separated immediately after blood was drawn from 19 healthy persons, 11 nonatherosclerotic outpatients, 7 patients with

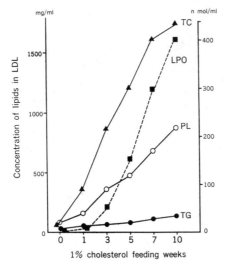

FIGURE 3. Weekly changes of each lipid in LDL after 1% CH feeding in rabbits. N = 8.

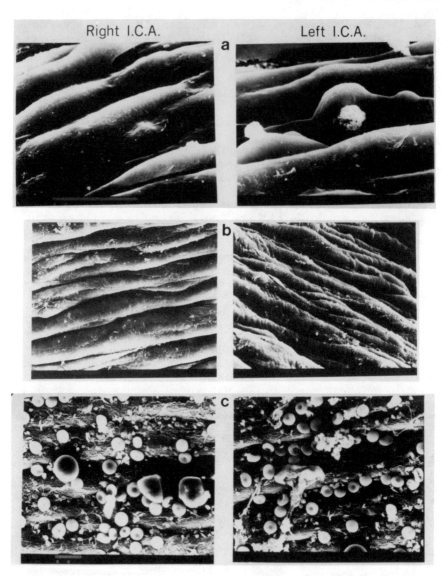

FIGURE 4. Scanning electron microscopic findings of internal carotid artery (ICA) after infusion with **(a)** saline solution, **(b)** normal LDL, and **(c)** 1% cholesterol feeding LDL. The infusion was carried out in the *left* carotis communis.

angina pectoris, and 22 patients with old myocardial infarction diagnosed by coronary angiography. Lipids were extracted from LDL from each patient by Bligh-Dyer's method and TLCs were performed.

10) The quantitation of lipids from TLC was estimated by charring method.

11) To investigate the changes in LDL-CH and LDL-apo B by probucol treatment, 23

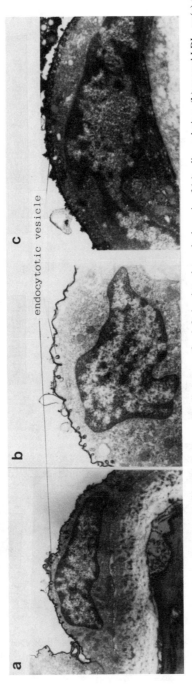

FIGURE 5. Transmission electron microscopic findings of basilar artery after infusion into the auricular vein of (**a**) saline solution, (**b**) normal LDL, or (**c**) 1% cholesterol feeding LDL. (a) × 72,000; (b) and (c) × 140,000.

LDL :

Free cholesterol $(387 = MW)$ 1
Ester cholesterol $(667 = MW)$ 4 $\left.\right\}$ average M.W. $\fallingdotseq 611$

ApoB M.W.   : $30 \times 10^{4} \sim 60 \times 10^{4}$

<u>1% cholesterol feed</u>

OW ApoB : cholesterol $\fallingdotseq 1 : 120 \sim 240$

2W ApoB : cholesterol $\fallingdotseq 1 : 600 \sim 1200$

5W ApoB : cholesterol $\fallingdotseq 1 : 700 \sim 1400$

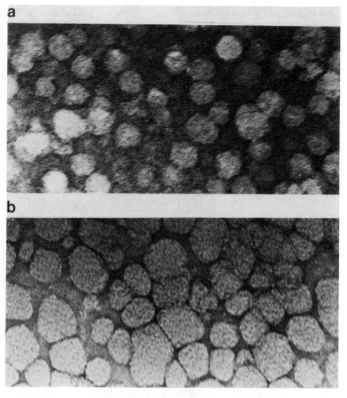

FIGURE 6. Apo B and cholesterol ratio in LDL (*above*), and molecular size of (**a**) normal LDL and (**b**) 1% cholesterol feeding LDL by transmission electron microscopy (negative staining).

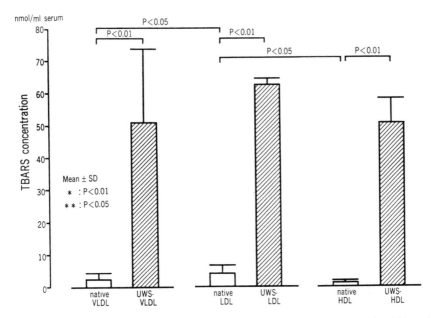

FIGURE 7. Concentration of thiobarbituric acid reactive substance (TBARS) in native LDL and UWS-lipoprotein.

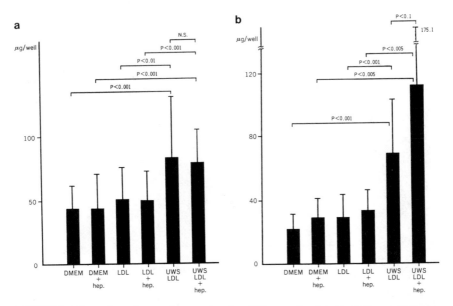

FIGURE 8. Mice peritoneal macrophages and various LDLs were incubated in Dulbecco minimum essential medium (DMEM) at 37°C for 48 hours. Thereafter, the amount of **(a)** protein and **(b)** cholesteryl ester in macrophages were measured.

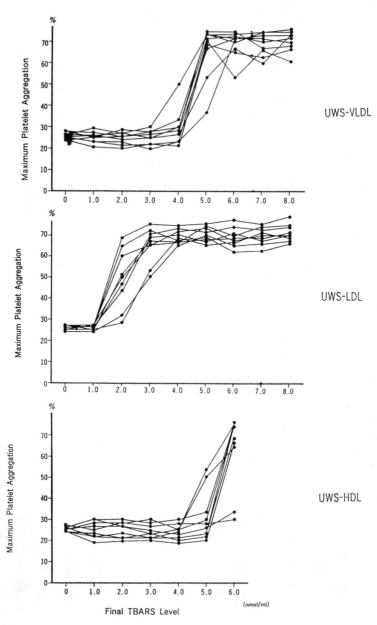

FIGURE 9. The effect of modified lipoprotein on ADP-induced platelet aggregation by each TBARS concentration.

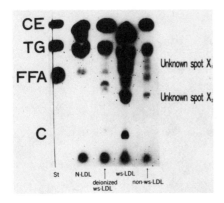

FIGURE 10. Thin layer chromatography (TLC) profiles of various lipoproteins.

male rabbits were used; group 1 consisting of 8 rabbits fed standard feed + 1% CH; group 2, 7 rabbits fed the same diet as in group 1 + 1% probucol, and group 3, 8 rabbits fed group 1 diet + 2% probucol.

Results

1) TBARS concentrations in UWS-LDL were tremendously higher than those in native LDL as shown in FIGURE 7. The TBARS concentrations in UWS-VLDL and UWS-HDL were also higher than those in native VLDL and native HDL.

2) To investigate the biological functions of UWS-LDL, protein and cholesteryl ester in mice peritoneal macrophages were measured after incubation with normal LDL or UWS-LDL. As shown in FIGURE 8, UWS-LDL was clearly internalized into macrophages although native LDL was not.

Furthermore, platelet aggregabilities were measured by Born's method before and after the addition of UWS-VLDL, UWS-LDL, or UWS-HDL. As shown in FIGURE 8, the enhancement of platelet aggregabilities was strongest in UWS-LDL among UWS-lipoproteins.

3) To clarify the differences between native LDL and various UWS-lipoproteins, TLCs of lipids extracted from native LDL and UWS- LDL were carried out.

As shown in FIGURE 10, cholesteryl ester (CE), TG, free fatty acid (FFA), free cholesterol (FC), and PL from normal LDL (N-LDL) were stained in iodine vapors. From UWS-LDL two additional spots, which were not seen in normal LDL, were stained; one between CE and TG on TLC and the other between TG and FFA. We named the former "spot X_1" and the latter "spot X_2."

However, if ethylene diamine tetra acetic acid 2Na (EDTA) or butyric acid hydroxy toluene (BHT) was added to the tap water when dialysis was performed to detect the formation of UWS-LDL from native LDL, spot X_1 did not appear on the TLC. Accordingly, it was considered that the formation of spot X_1 in UWS-LDL was caused by the oxidation of the native LDL. When TLC was performed by using another solvent (FIG. 10) the results were the same. Furthermore, spot X_1 was not found from UWS-VLDL, but a small spot X_1 was found from USW-IDL (FIG. 11).

To investigate further the nature of spot X_1, each lipid which was scraped from the TLC of the native LDL was oxidized by 10 μM Cu^{++} for 12 hours at 37°C. Thereafter, re-TLC of each oxidized lipid was carried out.

As shown in FIGURE 12, spot X_1 was only recognized on the TLC of oxidates of CE.

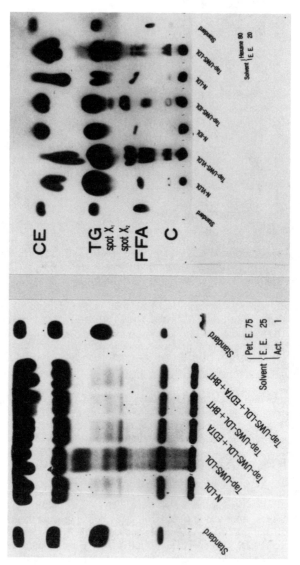

FIGURE 11. TLC profiles of lipids in modified lipoproteins.

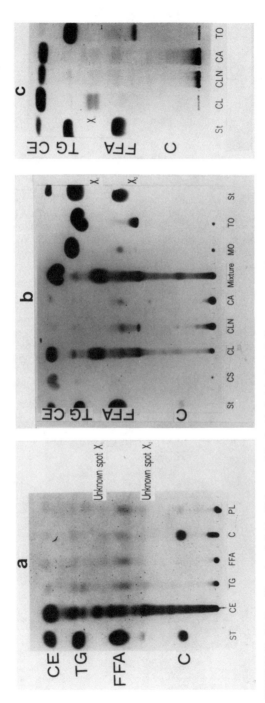

FIGURE 12. TLC profiles of each lipid which was oxidized with Cu^{++}. Each lipid was taken out from lipids included in normal LDL on TLC and thereafter each lipid was oxidized with Cu^{++} (**a**). Various cholesteryl esters which were oxidized with Cu^{++} were developed on TLC. (**b**) Cholesteryl stearate (CS), cholesteryl linolate (CL), cholesteryl linolenate (CLN), cholesteryl arachidonate (CA), methyl oleate (MO), and trioleate (TO) were oxidized with Cu^{++} (10 μM). (**c**) Oxidation with 1 μM Cu^{++}.

Therefore, many CE such as cholesteryl stearate, cholesteryl linolate, cholesteryl lino-lenate, cholesteryl arachidonate, and trioleate were oxidized with Cu^{++} by the same method. As shown in FIGURE 12, spot X_1 was only recognized on the TLC of the oxidate of cholesteryl linolate.

To investigate the character of the UWS-LDL, Bio-gel A-150 column chromatography and agarose gel electrophoresis of native LDL and UWS-LDL were carried out as shown in FIGURE 13.

The molecular size by Bio-gel A-150 column chromatography and the movement by agarose gel electrophoresis from the origin were almost the same between native LDL and UWS-LDL.

4) Modified LDLs with peroxidized cholesteryl linolate were not recognized in healthy young persons and nonatherosclerotic outpatients. But as shown in FIGURE 14, they were recognized in patients with angina pectoris, and they were clearly visible in patients with myocardial infarction. Spot X_1 was recognized in 43% of the patients with angina pectoris and 72% of the patients with old myocardial infarction.

The ratios of the optical density of spot X_1 to that of cholesteryl ester are shown in FIGURE 15. The ratios of spot X_1 to CE in descending order are as follows: old myocardial infarction, angina pectoris, nonatherosclerotic outpatients, healthy young persons.

5) From the above results, modified LDL with peroxidized cholesteryl linolate was considered as an important risk indicator for atherosclerotic diseases. Thus, as the next step an attempt was made to examine whether probucol and soycream treatment can prevent the formation of spot X_1.

LDL-CH levels increased markedly during the 10 weeks of CH feeding, and probucol treatment (both 1 and 2%) did not affect the levels of LDL-CH (FIG. 16). LDL-apo B levels were higher in the probucol-treated group up to 5 weeks after the CH feeding but this difference disappeared after 7 weeks. LDL-LPO levels did not change during the 10 weeks of standard feeding. They increased tremendously when 1% CH was added to the

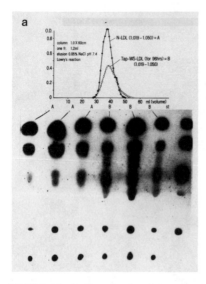
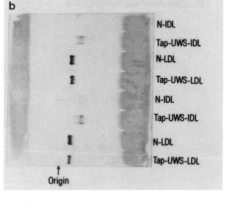

FIGURE 13. Profiles of various lipoproteins by **(a)** Bio-Gel A 150 column chromatography and **(b)** agarose gel electrophoresis.

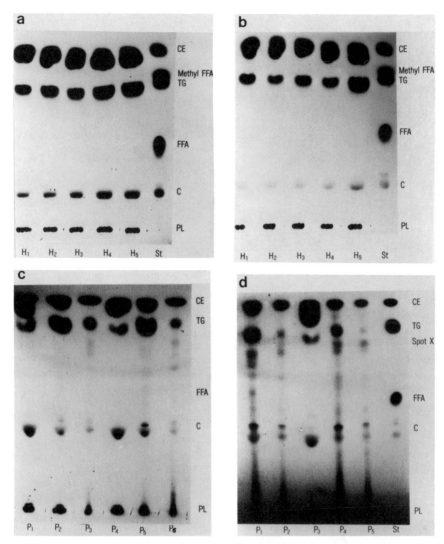

FIGURE 14. TLC profiles of native LDL separated from (**a**) young healthy persons (19 years old), (**b**) healthy outpatients without sclerotic disease (30–53 years old), (**c**) patients with angina pectoris, and (**d**) patients with myocardial infarction. H, healthy person; P, patient.

feed. However, when probucol or soycream was added to the 1% CH feed this increase was almost completely suppressed (TABLE 2).

Three kinds of native LDLs separated from 1% CH-fed rabbits, 1% CH + 1% or 2% probucol-fed rabbits, and 1% CH + 10% soycream-fed rabbits were dialyzed into filtered tap water for 96 hours to investigate their peroxidizability. As shown in FIGURE 17, although spot X_1 was recognized in 1% CH LDL, it was not visible on TLC on soycream LDL and probucol LDL.

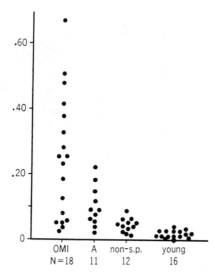

FIGURE 15. Optical density (O.D.) of spot X_1/O.D. of CE ratio (charring method) was shown in old myocardial infarction (OMI), angina pectoris (A), nonsclerotic patients (Non-s.p.), and young healthy persons.

Discussion

Many epidemiological studies have been reported[17,18] dealing with the prevention of ischemic heart diseases. In these studies several risk factors are pointed out; for example, hypercholesterolemia, hypertension, diabetes mellitus, smoking, and obesity. They emphasized that it is important to keep low LDL-CH and high HDL-CH for the prevention

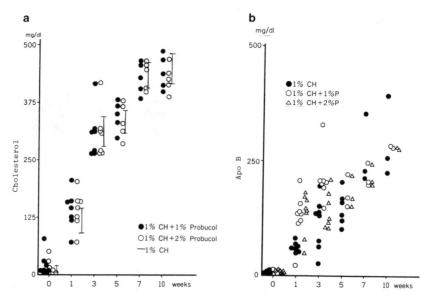

FIGURE 16. Effect of probucol on **(a)** LDL-cholesterol and **(b)** LDL-apo B in rabbits that were fed with 1% CH feeding during 10 weeks.

TABLE 2. Changes in LDL-LPO Fed Various Diets in Rabbits: Effect of Each Feed on LPO[a]

Feed	Weeks					
	0	1	3	5	7	10
St	0.62 ± 0.21	0.69 ± 0.24	0.72 ± 0.18	0.81 ± 0.24	0.80 ± 0.18	0.72 ± 0.38
St + 1% CH	0.59 ± 0.21	16.8 ± 10.1	124.4 ± 77.8	67.0 ± 24.0	300.4 ± 124.0	404.2 ± 170
St + 1% CH + 1% P	0.62 ± 0.3	3.21 ± 2.8	5.26 ± 1.91	6.62 ± 2.18	6.25 ± 0.83	7.18 ± 1.32
St + 1% CH + 2% P	1.01 ± 0.92	7.41 ± 7.3	6.65 ± 2.5	7.71 ± 1.92	15.8 ± 10.2	8.78 ± 2.10
St + 1% CH + 10% Soy	0.88 ± 0.32	7.24 ± 0.28	0.82 ± 0.38	7.12 ± 0.28	7.28 ± 3.21	6.98 ± 1.92

[a]nmol/ml; mean ± SD; n = 8. St, standard; CH, cholesterol; P, probucol; Soy, soycream.

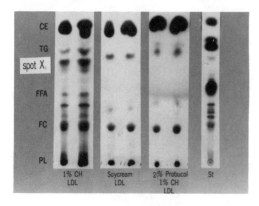

FIGURE 17. Effect of soycream and probucol on peroxidation in rabbits.

and treatment of atherosclerosis. Recently, Steinberg[5] and Kita[6] reported that reducing LPO was more important for the prevention of formation of atherosclerotic lesion than reducing LDL-CH in animal experiments. Thus, it seems uncertain what is most important for the prevention and treatment of atherosclerosis.

In this paper, possible ways to prevent and treat atherosclerosis are discussed from the view point of the composition and physical character of the LDL. Extensive atherosclerotic lesions can be produced in arteries of rabbits by CH feeding but the administration of soycream or probucol prevents the development of atheroma. In these animals CH feeding made the LDL-CH/LDL-apo B ratio markedly increase, and the addition of soycream in the CH feed made the ratio decrease. Also, the LDL-CH/LDL-apo B ratio in the patients with ischemic heart diseases was higher than that in healthy persons. In CH-fed rabbits probucol administration did not change their increased LDL-CH levels but it clearly suppressed the levels of increased LDL-LPO and the formation of atheroma. Therefore, these results suggest that the reduction of the LDL-CH/LDL-apo B ratio and LDL-LPO are important for the prevention and treatment of atherosclerosis.

The experiment for endothelial cell injuries was carried out in rabbits *in vivo*. Normal LDL and 1% CH LDL were separated ultracentrifugally and dialysed into saline solution. These two LDLs were diluted to the concentration of the normal plasma CH level of the rabbit by saline solution. Thus, there were no differences in CH and LPO levels between the diluted normal LDL and the diluted 1% CH LDL. These two kinds of diluted LDLs were infused into rabbit artery or vein. The infusion of the diluted normal LDL did not cause endothelial cell injuries, but the infusion of the diluted 1% CH LDL did cause clear endothelial cell injuries.

In the experiment described above the LDL-LPO level appeared to be important in preventing the formation of atherosclerotic lesions, but in the experiment just described both LDL-CH level and LDL-LPO level did not seem to be important for endothelial cell injuries. How do we reconcile these apparently contradictory results? In another experiment we found that the LDL-CH/LDL-apo B ratio and molecular size of the diluted 1% CH LDL were markedly greater than those of the diluted normal LDL.

Thus, when we combine the results of those several experiments it may be reasonable to conclude that the reduction in the LDL-CH/LDL-apo B ratio and molecular size of LDLs are more important than LDL-CH level or LDL-LPO level for the prevention or treatment of atherosclerosis produced by CH feeding.

In Experiment II, modified LDL with peroxidized cholesteryl linolate was investigated for its biological functions.

LDL with peroxidized cholesteryl linolate showed enhancement of platelet aggregation, and internalization into macrophages. The modified LDL did not differ from the native LDL in its molecular size and in the movement by agarose gel electrophoresis. Therefore, even if such modified LDL do exist *in vivo*, it will be impossible to prove its existence except to show the presence of peroxidized cholesteryl linolate in the native LDL.

We estimated the presence of the peroxidized cholesteryl linolate in the native LDL in 43% of the patients with angina pectoris and in 72% of the patients with old myocardial infarction. In addition, the ratio of peroxidized cholesteryl linolate to cholesteryl ester in patients with myocardial infarction was much greater than in healthy persons. Thus, the modified LDL was considered as an important risk indicator in ischemic heart diseases.

With the above results in mind, the oxidizability of separated LDLs was studied in the presence of divalent metal ion and oxygen. In this study 1% CH LDL, 1% CH + 10% soycream LDL and 1% CH + 1% probucol or 2% probucol LDL were separated from rabbits after 5 weeks of feeding. And they were dialysed into filtered tap water for 96 hours.

Peroxidized cholesterol linolate was estimated only from 1% CH LDL; it was not recognized from LDLs separated from rabbits given soycream or probucol. This suggests that the presence of peroxidized cholesteryl linolate plays an important role for prevention and treatment of atherosclerosis.

CONCLUSION

LDLs with a high ratio of cholesterol to apo B, and LDL with peroxidized cholesteryl linolate appear to atherogenic. But LDLs with normal or low ratio of cholesterol to apo B, and LDL without peroxidate seem not to be atherogenic.

Accordingly, conversion of atherogenic LDLs to nonatherogenic LDLs may be important for the prevention and treatment of atherosclerosis caused by dyslipoproteinemia.

REFERENCES

1. MILLER, N. E. 1987. Association of high-density lipoprotein subclasses and apolipoproteins with ischemic heart disease and coronary atherosclerosis. Am. Heart J. **113:** 589–597.
2. CASTELLI, W. P., P. W. F. WILSON, D. LEVY, & K. ANDERSON. 1989. Cardiovascular risk factors in the elderly. Am. J. Cardiol. **63:** 12H–19H.
3. BLATON, V. H. & B. DECLERG. 1984. Plasma lipoprotein changes by diet. Effect on progression and regression of arterial lesions in nonhuman primates. *In* Regression of Atherosclerotic Lesions. M. R. Malinow & V. H. Blaton, Eds. 105–120. NATO ASI Series.
4. OLSSON, A. G., V. ERIKSON, G. HELMIUS, A. HEMMINGSSON & G. RUHN. 1984. Regression of femoral atherosclerosis in humans: Methodological and clinical problems associated with studies on femoral atherosclerosis development as assessed by angiograms. *In* Regression of Atherosclerotic Lesions. M. R. Malinow & V. H. Blaton, Eds. 311–328. NATO ASI Series.
5. STEINBERG, D., D. SCHWENKE & T. E. CAREW. 1988. The antioxidant effect of probucol in 'relation to arterial LDL metabolism. *In* Modified Lipoproteins—Satellite Meeting (8th International Symposium on Atherosclerosis-Venice). 35–38. CIC Edizioni International.
6. KITA, T., Y. NAGANO, M. YOKODE, K. ISHI, N. KUME, A. OOSHIMA, H. YOSHIDA & C. KAWAI. 1987. Probucol prevents the progression of atherosclerosis in Watanabe heritable hyperlipidemic rabbit, an animal model for familial hypercholesterolemia, Proc. Natl. Acad. Sci. USA **84:** 5928–5931.
7. HAVEL, R. J., H. A. EDER & J. H. BRAGDON. 1955. The distribution and chemical composition of ultra centrifugally separated lipoproteins in human serum. J. Clin. Invest. **51:** 1486–1494.
8. KANAZAWA, T., C. D. HUA, O. KOMATSU, K. ONODERA & Y. OIKE. 1989. Experimental

study on the pathogenesis of cerebral infarction in rabbits by injecting sephadex G-75 (Part I)—Hourly pathological changes of cerebral tissue due to ischemia. Jpn. J. Stroke **11:** 337–346.

9. NONOMURA, S. 1982. A method of negative staining. The Method for Observation of Electron Microscope. H. Akabori, Ed. 136–145. Maruzen LTD.

10. KANAZAWA, T., M. IZAWA, H. MURAOKA, K. ONODERA & H. METOKI. 1981. The method of fractionation of ultra-water soluble and non-water soluble lipoproteins from serum, and the significances of these lipoproteins in stroke. Jpn. J. Stroke **3:** 243–249.

11. OHKAWA, H., N. OHISHI & K. YAGI. 1978. Reaction of linoleic acid hydroperoxide with thiobarbituric acid. J. Lipid Res. **19:** 1053–1057.

12. ADAMS, D. O. 1979. Macrophages. Methods Enzymol. **108:** 494–506.

13. LOWRY, O. H., N. J. ROSEBROUGH, A. L. FARR & R. J. RANDALL. 1951. Protein measurement with the Folin-phenol reagent. J. Biol. Chem. **193:** 265–275.

14. KRITCHEVSKY, D., L. M. DARIDSON, H. K. KIM & S. MALHOTRA. 1973. Quantitation of serum lipids by a simple TLC-charring method. Clin. Chim. Acta **46:** 63–68.

15. BLIGH, E. G. & W. J. DYER. 1959. A rapid method of total lipid extraction and purification. Can. J. Biochem. Physiol. **37:** 911–917.

16. IZAWA, M., T. KANAZAWA, H. KANEKO, Y. HOSHI, A. MIKUNIYA, K. ONODERA, H. METOKI, Y. SHIMANAKA, R. KAWAHARA, C. NIHEI & Y. OIKE. 1985. Potentiation of platelet aggregation induced by several kinds of aggregating agents. J. Jpn. Atheroscler. Soc. **13:** 89–97.

17. GOTTO, A. M. 1979. Status report : plasma lipids, lipoproteins, and coronary artery disease. *In* Atherosclerosis Review. R. Paoletti & A. M. Gotto, Eds. Vol. **4:** 17–28. Raven Press. New York, NY.

18. EPSTEIN, F. H., B. KANNEL, N. KLIMOV & T. W. MEADE. 1987. Relation of risk factors to clinical events. *In* Atherosclerosis Biology and Clinical Science. A. G. Olsson, Ed. 381–388. Churchill Livingstone.

Production of Apolipoprotein E-Rich LDL by the Liver

The Effect of Dietary Cholesterol and Some Lipid Lowering Agents[a]

TAMIO TERAMOTO, TERUHIKO MATSUSHIMA,
YUKIO HORIE, AND TSUYOSHI WATANABE

First Department of Internal Medicine
Faculty of Medicine
University of Tokyo
7-3-1 Hongo, Bunkyo-ku
Tokyo 113, Japan

INTRODUCTION

Plasma LDL is largely derived from the catabolism of plasma VLDL,[1,2] but it remains to be established whether the liver is a direct source of plasma LDL. Hepatic secretion of LDL was reported in the state of hypercholesterolemia and cholesterol feeding, which are considered to play a role in atherogenesis.[3-5]

Previously, using Japanese monkey liver, we showed that the liver secreted two types of LDL, apo E-LDL composed of only apo E with respect to apoprotein moiety, and apo B,E-LDL composed of apo B and apo E.[6] In the report we showed that cholesterol feeding induced a decrease in LDL-apo B100 and an increase in LDL-apo E, resulting in an apo E-rich LDL. Cholesterol feeding is one of factors that induce atherosclerosis. Therefore, it is important to study the role of hepatic LDL in lipoprotein metabolism and atherogenesis, and to learn the mechanism of the effects of dietary cholesterol.

In this study we conducted rat liver perfusions to elucidate the mechanism with use of HMG Co A reductase inhibitor (CS-514), which suppresses a hepatic cholesterogenesis,[7] and Kampo medicine (Daisaikoto), which suppresses hepatic accumulation of cholesterol.

METHOD

All animals for liver perfusion studies were Wistar male rats (bodyweight 200 g) maintained on a chow diet low in fat and cholesterol, and were fasted overnight before being killed. Three groups of male Wistar rats were established according to the composition of diet as follows. 1) Normal control group; 0.09% cholesterol, 2) Cholesterol group; 2% cholesterol, 25% lard, and 1% cholic acid, 3) Test group; 5 mg/g of Daisaikoto extract was added to the cholesterol diet. Animals were fed the diet for 7 days before being sacrificed. The control group was divided into two groups. In one group CS-514 was added to the perfusate to give a final concentration of 50 ng/ml; in the other group CS-514 was eliminated from the perfusate. The method of liver perfusion was reported elsewhere[8] with the use of a silastic tubing instead of a glass column as an oxygenator

[a]This work was supported by the Sankyo Foundation of Life Science.

according to the method of Hamilton et al.[9] Recirculating perfusion was established with 50 ml of the perfusate, to which 0.1 mCi of ^{3}H-phenylalanine was added. In some perfusions, ^{35}S-methionine was added instead of ^{3}H-phenylalanine in the perfusate to see the perfusate apolipoprotein profile by fluorography. After perfusion for 60 min, the perfusate was discarded as a washout perfusion and replaced with a fresh perfusate including the same concentration of ^{3}H-phenylalanine, and recirculating perfusion was continued for 150 min. At the termination of the perfusions, the red blood cells were removed from the perfusate, and a preservative solution was added to the perfusate to give a final concentration of 0.01% NaN_3, 0.05% EDTA, 0.005% gentamycin, and 1 mM phenylmethyl sulfonyl fluoride (PMSF).

Lipoproteins were separated into 3 fractions based on the density as following: d <1.006 g/ml; d, 1.019–1.050 g/ml, and d, 1.063–1.21 g/ml, by sequential ultracentrifugation flotation according to the method of Havel et al.[10]

Polyacrylamide gel electrophoresis in the presence of sodium dodecyl sulfate (SDS-PAGE) was performed in 1.0-mm-thick slab gel.[11]

For measurement of the radioactivity in each apolipoprotein, the corresponding band was excised from the electrophoretic gels, and was counted in a toluene scintillator.

Plasma lipid were assayed by the enzymatic method. Hepatic cholesterol was measured by the method of Searcy,[12] and the triglyceride with use of Triglyceride test Wako^R.[13]

RESULTS

Incorporation rate of the precursor amino acid into the proteins was constant until the end of perfusion, indicating that hepatic synthesis of the proteins was active during 210 min in vitro perfusion.

Apolipoproteins of perfusate VLDL and LDL were heavily labeled with radioactive precursor (^{35}S-methionine) as shown in FIGURE 1. The fluorography of the perfusate lipoproteins indicates the newly synthesized apolipoproteins in each lipoprotein. In both of the VLDL and the LDL most heavily labeled apolipoproteins were apo E, apo B100 and apo B48, though the distribution of radioactivity was clearly discriminated between the VLDL and the LDL.

TABLE 1 represents the distribution of radioactivity among the lipoproteins. There was no significant difference in the protein synthesis among the control, cholesterol, and CS-514 groups, though VLDL was increased and LDL was decreased in the cholesterol group, significantly. When CS-514 was added to the perfusate, VLDL was increased slightly but no difference in the LDL was observed.

Distribution of the radioactivities to each apolipoprotein are shown in TABLE 2. The results are represented as the ratio of each apoprotein to total radioactivities. Apo E was increased in VLDL by both cholesterol feeding and the addition of CS-514, while apo B100 was decreased markedly and apo E was increased in LDL by cholesterol feeding but not by addition of CS-514.

FIGURE 2 shows the effect of dietary cholesterol and CS-514 on the incorporation of ^{14}C-acetate into hepatic cholesterol, and revealed that both the dietary cholesterol and CS-514 suppressed hepatic cholesterogenesis to 1/4 and 1/6 of the control, respectively.

When Daisaikoto was added to the cholesterol diet, plasma cholesterol level was decreased and HDL-cholesterol level was increased significantly compared to the cholesterol group as shown in FIGURE 3 and TABLE 3. The increase in hepatic cholesterol level induced by cholesterol feeding was suppressed in the Daisaikoto group, as shown in FIGURE 4.

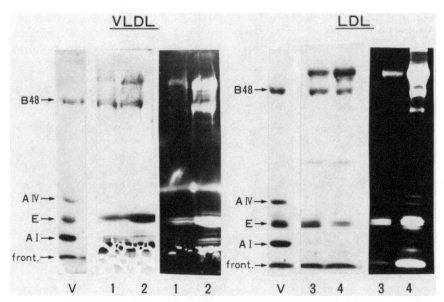

FIGURE 1. Fluorography of apolipoproteins produced by the perfused rat liver. The rat livers were perfused *in vitro* as described in the text. Apolipoproteins were separated by SDS-PAGE. The gels were immersed in En[3]Hance, dried, and exposed to X-ray film for several days at −80°C. V: rat lymph VLDL; 1,3: perfusate VLDL and LDL from the first 60 min, respectively; 2,4: perfusate VLDL and LDL from the latter 150 min, respectively. The *left lanes* are protein staining and the *right lanes* are their fluorography.

The liver perfusion study of the Daisaikoto group revealed that LDL production, which was suppressed by cholesterol feeding, was enhanced by Daisaikoto, though VLDL production was not affected. The effects of Daisaikoto on the secretion of apolipoproteins are shown in TABLE 4, and revealed that Daisaikoto induced the increase in apo B100 and the decrease in apo E compared to the cholesterol group in the fraction of the LDL.

DISCUSSION

We showed that apo B of the perfusate VLDL and LDL was heavily labeled with the precursor amino acid, suggesting that newly synthesized apo B is secreted in association

TABLE 1. Effect of Dietary Cholesterol and HMG Co A Reductase Inhibitor on Lipoprotein Secretion from Perfused Rat Livers[1]

	Control (10)	Cholesterol-Fed (8)	HMG Co A Reductase Inhibitor (5)
VLDL	0.315 ± 0.19	0.914 ± 0.52*	0.576 ± 0.16*
LDL	0.273 ± 0.12	0.125 ± 0.07**	0.336 ± 0.16
HDL	0.122 ± 0.05	0.053 ± 0.05*	0.208 ± 0.05*

[a]Mean ± SD; *$p < 0.05$; **$p < 0.01$. Secretion rate of newly synthesized lipoproteins was estimated by incorporation of ^{3}H-phenylalanine into each lipoprotein. The results are represented as the percentage of lipoprotein radioactivity to total TCA precipitable radioactivities. The numbers in parentheses are the number of experiments.

TABLE 2. Effect of Dietary Cholesterol and HMG Co A Reductase Inhibitor on Apolipoproteins Secreted by Perfused Rat Livers[a]

	Control (10)	Cholesterol-Fed (8)	HMG Co A Reductase Inhibitor (5)
VLDL			
B100	22.3 ± 12.4	28.6 ± 21.5	27.6 ± 10.7
B48	35.4 ± 21.7	13.5 ± 8.1*	37.5 ± 7.9
E	6.8 ± 3.5	15.4 ± 7.5*	12.2 ± 3.6*
A-I	2.03 ± 1.4	8.8 ± 7.5*	2.3 ± 1.1
SMP	33.4 ± 17.1	33.7 ± 12.4	21.0 ± 7.3
LDL			
B100	50.7 ± 18.5	27.1 ± 21.8*	53.0 ± 7.1
B48	22.5 ± 8.3	19.0 ± 11.0	23.9 ± 7.7
E	6.75 ± 4.7	17.9 ± 4.4***	9.48 ± 7.4
A-I	2.19 ± 2.32	3.70 ± 2.4	4.98 ± 4.2
SMP	18.1 ± 16.0	32.4 ± 21.7	8.44 ± 2.7
HDL			
B48	63.3 ± 27.1	53.4 ± 23.3	50.9 ± 21.7
E	5.76 ± 5.0	15.3 ± 10.3	9.53 ± 7.1
A-I	8.56 ± 6.7	7.54 ± 4.1	12.7 ± 5.1
SMP	22.3 ± 17.8	23.8 ± 13.9	26.9 ± 13.0

[a]Mean ± SD; *$p < 0.05$; **$p < 0.01$; ***$p < 0.001$. To estimate the incorporation of radioactive amino acid into each apolipoprotein of lipoproteins, the corresponding band on the SDS-PAGE was cut out, added NCS (Amersham) diluted 9:1 with water, heated for 2 hr at 50°C. Samples were counted in a toluene scintillator (PPO 4 g/L, POPOP 0.1 g/L in toluene). SMP: small molecular proteins. The results are expressed by the ratio of apoprotein radioactivity to the lipoprotein radio-activities.

with VLDL and LDL. Since apo B is essential for secretion of triglyceride-rich lipoproteins and is not transferred from other lipoproteins, labeled apo B in LDL fraction indicates that newly synthesized apo B is secreted in association with LDL particles. Although it remains to be established whether the liver is a direct source of plasma LDL,[14–18] we showed that a part of LDL are derived from the liver.

The aim of our studies is to elucidate the mechanism by which dietary cholesterol induced the decrease in apo B100 and the increase in apo E of LDL, which were observed in the monkey liver perfusion. In this study we confirmed these evidences with use of rat liver perfusion.

Since there is a possibility that apo B100 was distributed to VLDL from LDL because of enhancement of VLDL production by cholesterol feeding, we tested the effect of fatty

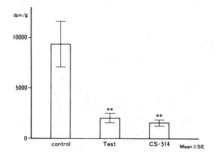

FIGURE 2. Effect of dietary cholesterol and HMG Co A reductase inhibitor on hepatic synthesis of cholesterol. The livers from the rats fed cholesterol diet (Test) were perfused with addition of ^{14}C-acetate, and the incorporation into hepatic cholesterol was estimated as a cholesterogenesis. In the case of HMG Co A reductase inhibitor, CS-514 was added to the perfusate together with ^{14}C-acetate, and the incorporation of ^{14}C-acetate into cholesterol was counted after perfusion.

TABLE 3. Effect of Dietary Cholesterol and Daisaikoto on Lipoproteins Secreted by Perfused Rat Livers[a]

	Control (4)	Cholesterol-Fed (5)	Daisaikoto (5)
VLDL	0.376 ± 0.33	0.830 ± 0.30	0.800 ± 0.16*
LDL	0.215 ± 0.14	0.114 ± 0.04*	0.182 ± 0.08
HDL	0.154 ± 0.15	0.029 ± 0.02**	0.05 ± 0.02**

[a]Mean ± SD; *p <0.05; **p <0.01. Secretion rate of newly synthesized lipoproteins was estimated by incorporation of ^{3}H-phenylalanine into each lipoprotein. The results are represented as the percentage of lipoprotein radioactivity to total TCA precipitable radioactivities. The numbers in parentheses are the number of experiments.

acid load, which induced overproduction of VLDL, on hepatic secretion of apolipoprotein, and found that neither decrease in apo B100 nor increase in apo E of the LDL were observed (data not shown).

The major effects of cholesterol diet are a suppression of hepatic cholesterogenesis and a cholesterol accumulation in the liver. So we conducted two types of liver perfusion experiments.

When HMG Co A reductase inhibitor was added to the perfusate, apo B100 in LDL was not decreased, although cholesterogenesis was suppressed to the degree comparable to cholesterol feeding as observed in FIGURE 2.

When Daisaikoto was added to the diet together with cholesterol, the cholesterol accumulation in the liver was diminished and the decrease in LDL-apo B100 was also diminished, suggesting that hepatic production of apo B100 and apo E in LDL is regulated by hepatic cholesterol level but not by the level of cholesterogenesis.

Mazzone *et al.* reported that mouse peritoneal macrophages loaded with cholesterol

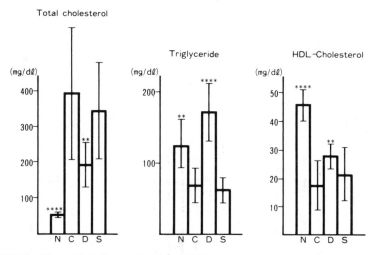

FIGURE 3. Effect of Daisaikoto on the plasma lipid levels. Daisaikoto and Saikokaryukotuboreito were added to the diet together with cholesterol as described in the text for 7 days. N: normal control; C: cholesterol diet; D: cholesterol diet plus Daisaikoto; S: cholesterol diet plus Saikokaryukotuboreito, Mean ± SD; **p <0.01; ****p <0.001.

TABLE 4. Effect of Daisaikoto on Apolipoproteins Secreted by Perfused Rat Livers[a]

	Control (4)	Cholesterol-Fed (5)	Daisaikoto (5)
VLDL			
B100	47.5 ± 30.3	42.8 ± 5.5	34.4 ± 14.5
B48	22.3 ± 12.1	26.0 ± 5.4	23.8 ± 8.4
E	7.7 ± 4.9	10.1 ± 2.1	8.2 ± 3.3
LDL			
B100	52.3 ± 6.0	37.8 ± 5.5**	51.8 ± 10.7
B48	25.6 ± 3.6	18.5 ± 5.0*	22.8 ± 7.4
E	5.3 ± 2.4	12.1 ± 2.0**	4.9 ± 0.9
HDL			
B48	51.8 ± 8.5	24.8 ± 10.5**	31.5 ± 19.5
E	13.4 ± 3.0	30.7 ± 7.1**	32.7 ± 13.7
A-I	9.3 ± 2.5	20.1 ± 3.5	15.6 ± 9.2

[a]Mean ± SD; *p <0.05; **p <0.01; ***p <0.001. To estimate the incorporation of radioactive amino acid into each apolipoprotein of lipoproteins, the corresponding band on the SDS-PAGE was cut out, added NCS (Amersham) diluted 9:1 with water, heated for 2 hr at 50°C. Samples were counted in a toluene scintillator (PPO 4 g/L, POPOP 0.1 g/L in toluene). SMP: small molecular proteins. The results are expressed by the ratio of apoprotein radioactivity to the lipoprotein radio-activities.

show an increase in apo E biosynthesis and in mRNA levels.[19] However, with respect to apo B the intracellular regulation mechanism remained to be elucidated.[20,21] Our observations indicate that the intracellular cholesterol level is one of the regulatory factors of LDL-apo B100 secretion besides the regulatory factors of apo E secretion.

Taken together, cholesterol load on the liver induced an increase in apo E and a decrease in apo B of LDL, consequently apo E-rich LDL. Such apo E-rich LDL may play a role in atherogenesis. The *in vivo* metabolism and specific atherogenic potency of apo E-rich LDL is under investigation.

SUMMARY

We reported previously that cholesterol feeding induced an increase in hepatic secretion of VLDL and a decrease in that of LDL, especially LDL-apo B100, using monkey

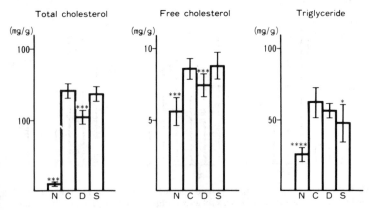

FIGURE 4. Effect of Daisaikoto on the hepatic lipid levels. Abbreviations as in FIGURE 3. Mean ± SD; *p <0.05; ***p <0.005; ****p <0.001.

liver perfusion.[6] In the present study we conducted rat liver perfusion using the HMG Co A reductase inhibitor (CS-514) and Kampo medicine (Daisaikoto) to elucidate the mechanism of the effect of dietary cholesterol on hepatic lipoprotein and apolipoprotein synthesis.

Although the secretion of VLDL was increased by cholesterol feeding, that of LDL and especially of apo B100 of LDL were markedly decreased, and apo E of the LDL was increased as observed in the monkey liver perfusion experiments. The effect of CS-514 was clearly different from the effect of dietary cholesterol in spite of the suppression of hepatic cholesterogenesis which was comparable to that induced by cholesterol feeding, suggesting that the decrease in secretion of LDL-apo B100 induced by the dietary cholesterol is not due to suppressed cholesterogenesis. Daisaikoto, which was added to the diet together with cholesterol, diminished the effects of dietary cholesterol on the plasma and hepatic cholesterol levels. When the liver treated with Daisaikoto was perfused, the effect of dietary cholesterol on the production of lipoprotein and apolipoprotein was markedly diminished.

This evidence indicates that the decrease in LDL-apo B100 and the increase in apo E were mediated by the hepatic cholesterol level.

ACKNOWLEDGMENT

We wish to thank Miss A. Tajima for her expert technical support.

REFERENCES

1. SIGURDSSON, G., A. NICOLL & B. LEWIS. 1975. J. Clin. Invest. **56:** 1481–1490.
2. EISENBERG, S., D. W. BILHEIMER, R. I. LEVY *et al.* 1973. Biochim. Biophys. Acta **326:** 361–377.
3. JANUS, E. D., A. NICOLL, R. WOOTTON *et al.* 1980. Eur. J. Clin. Invest. **10:** 149–159.
4. PACKARD, C. J., L. MCKINNEY, K. CARR *et al.* 1983. J. Clin. Invest. **72:** 45–51.
5. JOHNSON, F. L., R. W. ST. CLAIR & L. L. RUDEL. 1983. J. Clin. Invest. **72:** 221–236.
6. TERAMOTO, T., H. KATO, M. KINOSHITA *et al.* 1987. Eur. J. Clin. Invest. **17:** 522–529.
7. TSUJITA, Y., M. KURODA, Y. SHIMADA *et al.* 1986. Biochim. Biophys. Acta **877:** 50–60.
8. JONES, L. A., T. TERAMOTO, D. JUHN *et al.* 1984. J. Lipid Res. **25:** 319–335.
9. HAMILTON, R. L., M. N. BERRY, M. C. WILLIAMS *et al.* 1974. J. Lipid Res. **15:** 182–186.
10. HAVEL, R. J., H. A. EDEL & J. H. BRAGDON. 1955. J. Clin. Invest. **34:** 1345–1453.
11. LAEMMLI, U. K. 1970. Nature (London) **227:** 680–685.
12. SEARCY, R. L. *et al.* 1960. Clin. Chim. Acta **5:** 192–199.
13. FLETCHER, M. J. 1968. Clin. Chim. Acta **22:** 393–397.
14. SWIFT, L. L., P. D. SOULE & V. S. LEQUIRE. 1982. J. Lipid Res. **23:** 962–971.
15. NOEL, S. P., L. WONG, P. J. DOLPHIN, L. DORY & D. RUBINSTEIN. 1979. J. Clin. Invest. **64:**674–683.
16. GUO, L. S. S., R. L. HAMILTON, R. OSTWALD & R. J. HAVEL. 1982. J. Lipid Res. **23:** 543–555.
17. NAKAYA, N., B. H. CHUNG, J. R. PATSCH & O. D. TAUNTON. 1977. J. Biol. Chem. **252:** 7530–7533.
18. JOHNSON, F. L., L. L. SWIFT & L. L. RUDEL. 1987. J. Lipid Res. **28:** 549–564.
19. MAZZONE, T., H. GUMP, P. DILLER *et al.* 1987. J. Biol. Chem. **262:** 11657–11662.
20. DAVIS, R. A., J. R. BOOGAERTS, R. A. BORCHARDT *et al.* 1985. J. Biol. Chem. **260:** 14137–14144.
21. CRAIG, W. Y., R. NUTRIK & A. D. COOPER. 1988. J. Biol. Chem. **263:** 13880–13890.

Retardation of Atherogenesis and Other Effects of a Fish Oil Additive to a Hyperlipidemic Diet for Swine

W. A. THOMAS,[a] D. N. KIM,[a] AND J. SCHMEE[b]

.[a]Department of Pathology
Niel Hellman Research Building
Albany, New York 12208
and
[b]Statistical Unit
Union College
Union Street
Schenectady, New York 12308

INTRODUCTION

Greenland Eskimos consuming large quantities of fish have been reported to have a low incidence of coronary heart disease.[1] Low incidence of deaths from coronary atherosclerosis have also been found in Japan particularly among groups with high fish intake.[2] A 20-year mortality study carried out in a Dutch population has shown a dose response relation between fish consumption and the incidence of coronary deaths with as little as two fish meals a week seeming to provide some protection.[3]

Attention has been focussed on the fish oils in the fish diets and particularly on the major omega-3 fatty acids found in fish oil which are eicosapentaenoic acid (EPA) and docosahexaenoic acid (DHA). A considerable body of indirect evidence has accumulated suggesting that these omega-3 fatty acids are the active ingredients re atherosclerotic heart disease. Numerous clinical studies have been carried out in man on the effects of fish oils on lipids, platelet functions, eicosonoid metabolism, and other systems and these have been summarized recently in an excellent review by Harris.[4] These clinical studies in man cannot of course provide any direct evidence on the effect of fish oil on atherogenesis. Recent trials involving practical amounts of fish oil have shown a hypotriglyceridemic effect, little or no effect on total cholesterol, and in several trials an increase in LDL cholesterol. Other studies have also shown reduced platelet aggregability and reduction in some eicosonoid metabolites.

Studies in experimental animals of the effects of fish oil on atherogenesis in cholesterol-fed animals are of interest. In nonhuman primates Davis et al.[5] have shown retardation of atherogenesis but with a marked hypocholesterolemic effect not usually seen in man. In rabbits results have been controversial. Thiery and Seidel[6] reported an increase in atherogenesis which they suggested might be associated with lipid peroxidation. Zhu et al.[7] reported a decrease in atherogenesis in rabbits with no significant change in plasma cholesterol levels. Weiner et al.[8] carried out studies in swine subjected to balloon catheter endothelial denudation of a coronary artery and a high saturated fat, high cholesterol diet containing sodium cholate for six months with and without a cod liver oil additive. They

TABLE 1. Features Studied in the Swine

Atherosclerotic lesions
Lipoproteins
Monocyte/macrophages
TBARS
Arachidonic acid metabolites
Platelets

found a marked reduction in atherogenesis without a significant change in plasma cholesterol levels which they thought might be associated with a reduction in thromboxane A_2 levels produced by the fish oil. We have carried out studies in swine similar to those of Weiner *et al.* except that the animals were not subjected to balloon catheter endothelial denudation nor given dietary cholesterolemic enhancers such as sodium cholate but only saturated fats (butter) and cholesterol with and without a fish oil (cod liver oil) additive for 4 months.[9] We too found a dramatic retardation of atherogenesis produced by the fish oil additive with only a modest reduction in plasma cholesterol levels and an actual increase in LDL cholesterol. We are engaged in carrying out a series of studies on various features in these swine. These will be discussed as listed in TABLE 1.

Most of the specific data that we shall present in this and subsequent sections is from our initial experiment but we have subsequent studies in various stages of completion that confirm the initial results and provide supplementary data. The design of the experiment is shown in FIGURE 1. The diets that we used are in TABLE 2. The ingredients of note in the atherogenic diet (BT) are the saturated fats and the cholesterol. The treatment diet (BT + FO) has 30 ml of cod liver oil added to the BT diet and thus contains 270 more kilocalories. The swine were about two months of age at the outset and were sacrificed at four months on diet.

Retardation of Atherosclerotic Lesion Development in Hyperlipidemic Swine by a Fish Oil Additive

Quantitative assessments of extent and quality of atherosclerotic involvement were made in our studies at selected anatomically defined sites as shown in FIGURE 2 on standardized cross sectional microscopic sections with data being analyzed by computer. The features quantified included: (1) average intimal area occupied by lesion (or, in mash-fed controls, normal intimal cellular masses also known as cushions), which provided and index of size, (2) percent of lesion area occupied by necrotic residual including

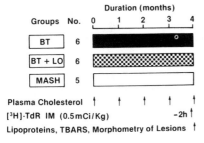

FIGURE 1. Experimental Design. Young male Yorkshire swine were fed the three respective diets for 4 months. Determinations of plasma cholesterol were performed at times indicated by *upward arrow*. Terminally 2 hours before sacrifice swine were given [³H]-Tdr 0.5 mCi/Kg intramuscularly. Lipoprotein fractions, TBARS determinations, and morphometry of atherosclerotic lesions were also carried out[9] terminally.

TABLE 2. Composition of Daily Diets[a]

	Mash[b]	Hyperlipidemic Butter Diet (g)	BT plus Fish Oil (BT + FO) (g)
Mash	700	—	—
Corn oil	—	10	10
Butter	—	90	90
Cod liver oil[c]	—	—	30
Corn starch	—	200	200
Casein[d]	—	130	130
Alphacel[e]	—	64	64
Salt mix	—	4	4
Vitamin mix	—	4	4
Cholesterol	—	10	10
Total	700	512	542
Total calories (Kcal)	2170	2170	2440
% Calories as:			
Fat	9.5	41.5	48.0
Protein	16.5	21.6	19.2
Carbohydrates	74.0	36.9	32.8

[a]Based on Kim et al.[9]

[b]Hog Mash, Agway, Syracuse, NY.

[c]USBC, Cleveland, OH. Cat #13768. Total amount of Omega-3 fatty acids in cod liver oil as calculated is 7.5 g (3.6 g eicosapentaenoic acid, 3.6 g docosahexaenoic acid, 0.3 g linolenic acid). According to the supplier's information, this product meets all requirements of U.S.P. XXI/NF XVI even though it is sold for research use only. No added antioxidants. Contains vitamin A 1000 USP units/g and vitamin D 100 USP units/g.

[d]90% protein.

[e]Cellulose type fiber.

calcium, (3) the average number of intimal nuclear profiles per cross section (Np/Cx) providing an index of lesion cell numbers, (4) percentage of lesion cells that were smooth muscle cells (SMC) or monocyte/macrophages (M/MØ) determined by a monoclonal antibody staining technique, and (5) tritiated thymidine labeling indices of each cell type providing an index of lesion proliferative activity.

Swine fed the atherogenic BT diet developed extensive early lesions at all sites that were studied. The addition of fish oil (BT + FO diet) resulted in dramatic retardation of lesion development at all sites including sizes, cell numbers (Np/Cx), and extent of necrosis. Microscopic sections of the left anterior descending artery (LAD) from BT, BT + FO and control mash (MA) groups are illustrated in FIGURES 3, 4, and 5. In FIGURE 6 we show bar graphs comparing lesion cell numbers (Np/Cx) in the BT and BT + FO groups at all sites. A graph of lesion areas and necrosis (not shown) provides similar contrasts. The retardation in lesion development produced by fish oil additive is dramatic. Reduction in lesion sizes ranged from 71 to 94%.

The retardation effect on lesion development is similar to that reported in swine earlier by Weiner et al.[8] and to that reported by Davis et al.[5] in Rhesus monkeys. Hollander et al.[10] reported similar retardation in the aorta and carotids of Cynomolgus monkeys but not at the carotid bifurcation. In rabbits Zhu et al.[7] showed retardation of lesion development by fish oil while Thiery and Seidel[6] showed acceleration. In man no data are available regarding the effects of fish oil on atherosclerotic lesion development.

Plasma Cholesterol Levels and Lipoprotein Patterns

Plasma cholesterol levels in the swine experiment being summarized are presented in TABLE 3 in various categories. The total mean plasma cholesterol level was modestly though significantly higher in the untreated hyperlipidemic BT group than in the BT + FO group given the fish oil additive. However, this difference would not seem to be sufficient to account for the marked difference in lesion development unless we are dealing with a critical level phenomenon. The LDL cholesterol (in the swine from 1.020 to 1.090 g/ml and excluding the HDL_c studied by Mahley and Wiesgraber[11,12]) was significantly higher in the fish oil-treated BT + FO group. The LDL fraction in these hyperlipidemic swine can be divided into a component containing both apolipoproteins (apo) B and E and the conventional component containing only apo B as will be explained subsequently. TABLE 3 shows that the cholesterol in the conventional apo B only LDL component is far greater in the BT + FO swine given the fish oil than in untreated BT groups. Thus popular wisdom that favors LDL as the most atherosclerotic lipoprotein component would predict greater lesions in the group given the fish oil, and yet we know that the lesions were far larger in the BT group *not* receiving the fish oil.

Terminally fasting plasma was obtained and separated by density gradient ultracentrifugation, Pevikon block electrophoresis, and immunoelectrophoresis. Apoprotein B, A-I, E, and C contents were determined by polyacrylamide gel electrophoresis and densitometry of gels stained with Coomassie blue. HDL_c was separated from LDL by Pevikon block electrophoresis. LDL was divided into an apo B,E-containing component and

TABLE 3. Cholesterol Contents of Plasma and Various Lipoprotein Fractions and TBARS Levels of Swine Fed BT and BT + FO Diets for 4 Months[a]

	Mash (N = 5)	BT (N = 6)	BT + FO (N = 6)	BT vs BT + FO p Values[e]
Plasma-CH (mg/dl)	73 ± 5[b]	816 ± 64	629 ± 14	0.02
VLDL-CH (mg/dl)	1.7 ± 0.5	49 ± 20[c]	5 ± 1	0.04
IDL-CH	1.4 ± 0.4	170 ± 47	21 ± 5	0.02
LDL without HDL_c-CH	28 ± 2	428 ± 45	522 ± 17	0.04
HDL_2-CH	13 ± 2	53 ± 9	49 ± 23	NS
HDL_3-CH	16 ± 2	25 ± 11	15 ± 2	0.03
HDL_c-CH	1.4 ± 0.5	90 ± 10	12 ± 3	0.0004
LDL (B,E)-CH (mg/dl)	[d]	269 ± 27	177 ± 15	0.01
LDL (B)-CH	—	158 ± 29	344 ± 15	0.0005
LDL_1 (B,E)-CH	—	241 ± 22	143 ± 16	0.003
LDL_1 (B)-CH	—	77 ± 16	121 ± 19	NS(0.06)
LDL_2 (B,E)-CH	—	28 ± 5	34 ± 7	NS
LDL_2 (B)-CH	—	82 ± 20	223 ± 26	0.0005
B,E LP [IDL + LDL (B,E)]-CH	—	439 ± 65	198 ± 17	0.005
All B,E LP [VLDL + IDL + LDL (B,E)]-CH	—	488 ± 84	204 ± 17	0.005
TBARS umoles/L	1.01 ± 0.08	1.28 ± 0.09	1.98 ± 0.20	0.005

[a]Based on Kim *et al.*[9]

[b]Mean ± standard error of mean.

[c]In 5 of 6 swine the VLDL was almost entirely beta-VLDL in contrast to BT + FO values which include no beta VLDL.

[d]Not determined.

[e]One-tailed Student *t* test.

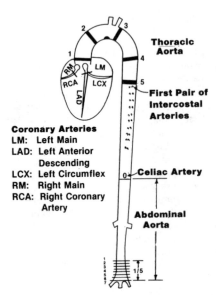

Coronary Arteries
LM: Left Main
LAD: Left Anterior
        Descending
LCX: Left Circumflex
RM: Right Main
RCA: Right Coronary
        Artery

FIGURE 2. Tissue sampling for morphometry, autoradiography, and immunohistochemistry. For the abdominal aorta, the distal 1/5 measuring from celiac artery to trifurcation was divided into 7 rings of equal length. For thoracic aorta, 5 segments were obtained. For coronary arteries, as many as possible 2-mm-long segments were cut from LM and RM, and 5 such segments were obtained from LAD, LCX, and RCA. Segment #6 of the abdominal aorta, segment #5 of thoracic aorta, and the LM segment nearest to the bifurcation were used for immunohistochemical identification of monocyte/macrophages using monoclonal antibody. (From Kim *et al.*[9] Reprinted by permission from *Atherosclerosis*.)

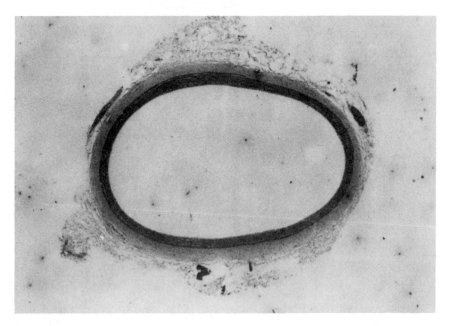

FIGURE 3. A cross section of proximal LAD from a swine fed a low fat, low cholesterol mash diet. H & E stain.

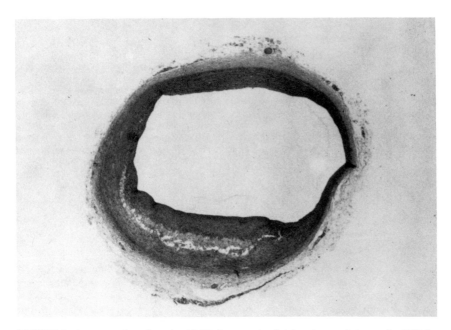

FIGURE 4. A cross section of proximal LAD from a swine fed the atherogenic butter diet (BT) for 4 months without fish oil additive. H & E stain.

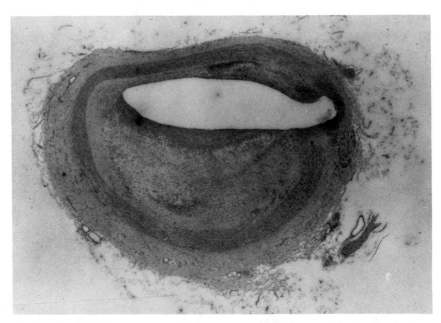

FIGURE 5. A cross section of proximal LAD from a swine fed the BT diet with fish oil additive for 4 months. H & E stain.

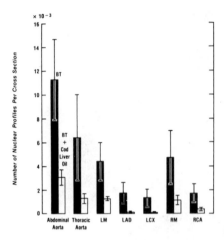

FIGURE 6. Mean number of nuclear profiles per cross section (with ± standard error of mean) of various aortic and coronary artery sites of swine fed butter diet (BT) (*darkshaded bars*) and butter plus cod liver oil (BT + FO) (*white bars*) for 4 months. The differences between the two groups are significant at all sites.[9]

an apo B only component by immunoelectrophoresis in the gel containing anti-apo E antisera. In FIGURES 7, 8, and 9 we show optical density scans and rocket immunoelectrophoresis patterns from representative swine fed respectively the low fat, low cholesterol control mash diet, the atherogenic BT diet, or the BT + FO diet with the fish oil

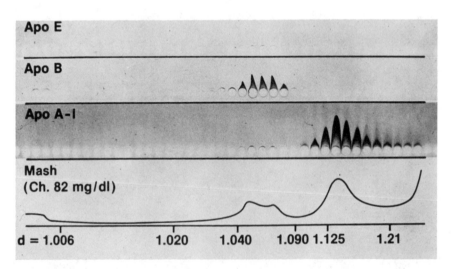

FIGURE 7. Optical density scan at 280 nm during the fractionation of the density gradient tubes after ultracentrifugation of plasma of mash-fed swine with terminal cholesterol of 82 mg/dl. Swine LDL extends up to d = 1.090 g/ml. Two peaks are clearly shown in the LDL region. The lower of the two peaks corresponds to lipoprotein (a) [Lp(a)].

additive. In FIGURE 10 we show a direct comparison of the optical density scans from FIGURES 8 and 9. In the hyperlipidemic swine it can be seen that the separation between the d = 1.006–1.020 g/ml IDL and the 1.020–1.090 g/ml LDL has become obscured. Further study of this showed that the fraction above 1.020 and especially the portion from 1.020 to 1.040 contained a great deal of lipoproteins containing both apo B and apo E (as in IDL and VLDL) which we have chosen to call apo B,E LDL to distinguish it from the associated conventional apo B only LDL.

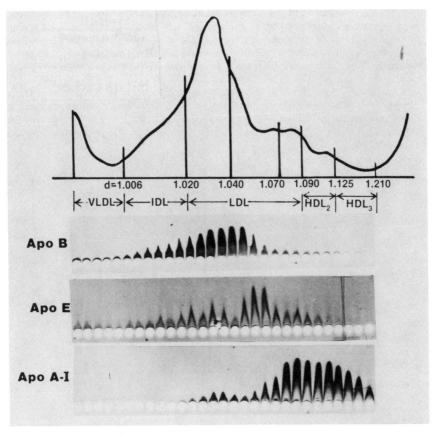

FIGURE 8. Optical density scan at 280 nm during the fractionation of the density gradient tubes after ultracentrifugation, and rocket immunoelectrophoresis patterns of the fractions for apo B, A-I, and E of a swine fed the butter (BT) diet for 4 months with a terminal cholesterol of 802 mg/dl.[9]

In our view the most significant point to note in comparing the BT and BT + FO patterns is the marked shift produced by fish oil away from VLDL, IDL, and the portion of LDL rich in the apo B,E-containing component toward the conventional apo B only LDL. In FIGURE 11 bar graphs are shown of mean data for all of the swine in the two hyperlipidemic groups. This confirms the marked shift that has been produced by the fish oil additive from apo B and E-containing lipoproteins to those containing apo B only.

Looking back at TABLE 3 one can see how this is reflected in quantities of plasma cholesterol in apo B,E and apo B only lipoproteins in the two hyperlipidemic groups.

In TABLE 4 we show some correlation coefficients for various lipoprotein fractions and an index for lesion extent (Np/Cx). There is a highly significant positive correlation between apo B,E-containing lipoproteins and lesion extent whether the fractions are taken individually or grouped. In contrast there is a negative correlation for apo B only LDL and lesion extent probably because apo B,E and apo B only lipoproteins are negatively correlated.

We have concluded from these results (supported by confirmatory data from subsequent experiments) that it is likely that apo B,E-containing lipoproteins are far more atherogenic than those containing apo B only. The levels of HDL_c, and HDL_3 in these swine were sharply reduced by the fish oil additive, and HDL_2 was relatively unchanged. In spite of these findings, which popular wisdom would view as pro-atherogenic, atherosclerotic lesion growth was markedly retarded.

Rudel et al.[13] have shown in nonhuman primates that there is a correlation between lipoprotein particle size and degree of atherogenicity with the larger particles being more atherogenic. Parks and Bullock[14] have shown that the LDL in nonhuman primates fed fish oil are smaller than when saturated fat is fed. St. Clair et al.[15,16] have shown in vitro that

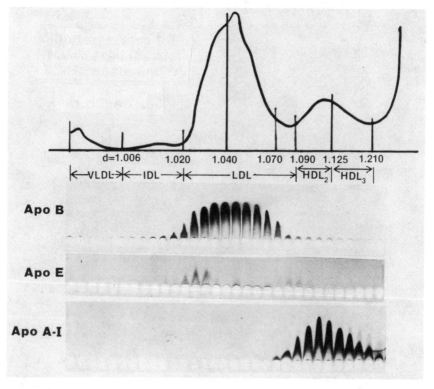

FIGURE 9. Optical density scan at 280 nm during the fractionation of the density gradient tubes after ultracentrifugation, and rocket immunoelectrophoresis patterns of the fractions for apo B, A-I, and E of a swine fed butter plus fish oil (BT + FO) for 4 months with a terminal cholesterol of 688 mg/dl.[9]

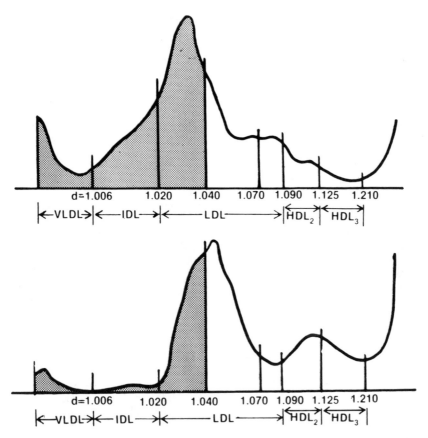

FIGURE 10. Direct comparison of optical density scans from FIGURES 8 and 9. The *upper figure* is from a butter (BT) swine with terminal plasma cholesterol of 802 mg/dl. The *lower figure* is from a butter plus fish oil swine with a plasma cholesterol of 688 mg/dl. Note markedly higher levels in lipoproteins of densities lower than 1.040 g/ml (VLDL, IDL, and LDL of lower densities; *dotted areas*) in the BT swine.

larger LDLs have a much greater affinity for cell surface bonding sites than smaller ones. They suggest that this might be because of the greater apo E content of large particles. Apo E has a much greater affinity for the B,E (LDL) receptor than does apo B. These studies might help explain the putatively greater atherogenicity of the apo B,E lipoproteins.

Monocyte/Macrophages (M/MØ)

The principal cell types in the atherosclerotic lesions in the swine are smooth muscle cells (SMC) and monocyte/macrophages (M/MØ). We were able to distinguish them on morphological grounds and by the use of a monoclonal antibody technique. The numbers of total lesion cells of both types were greatly reduced by the fish oil additive and in about the same proportions.

The tritiated thymidine labeling indices (LI) which provide an index of proliferative activity could be determined for each cell type separately using a monoclonal antibody technique for identification. The LIs for the lesion SMC were elevated in the swine fed the atherogenic diet as has been demonstrated previously and were not demonstrably affected by the fish oil additive. The lesion M/MØ had LIs almost as high as those of the SMC. Thus M/MØ are being supplied by mitotic activity as well as by infiltration of monocytes from the blood stream. A similar observation was made by Rosenfeld et al.[17] in monkeys.

We also carried out by scanning electron microscopy a study of the number of monocytes attached to the endothelium per unit area using the LAD coronary as the sample site (FIG. 12). The number was found to be considerably increased over lesions by the atherogenic diet as compared to control mash values. It was significantly decreased by the fish oil additive both in toto and per unit area but not to control mash levels (TABLE 5). These values correlated significantly with apo B,E lipoproteins in the blood.

Foxall et al.[18] carried out in vitro studies of attachment of monocytes to endothelial cell cultures using blood from swine fed either butter, fish oil or safflower oil for a year. In contrast to our in vivo results they found greater attachment with fish oil blood than with the butter. The difference in results is perhaps due to a chemotactic factor being produced in the lesions in our in vivo study. Also they were using the fish oil as a total substitution and not as an additive. Gerrity's[19] results also suggest a chemotactic factor. Rogers and Karnovsky[20] carried out a study in rats of monocyte attachment to the aorta comparing safflower oil and fish oil diets (which in pertinent diets also contained cholic acid with or without thiouracil). They found larger numbers attached with fish oil than with safflower oil but they did not compare with saturated fat diets such as butter and they used the fish oil as a total substitution and not as an additive.

Plasma Levels of Thiobarbituric Acid Reactive Substances (TBARS)

The significance of these substances is rather controversial but they are thought by many to provide some index of peroxidative activity. In a study in hyperlipidemic rabbits Thiery and Seidel[6] found an increase in lesion areas associated with a fish oil diet. They

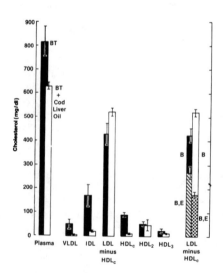

FIGURE 11. Mean cholesterol concentrations in plasma and various lipoprotein fractions separated by ultracentrifugation, Pevikon block electrophoresis and immunoelectrophoresis in swine fed either butter (BT) or butter plus fish oil (BT + FO) diet for 4 months. Total cholesterol concentrations in plasma, VLDL, IDL, and HDL_c are significantly higher in the BT group. In the fraction LDL minus HDL_c, the cholesterol level is significantly higher in the fish oil group. On the *right side* of the figure, LDL minus HDL_c, for both BT (*left bar*) and BT + FO (*right bar*) diet groups are repeated to show that apo B,E LDL is higher in the BT group, and that apo B LDL is higher in the BT + FO group. VLDL and IDL contain apo B,E lipoproteins with larger molecules.[9]

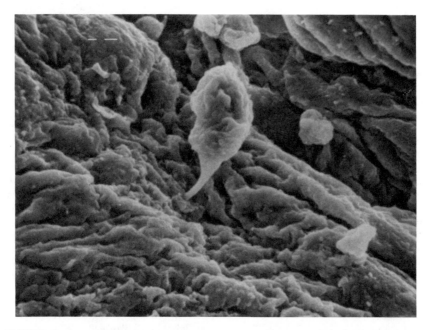

FIGURE 12. Scanning electron micrograph of a monocyte with an elongated cell body anchored in the wall. There is no denudation of the endothelium. BT swine. 3700 ×.

also found an increase in plasma TBARS as compared with a saturated fat diet. They suggested that the increased lesion areas and the TBARS might be related.

In our study in swine we measured levels of plasma TBARS. They were not elevated by the BT diet alone but were increased about twofold by the fish oil additive. In spite of this lesion development was greatly retarded.

Thromboxane, Prostacyclin, and Leukotriene B_4

Arachidonic acid (AA) serves as a substrate for cyclooxygenase and lipoxygenase to produce a variety of prostaglandins, leukotrienes, and other products that are important in inflammatory responses and in regard to platelet activity. Eicosapentaenoic acid (EPA) from fish oils competes as a substrate with AA and results in slightly different products some of which are as active as those derived from AA and others less active. Three AA derivatives that have received considerable attention are thromboxane (TXA_2 from AA, and TXA_3 from EPA), prostacyclin (PGI_2 from AA and PGI_3 from EPA) and leukotriene B_4 (LTB_4 from AA and LTB_5 from EPA).[21]

TXA_2 derived mostly from platelets is a promoter of platelet aggregation. TXA_3 is virtually inactive in this regard.[22] A fish oil-containing diet would be expected to reduce TXA_2 and associated platelet aggregatory activity and this has been shown to be the case in man and experimental animals. Rather unexpectedly we found in our swine that serum levels of TXB_2 (a more stable derivative of TXA_2 used as an index for TXA_2) was reduced by the atherogenic BT diet even without the addition of fish oil over levels in control mash fed swine. However, levels were reduced still further by the addition of fish oil. TXB_3 has not as yet been measured but since it is considered relatively inactive it is of little interest.

PGI_2 (from AA, derived mostly from vessel walls) is an inhibitor of platelet aggregation and much has been made of the need for a proper balance between TXA_2 and PGI_2 in platelet aggregation. PGI_3 (from EPA) is considered to be as active as PGI_2. PGI_2 also has a number of other functions which may be important in relation to atherogenesis. These were discussed at some length by Moncado and Radomski[2] at the First Saratoga Conference on Atherosclerosis. One of the more interesting is a "cytoprotective" activity which might play a role in reducing the necrotizing feature in atherogenesis. In our swine we measured serum levels of 6-keto PG F1 Alpha, (a stable derivative of PGI_2 which is used as an index for PGI_2) and found that the atherogenic BT diet alone resulted in a decrease over levels in swine on a control mash diet. Levels were reduced significantly more by the fish oil additive. We have not as yet measured levels of any index of PGI_3 in the swine. In humans on a western (?atherogenic) diet the effect of a fish oil additive has been studied on both PGI_2 and PGI_3. The combined total of the two has been shown to be elevated over the PGI_2 level on the western diet without fish oil. We would expect the effect to be similar in the swine. If this is the case the prostacyclin-thromboxane balance is probably being shifted toward the prostacyclin side. This shift could play a significant role in reducing the inflammatory reactions and the effect of platelet products such as PDGF that might contribute to the severity of the atherogenic process.

Leukotriene B_4 is derived from arachidonic acid via the lipoxygenase pathway. It is a chemotactic agent which should attract monocytes. Serum levels are reduced by the BT atherogenic diet and still further by the fish oil additive. Levels of LTB_5 from EPA have not been measured but this compound is considered to be relatively inactive.

It is too early to interpret these results on products related to inflammation and platelet activity in any precise fashion. If, as we believe, atherogenesis is mainly a reaction to injury, they may be key factors in accounting for the retarding effect of the fish oil on atherogenesis. The relation between these elements and changes in lipoprotein patterns is another unknown.

TABLE 4. Correlation Coefficients (r) for Apo B,E and Apo B-Containing Lipoproteins with Lesion Np/Cx for 12 Swine (BT and BT + FO) of TABLES 2 and 3[a]

	Lesion Np/Cx			
Lipoprotein Cholesterol Values	Abd. Aorta r	Thor. Aorta r	Left Main Coronary r	LAD Coronary r
B,E [IDL + LDL (B,E)]-CH	0.927	0.814	0.940	0.973
All B,E LP-CH	0.931	0.838	0.916	0.907
VLDL-CH	0.871	0.872	0.821	0.872
IDL-CH	0.908	0.868	0.861	0.945
LDL (B,E)-CH	0.805	0.593	0.889	0.614
LDL (B)-CH	−0.574	−0.402	−0.167	−0.638

[a]With n = 12 all r values greater than ± 0.497 are significant at least at the $p < 0.05$ level so that most of the values above are highly significant. The significant negative correlations with LDL(B)-CH disappear when we use partial correlation coefficients to fix for LDL(B,E)-CH due to the negative correlation between LDL(B)-CH and LDL(B,E)-CH. This suggests that LDL(B)-CH has a neutral effect on atherogenesis. However, the positive correlations with LDL(B,E)-CH generally remain highly significant, even when using LDL(B)-CH as a covariate. (Based on Kim et al.[9])

TABLE 5. Number of Monocytes Attached per Square Millimeter (mm^2) of Endothelial Surface of the Left Anterior Descending (LAD) Coronary Artery as Determined by Scanning Electron Microscopy

Attached Cells per mm^2	MA (N = 5)	CT (N = 5[a])	BT + FO (N = 5[a])
Over lesions[b]	69 ± 8	570 ± 111	264 ± 56
Not over lesions[c]	115 ± 48	85 ± 8	143 ± 31

[a]One specimen in each of these two groups was not suitbale for scanning electron microscopy counting.

[b]One sided significance values for: over lesions—BT vs MA (p <0.003), BT vs BT + FO (p <0.01), BT + FO vs MA (p <0.02).

[c]Not over lesions—no significant differences among the 3 groups.

Platelet Numbers and Aggregation Features

Ross[23] and others have done extensive studies on the effect of platelet derived growth factor (PDGF) on arterial smooth muscle cell (SMC) proliferation *in vitro*. Increased availability of PDGF in the arterial intima could be a factor in accounting for the SMC proliferative component in atherogenesis. In man platelet aggregatory activity and platelet counts have been shown to be decreased by fish oil. Whether this is associated with decreased availability of PDGF in the arterial intima is not known. The perturbations in platelet activity produced by the fish oil also raises the possibility of harmful effects in man although these have not been proved in man. Eskimos and Japanese, who are heavy fish eaters, are thought to have higher incidences of cerebral hemorrhage than more moderate fish-eating populations. However, many factors are involved in cerebral hemorrhage and a fish oil effect on platelets is not necessarily a component. Nonetheless, this aspect needs to be investigated thoroughly.

We have only beginning studies on platelets in our swine. We have studied blood platelet counts only up to three months on diets and found no significant change. We have studied platelet aggregation up to three months. Rather unexpectedly we found that low dose collagen-induced platelet aggregation was reduced over control values by the atherogenic BT diet alone as early as one week after starting and that the addition of fish oil produced no further change even at four months. This aspect clearly needs much more study.

SUMMARY AND CONCLUSIONS REGARDING SOME EFFECTS OF FISH OIL IN SWINE

1. A fish oil additive markedly retards the development of atherosclerosis in swine fed a highly atherogenic diet.
2. The modest reduction in the very high plasma cholesterol levels produced by the fish oil additive does not seem sufficient to account for the dramatic effect on lesion development and sophisticated statistical analyses supports this conclusion.
3. The fish oil additive produces marked changes in the distribution of lipoprotein fractions in the blood of the hyperlipidemic swine.
   a. Conventional LDL containing only apo B is increased considerably.
   b. VLDL, IDL, and LDL containing apo B and E are markedly decreased.
   c. HDL_c found in the LDL density region is decreased.
   d. HDL_2 and HDL_3 are either unchanged or decreased.

4. We conclude that the apo B and E-containing lipoproteins (VLDL, IDL, and part of LDL) are probably more atherogenic than conventional apo B only LDL and that the reduction in HDL has no serious consequences.
5. The cell types in the atherosclerotic lesions in the swine fed the diets we used were almost entirely smooth muscle cells and monocyte/macrophages at four months on diet often in about equal numbers; the fish oil additive:
   a. Reduced the numbers of each cell type proportionately.
   b. Did not reduce the tritiated thymidine labeling indices of either cell type which were elevated above controls for each.
   c. Reduced the number of monocytes attached to endothelium over lesions which were elevated over control values by the atherogenic BT diet.
6. Levels of thiobarbituric acid reactive substances were doubled in the blood by the fish oil but this did not prevent retardation of lesion development.
7. Serum levels of markers for several arachidonic acid (AA) metabolites were reduced by the atherogenic BT diet and still further by the fish oil additive including both cyclooxygenase and lipoxygenase products related to inflammation and platelet activity; these included:
   a. Thromboxane A_2 (TXA_2) which is a pro-aggregatory factor for platelets.
   b. Prostacyclin (PGI_2) which is an anti-aggregatory factor for platelets and a "cytoprotective" agent.
   c. Leukotriene B_4 which is a chemotactic factor for leukocytes.
8. The finding that serum levels of the arachidonic acid products were reduced by the atherogenic diet alone (over values in control swine fed low fat, low cholesterol diets) was unexpected and needs further study for significance and explanation.
9. The further reduction of above levels by the fish oil additive is probably because of substrate competition with AA by eicosapentaenoic acid (EPA); the EPA-derived counterparts of the AA products have not been measured in our swine and are of special interest in the case of prostacyclin where the EPA counterpart is known to be as active as the AA product.
10. Low dose collagen-induced platelet aggregation *in vitro* was reduced over control values by the atherogenic BT diet alone but no further by the fish oil additive.
11. The results with the platelets are probably linked to the results with AA metabolites and require further study for explanation and significance.
12. The swine showed no excessive bleeding or other recognized ill effects from the fish oil additive, but this aspect also requires much further study.

REFERENCES

1. BANG, H. O., J. DYERBERG & H. M. SINCLAIR. 1980. The composition of Eskimo food in North Western Greenland. Am. J. Clin Nutr. **33:** 2657–2661.
2. KAGAWA, Y., M. NISHIZAWA, M. SUZUKI *et al.* 1982. Eicosapolyenoic acid of serum lipids of Japanese islanders with low incidence of cardiovascular diseases. J. Nutr. Sci. Vitaminol. (Tokyo) **28:** 441–453.
3. KROMHOUT, D., E. B. BOSSCHIETER & C. D. L. COULANDER. 1985. The inverse relation between fish consumption and 20-year mortality from coronary heart disease. N. Engl. J. Med. **312:** 1205–1209.
4. HARRIS, W. S. 1989. Fish oils and plasma lipid and lipoprotein metabolism in humans: a critical review. J. Lipid Res. **30:** 785–807.
5. DAVIS, H. R., R. T. BRIDENSTINE, D. VESSELINOVITCH & R. W. WISSLER. 1987. Fish oil inhibits development of atherosclerosis in Rhesus monkeys. Arteriosclerosis **7:** 441–449.
6. THIERY, J. & D. SEIDEL. 1987. Fish oil feeding results in enhancement of cholesterol-induced atherosclerosis in rabbits. Atherosclerosis **63:** 53–56.

7. ZHU, B. Q., D. L. SMITH, R. E. SIEVERS, W. M. ISEMBERG & W. W. PARMLEY. 1988. Inhibition of atherosclerosis by fish oil in cholesterol fed rabbits. J. Am. Coll. Cardiol. **12:** 1073–1078.

8. WEINER, B. H., I. S. OCKENE, P. H. LEVINE, H. F. CUENOUD, M. FISHER, B. F. JOHNSON, A. S. DAOUD, J. JARMOLYCH, D. HOSMER, M. H. JOHNSON, A. NATALE, C. VAUDREUIL & J. J. HOOGASIAN. 1986. Inhibition of atherosclerosis by cod-liver oil in a hyperlipidemic swine model. N. Engl. J. Med. **315:** 841–846.

9. KIM, D. N., H. -T. HO, D. A. LAWRENCE, J. SCHMEE & W. A. THOMAS. 1989. Modification of lipoprotein patterns and retardation of atherogenesis by fish oil supplement to a hyperlipidemic diet for swine. Atherosclerosis **76:** 35–54.

10. HOLLANDER, W., S. HONG, B. J. KIRKPATRICK, A. LEE, M. COLOMBO & S. PRUSTY. 1987. Differential effects of fish oil supplementation in atherosclerosis. Arteriosclerosis **7:** 527a.

11. MAHLEY, R. W. 1985. Atherogenic lipoproteins and coronary artery disease: concepts derived from recent advances in cellular and molecular biology. Circulation **72:** 943–948.

12. MAHLEY, R. W. & K. H. WEISGRABER. 1974. Canine lipoproteins and atherosclerosis. I. Isolation and characterization of plasma lipoproteins from control dogs. Circ. Res. **35:** 713–721.

13. RUDEL, L. L., M. G. BOND & B. C. BULLOCK. 1985. LDL heterogeneity and atherosclerosis in nonhuman primates. Ann. N.Y. Acad. Sci. **454:** 248–253.

14. PARKS, J. S. & B. C. BULLOCK. 1987. Effect of fish oil versus lard diets on the chemical and physical properties of low density lipoproteins of non human primates. J. Lipid Res. **28:** 173–182.

15. ST. CLAIR, R. W., J. J. MITSCHELEN & M. LEIGHT. 1980. Metabolism by cells in culture of low density lipoproteins from hypercholesterolemia. Biochim. Biophys. Acta **618:** 63–79.

16. ST. CLAIR, R. W., P. GREENSPAN & M. LEIGHT. 1983. Enhanced cholesterol delivery to cells in culture by low density lipoproteins from hypercholesterolemic monkeys. Correlation of cellular cholesterol accumulation with low density lipoprotein molecular weight. Arteriosclerosis **3:** 77–86.

17. ROSENFELD, M. E., P. GOODWIN, K. JONAS & R. ROSS. 1987. Frequency and spatial distribution analyses of cellular proliferation in atherosclerotic lesions of WHHL and fat-fed rabbits using digital image analysis. Arteriosclerosis **7:** 528a.

18. FOXALL, T. L., G. T. SHWAERY & A. H. PARSONS. 1988. A long term study of effects of lipid saturation on platelet and monocyte functions. Arteriosclerosis **8:** 557a.

19. GERRITY, R. G. 1986. Cellular events in early atherogenesis in swine. *In* Swine in Biomedical Research. Vol. 3. M.E. Tumbleson, Ed. 1497–1509. Plenum Press. New York, NY.

20. ROGERS, K. A. & M. J. KARNOVSKY. 1988. Dietary fish oil enhances monocyte adhesion and fatty streak formation in the hypercholesterolemic rat. Am. J. Pathol. **132:** 382–388.

21. LEE, T. H., R. L. HOOVER, J. D. WILLIAMS, R. I. SPERLING, J. RAVALESE, III, B. W. SUPUR, D. R. ROBINSON, E. J. COREY, R. A. LEWIS & K. F. AUSTEN. 1985. Effect of dietary enrichment with eicosapentaenoic and docosahexaenoic acids on *in vitro* neutrophil function. N. Engl. J. Med. **312:** 1217–1224.

22. MONCADA, S. & M. W. RADOMSKI. 1985. The problems and promise of prostaglandin influences in atherogenesis. Ann. N.Y. Acad. Sci. **454:** 121–130.

23. ROSS, R. & D. F. BOWEN-POPE. 1985. Platelets, macrophages, endothelium, and growth factors. Ann. N.Y. Acad. Sci. **454:** 254–260.

Eicosapentaenoic Acid and Apoplexy

Influence of EPA Loading on SHRSP

T. YASUGI, T. TOCHIHARA, T. FUJIOKA, S. KATO, E. SAITO,

E. MITSUI, T. ITO, T. UENO, H. KANNO, T. YAMADA,[a]

I. SAKURAI,[a] N. SAITO,[b] AND T. IWAI[b]

Second Department of Medicine
[a]Second Department of Pathology
Nihon University School of Medicine
30-1 Ohyaguchi-Kamimachi Itabashi-ku
Tokyo 173, Japan
and
[b]Tokyo Laboratory
Kowa Company, Ltd.
2-17-43 Noguchi-cyo Murayama-shi
Tokyo 189, Japan

Since it has been reported that eicosapentaenoic acid (EPA) has a favorable effect on the incidence of myocardial infarction,[1] much interest is focused on EPA including fish oils. However, it is well known that one of the main causes of death in Eskimos is cerebral bleeding, which might be related to the reduction of platelet aggregation. The purpose of this study is to investigate whether EPA plays an important role in the incidence of cerebral bleeding in the stroke-prone spontaneously hypertensive rat (SHRSP).

EPIDEMIOLOGICAL BACKGROUND IN JAPANESE[2]

Death rates by myocardial infarction and apoplexy have been studied in Tokyo and Higashi Izu (a typical fishing village). The death rates by both myocardial infarction and apoplexy were higher in Tokyo than in Higashi Izu. This was thought to be related to the higher incidence of hyperlipidemia (Type IIa and IIb) in Tokyo. Although the main cause of death in the apoplexy cases in Tokyo was cerebral infarction, it was cerebral bleeding in Higashi Izu. In connection with this, it was of interest that the incidence of hyper-EPAemia (arbitrarily designated as values over the mean + 1 SD of the levels in Tokyo) was significantly higher in Higashi Izu than in Tokyo, though the incidences of hypertension were almost similar in the both places.

These results indicate that a population taking a high amount of animal fat has a high serum cholesterol level and a high incidence of arteriosclerotic vascular disease; whereas a population taking a high amount of EPA has a high serum EPA level and a high incidence of cerebral bleeding.

ANIMAL EXPERIMENT

Dose Response Study

Subjects and Methods

Forty-eight 12-week-old male SHRSP, F-65, were bred under the barrier system, where temperature and humidity were maintained at $23 \pm 2°C$ and $60 \pm 10\%$. Basic

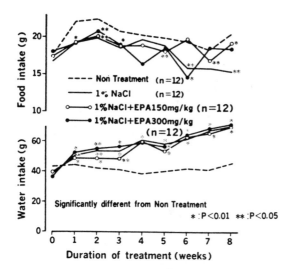

FIGURE 1. Food and water intake in salt-loaded SHRSP treated with EPA for 8 weeks (12 to 20 weeks old).

feeding pellet was sterilized by high pressured steam. The nontreatment group was given ultraviolet sterilized tap water, and the others were given 1% saline by water supply bottle. Then all subjects were subdivided into 4 groups as follows; a nontreatment group fed by basic pellet, a 1% NaCl group by basic pellet and 1% saline, an EPA 150 mg/kg group by basic pellet containing 150 mg/kg of EPA and 1% saline, and an EPA 300 mg/kg

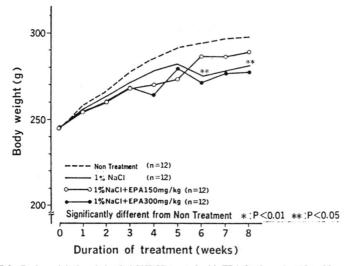

FIGURE 2. Body weight in salt-loaded SHRSP treated with EPA for 8 weeks (12 to 20 weeks old).

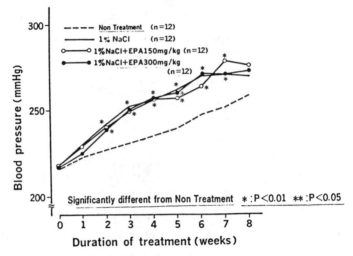

FIGURE 3. Blood pressure in salt-loaded SHRSP treated with EPA for 8 weeks (12 to 20 weeks old).

group by basic pellet containing 300 mg/kg of EPA and 1% saline. Each group included 12 subjects. Administered EPA was 91.7% pure ethylester (Nippon Yushi Co., Ltd.).

During the experimental period, body weight, intake amounts of feeding pellet, and water were measured every day. Systolic blood pressure was measured once a week by the tail cuff method.

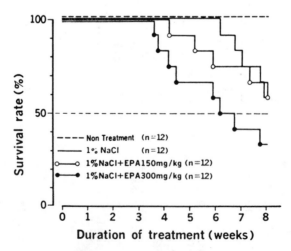

FIGURE 4. Survival rate in salt-loaded SHRSP treated with EPA for 8 weeks (12 to 20 weeks old).

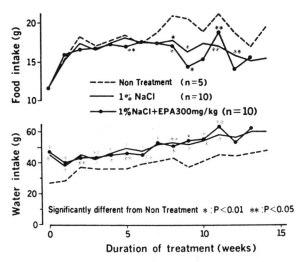

FIGURE 5. Food and water intake in salt-loaded SHRSP treated with EPA for 14 weeks (6 to 12 weeks old).

Results

1) Food and water intake. No significant differences were observed between each group except for the nontreatment group (FIG. 1).

2) Body weight. No significant differences existed between each group except for the nontreatment group (FIG. 2).

3) Blood pressure. Blood pressure was almost identical among the 3 groups except for the nontreatment group (FIG. 3).

4) Survival rate. There was no apoplexy case in the nontreatment group during the

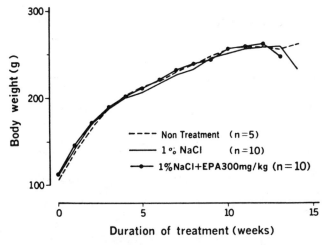

FIGURE 6. Body weight in salt-loaded SHRSP treated with EPA for 14 weeks (6 to 20 weeks old).

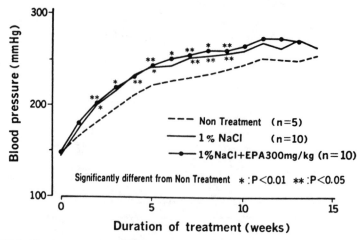

FIGURE 7. Blood pressure in salt-loaded SHRSP treated with EPA for 14 weeks (6 to 20 weeks old).

experimental period. In the 1% NaCl group, apoplexy appeared at the middle of the 6th experimental week. In the EPA 150 mg/kg group, apoplexy occurred during an earlier phase than in the former group, namely in the middle of 4th week. But, survival rates at the 8th experimental week in the both groups were similar. Apoplexy already appeared within the 3rd week, and the survival rate was very low (around 30%) in the EPA 300 mg/kg group. In this study, all of the apoplexy cases were of cerebral bleeding (FIG. 4).

5) These results suggest that EPA affects the incidence of cerebral bleeding and reduces the survival rate without effects on body weight and blood pressure. Dose response clearly exists with regard to the effect of EPA.

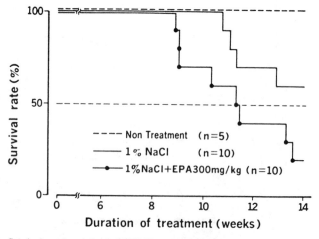

FIGURE 8. Survival rate in salt-loaded SHRSP treated with EPA for 14 weeks (6 to 20 weeks old).

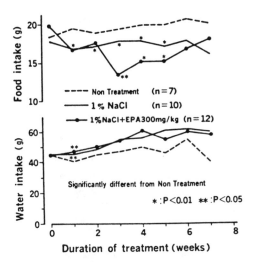

FIGURE 9. Food and water intake in salt-loaded SHRSP treated with EPA for 8 weeks (12 to 20 weeks old).

Studies in the Young Generation of SHRSP

Subjects and Methods

Thirty-two 6-week-old male SHRSP F-66, were subjected. Basic breeding conditions were similar to the above experiment. The subjects were subdivided into four groups as follows: the before-treatment group (n = 7) were sacrificed at the start of the experiment, the nontreatment group (n = 5) were fed basic pellet and tap water, the 1% NaCl group

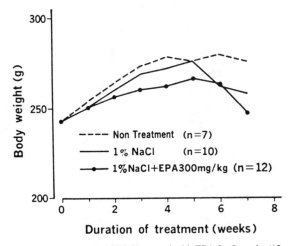

FIGURE 10. Body weight in salt-loaded SHRSP treated with EPA for 8 weeks (12 to 20 weeks old).

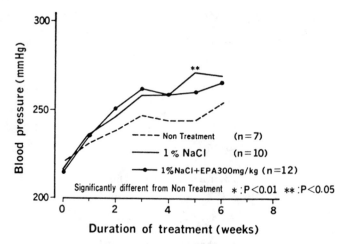

FIGURE 11. Blood pressure in salt-loaded SHRSP treated with EPA for 8 weeks (12 to 20 weeks old).

(n = 10) basic pellet and 1% saline, the EPA 300 mg/Kg group basic pellet containing 300 mg/kg of EPA and 1% saline.

Serum lipids were determined by enzymatic methods, malondialdehyde (MDA) by TBA method, and FFA by gas chromatography.

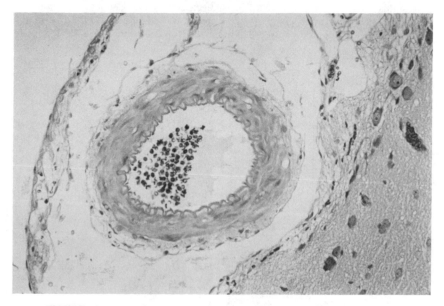

FIGURE 12. Cerebral small artery (1% NaCl-loaded group); HE staining. ×200.

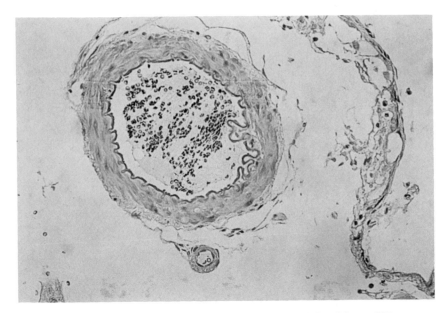

FIGURE 13. Cerebral small artery (EPA-loaded group); HE staining. ×200.

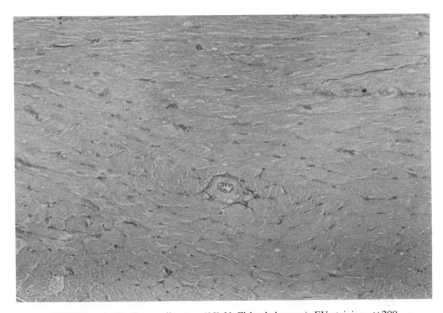

FIGURE 14. Cardiac small artery (1% NaCl-loaded group); EV staining. ×200.

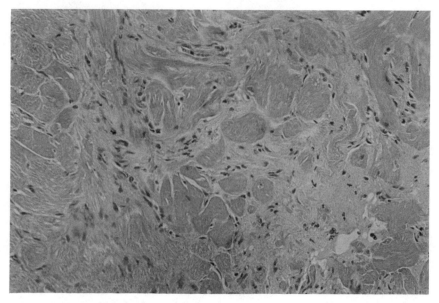

FIGURE 15. Myocardium (EPA-loaded group); HE staining. × 200.

Results

1) Food and water intake. No differences were observed between the groups except for the nontreatment group (FIG. 5).

2) Body weight was similar in all 3 groups (FIG. 6).

3) Blood presure was similar between the 1% NaCl and the EPA 300 mg/kg groups except for the nontreatment group (FIG. 7).

4) Survival rate. There was no case of apoplexy in the nontreatment group. In the 1% NaCl group, apoplexy occurred at the 11th experimental week and the survival rate at the

TABLE 1. Serum Fatty Acid Composition in Salt-Loaded SHRSP Treated with EPA for 14 Weeks (6 to 20 Weeks Old)[a]

| | Before (n = 7) | Nontreatment 6 WN (n = 5) | 1% NaCl 6 WC | | 1% NaCl + EPA 300 mg/kg 6 WE | |
			APO (−) (n = 5)	APO (+) (n = 1)	APO (−) (n = 2)	APO (+) (n = 8)
C16:0	21.9 ± 0.9	15.3 ± 2.5	15.4 ± 2.5	13.8	17.5 ± 1.4	19.2 ± 1.9
C18:0	11.9 ± 2.0	3.4 ± 1.0	3.4 ± 0.2	2.8	2.8 ± 0.5	2.8 ± 0.4
C18:1	7.1 ± 0.7	3.9 ± 0.4	4.1 ± 0.8	2.3	4.9 ± 0.7	7.3 ± 1.3
C18:2	18.6 ± 0.9	20.7 ± 1.4	18.9 ± 3.0	16.6	20.9 ± 1.7	26.1 ± 2.8
C18:3	0.1 ± 0.0	0.3 ± 0.4	0.1 ± 0.1	0.7	0.3 ± 0.3	0
C20:4	29.6 ± 2.1	42.4 ± 2.4	40.0 ± 4.6	45.3	35.8 ± 4.4	27.2 ± 6.3
C20:5	0.6 ± 0.2	1.0 ± 0.2*	0.8 ± 0.3	0.9	2.5 ± 0.6*	2.0 ± 0.2*
C22:6	3.7 ± 1.5	5.8 ± 0.2	7.5 ± 3.8	12.5	5.2 ± 0.8	7.6 ± 0.1

[a]Mean ± SD (%).

*$P < 0.01$ (vs before); differences between 1% NaCl + EPA 300 mg/kg and nontreatment, between 1% NaCl + EPA 300 mg/kg and 1% NaCl are statistically significant.

TABLE 2. Serum Lipids, TxB2, and MDA Levels in Salt-Loaded SHRSP Treated with EPA for 14 Weeks (6 to 20 Weeks Old)[a]

	Before (n = 7)	Nontreatment 6 WN (n = 5)	1% NaCl 6 WC		1% NaCl + EPA 300 mg/kg 6 WE	
			APO (−) (n = 5)	APO (+) (n = 2)	APO (−) (n = 5)	APO (+) (n = 2)
TC (mg/dl)	37.3 ± 4.1	53.8 ± 13.2*	79.7 ± 52.2*	146.6 ± 56.4*	51.8 ± 6.9*	189.7 ± 21.7**
TG (mg/dl)	19.2 ± 6.2	19.5 ± 3.6	21.2 ± 9.4	162.4 ± 64.1*	20.8 ± 5.5	273.7 ± 118.3*
PL (mg/dl)	70.2 ± 4.1	103.6 ± 8.9*	120.2 ± 50.4*	228.8 ± 98.0*	93.1 ± 5.6*	302.7 ± 43.5*
HDL-C (mg/dl)	32.6 ± 5.0	47.0 ± 3.8*	56.5 ± 28.7	100.2 ± 10.5	30.4 ± 23.6	99.9 ± 4.4*
FFA (mEq/l)	974.2 ± 196.5	530.0 ± 126.8	521.2 ± 271.2	527.4 ± 577.4	679.8 ± 32.2	1708 (n = 1)
TxB2 (pg/ml)	68.6 ± 8.8	30.3 ± 6.4	52.2 ± 0.9	—	41.6 ± 15.7*	29.6 ± 9.3*
MDA (mM/ml)	3.8 ± 0.4	8.1 ± 0.4	6.4 ± 2.7	3.3 ± 0.6	8.0 ± 1.0*	5.7 ± 1.2*

[a]Mean ± SD (%).
*$P < 0.01$ (vs before); **$P < 0.05$ (vs before).

end of the experiment (after 14 weeks treatment) was around 60%. In the EPA 300 mg/kg group, apoplexy appeared at the 8th experimental week and the survival rate was around 20%. All of the apoplexy cases were cerebral bleeding (FIG. 8).

5) Serum fatty acid compositions. During the experimental periods, decrease of C18:0 and increases of C16:0 and C20:4 in all groups were noticed. In the EPA 300 mg/kg group, C20:5 significantly increased and C20:4 decreased. And there were no differences in the serum fatty acid compositions between the groups with apoplexy and without apoplexy (TABLE 1).

TABLE 3. Serum Fatty Acid Composition in Salt-Loaded SHRSP Treated with EPA for 8 Weeks (12 to 20 Weeks Old)[a]

	Before (n = 7)	Nontreatment 12 WN (n = 6)	1% NaCl 12 WC		1% NaCl + EPA 300 mg/kg 12 WE	
			APO (−) (n = 16)	APO (+) (n = 6)	APO (−) (n = 8)	APO (+) (n = 16)
C16:0	21.9 ± 0.9	18.3 ± 1.2	16.8 ± 1.4	18.0 ± 0.5	18.7 ± 0.1	19.2 ± 2.3
C18:0	11.9 ± 2.0	4.3 ± 1.5	5.3 ± 3.2	5.2 ± 1.1	11.3 ± 0.1	6.2 ± 2.6
C18:1	7.1 ± 0.7	4.9 ± 1.7	5.3 ± 0.4	6.7 ± 0.9	6.1 ± 0.1	7.0 ± 2.4
C18:2	18.6 ± 0.9	24.1 ± 2.4	22.3 ± 2.4	21.3 ± 2.2	18.0 ± 1.1	22.2 ± 1.5
C18:3	0.1 ± 0.0	0.4 ± 0.3	0.8 ± 0.2	0.9 ± 0.3	0.1 ± 0.0	0.5 ± 0.3
C20:4	29.6 ± 2.1	38.3 ± 3.3	38.4 ± 5.7	34.3 ± 2.9	32.7 ± 0.8	30.1 ± 7.0
C20:5	0.6 ± 0.2	1.1 ± 0.2*	1.0 ± 0.3*	0.8 ± 0.4	1.9 ± 0.4*	2.0 ± 1.1*
C22:6	3.7 ± 1.5	5.2 ± 0.7	5.9 ± 1.2	9.7 ± 0.7	4.9 ± 0.4	8.7 ± 1.9

[a]Mean ± SD (%).
*$P < 0.01$ (vs before); differences between 1% NaCl + EPA 300 mg/kg and nontreatment, between 1% NaCl + EPA 300 mg/kg and 1% NaCl are statistically significant.

TABLE 4. Serum Lipids, TxB2, and MDA Levels in Salt-Loaded SHRSP Treated with EPA for 8 Weeks (12 to 20 Weeks Old)[a]

| | Before (n = 7) | Nontreatment 12 WN (n = 6) | 1% NaCl 12 WC | | 1% NaCl + EPA 300 mg/kg 12 WE | |
			APO (−) (n = 16)	APO (+) (n = 6)	APO (−) (n = 8)	APO (+) (n = 16)
TC (mg/dl)	32.6 ± 5.0	49.7 ± 4.2*	49.4 ± 8.1*	158.3 ± 10.5*	72.4 ± 26.5**	152.1 ± 38.2**
TG (mg/dl)	19.2 ± 6.2	16.0 ± 3.5	24.2 ± 6.7	114.5 ± 22.0*	26.7 ± 9.8	123.8 ± 72.1**
PL (mg/dl)	70.2 ± 4.1	9.12 ± 0.2*	110.8 ± 2.13**	243.2 ± 27.6*	119.3 ± 32.0*	214.7 ± 42.5*
HDL-C (mg/dl)	32.5 ± 3.8	40.0 ± 1.2	44.0 ± 22.3	87.5 ± 4.8*	53.5 ± 12.2*	63.8 ± 28.0
FFA (mEq/l)	974.2 ± 196.5	677.7 ± 5.8	662.7 ± 77.1	737.6 ± 295.0	652.5 ± 87.3	619.2 ± 187.0**
TxB2 (pg/ml)	68.6 ± 8.8	52.2 ± 1.0	47.5 ± 9.7	10.3	29.4	38.2 ± 18.6
MDA (mM/ml)	3.8 ± 0.4	7.9 ± 0.6**	7.9 ± 1.1*	8.2 ± 1.8*	6.3 ± 1.0**	6.4 ± 2.0

[a]Mean ± SD (%).
*$P < 0.01$ (vs before); **$P < 0.05$ (vs before).

6) Serum lipids, TxB2 and MDA. In all 4 groups, serum lipid levels such as TC, TG, PL, and HDL-C showed the tendency to increase compared to the levels in the before-treatment group. There were no clear differences among the 3 groups. However, significant increases of the lipid levels existed in the apoplexy cases both in the 1% NaCl and the EPA 300 mg/kg groups. TxB2 and MDA levels did not show significant differences between the 1% NaCl and the EPA 300 mg/kg groups (TABLE 2).

7) In this study, as in the dose response study, administration of EPA caused apoplexy in the early phase of the experiment and reduced the survival rate significantly without effecting body weight and blood presure. EPA did not remarkably affect the seum lipid levels except for the increase of C20:5 and the decrease of C20:4 in the serum fatty acid composition. Also, EPA did not affect TxB2 and MDA levels. These results suggest that the effect of EPA on the incidence of apoplexy does not relate to blood pressure, serum

TABLE 5. Incidence of Clinical Symptoms with Apoplexy in Salt-Loaded SHRSP Treated with EPA

	Before	Nontreatment	1% NaCl	1% NaCl EPA 300 mg/kg
Dose response study	(−)	0/12	5/12	8/12
Salt-loaded SHR treated with EPA for 14 weeks (6 to 20 weeks old)	0/7	0/5	5/10	8/10
Salt-loaded SHR treated with EPA for 8 weeks (12 to 20 weeks old)	0/7	1/6	3/10	9/12

lipids, prostaglandin, or lipid peroxide. The significant increases of serum lipid levels in the apoplexy cases should be influenced by catecholamine released by the stress of the stroke.

TABLE 6. Pathological Findings in Salt-Loaded SHRSP Treated with EPA

	Brain Artery	Brain Paren-chyma	Coro-nary Ar-tery	Myo-car-dium	Renal Ar-tery	Aorta		Brain Artery	Brain Paren-chyma	Coro-nary Artery	Myo-car-dium	Renal Artery	Aorta
B1	−	−	−	−	−	−	12WN1	−	−	+	−	−	−
B2	−	−	−	−	−	−	12WN2	+	+	−	−	+	+
B3	+	−	−	−	−	−	12WN3	+	+	+	−	−	−
B4	−	−	−	−	−	±	12WN4	−	−	−	−	±	±
B5	−	−	−	−	−	−	12WN5	+	−	−	−	±	−
B6	+	−	−	−	−	−	12WN6	−	+	−	−	−	+
B7	−	−	−	−	±	−	12WC1	−	−	−	±	−	±
							12WC2	+	−	−	−	+	−
6WN1	+	−	+	−	−	−	12WC3	−	−	−	−	+	−
6WN5	−	−	−	−	−	−	12WC4	−	+	−	−	±	−
6WN6	−	−	−	−	+	±	12WC5	+	−	−	−	±	−
6WC1	−	−	−	+	±	−	12WC6	−	−	*	*	±	−
6WC2	−	−	+	−	±	+	12WC7	−	+ +	−	+	±	−
6WC3	+	+ +	−	−	±	−	12WC8	−	+ +	+	−	+	−
6WC4	−	−	−	−	±	−	12WC9	−	−	−	−	±	−
6WC5	−	+	−	−	±	+	12WC10	−	−	−	+	+	−
6WC6	−	+	*	*	±	−	12WE1	+	−	−	±	±	−
6WC7	−	−	−	±	±	−	12WE2	−	−	−	±	±	−
6WC8	−	−	−	−	±	±	12WE3	+	−	+	−	±	−
6WC10	−	−	−	−	±	−	12WE4	−	−	−	−	±	−
6WE1	−	−	*	*	−	±	12WE5	+	−	−	−	±	−
6WE2	+	−	−	+ +	−	−	12WE6	−	−	−	±	±	−
6WE3	−	−	−	−	−	−	12WE7	+	+ + +	−	−	−	−
6WE4	−	−	+	+	−	−	12WE8	−	+	−	−	+	−
6WE5	+	−	−	−	±	±	12WE9	+	+	−	+	+	±
6WE6	−	−	−	+	−	−	12WE10	+	+ + +	−	+	±	−
6WE7	−	−	−	−	±	±	12WE11	+	+	−	±	±	±
6WE8	−	−	−	±	±	−	12WE12	−	−	−	−	+	+
6WE11	−	+	−	+	−	±							
6WE12	−	+	−	−	±	−							

*Not investigated.

Studies in the Aged Generation of SHRSP

Subjects and Methods

Twenty-eight 12-week-old male SHRSP were subjected. The breeding condition was similar to that in the previous experiments. The subjects were subdivided as follows: the nontreatment group ($n = 6$) was fed basic feeding pellet, the 1% NaCl group ($n = 10$) basic pellet, and the 1% saline and EPA 300 mg/kg group ($n = 12$) basic pellet containing 300 mg/kg EPA and 1% saline. The before-treatment group was the same as in the young generation study. Chemical methods were also the same. Survival rate was not investi-

TABLE 7. Score of Lesions in Salt-Loaded SHRSP Treated with EPA[a]

	Brain Artery	Brain Parenchyma	Coronary Artery	Myocardium	Renal Artery	Aorta
Before (n = 7)	0.6	0	0	0	0.1	0.1
Nontreatment (n = 9)	0.9	0.7	0.7	0	0.7	0.6
1% NaCl (n = 19)	0.3	0.9	0.2	0.4	1.2	0.3
1% NaCl + EPA 300 mg/kg (n = 22)	0.8	1.0	0.2	0.9	0.8	0.4

[a]Scores were designated as follows: zero points, no lesions; one point, minimal lesion ($\pm$); two points, mild lesion ($+$), four points, moderate lesion ($++$); and six points, severe lesion ($+++$), and total points were divided by case numbers. The table included results from the young and the aged groups.

gated in this study, since some of subjects were sacrificed during the experiment to investigate the pathological change.

Results

Results obtained from this study were nearly consistent with those from the young generation study (FIGS. 9, 10, 11; TABLES 3,4).

Pathological Study Overall

Subjects and Methods

In this study, all animals in the young and aged generation studies, except 3 sacrificed during the experiments were investigated, so that total number was 57. Cerebral bleeding,

TABLE 8. Frequiencies of Hyper, Normo and HypoEPAemia in Tokyo and Higashi Izu[a]

	Tokyo	Higashi Izu
Serum EPA levels (mean $\pm$ SD nmol/ml)	148.8 $\pm$ 71.1	180.7 $\pm$ 90.0
Frequencies		
HyperEPAemia[b] >220 nmol/ml	15.7%	24.4%
NormoEPAemia 78–220 nmol/ml	70.1%	59.3%
HypoEPAemia[c] <78 nmol/ml	14.2%	16.3%

[a]Serum EPA levels of SHRSP: EPA loaded (300 mg/kg/day), 236.1 $\pm$ 134.2 nmol/ml; control, 27.8 $\pm$ 1.4 nmol/ml.
[b]HyperEPAemia: mean $+$ 1 SD of Tokyo.
[c]HypoEPAemia: mean $-$ 1 SD of Tokyo.

including subarachnoideal and intracranial, were examined macroscopically. Middle cerebral artery, cerebral small arteries, cerebral parenchyma, coronary artery, myocardium and cardiac small arteries, renal artery, and aorta were studied microscopically.

Results

1) Incidence of clinical symptoms with apoplexy. TABLE 5 shows the incidences of cerebral bleeding in each study including the dose response study. It is obvious that incidence of the disease is markedly high in the EPA-loaded groups.

2) Pathological findings and scores of lesions. TABLE 6 shows pathological findings of the arteries and tissues, and TABLE 7 shows scores of lesions, in which was included the consideration of severity. Changes in brain arteries and brain parenchyma did not differ much in the nontreatment, the 1% NaCl, and the EPA-loaded groups. However, incidence and severity were higher in the EPA-loaded aged group than in the other groups. Pathological change in the myocardium was clearly high in the EPA-loaded group. Changes in coronary artery, renal artery, and aorta were not different between the EPA-loaded group and the 1% NaCl group.

FIGURE 12 shows the typical change of cerebral arteries in 1% NaCl groups. Changes such as intimal edema were slight and slight edema existed in the infra-internal elastic lamina. FIGURE 13 shows the typical change in the EPA-loaded groups. Irregularity and fragility of internal elastic lamina and edema in the intima were significant as compared with those in the 1% NaCl groups.

FIGURE 14 shows the typical change of cardiac small artery in the 1% NaCl-loaded groups. Structure of the artery was well preserved. However, minimal fibrosis of myocardium was observed around the small arteries. FIGURE 15 shows that of the EPA-loaded group. Significant fibrosis around the arteries was frequently observed compared with the 1% NaCl-loaded group. Those changes in the brain, cerebral arteries, and heart indicate that hypertensive changes may be stressed by EPA administration.

DISCUSSION

In the present study, loading of EPA to SHRSP caused an increase in cerebral bleeding and reduced survival rate even in the young generation without influence on blood pressure. The results of this study and of previous epidemiological studies clearly indicate that taking too much EPA to protect ischemic heart disease may be very dangerous, increasing the chance that cerebral bleeding might occur. It seems that favorable effects of EPA on ischemic heart disease were brought by inhibition of platelet aggregation; but there was no direct effect on the arteries, since EPA did not show any advantage to the coronary artery in this study. EPA will also have a beneficial effect in the development of atherosclerosis via lipid metabolism, since intake of polyunsaturated fatty acid such as EPA reduces the intake of saturated fatty acid. Now, what is the critical level of EPA and what is the desirable amount of EPA to take. At the present time, there are no answers to those questions. But, there are some data. TABLE 8 shows the frequencies of the EPAemias from the epidemiological Tokyo and Higashi Izu study and the mean level of EPA from the present study. It is of interest that there exists a great approximation between the starting point of arbitrarily designated hyperEPAemia (over 220 nmol/ml) and the mean serum level of EPA-loaded SHRSP (236 nmol/ml). Thus, the authors would like to propose the 220 nmol/ml of EPA as an upper limit of the serum level and 1.0–2.0 grams daily (the amount between the means of Tokyo and Higashi Izu) as the amount of

EPA intake to maintain the serum EPA level properly. It should be stressed that EPA significantly increases fibrosis in the myocardium. The clinical meaning of this change is still unknown. It will be very important to clarify this point. Further study continues in our laboratory.

CONCLUSION

EPA may play a favorable role in preventing the incidence of myocardial infarction. However, an excess amount of EPA increases the incidence of cerebral bleeding and reduces the survival rate. Also, EPA may lead to fibrosis in the myocardium. Further study is needed to search for the proper serum level and the proper amount of intake, and to find the clinical meaning of the changes in the heart.

REFERENCES

1. DYERBERG, J., H. O. BANG & N. HJORNE. 1975. Fatty acid composition of the plasma lipids in Greenland Eskimos. Am. J. Clin. Nutr. **28:** 958–966.
2. YASUGI, T. 1986. Serum lipid levels and incidences of ischemic arteriosclerotic diseases in Japanese population through the past 30 years, with special reference on serum lipids and eicosapentaenoic acid levels. Atherosclerosis **7:** 55–59.

High Density Lipoproteins and Prevention of Experimental Atherosclerosis with Special Reference to Tree Shrews

SHE MING-PENG, XIA REN-YI, RAN BI-FANG,
AND WONG ZONG-LI

Department of Pathology
Institute of Basic Medical Sciences
Chinese Academy of Medical Sciences
and
Faculty of Basic Medicine
Peking Union Medical College
Beijing 100730, China

It is known from data from epidemiological surveys and laboratory investigations that hypercholesterolemia, unreasonable dietary collocation, smoking, and hemodynamic changes are the main risk factors in atherogenesis.[1] In order to decrease further the incidence of atherosclerosis or to postpone the course of its progression, it seems important to adopt measures including increasing the polyunsaturated fatty acids intake and reducing the saturated fatty acids. Additionally, data from current literatures points to the possibility of regression of atherosclerotic plaque.

It has been noticed for years that a negative correlation is present between the mortality rate from ischemic heart disease (atherosclerosis) and the serum high density lipoproteins (HDL) level.[2] The main component of HDL is apo A_1 (70% $\pm$) and data of experiments *in vitro* also indicated that HDL inhibit: the penetration rate of LDL through the intima; the combination rate of LDL with endothelial cells; and the synthesis of aminoglycans in stroma by smooth muscle cells.[3,4] So that, studying the role of HDL in those processes of intake, transportation, and degradation of lipid in the arterial wall as well as in liver is still necessary in clarifying the mechanism involved, including particularly, the retardation of atheromatous plaque development.

The Role of Serum HDL in the Development of Atheromatous Plaques in Tree Shrews[5,6]

Tree shrews (tupaia belangera yunalis) are known as the lowest class of primates. Their serum cholesterol level is close to that of healthy humans (192.9 $\pm$ 47.2 mg/dl), while in their serum protein, α-lipoproteins (HDL) comprise 70–75% and β-lipoproteins (LDL) 25–30%. The animals used were reared in Yunnan Province of the south-western part of China for 3 months after being caught and then, were transfered to Beijing for a further 7-month period of adjustment and stabilization before the experiment commenced. 3 experiments were carried out in studying the effect of HDL and each lasted a total of 242 days (8 months). The regular diet was 20 gm/animal/day of steamed cake consisting of vitamins, fish and bone powders and corn flour. In addition, 20 grams of apple was given/animal/day and ¼ egg and 30 gm rabbit meat or beef meat were given per animal twice per week. Apart from the regular diet, the experimental animals each received orally 5 gm of a mixed ration containing 0.2 gm cholesterol 6 times per week through the whole course of the experiment. The composition of the mixed ration per 100 grams was: cholesterol (C.P.) 4 gm, yolk powder 20 gm, pork lard 15 gm, and corn flour 61 gm. Blood samples were taken for lipid analysis before the experiment and by the end of the 8th, 24th (or 28th), and 32nd week. Tissue blocks from aortae, livers, and kidneys were taken for light and electronic microscopy.

First Experiment

Twenty-two tree shrews were used (mean body weight 132.5 ± 17.4 gm). Twelve animals were used for the experiment (one died in the 16th week after collecting of blood sample) and 10 for controls. Serum cholesterol was raised to 349.2 ± 99.5 mg/dl by the end of the 8th week and the mean value of the control group was 142.5 ± 31.2 mg/dl. α-lipoproteins of animals in the experimental group were known to be 75.0 ± 7.1% of the serum total lipoproteins at the beginning and 69.3 ± 4.2% by the end of the experiment, even with hypercholesterolemia, and the values of the control animals were 75.5 ± 7.1%. The incidence of atheromatous plaque development was 9% (1/11 animals), but was zero in animals of the control group.

Second Experiment

Twenty-five animals were used. Ten animals were used for each experimental or control group, respectively, and in addition, 5 more tree shrews were used as the 3rd group with a special ration of 0.2 gm cholesterol plus 0.1–0.2 mg tabazole/animal/day in order to lower the thyroid activity. By the end of the 32nd week, both HDL and HDL-cholesterol of all 15 animals of the cholesterol feeding and cholesterol plus tabazole groups again kept a high percentage of α-lipoproteins very similar to those shown in the control group (TABLE 1). The incidence of atheromatous lesions was zero in all 15 experimental animals (FIG. 1).

Third Experiment

Fifty animals were divided into 5 groups, 10 for each. Animals of three groups were fed with a high cholesterol ration as mentioned above. Among them, 10 animals received a daily high carbohydrate diet (high sugar content) instead of the regular ration, and another 10 animals, besides being subjected to the daily cholesterol intake, were reared in smaller cages (equivalent to 1/6 capacity of the original cages) in order to limit their physical activities. Animals of the remaining two groups were left as controls (TABLE 2).

TABLE 1. Changes of Serum Lipids by the End of Experiment 2

Groups	No. of Animals	HDL-CH (mg/dl)	Total CH (mg/dl)	HDL-CH/ Total CH (%)	Lipo./ Total Lipo. (%)	β-Lipo./ Total Lipo. (%)
Cholesterol	10	159.4 ± 53.2	271.2 ± 161.6	64.9 ± 14.3	74.1	25.9
Cholesterol + tabzole	5	164.7 ± 32.8	227.6 ± 52.7	75.5 ± 6.4	67.0	33.0
Controls	10	92.8 ± 22.7	147.3 ± 33.9	63.2 ± 7.8	70.5	29.5

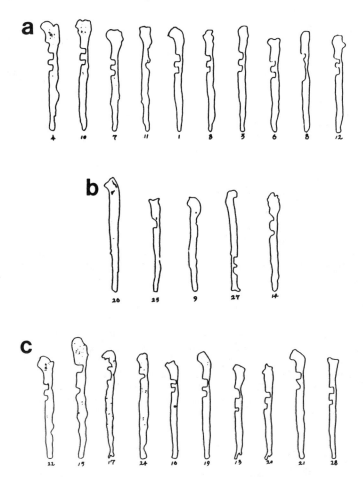

FIGURE 1. Lipid deposition in aortic intima of tree strews in different groups (experiment 2): **(a)** cholesterol, **(b)** tabazole + cholesterol, and **(c)** control.

Results obtained by the end of the experiment were similar to those of the previous 2 experiments. The incidence of atheromatous plaques was 1 in 30 experimental animals.

Among the 56 tree shrews in all the experimental groups of the 3 successive experiments, an important point is that the incidence of gall stone formation was very high (48–80% just by gross examination), and 99% of the composition was cholesterol analyzed by chemical assay and X-ray defraction examination. However, no gall stone was found in the control animals. This indicated that most of the cholesterol absorbed seemed to be transfered into the liver through HDL in a cholesterol ester form and was excreted later via the bile duct after degradation had taken place in liver.

Effect of HDL on Lipid Uptake and Transportation of Cells of the Arterial Wall

Endothelial cells, smooth muscle cells, monocytes, fibroblasts, and platelets are known to be the main participants in the process of atheromatous plaque development.

TABLE 2. Comparison of Serum Lipid Levels at the End of the 32nd Week in Experiment 3 (mg/dl ± SD for Serum Lipids)

Groups	HDL-CH	Total CH	HDL-CH/ Total CH (%)	α-Lipo.	α-lipo./Total Lipo. (%)
Cholesterol	146.0 ± 45.0 (8)	185.0 ± 59.0 (8)	79.0 ± 5.0 (8)	123.0 ± 47.0 (8)	81.0 ± 4.0 (7)
Cholesterol + high carbohydrate	199.0 ± 37.0 (6)	257.0 ± 39.0 (7)	78.0 ± 5.0 (6)	127.0 ± 41.0 (7)	88.0 ± 3.0 (4)
Cholesterol + limited activity	169.0 ± 35.0 (9)	229.0 ± 57.0 (9)	74.0 ± 9.0 (9)	130.0 ± 64.0 (9)	77.0 ± 7.0 (9)
Limitation of activity	98.0 ± 77.0 (7)	126.0 ± 25.0 (7)	78.0 ± 5.0 (7)	64.0 ± 25.0 (7)	77.0 ± 6.0 (7)
Controls	107.0 ± 20.0	136.0 ± 19.0	78.0 ± 5.0	106.0 ± 32.0	79.0 ± 5.0

Tabazole used in experiment 2 for inhibition of thyroid is 0.1–0.2 mg/animal/day for a total of 242 days.

Cell interaction and reactions of various mediators definitely influence the lipid metabolism of these cells. Furthermore, HDL also play an important role on these activities.

Promoting Effect of HDL on Monocyte Migration Activity in Vitro[7]

A chemotactic chamber was designed as shown in FIGURE 2. A thin layer of intima preparation (from rabbit's aorta) was placed at the site between the upper and lower chambers of the device. Laboratory data showed that HDL promoted the adherence rate (after 1 hour incubation at 37°C) and the penetration rate (after 4 hours incubation at 37°C) of the ^{51}Cr labelled monocytes, which were isolated from the rabbit's anticoagulated blood. The increased range was 106% for the adherence and 74% for the penetration rate compared to controls (FIG. 3).

Promoting Effect of HDL on the Cholesterol Clearance Rate of Smooth Muscle Cells[8]

HDL in various concentrations promoted the clearance rate of smooth muscle cells from either rabbit's or tree shrew's aortae, respectively, on ^{3}H-cholesterol (TABLE 3, FIGS. 4,5). Additionally, a cross effect, *i.e.*, no species specificity, was obtained between rabbit's HDL on tree shrew's SMC or vice versa. Data also indicated that there was a

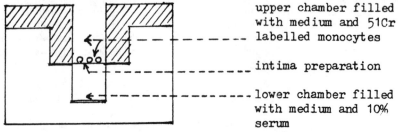

upper chamber filled with medium and 51Cr labelled monocytes

intima preparation

lower chamber filled with medium and 10% serum

FIGURE 2. Sketch of the chemotactic chamber.

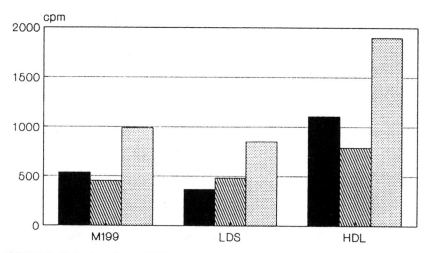

FIGURE 3. Promoting effect of HDL on monocyte migration activity *in vitro* (51Cr cpm). *Filled columns,* adherence; *hatched columns,* penetration; *dotted columns,* adherence + penetration. LDS, lipid deficiency serum.

negative correlation between the promoting ability of the cholesterol clearance effect of HDL isolated from hypercholesterolemia serum (from either rabbits or tree shrews) and the amount (%) of cholesterol combined with HDL.

Since tree shrews are resistant to the development of experimental atherosclerosis, the interesting point is that even the serum cholesterol level had been raised to 3 times higher

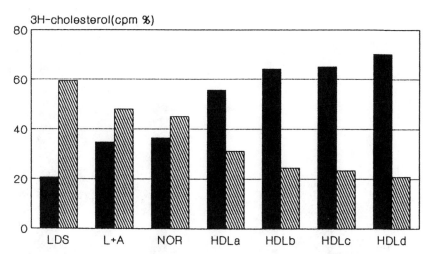

FIGURE 4. Amount of ^{3}H-cholesterol released from cultured SMC of tree shrews. *Filled columns,* cpm in medium; *hatched columns,* cpm in cells. LDS, lipid deficiency serum; L + A, LDS + calf albumin; HDLa, HDL 0.5 mg/ml medium; HDLb, HDL 1.0 mg/ml medium; HDLc, HDL 1.5 mg/ml medium; HDLd, HDL 2.0 mg/ml medium.

TABLE 3. Release of ³H-Cholesterol from Cultured SMC by HDL of Tree Shrew (cpm %)

Acceptors in Medium	In Medium			In Cell		
	Exp. 1	Exp. 2	Mean	Exp. 1	Exp. 2	Mean
HDL 2.0 mg/ml	75.00	65.40	70.20 ± 6.78	18.65	23.00	20.82 ± 3.07
HDL 1.5 mg/ml	68.25	61.73	64.99 ± 4.61	21.73	25.00	23.36 ± 2.31
HDL 1.0 mg/ml	67.80	60.54	64.17 ± 5.13	23.81	25.00	24.40 ± 0.85
HDL 0.5 mg/ml	59.32	51.87	55.65 ± 5.19	32.20	30.00	31.12 ± 1.55
Normal serum	40.14	32.65	36.40 ± 5.29	46.00	44.00	45.00 ± 1.41
LDS + albumin	37.00	32.58	34.79 ± 3.12	47.00	49.00	48.00 ± 1.40
LDS	19.00	22.00	20.60 ± 2.26	61.00	58.00	59.50 ± 2.12

than that before the experiment in tree shrews. However, the percentage of phospholipid in serum was still kept at the same level as before. Contrast to that, the percentage of phospholipid in rabbits was markedly reduced in the hypercholesterolemic serum (TABLE 4). Possibly, maintaining a high phospholipid percentage during hypercholesterolemia is one of the essential factors inhibiting the development of atheromatous lesions in tree shrews.

Inhibitory Effect of HDL on LDL or Ac-LDL Degradation in Rabbit's Endothelial Cells[11]

Either rabbit's serum HDL or apo A₁ was added to the culture media, respectively, for detecting its inhibitory effect on the degradation rate of LDL or Ac-LDL by the endothelial cells. Data indicated that only less than 20% of the degradation was decreased when the concentration of HDL used was 10-fold larger than the amount of ^{125}I-LDL used. On the other hand, no inhibitory effect was obtained on ^{125}I-Ac-LDL by HDL.

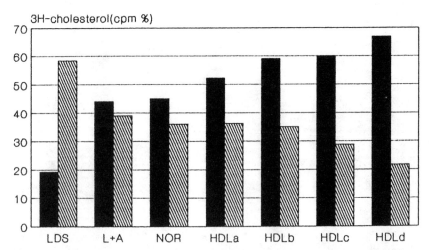

FIGURE 5. Amount of ³H-cholesterol released from cultured SMC of Rabbits (abbreviations as in FIGURE 4).

TABLE 4. Analysis of Serum Lipids with Thin Layer Chromatography (%)

	Total Cholesterol	Triglyceride	Phospholipid
Tree shrews:			
Normal serum	61.65	29.05	9.28
Hyperlipemic serum	89.67	0.47	9.80
Rabbits:			
Normal serum	65.00	24.77	9.99
Hyperlipemic serum	83.00	13.55	3.40

Similarly, serum apo A_1 also produced no inhibitory effect on the degradation rate of LDL or Ac-LDL in the cultured endothelial cells (FIG. 6).

Characterization of HDL Binding Sites in Cultured Smooth Muscle Cells[10]

Cultured smooth muscle cells from rabbit's aorta were studied with ^{125}I labelled rabbit's serum HDL_3. Saturation curves measured at 4°C showed the presence of two different components: the low affinity nonsaturable binding portion and the high affinity binding portion (Kd about 5.6×10^{-8} mol/L and B_{max} about 0.321 μg/ml cell protein). Scatchard analyses of the high affinity binding portion suggest the presence of a single class of binding sites. Binding of rabbit's HDL_3 on cultured smooth muscle cells was relatively resistant to trysin and pronase, and this behavior independent of Ca^{2+}. The binding rate of ^{125}I-HDL_3 on smooth muscle cells was highest at 4°C and the optimal pH was 2. Presence of a high concentration of apo A_1 reduced 50% of the binding rate of ^{125}I-HDL_3. ^{125}I labelled HDL_3 being pretreated (blocked) with rat antirabbit apo A_1 IgG in different concentrations lost 70% of its original binding rate with the smooth muscle cells (FIGS. 7,8). Besides, if HDL_3 from either rabbit's or tree shrew's sera had been conjugated with the binding sites of smooth muscle cells from the same species beforehand and the cell sections were incubated together with solution containing gold chloride granules being already labelled with either protein A or sheep antimouse IgG antibody, respectively. These binding sites could be displayed clearly under an electronic microscope. Clusters of gold granules indicating the binding sites of HDL_3 were obtained on the cell surface (FIG. 9). All these results supported the idea that either rabbit's or tree shrew's smooth muscle cells possess specific binding sites for apo E free HDL, which recognizes apo A_1 as a ligand.

Inhibitory Effect of HDL-Lipoproteins on the Development of Atherosclerosis in Rabbits[12,13]

Apolipoproteins (mainly apo A_1) were isolated by using the dextran sulfate concentration method and gradient ultracentrifugation from about 100 liters of rabbit's serum for

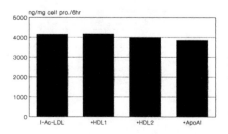

FIGURE 6. Effect of HDL & apo A_1 on ^{125}I-Ac-LDL degradation in rabbit aortic EC.

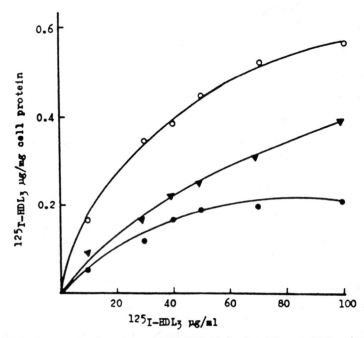

FIGURE 7. Concentration-dependence of rabbit HDL, binding by rabbit aortic SMC at 4°C for 1 hr. SMC was incubated with increasing amounts of ^{125}I-HDL$_3$ in the absence (○) or presence (▲) of excess apolipoprotein A$_1$ (1 mg/ml). Specific binding related to apo A$_1$ (●) is the difference between the binding in the absence and that in the presence of excess unlabelled apo A$_1$.

studying the inhibitory effect on atherosclerosis development in rabbits. Two successive experiments were carried out and a total of 36 New Zealand white rabbits were used. Cholesterol 0.5 gm/kg body weight was given to each rabbit of the experimental groups for 4 weeks accompanied by administration of HDL-apolipoproteins with a dosage of 3 mg/kg b.w. three times per week intravenously. All of the animals were sacrified by the end of the 12th week of the experiment. In the second experiment, cholesterol 0.2 mg/kg body weight was given to the experimental group animals in the first 4 weeks and the cholesterol amount was reduced to 0.1 mg/kg b.w. 6 times per week afterwards until the end of the experiment (altogether 12 weeks). Other measures were similar to those

TABLE 5. Lipid Deposition in the Aortic Intima of Rabbits in Different Groups (Experiment 1)

Groups (No. of Animals)	Lipids in Intima (mg/gm wet wt.)		
	Total CH	CH Ester	Free CH
Cholesterol control (6)	16.5 ± 4.8	8.9 ± 2.0	7.6 ± 2.9
Experimental (6)	6.7 ± 9.4 (P <0.05)	3.8 ± 5.6 (P <0.05)	2.9 ± 3.8 (P <0.05)
Blank control (6)	1.7 ± 0.1 (P <0.01)	0.6 ± 0.2 (P <0.01)	1.2 ± 0.1 (P <0.001)

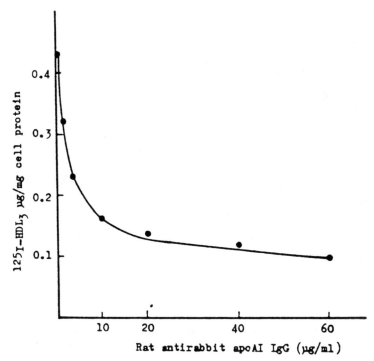

FIGURE 8. Binding of ^{125}I-HDL$_3$ by rabbit aortic SMC after ^{125}I-HDL$_3$ was blocked by different concentrations of rat antirabbit apo A$_1$ IgG. Each point represents the mean value of two duplicate determinations (232.6 cpm/ng ^{125}I-HDL$_3$).

adopted in the previous experiment. By the end of these two successive experiments, the lipid content in aortic intima, the area of atheromatous lesion or fatty streak involved, the lipid deposition in intima morphologically, as well as the thickness of the atheromatous plaques were lower in animals of the apolipoprotein-receiving groups in comparison with those of the cholesterol control groups (TABLES 5, 6; FIG. 10). Data from these experiments clarified that apolipoproteins (mainly apo A$_1$) in HDL are the main factors acting on the inhibitory effect against atheromatous plaque formation. Owing to the small number of animals used and the difference of individual response, no statistical significance

TABLE 6. Lipid Deposition in the Aortic Intima of Rabbits in Different Groups (Experiment 2)

Groups (No. of Animals)	Lipids in Intima (mg/gm wet wt.)		
	Total CH	CH Ester	Free CH
Cholesterol control (6)	9.21 ± 5.9	6.4 ± 4.6	2.9 ± 1.6
Experimental (6)	4.3 ± 1.7	2.6 ± 1.1	1.8 ± 0.9
Blank control (6)	1.0 ± 0.3	0.2 ± 0.2	0.8 ± 0.3

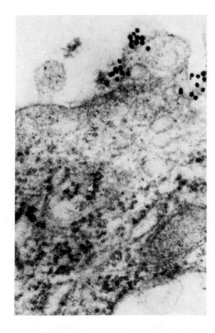

FIGURE 9. Clusters of gold granules on the cell surface of tree shrew's SMC (binding sites of HDL). ×30 K ×1.5. Granule diameter 10 nm.

was obtained on lipid deposition in intima between the experimental (apo A_1-receiving) and the experimental control (cholesterol control) groups in experiment 2.

Promotion of the Cholesterol Clearance Effect of Smooth Muscle Cells by Apo A_1/Phospholipid Liposomes[14]

Based on the laboratory data of the previous experiments, the inhibitory effect of apo A_1 alone is not so strong in the development of atheromatous plaques as that of HDL. It seems necessary to make further investigation to detect new combinations of apolipoproteins with other agents. Liposome is known to be one. Apo A_1 combining with a synthetic phospholipid—dipalmitoylphosphorycholine (DPPC) was tried particularly to make clear its effectiveness and stability. Apo A_1/DPPC was prepared with a ratio of 1 : 2.5 (w/w) by using either rabbit's apo A_1 (Rlip1) or apo A_1 from tree shrew (Tlip1), respectively. Additionally, another form of liposome, Apo A_1/DPPC/cholesterol was prepared under a

TABLE 7. Clearance of ^{3}H-Cholesterol from Tree Shrew SMC by Apo A_1/DPPC Liposome[a]

	^{3}H-Cholesterol Released (cpm %)		
	Exp. 1	Exp. 2	Mean
T LDS	16.32	14.92	15.62
T apo A_1	20.45	23.83	22.14
DPPC	21.41	24.84	23.13
T lip1	32.42	31.92	32.17
T lip2	32.81	32.92	32.87

[a]TLDS, tree shrew lipid deficiency serum; T lip1, tree shrew apo A_1/DPPC; T lip2, tree shrew apo A_1/DPPC/cholesterol.

ratio of 1 : 2.5 : 0.12 (w/w) with Apo A_1 isolated either from rabbit's (Rlip2) or tree shrew's sera (Tlip2). Results indicated that both apo A_1DPPC and apo A_1/DPPC/cholesterol liposomes from either rabbit's or tree shrew's sera gave a very strong effect in activating LCAT. These liposomes also markedly promoted the clearance effect of smooth

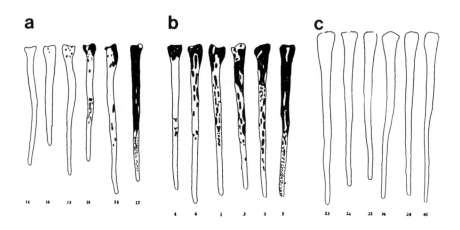

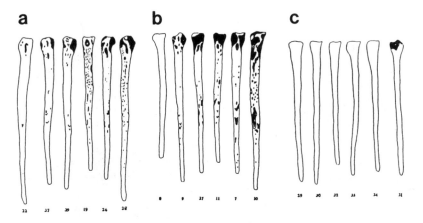

FIGURE 10. Lipid deposition in aortic intima of rabbits in different groups. Experiment 1, *above;* experiment 2, *below.* (**a**) Experimental group; (**b**) experimental controls; (**c**) controls.

muscle cells on ^{3}H-cholesterol (TABLE 7; FIG. 11) and which was much stronger than that exerted by lipid deficiency serum, or DPPC or apo A_1 alone.

Besides, liposomes prepared with apo A_1 from either rabbit's or tree shrew's sera also possess a cross effect in promoting cholesterol clearance rate of the smooth muscle cells

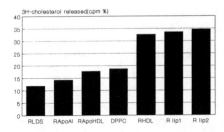

FIGURE 11. Clearance of ^{3}H-cholesterol from rabbit SMC by apo A_1/DPPC liposome. RLDS, rabbit lipid deficiency serum; DPPC, dipalmitoylphosphorylcholine; R lip1, rabbit apo A_1/DPPC liposome; R lip2, rabbit apo A_1/DPPC/cholesterol liposome.

isolated from different species of animals (FIG. 12), *i.e.*, liposomes of tree shrew's apo A_1 promoted the cholesterol clearance rate of rabbit's smooth muscle cells, and vice versa.

In conclusion, so far as we know, the role of HDL in preventing the development of atheromatous plaques is multifactorial. It involves various links concerning lipid uptake, esterification, transportation, and degradation. Moreover, the inhibitory effect of apo A_1 on the progression of atherogenesis, even though not strong enough, is very important. One must carry on further study to clarify the essential factors required for strengthening its action and the machanism involved, which might provide more information in searching for new measures of retarding the development or in promoting the regression process of atherosclerotic plaque in the future.

SUMMARY

According to data obtained from epidemiological and experimental survey, serum HDL level is known to be correlated conversely with the incidence of atherosclerosis. Experimental data collected in this article explained part of its mechanism, which is described in four parts as follows:

1. The result of 3 successive experiments on experimental atherosclerosis in tree shrews (total of 96 animals available including 40 as the controls) showed that the serum HDL level had been kept persistantly to 69–88% of the total serum lipoproteins even after a high cholesterol intake for 32 weeks. The incidence of atheromatous lesions developed was only 0–9%, but the incidence of gall stone was very high, 48–84% by gross examination by the end of these experiments.
2. HDL are also capable of (1) promotion of monocyte migration activity; (2) enhancement of cholesterol clearance rate of aortic smooth muscle cells originally isolated from either rabbits or tree shrews; (3) inhibition of 20% of LDL degradation but with no inhibitory effect obtained on Ac-LDL degradation in the en-

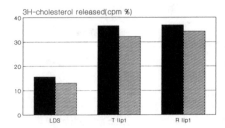

FIGURE 12. Cholesterol clearance of apo A_1/DPPC from different species of animals on SMC. *Filled columns,* tree shrew; *hatched columns,* rabbit. T lip1, tree shrew apo A_1/DPPC liposome; R lip1, tree shrew apo A_1/DPPC liposome.

dothelial cells; (4) presence of specific binding sites for apo E free HDL on the surface of aortic smooth muscle cells from either rabbits or tree shrews which recognizes apo A_1 as a ligand.

3. Data from 2 successive experiments in rabbits showed that HDL lipoproteins (mainly apo A_1) possess an inhibitory effect on the development of atheromatous plaques, but not a very strong one.

4. The colesterol clearance effect of smooth muscle cells was markedly enhanced by apo A_1/phospholipid liposomes (the apo A_1 used was isolated from either rabbit's or tree shrew's serum) *in vitro*.

REFERENCES

1. SCHETTLER, G: 1989. 8th international symposium on atherosclerosis. J. Int. Soc. Fed. Cardiol. **2:** 3.
2. MILLER, GJ, *et al.* 1975. Plasma high density lipoprotein concentration and development of ischemic heart disease. Lancet **1:** 16.
3. EISENBERG, S. 1984. High density lipoprotein metabolism. J Lipid Res. **25:** 1017.
4. BADIMEN, JJ *et al.* 1987. High and very high density lipoprotein administration inhibits progression of atherosclerotic lesions in cholesterol-fed rabbits. Atherosclerosis **7:** 522a.
5. SHE MING-PENG *et al.* 1983. The effect of alpha-lipoproteins in preventing atheromatous plaques in tree shrews with induced hypercholesterinemia. Sino-Jpn. J. Allergol. Immunol. **1:** 66.
6. SHE MING-PENG *et al.* 1988. Experimental atherosclerosis in tree shrews. J. Nutr. Sci. Vitaminol. **34:**(Spec. Suppl.): 439.
7. LING YUN, XIA REN-YI & WONG ZONG-LI. 1987. The influence of high density lipoproteins (HDL) on adherence and penetration abilities of monocytes against the intima preparation. Abstract of the 2nd Congress on Atherosclerosis in China 1987. 33.
8. DONG LI-MING & XIA REN-YI. 1989. Study on cholesterol clearance effect of high density lipoproteins (HDL) on smooth muscle cells. Natl. Med. J. China. In press.
9. XU QING-BO *et al.* 1988. Distribution of the binding sites of LDL and HDL on rabbits' aortae with double-labelling immunogold technique. Sino-Jpn. J. Allergol. Immunol. **4:** 463.
10. XU QING-BO *et al.* 1989. Characterisation of HDL binding sites and its ligand in cultured smooth muscle cells of rabbit's aorta. (Abstract) The 8th International Congress of Atherosclerosis, October 1988. P. 754. Chin. Med. J. **102:** 469.
11. LIN JIE *et al.* Investigation on uptake and degradation of low density lipoproteins (LDL and Ac-LDL) by rabbit's endothelial cells. Not yet published.
12. RAN BI-FANG *et al.* 1989. The inhibitory effect of apolipoproteins in HDL on experimental atherosclerosis in rabbits. (Abstracts) 34th Scientific Meeting of the Royal College of Pathologists of Australasia, September 1989, Hong Kong.
13. REN BI-FANG *et al.* 1989. Study on the inhibitory effect of rabbit's HDL-lipoproteins on experimental atherosclerosis. Chin. J. Pathol. **18:** 257.
14. CAI CHUN-BO & XIA REN-YI. 1990. Study on the clearance effect of apo A_1/phospholipid liposomes on cholesterol from smooth muscle cells *in vitro*. Chin. J. Pathol. **19.** In press.

The Effect of Dietary Oils on Tissue-Specific Expression of Apo A-1 mRNA in the Rat

HIROSHIGE ITAKURA, AKIYO MATSUMOTO, SATOSHI
NAGANAWA, NAOHISA OHKUSHI, HIROSHI ITOH, AND
SHINJI IKEMOTO

Department of Clinical Nutrition
National Institute of Health and Nutrition
1-23-1 Toyama, Shinjuku-ku
Tokyo 162, Japan

INTRODUCTION

Epidemiological studies suggest that replacement of saturated fatty acids in the diet by polyunsaturated fatty acids reduces the incidence of coronary heart disease.[1] Polyunsaturated fatty acids of the n-3 series enriched in some types of fish oil may have some beneficial actions compared with polyunsaturated fatty acids of the n-6 series found in vegetable oils. Effects of the n-3 polyunsaturated fatty acids on HDL-cholesterol levels have been inconsistent. Many factors help determine HDL-cholesterol levels. In this report, we studied the effects of different kinds of fatty acids on the amount of expression of the apo A-I gene.

EXPERIMENTAL PROCEDURE

Animals and Diets

Fourteen groups of ten male, eight-weeks-old, Spague-Dawley rats were fed ad libitum for four weeks. The diet of each group contained different kinds of 10% oil with or without 0.5% cholesterol. The kind of fatty acids were as follows: soybean oil, safflower oil, codfish oil, sardine oil, beef tallow, lamprey oil, and a mixture of beef tallow and EPA (70% purified).

Analysis of Messenger RNA

Each tissue from the rats was frozen immediately after excision. Total RNAs were isolated by the guanidium thiocyanate method of Chirgwin *et al.*[2] Then, the RNA was treated with 1 M glyoxal at 50°C for 1 hour. After treatment, the RNA was electrophoresed on 1% agarose gel in 10 mM phosphate buffer (pH 7.0). Then, the RNA was transferred to a nylon membrane and hybridized with ^{32}P-labeled cDNA probes. The amount of mRNA from the autoradiogram was measured with a densitometer.

352

TABLE 1. Plasma Lipids of Rats Fed Normal (-ch) and High-Cholesterol (+ch) Diets

	T-ch (mg/dl)		HDL-ch (mg/dl)		TG (mg/dl)	
	−ch	+ch	−ch	+ch	−ch	+ch
Soybean	71.67	127.7	66.1	49.6	271.0	268.0
	± 8.2	± 43.6	± 10.2	± 9.2	± 175.7	± 101.0
Safflower	72.8	155.9	66.7	53.7	205.2	188.2
	± 7.0	± 21.0	± 7.1	± 13.3	± 67.5	± 75.5
Codfish	85.2	134.4	54.2	38.4	186.4	130.8
	± 15.5	± 42.2	± 9.4	± 5.6	± 69.1	± 29.3
Sardine	59.9	118.7	42.9	41.5	102.9	121.4
	± 7.9	± 34.9	± 12.8	± 5.7	± 16.7	± 20.9
Beef tarrow	79.6	384.2	57.1	28.1	202.3	122.2
	± 11.5	± 60.5	± 6.4	± 4.8	± 56.3	± 37.6
Lamprey	70.0	114.8	39.0	38.8	106.4	124.6
	± 14.9	± 32.6	± 6.3	± 8.6	± 13.1	± 29.1
EPA + beef	59.1	205.0	30.2	25.4	75.6	92.4
	± 14.4	± 34.6	± 6.3	± 8.2	± 6.7	± 25.4

RESULTS

Serum cholesterol levels were increased in the beef tarrow groups (TABLE 1). No differences in serum cholesterol levels were found in the vegetable oil, fish oil and mixture of EPA and beef tarrow groups. HDL-cholesterol levels in these groups were almost the same, but the levels in the vegetable oil groups were slightly higher than in the beef tarrow and beef tarrow with EPA.

The amounts of apo A-I mRNA in the liver were observed to be suppressed in the sardine oil and lamprey oil groups (TABLE 2). The amount of apo A-I mRNA in the beef tarrow with EPA group was lower than in the beef tarrow group. In the intestine, sardine oil did not suppress the expression of the apo A-I gene.

The fatty acid composition of the rat liver was changed depending on the supplemented oils (TABLE 3). Concentrations of EPA and DHA were elevated in the sardine oil, lamprey oil and beef tarrow with EPA groups. Linoreic acid was increased in the soybean and safflower oil groups. The amount of apo A-I mRNA measured by densitometer was correlated with the amount of EPA or DHA in the liver (FIG. 1).

TABLE 2. Densitometric Comparison of the Expression of Apo A-I mRNA

	Liver		Intestine	
	−ch	+ch	−ch	+ch
Soybean	1.0	1.0	1.0	1.0
Safflower	1.12	0.92	0.93	1.00
Codfish	1.13	0.84	0.83	1.00
Sardine	0.85	0.36	0.99	1.18
Beef tarrow	1.50	1.44	1.18	0.75
Lamprey	0.61	0.26	0.51	1.18
EPA + beef	0.87	0.48	1.12	0.59

TABLE 3. Fatty Acid Composition of Rat Liver (High-Cholesterol Diet)

	C14:0	C16:0	C16:1	C18:0	C18:1	C18:2	C18:3	C20:4	C20:5	C22:6
Soybean	1.2	17.7	9.9	3.9	27.8	25.7	3.4	5.5	0.4	1.1
Safflower	1.0	19.3	7.8	3.4	23.7	34.3	1.3	5.1	—	0.3
Codfish	1.6	21.4	12.2	3.0	41.1	4.3	4.4	2.6	2.3	2.4
Sardine	3.4	22.7	9.4	3.2	20.7	2.8	1.7	2.7	5.0	10.3
Beef tarrow	1.3	27.3	8.9	7.3	42.1	3.4	0.5	4.2	0.2	1.3
Lamprey	3.0	25.2	9.4	6.5	23.6	4.5	1.9	2.9	4.1	11.0
EPA + beef	5.2	18.0	4.7	10.5	24.4	8.8	1.1	6.7	7.4	6.3

DISCUSSION

HDL is one of the major plasma lipoproteins and is thought to play an important role in preventing atherosclerosis. Epidemiological studies have identified that decreased HDL levels are associated with increased risk of coronary heart diseases. Thus it is important to understand the factors which determine the levels of plasma HDL. Apo A-I is a major constituent of HDL, and apo A-I production may be important in the regulation of plasma HDL concentrations. Fatty acids are known to be important dietary factors. High intake of saturated fatty acid is known to induce hypercholesterolemia.

In this study, we observed the effect of different kinds of fatty acids on the expression of apo A-I messenger RNA in the liver and intestine. The amounts of apo A-I messenger RNA in the liver were suppressed in the fish oil groups and were shown to be negatively associated with the percentage amount of EPA and DHA. However, in the intestine, expression of apo A-I was not suppressed by fish oils.

In conclusion, tissue-specific expression of apo A-I mRNA was different from or-

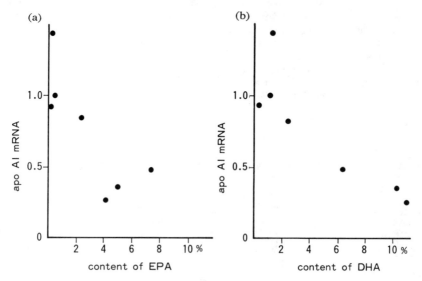

FIGURE 1. Correlation with the content of EPA **(a)** and DHA **(b)** and the amount of apo A-1 mRNA in the liver.

gans. n-3 Fatty acids such as EPA and DHA may suppress the expression of apo A-I RNA especially in the liver.

REFERENCES

1. PHILLIPSON, B. E. *et al*. 1985. Reduction of plasma lipids, lipoproteins, and apoproteins by dietary fish oils in patients with hypertriglyceridemia. N. Engl. J. Med. **312:** 1210.
2. CHIRGWIN, J. A. *et al*. 1979. Isolation of biologically active ribonucleic acid from sources enriched in ribonuclease. Biochemistry **18:** 5294.

Antiplatelet Therapy for Atherosclerotic Disorders

FUJIO NUMANO, YUKIO KISHI, TAKASHI ASHIKAGA,
TAKAHIRO KOBAYASHI, KENTARO SIMOKADO, FUJIE
NUMANO, AND MICHIYOSHI YAJIMA

Tokyo Medical and Dental University
Department of Internal Medicine
1-5-45 Yushima, Bunkyo-ku
Tokyo 113, Japan

Modern studies on atherogenesis have been focused on vascular injury and the following phenomenon induced by an imbalance between blood cells and the vascular wall. In this case, vascular injury does not always mean morphological changes in the endothelial line but rather the physiological and metabolic impairment of the endothelial cells, because such vascular injury results in the entry of plasmal flow into the vascular wall, following various cellular responses in the vessel wall to initiate atherosclerosis.[1-3]

Among many factors causing vascular injury, aggregated platelets adhering to the surface of the endothelial lines and/or to the rough surface stripped off endothelial cells have been intensively studied as the key phenomenon to initiate and to perpetuate vascular injury into the atherosclerotic lesions.[4-6]

In fact, sometimes platelets have been encountered adhering to the endothelial line, and various substances such as serotonin, histamine, adenosine diphosphate, and thromboxane A_2 were found to be released, which accelerate platelet aggregation causing the endothelial line to induce morphological changes. Platelet-derived growth factor (PDGF) released from activated platelets induces the proliferation of macrophages invaded into the subendothelial layer of the arterial wall and leads to the immigration and the proliferation of smooth muscle cells from the media to the subendothelial layer.[1,6-8]

Activated Platelets and Vascular Injury

Our experimental *in vivo* and *in vitro* studies demonstrate the positive interaction of activated platelets on vascular endothelial cells.

FIGURE 1 shows the vascular injury observed in the coronary artery of a rabbit to which thromboxane A_2 was administered by cathether into the coronaries. Thromboxane A_2 was obtained by the mixture of 30μg of PG H_2 and 5mg of microsome protein obtained from cow platelets.[9] Typical edematous change was observed in the subendothelial layer of the coronaries. Electronmicroscopic studies demonstrated contracted and swollen endothelial cells with edema at the subendothelial and upper part of the medial layer as shown in FIGURE 2. These *in vivo* studies suggest that activated platelets will induce damage to endothelial cells resulting in vascular injury.

Our *in vitro* study, shown in FIGURE 3, also confirmed the direct injury of endothelial cells by the activated platelets.[10]

Endothelial cells isolated from fetal bovine aorta were preincubated with [³H]adenine at a concentration of 0.2 M for 3 hours. Activated platelets were prepared by incubating the washed human platelets suspension with 10 μg/ml of collagen or by sonication for 20

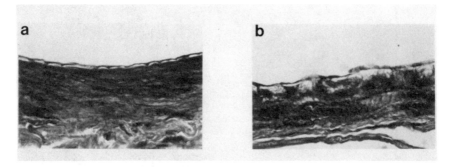

FIGURE 1. Vascular Injury in coronary artery of rabbits challenged by Thromboxane A_2 **(a)** Control; **(b)** injured coronaries. Stained by Azan Mallory's method. $\times$ 1,000.

sec. The [^{3}H]adenine incorporated endothelial cells were incubated with platelet suspension with or without collagen or platelet lysate for 2 hours at 37°C.

[3H]adenine release was calculated as the ratio of radioactivity in the medium to the total activity initially taken up by the cells. Thus, the degree to which the endothelial cells were damaged by activated platelets was calculated. Sonicated platelets exhibited the highest radioactivity from [3H]adenine release, followed in turn by collagen-activated-platelet and untreated-platelet suspensions. These three values were all significantly higher than that of controls. The release of [3H]adenine by activated platelets increased according to the number of platelets and to the time of incubation.

FIGURE 4 shows substances that can prevent endothelial cells from platelet-induced damage. Cultured endothelial cells were pretreated with these agents for 10 minutes before they were incubated with collagen-activated platelet suspension.

Methysergide, a serotonin antagonist (10^{-6} M), ONO3708, a thromboxane A^2 antagonist (10^{-5} M), ZK36374, a prostacycline analogue (10^{-6} M) all prevented endothelial cells from platelet-induced damage to some degree. However, 10^{-3} M IBMX, a phosphodiesterase inhibitor combined with 10^{-6} M ZK3674 protected the endothelial cells from damage almost completely.

These data suggest that the protection of endothelial cells from platelet adhesion will be available for the prevention of atherosclerosis and that the intervention whereby the

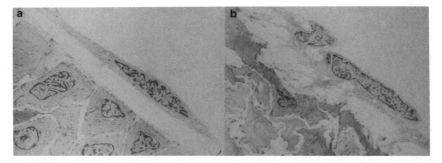

FIGURE 2. Vascular injury in coronary artery of rabbit given thromboxane A_2. **(a)** Control; **(b)** vascular injury. $\times$ 1,000.

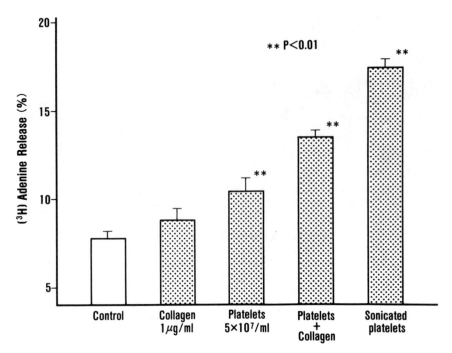

FIGURE 3. [³H] Adenine release from endothelial cells.

endothelial cells accumulate cyclic AMP may achieve the protection of endothelial cells from platelet-induced vascular injury. Cyclic AMP is currently considered to be an inhibitory modulator of intracellular calcium, a factor which might be associated with cell change.[11]

Cyclic Nucleotides and Endothelial Cells

Cyclic nucleotides are the intracellular secondary messengers to various hormones and amines by which the physiological tone of vessel wall is controlled. Recent studies have elucidated the fact that EDRF and prostacyclin in endothelial cells play important roles in keeping physiological vascular tone, as both were found to effect the vessel wall by changing the metabolism of cyclic nucleotides.[12-14]

In fact, endothelial cells seem to possess a characteristic metabolism of cyclic nucleotides different from that in smooth muscle. TABLE 1 summarizes the cyclic AMP (cAMP) and cyclic GMP (cGMP) contents in cultured endothelial cells and smooth muscle cells taken from pig coronary arteries. Endothelial cells contain 10 times as much cAMP, significantly higher than cGMP. On the other hand, smooth muscle cells contain levels of cGMP similar to that in endothelial cells ($p < 0.001$). Thus, the A/G ratio is statistically higher in endothelial cells than in smooth muscle cells (16.67 ± 2.8 (EC) vs 3.42 ± 0.78 (SM); $p < 0.01$).

FIGURE 5 shows the dilution pattern of phosphodiesterase (PDE) separated by affinity column chromatography. In endothelial cells, high activity of type III (cAMP PDE) and very low activity of type I (cGMP PDE) were found. In contrast, smooth muscle cells revealed high activity of type I (cGMP PDE).[15]

Vascular injury is known to induce change in cyclic nucleotide metabolism. The authors have reported that in the rabbit challenged with epinephrine and/or angiotensin, the content of cyclic AMP in the intima of the aorta decreased significantly compared with that of controls,[5,16] and that progression of experimentally induced atherosclerosis is associated with the gradual decrease in cAMP levels and the increased activity of cAMP PDE in rabbits fed a cholesterol diet.[17,18] Perhaps lower levels of cAMP may cause the easy contraction of endothelial cells to increase plasmal flow into the arterial wall and the proliferation of intimal cells to develop atheromatous lesions. Gryglewski stressed the important roles of cyclic AMP in the progression and regression of atherosclerosis.[19] Jurakova[20] and Lundholm[21] also reported a fall in cyclic AMP in the atherosclerotic aorta of the rat and pig. Tertov in his culture study observed that an increase of intracelluler cyclic GMP and a fall in the cyclic AMP level can stimulate the proliferative activity of the aortic wall, whereas increased cyclic AMP concentration leads to the inhibition of cell division.[22] At the same time he pointed out that a rise in intracelluler cyclic AMP can stimulate the hydrolysis of cellular lipid. Hajaar confirmed that prostacyclin accelerates the hydrolyzation of cholesterol ester in the vascular wall,[23,24] which is known by its increasing effect of cAMP.[25]

Antiplatelet Therapy

The above survey may suggest antiplatelet therapy as the remedy not only for thrombotic disorders but also for atherosclerotic diseases.[26–28]

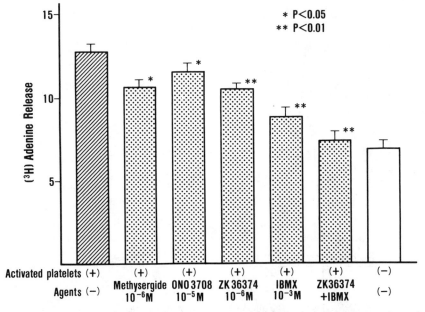

FIGURE 4. Prevention of endothelial cells from activated platelet-induced damage by various substances. The agents were applied 10 min before addition of activated platelet suspension.

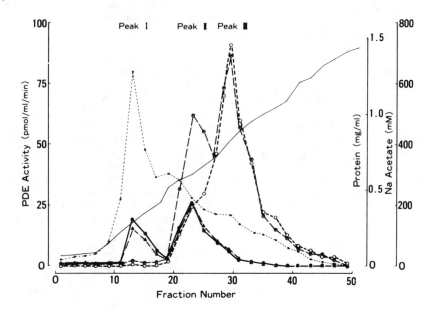

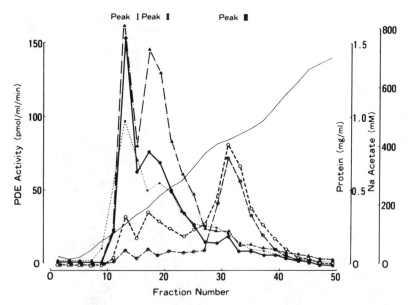

FIGURE 5. The dilution pattern of phosphodiesterase.

TABLE 1. Levels of Cyclic Nucleotides in the Cells of the Vascular Wall[1]

	Cyclic AMP (pmol/mg Protein)	Cyclic GMP (pmol/mg Protein)	A/G
Endothelial cells (N = 4)	5.31 ± 0.62	0.529 ± 0.057	10.67 ± 2.18
Smooth muscle cells (N = 6)	7.10 ± 0.87	2.31 ± 0.30*	3.42 ± 0.78**

[a]Mean ± SE. *p <0.001; ** p <0.01.

In Japan, many agents have been clinically evaluated or used as antiplatelets as shown in TABLE 2. Many of these agents are known pharmacologically for their marked effect on cAMP level in platelets and/or endothelial cells.

Phthalozinol is a phosphodiesterase inhibitor synthesized by Shimamoto and Ishikawa[5,29] in 1976, and has been studied for its clinical effects on atherosclerotic disorders and/or neurological disorders.[30,31] Recently, Majokowski reported its therapeutic efficacy on patients with amyotrophic lateral sclerosis.[32]

Cilostazol is a derivative of quinokinone synthesized by Nishi *et al.* as an antithrombotic agent in 1975.[33] Pharmacological studies revealed its antiaggregatory effect on platelets by inhibiting their phosphodiesterase activity.[34,35] This agent has been on the market since 1988 in Japan as an antithrombotic. We recently reported on tis therapeutic effect on peripheral vascular disorders.[33]

Ticlopidine from France has been widely used in Japan as an antiplatelet. Its pharmacological effect is also achieved by inducing cAMP production.[37] The Canadian-American Ticlopidine study (CAT-study) recently reported its preventive effect against cerebral vascular disorders.[38]

The antipyretic agent, aspirin, is well known as a typical antiplatelet agent. The antithrombotic effect of aspirin has already been noticed early from extensive clinical experience before its antithromboxane A_2 effect was elucidated and since the first report by Cravan in 1953,[39] many clinical studies have been reported on the preventive action of aspirin on coronary and cerebral disorders.[26-28] Presently, its clinical effect for secondary prevention of coronary and cerebral thrombosis has been generally accepted.[40]

However, since the discovery of thromboxane A_2 and prostacyclin and the elucidation of their physiological function between platelets and the vascular wall, the mechanism of aspirin as an antithrombotic agent has been clarified. This caused much discussion on its dosage when prescribed clinically, because of the so-called aspirin dilemma and required careful monitoring for its long-term efficacy vs any negative side effects.

TABLE 2. Antiplatelet Drugs Used in Japan

Acetyl salicylic acid	(cyclooxigenase inhibitor)
Iloprost[a]	(PGI$_2$ analogue)
Prostaglandin E$_1$	(adenylate cyclase stimulator)
Ticlopidine	(adenylate cyclase stimulator)
Pyridinolcarbamate	(ATP increasing effect)
Phthalazinol[a]	(cAMP PDE inhibitor)
Cilostazol	(cAMP PDE inhibitor)
Bifemelane	(cAMP PDE inhibitor)
Milrinon[a]	(cAMP PDE inhibitor)
Dipyridamole	(cGMP PDE inhibitor)
Calan	(Ca^{++}/calmodulin PDE inhibitor)

[a]Under clinical study (Oct. 1989).

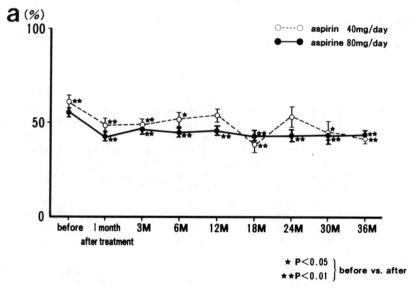

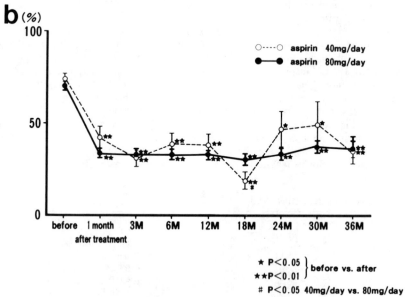

FIGURE 6. (a) Changes in ADP (3μM) induced platelet aggregation by aspirin treatment. **(b)** Changes in collagen (2μg/ml) induced platelet aggregation by aspirin treatment.

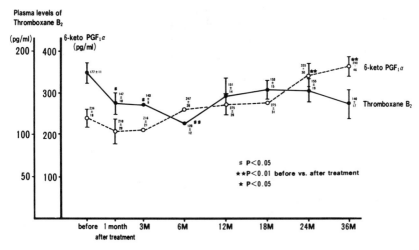

FIGURE 7. Changes in plasma prostanoids by a small dose of aspirin treatment.

Our previous studies on its dosage involving patients with Takayasu arteritis demonstrated the improvement in platelet aggregation by the prescription of a daily dose of 80 or 40 mg of aspirin, decreasing the plasma thromboxane B_2 level without any remarkable effect on 6-keto $PGF_{1\alpha}$ levels.[41]

From this background, we are now pursuing comparative clinical studies on the efficacy of 40- or 80-mg doses of aspirin for the secondary prevention of atherosclerotic disorders with 109 patients.[42] Already fifty-two patients have been treated for more than 3 years. FIGURE 6 shows changes in ADP-induced platelet aggregation over 3 years, with

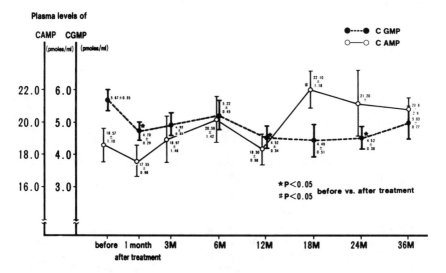

FIGURE 8. Changes in plasma cyclic nucleotide levels by a small dose of aspirin treatment.

the 40-mg regimen revealing fluctuating aggregative ability. FIGURES 7 and 8 reveal changes in plasma prostanoid and cyclic nucleotide levels in the 80-mg regimen. Under this treatment, plasma thromboxane B_2 levels steadily decreased during the first 6 months and then maintained low levels as compared with the level before treatment.

Furthermore, it should be noted that under the 80-mg regimen, the 6-keto PDG_1 level first decreased and then gradually increased to significantly higher levels than those before treatment.

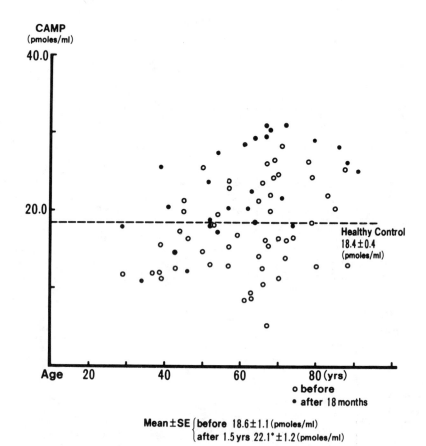

FIGURE 9. Plasma cAMP levels before (○) and 18 months after (●) aspirin (80 mg/day) treatment.

Parallel to these changes, cAMP also revealed significantly high levels in plasma after more than 2 years' treatment. These high levels of cAMP may reflect the good condition of a patient. In fact, as shown in FIGURE 9, these increasing higher levels of cAMP after treatment were observed at every age. The elucidation of this phenomenon induced by small doses of aspirin over a long term is our next research target.

SUMMARY

Recent studies have revealed the important roles of platelets in atherogenesis via vascular injury. Our *in vivo* and *in vitro* studies clearly demonstate that activated platelets directly inflict injury to vascular endothelial cells, which is associated with a decrease in intracellular cyclic AMP levels in vascular tissues.

Antiplatelet therapy is clinically important not only for the prevention of thrombotic episodes but also for the prevention of vascular injury and atherosclerosis. A small dose of aspirin (80 mg) induces clinically hypoaggregativeness of platelets with concomitantly decreased levels of thromboxane A_2 in plasma. Our clinical study involving more than 3 years of treatment with small doses of aspirin demonstrated favorable therapeutic effects characterized by hypoaggregation of platelets and increased levels of cAMP and 6-keto $PGF_{1\alpha}$ in plasma which will aid in the prevention of atherosclerosis.

REFERENCES

1. Ross, R. 1981. Atherosclerosis: A problem of the biology of arterial wall cells and their interaction with blood component. Arteriosclerosis **1:** 293–311.
2. Marcus, A. J., L. B. Safier, H. L. Ullman, N. Islam, M. J. Broekman, J. R. Falck, S. Fischer & C. Schacky. 1988. Platelets-neutrophil interaction. J. Biol. Chem. **265(5):** 2223–2229.
3. Davies, P. F. 1986. Biology of disease, vascular cell interaction with special references to the pathogenesis of atherosclerosis. Lab. Invest. **55:** 5–24.
4. Gimbrone, M. A. 1982. Interactions of platelets and leucocytes with various endothelium *in vitro* studies. Ann. N.Y. Acad. Sci. **401:** 171–183.
5. Numano, F. 1980. Chemotherapy of atherosclerosis. Jpn. Circ. J. **44:** 55–68.
6. Ross, R. 1986. The pathogenesis of atherosclerosis—an update. N. Engl. J. Med. **314:** 488–500.
7. Asada, Y., T. Hayashi & A. Suminyoshi. 1988. Vascular injuries induced by materials released from platelet-rich thrombus *in vitro*. Atherosclerosis **70:** 1–6.
8. Numano, F. 1981. Thromboxan A_2 and atherosclerosis. *In* Medicinal Chemistry Advances. F. G. 'de Las Heras & S. Vega, (Eds.) 131–140. Raven Press. New York, NY.
9. Numano, F., N. Yajima, K. Nishiyama, K. Shimokado, Fe. Numano, S. Sasagawa & K. Moriya. 1982. Effects of thromboxane A_2 injection on the rabbit coronary artery. Exp. Mol. Pathol. **37:** 118–132.
10. Kishi, Y. & F. Numano. 1989. *In vitro* study of vascular endothelial injury by activated platelets and its prevention. Athersclerosis **76:** 95–101.
11. Katz, A. M. & M. Reuter. 1979. Cellular calcium and cardiac cell death. Am. J. Cardiol. **44:** 188–195.
12. Furchgott, F. R. 1983. Roles of endothelium in response to vascular smooth muscle. Circ. Res. **53:** 557–573.
13. Moncada, S. 1982. Prostacyclin and arterial wall biology. Atherosclerosis **2:** 193–207.
14. Murad, F. 1986. Cyclic guanosine monophosphate as a mediator of vasodilation. Am. Soc. Clin. Invest. **78:**1–5.
15. Kishi, Y., T. Ashikaga & F. Numano. 1990. Phosphodiesterase in vascular endothelial cells. Adv. Second Messenger Phosphoprotein Res. S. J Strada & H. Hidaka, Eds. Vol. 24. Raven Press. New York, NY. In press.
16. Numano, F., T. Kuroiwa, K. Takano, *et al.* 1978. The effect of vascular injury caused by angiotensin II or cholesterol and epinephrine in phosphofructokinase, G-6-PDH and cyclic nucleotides in the rabbit's aorta. Artery **4:** 332–329.
17. Numano, F. 1979. Cyclic nucleotides and atherosclerosis. *In* Cyclic Nucleotides and Therapeutic Perspectives. G. Cehovis and G.A. Robinson, Eds. 137–146. Pergamon Press. Oxford.
18. Numano, F., H. Maezawa, T. Shimamoto & K. Adachi. 1976. Changes in cyclic AMP and

cyclic GMP phosphodiesterase in the progression and regression of experimental atherosclerosis. Ann. NY. Acad. Sci. **275:** 311–320.

19. GRYGLEWSKI, R. 1980. Prostaglandins, platelets and atherosclerosis. *In* CRC Critical Reviews in Biochemistry. 291–338.

20. JURUKEREA, A. & B. BOSHKOV. 1977. Cyclic adenosine monophosphate system in rat experimental atherosclerosis. Prog. Biochem. Pharmacol. **13:** 268–270.

21. LUMJHOLM, L., L. JACOBSSON & R. ANDERSSON. 1980. Relationship between cyclic AMP and protein synthesis in atherosclerotic pig aorta. *In* Vascular Neuro Effector Mechanism. J. A. Bevan, Ed. 257–259. Raven Press. New York, NY.

22. TERTOV, V. V., A. N. OREKHOV, S. A. KUDRYASHOV, *et al.* 1987.Cyclic nucleotides and atherosclerosis studies in primary culture of human aortic cells: Exp. Mol. Pathol. **47:** 377–389.

23. HAJAAR, D. P. 1985. Prostaglandins and cyclic nucleotides. Biochem. Pharmacol. **34(3):** 295–300.

24. HAJAAR, D. P. & WEKSLER, B. B. 1983. Metabolic activity of cholesterol esters in aortic smooth muscle cells is altered by PGI_2 and E_2. J. Lipid Res. **24:** 1176–1185.

25. DEMBINSKA-KIEC, A., W. RÜCKER & P. S. SCHÖNHÖFER. 1979. PGI_2 enhanced cAMP content in bovine coronary arteries in the presence of isobutylmethylxanthine. Naunyn–Schmiedeberg's Arch. Pharmacol. **308:** 107–110.

26. YUSUF, S. 1988. Overview of results of randomized clinical trials in heart disease. J. Am. Med. Assoc. **260:** 2259–2263.

27. DOUGLAS, A.S. 1983. Trials of antiplatelet drugs in coronary prevention. In Atherosclerosis. N. E. Miller, Ed. 77–90. Raven Press. New York, NY.

28. FITZGERALD, G. A., G. MAYO, P. PRICE & K. TAKAHARA. 1989. Aspirin in cardiovascular disease. *In* Biochemical Pharmacology and Clinical Trials. Prostaglandins in Clinical Research: Cardiovascular System. 97–106. Alan R. Liss, Inc. New York, NY.

29. ADACHI, A. & F. NUMANO. 1977. Phosphodiesterase inhibitor; their comparative effectiveness *in vitro* in various organs. Jpn. J. Pharmacol. **27:** 97–103.

30. SHIMAMOTO, T., H. MURASE & F. NUMANO. 1976. Treatment of senile dementia and cerebellar disorders with phthalazinol, cyclic AMP-increasing agent. Mech. Ageing Dev. **5:** 241–250.

31. SHIMAMOTO, T. 1977. Prevention and enhancement of regression of human atherosclerosis by modifying local factors. Atheroscler. Rev. **2:** 233–251. R. Paoletti & A. M. Gotto, Jr., Eds. Raven Press. New York, NY.

32. MAJKOWSKI, J. 1990. Long-term treatment of amyotrophic lateral sclerosis with phthalazinol. Adv, Second Messenger Phosphoprotein Res. S. J. Strada & H. Hidaka, Eds. Vol. 24. Raven Press. New York, NY. In press.

33. NISHI, T., *et al.* 1983. Studies on 2-oxoquinoline derivatives as blood platelet aggregation inhibitors I, alkyl 4-(2-oxo-1,2,3,4-tetra hydro-6-quinolyloxy) butyrates and related compounds. Chem. Pharmacol. Bull. **31:** 1151–1157.

34. KIMURA, Y., T. TANI, T. KANBE & K. WATANABE. 1985. Effect of cilostazol on platelet aggregation and experimented thrombosis. Arznei Forsch. Drug Res. **35:** 1144–1149.

35. TANAKA, T., T. ISHIKAWA, M. HAGIWARA, K. ONODA, H. ITO & H. HIDAKA. 1988. Effect of cilostazol, a selective cAMP phosphodiesterase inhibitor, on the contraction of vascular smooth muscle. Pharmacology **36:** 313–320.

36. NUMANO, F., Y. KISHI & T. ASHIKAGA. 1990. Clinical studies on phosphodiesterase inhibitor for cardiovascular disease. *In* Adv. Second Messengers Phosphoprotein Res. S. J. Strada & H. Hidaka, Eds. 24: Raven Press. New York, NY. In press.

37. ASHIDA, S. & Y. ABIKO. 1980. Inhibition of platelet aggregation by a new agent, ticlopidine. Thromb. Haemostasis **40:** 542.

38. NELSON, E. 1990. Current use of antiplatelet drugs in stroke syndromes in the USA. Ann. N.Y. Acad. Sci. This volume.

39. CLAVAN, L. L. 1953. Experiences with aspirin with nonspecific prophylaxis of coronary thrombosis. Miss. Valley Med. J. **75:** 38–44.

40. ANTIPLATELET TRIALISTS' COLLABORATION. 1988. Secondary prevention of vascular disease by prolonged antiplatelet treatment. Br. Med. J. **296:** 320–331.

41. NUMANO, F., Y. MARUYAMA, T. KOYAMA & FE. NUMANO. 1986. Antiaggregative aspirin dosage at the affected vessel wall. Angiology 37(**10**): 695–701.
42. NUMANO, F., Y. KISHI, T. OTA, R. MORIWAKI, J. MITANI, T. KUROIWA, N. FURUTA & F. NUMANO. 1989. Small dose aspirin treatment on vascular diseases. Thromb. Haemostasis **62**: 599.

Current Use of Antiplatelet Drugs in Stroke Syndromes in the USA

ERLAND NELSON

Department of Neurology
Lovelace Medical Center
University of New Mexico School of Medicine
Albuquerque, New Mexico 87108

It is my intention to focus on one of the important artherosclerotic disorders (the most important, to me as a neurologist) specifically, stroke syndromes, which are cerebral ischemic disorders and usually considered secondary to thromboembolism.

My interest in vascular disease and stroke is long-standing. Along with many colleagues, I spent a number of years on ultrastructural studies of innervation of arteries and capillaries, primarily of the brain (and heart).[1-3] Coincidentally, there were early transmission electron microscopic (TEM) observations on human intracranial artery aging and atherosclerosis.[4] Then, with the obvious advantage of scanning electron microscopy (SEM) in examining the endothelial surface, we reported a number of combined SEM-TEM investigations on experimental vascular ischemia, trauma, vasospasm, and atherosclerosis.[5-7]

Seeing that many antiplatelet drugs are widely used in other countries but are not available for clinical use in the USA, I shall limit this paper to a drug recently tested in two, large, North American trials, *i.e.,* ticlopidine hydochloride, to aspirin therapy, and, very briefly, to a few others used in the USA.

Ticlopidine is one of the newer and most promising of the antiplatelet drugs. It has been under worldwide investigation since the mid-1970s and is currently widely used in at least 45 countries. The exact mechanism of ticlopidine action is not completely known; however, it seems to act by strongly inhibiting ADP-induced platelet aggregation and aggregation brought on by several other inducers. It appears to interfere with ADP and fibrinogen receptor pathways on the platelet membrane, and does not inhibit cyclo-oxygenase or cyclic AMP phosphodiesterase.[8]

The two recent North American studies were: the Ticlopidine-Aspirin Stroke Study (TASS), and the Canadian American Ticlopidine Study (CATS).[8-10] They are similar in results and adverse effects, but differ significantly in design, patient populations, and methodology.

TASS set out to prove that ticlopidine was superior to aspirin, an already clinically established antiplatelet drug for patients with transient ischemic attacks (TIAs) or minor strokes. Some baseline data are shown in TABLE 1. TASS was designed to study patients at one end of the ischemic stroke spectrum, with early and/or mild symptoms. These quantities of medication were chosen because this dose of ticlopidine had been approved for marketing in Europe, and this dose of aspirin had been approved by both US and Canadian agencies for primary stroke prevention in males suffering from TIAs. The TASS study, using intent-to-treat analysis, showed that ticlopidine significantly reduced the risk of death from all causes or nonfatal stroke compared to aspirin, by a modest 12% with a *p*-value of 0.048. A reduction of risk of 21% for fatal or nonfatal stroke was more significant, with a *p*-value of 0.024. (FIGS. 1 and 2). The risk of death from all causes or nonfatal stroke was reduced by as much as 41% at the end of the first year, the year of greatest risk. In all of these analyses, ticlopidine was more effective than aspirin in females as well as males.

TABLE 1. Baseline Data for the Ticlopidine-Aspirin Stroke Study (TASS)

Inclusion Criteria	40 years of age or more TIA (including amaurosis fugax), RIND, or minor stroke, within 3 months of enrollment
Number of centers	56
Number of patients	3069
Duration of enrollment	4.3 years
Follow-up	2–6 years
Dose of medication	
Ticlopidine	250 mg twice daily
Aspirin	650 mg twice daily

CATS was begun in 1983 as an investigation of antiplatelet drugs for the secondary prevention of stroke, recognizing that stroke survivors also represented a high-risk population. Unlike the TASS program which considered a group already known to benefit from aspirin administration, there was no evidence that aspirin would be beneficial in this stroke survivor population. Thus, aspirin was unwarranted as a control agent and placebo was used. CATS considered patients at the other end of the ischemic stroke spectrum, and

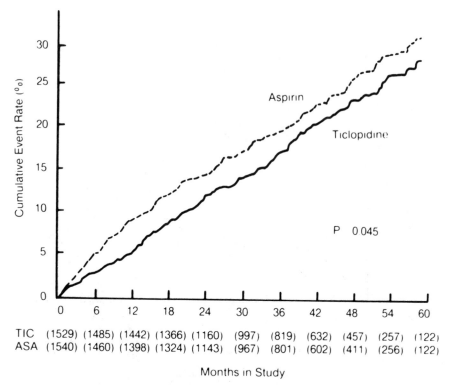

TIC	(1529)	(1485)	(1442)	(1366)	(1160)	(997)	(819)	(632)	(457)	(257)	(122)
ASA	(1540)	(1460)	(1398)	(1324)	(1143)	(967)	(801)	(602)	(411)	(256)	(122)

Months in Study

FIGURE 1. Cumulative event-rate curves for death from any cause or nonfatal stroke. *Values in parentheses* indicate the number of patients in the Ticlopidine and Aspirin Groups. TASS.

TABLE 2. Baseline Data for the Canadian American Ticlopidine Study (CATS)

Inclusion criteria	thromboebolic stroke within 1 week–4 months
Number of centers	23
Number of patients	1073
Duration of enrollment	3 years
Follow-up	mean of 24 months
Dose of medication	
Ticlopidine	250 mg twice daily
Placebo	identical capsules twice daily

included patients with a well-documented thromboembolic stroke within 1 week to 4 months prior to enrollment. Baseline data is shown in TABLE 2. Ticlopidine significantly reduced the risk of the primary endpoint of vascular death (cardiovascular or cerebrovascular in origin), nonfatal stroke, or nonfatal MI by 30.2% with a p-value of 0.006 in the efficacy analysis and by 23.3% (p = 0.020) in the intent-to-treat analysis. (FIGS. 3 and 4).

Adverse experiences were important and occurred in both the TASS and CATS trials, but more so in TASS, where aspirin was given (1300 mg/day), rather than the placebo

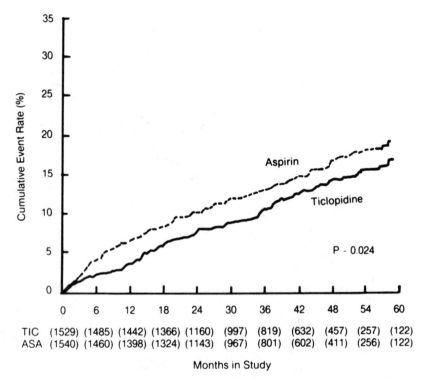

TIC	(1529)	(1485)	(1442)	(1366)	(1160)	(997)	(819)	(632)	(457)	(257)	(122)
ASA	(1540)	(1460)	(1398)	(1324)	(1143)	(967)	(801)	(602)	(411)	(256)	(122)

Months in Study

FIGURE 2. Cumulative event-rate curves for fatal or nonfatal stroke. *Values in parentheses* indicate the number of patients in the Ticlopidine and Aspirin Groups. TASS.

used in CATS (TABLE 3). The most common reactions that led to temporary reduction in dosage or discontinuation of therapy in those receiving ticlopidine were diarrhea, rash, and neutropenia, with the last being considered "serious" in ticlopidine patients (0.9%). All reversed after discontinuation of the drug, but one patient whose white count had recovered fully, died with an infection and renal failure one month later. All cases of neutropenia occurred within the first 3 months of beginning therapy, and the diarrhea and rash began to occur a few weeks after treatment had begun. Thus, careful monitoring, especially during the early months of therapy with ticlopidine is clearly required. In these, as in other clinical trials with this drug, there was an increase in total cholesterol. In the TASS trial, there was an increase in all lipoprotein fractions with the largest being in the very-low-density lipoprotein and the lowest in the low-density lipoprotein fractions.

To summarize the ticlopidine trials, the TASS study demonstrated that administration of ticlopidine resulted in a significant reduction of risk, especially of recurrence of fatal and nonfatal stroke in patients with a history of TIAs and minor strokes, as compared with

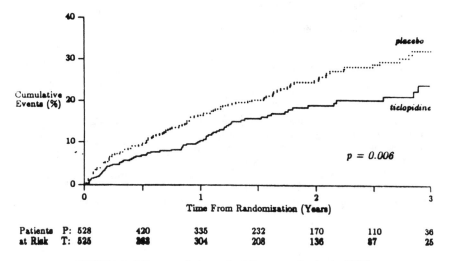

| Patients at Risk | P: | 528 | 420 | 335 | 232 | 170 | 110 | 36 |
| | T: | 525 | 363 | 304 | 208 | 136 | 87 | 25 |

FIGURE 3. Efficacy analysis: stroke, MI, or vascular death. CATS.

aspirin. CATS demonstrated even more convincingly a reduction in vascular death, non-fatal stroke or nonfatal myocardial infarction in patients surviving a completed stroke. Thus, for the first time, there appears to be an effective drug which is of benefit to both females and males, and for use in threatened stroke, and following a completed stroke.

The ability of aspirin to inhibit platelet function was established more than 20 years ago.[11] Since that time, there has been a host of reports, analyses (retrospective and prospective), and now meta-analyses. The largest and most recent of the meta-analyses comes from the Antiplatelet Trialists' Collaboration, who attempted an overview of all randomized trials of prolonged treatment with drugs whose principal purpose is inhibition of platelet aggregation, with aspirin being the one most extensively tested.[12,13] (Ticlopidine data were not available.) Patients studied included some 29,000 men and women with a history of stroke, TIA, MI, or unstable angina. This meta-analysis indicated that antiplatelet drugs reduced mortality secondary to vascular causes by about 15% (SD 4%). Nonfatal vascular events including MI or stroke were reduced by 30% (SD 4%). No

TABLE 3. Selected Adverse Experiences

Experience	Ticlopidine Group	Aspirin Group
Patients exposed to study medication[a]	1518	1527
Patients with any adverse experience	945 (62.3)	813 (53.2)
Diarrhea	310 (20.4)	150 (9.8)[b]
Dyspepsia	191 (12.6)	210 (13.8)
Nausea	169 (11.1)	156 (10.2)
Gastrointestinal pain	110 (7.2)	153 (10.0)[b]
Gastritis	13 (0.9)	26 (1.7)[b]
Gastrointestinal hemorrhage	7 (0.5)	21 (1.4)[b]
Peptic ulcer	12 (0.8)	45 (2.9)[b]
Rash	180 (11.9)	80 (5.2)[b]
Unicaria	30 (2.0)	5 (0.3)[b]
All hemorrhagic	137 (9.0)	152 (10.0)
Severe neutropenia	13 (0.9)	0 (0.0)[b]

[a]Eleven patients assigned to ticlopidine and 13 assigned to aspirin took no study medication before premature termination.
[b]Values are significantly different from those for the ticlopidine group ($p<0.05$).

significant difference was noted in nonvascular mortality. In 11 trials (n = 5,807) that specifically considered TIAs or minor strokes, antiplatelet drugs reduced nonfatal stroke by 24%. In 10 trials of patients with MI (n = 13,544), nonfatal stroke was reduced by 25% Thus, in these categories of patients, antiplatelet drugs are clearly indicated. In this same meta-analysis, the choice of antiplatelet drug was also considered. In those that compared aspirin with dipyridamole, no difference was detected and, in aspirin vs sulphinpyrazone, aspirin was favored. A recently published trial involving 60 consultant neurologists (approximately 1/3 of the total number working in the United Kingdom and Ireland) studying 2,435 patients with TIA or minor ischemic stroke, specifically compared aspirin 600 mg twice daily with aspirin 300 mg once daily. There was an 18% reduction of patients suffering nonfatal MI, nonfatal major stroke, vascular death, or

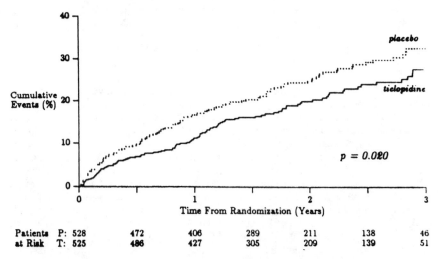

FIGURE 4. Intent-to-treat analysis: stroke, MI, or vascular death. CATS.

nonvascular death. There was no significant difference in reduction of endpoints comparing the 300 mg and 1200 mg daily doses, except for a decrease in gastrointestinal side-effects with the lower dose of aspirin.[14] Thus, the optimum dose for aspirin is not yet settled. The question of value of antiplatelet agents in stroke reduction in males seems reasonably resolved; however, in females, the case for utilization of aspirin (or sulfinpyrazone) is unclear. Somewhat surprisingly, the usefulness of antiplatelet drugs in patients following a completed stroke has not been extensively studied. To date, prospective reports using aspirin have failed to show significant benefit in reducing stroke recurrence.[15,16]

The question of primary stroke prevention by administration of aspirin to patients who had no prior history of either stroke or myocardial infarction had never been adequately studied. This has been specifically addressed by two large prospective studies, involving male physicians in the United States (n = 22,071) and in the United Kingdom (n = 5,139).[13,17,18] That part of the US study that utilized aspirin was randomized and double blinded, using aspirin at a 325 mg dose given on alternate days and tested against placebo. Aspirin as the treatment drug was terminated early because of what was perceived as a surprisingly large reduction of both fatal and nonfatal myocardial infarctions in those taking aspirin. Although there was no significant difference in total number of strokes, there was a significant increase in the disabling and fatal hemorrhagic strokes.* It should be noted that incidence of death from all cardiovascular causes was identical and unexpectedly low (0.08% per year). The British trial was unblinded and randomly compared groups on 300 mg or 500 mg aspirin, with the other half instructed to avoid aspirin or aspirin-containing products. There was no significant difference in total mortality or the incidence of nonfatal MI or stroke; although, as in the American Physician's Health Research Group Study, the frequency of hemorrhagic and disabling stroke was somewhat higher. Thus, the routine use of aspirin as a prophylactic agent to prevent stroke (without a prior history of vascular disease) is not generally recommended.

In a recently updated and practical guide to antithrombotic treatment of thromboembolic strokes to which this author has alluded several times previously in this paper, there is a careful examination and critical review of the recent and important literature on antiplatelet drug use.[13] Anticoagulant therapy for specific types of cardiac disease is also thoroughly considered in the same publication, but is beyond the scope of this paper.

In conclusion, I have summarized briefly the two recently completed, large scale trials in North America designed to test the effectiveness of ticlopidine in stroke patients. This is an antiplatelet agent with different properties and different methods of action than those possessed by aspirin, itself, proven a relatively safe and useful drug for ischemic brain syndromes. Ticlopidine decreases risk of TIAs and minor stroke as compared to aspirin, and also decreases the risk of recurrence of a previous stroke. It appears to be the definite drug of choice in women, where earlier studies with several different antiplatelet drugs, including aspirin, showed no proof of favorable effect.

The several important studies on the definite efficacy of aspirin in TIAs and mild strokes were reviewed, with the recent addition of meta-analysis. This analysis of several somewhat dissimilar studies appears to strengthen statistical power of the data, and provides new insights. The absence of a therapeutic effect by the next most commonly

*Note Added in Proof: Since preparation of this paper, the "Final report of the aspirin component of the ongoing physicians' health study" has been published. The increased risk associated with aspirin in the subgroup of moderate-to-severe or fatal hemorrhagic stroke observed previously was no longer statistically significant. (THE STEERING COMMITTEE OF THE PHYSICIAN'S HEALTH RESEARCH GROUP. 1989. Final report of the aspirin component of the ongoing physician's health study. N. Engl. J. Med. **321**(4): 129–135.)

used antiplatelet drugs, dipyridimole and sulfinpyrazone was reconsidered in meta-analyses, and a clearly favorable effect is still lacking.

The orderly, progressive relationship between biomedical research and clinical drug trials must continue in spite of their increased costs and complexities.

ACKNOWLEDGMENTS

Appreciation is expressed to Professor William K. Hass from the New York Medical Center, and to all of the members of the Ticlopidine Aspirin Stroke Study Group, and equally to Profesor Michael Gent from the Faculty of Health Sciences, McMaster University, and to all contributors to the Canadian American Ticlopine Study. Special thanks to the Syntex Research Corporation in Palo Alto, California and to their helpful, encouraging, and appropriately optimistic Dr. Basil A. Molony, Head of the Department of Antithrombotic Therapy. My dear wife, Constanza, also assisted me in several important ways.

REFERENCES

1. NELSON, E. & M. RENNELS. 1970. Neuromuscular contacts in intracranial arteries of the cat. Science **167:** 301–302.

2. RENNELS, M. & E. NELSON. 1975. Capillary innervation in the mammalian central nervous system. Am. J. Anat. **44:** 233–241.

3. FORBES, M. S. M. RENNELS & E. NELSON. 1977. Innervation of myocardial micro-circulation: terminal autonomic axons associated with capillaries and post-capillary venules in mouse heart. Am. J. Anat. **149:** 71–91.

4. FLORA, G., E. DAHL & E. NELSON. 1967. Electron microscopic observations on human intracranial arteries. Changes seen with aging and atherosclerosis. Arch. Neurol. **17:** 162–173.

5. NELSON, E., S. D. GERTZ, M. RENNELS, M. S. FORBES & O. BLAUMANIS. 1976. Ultrastructural changes in the arterial endothelium: possible relationship to atherosclerosis. *In* Cerebrovascular Diseases. P. Scheinberg, Ed. 97–109. Raven Press. New York, NY.

6. GERTZ, S. D., G. MERIN, R. C. PASTERNAK, M. S. GOTSMAN, O. R. BLAUMANIS & E. NELSON. 1978. Endothelial cell damage and thrombosis following partial coronary arterial constriction: relevance to the pathogenesis of myocardial infarction. Israel J. Med. Sci. **14**(3): 384–388.

7. NELSON, E., S. D. GERTZ, M.S. FORBES, M. L. RENNELS, F. P. HEALD, M. A. KAHN, T. M. FARBER, E. MILLER, M. M. HUSSAIN & F. L. EARL. 1976. Endothelial lesions in the aorta of egg yolk-fed miniature swine: a study by scanning and transmission electron microscopy. **25:** 208–220.

8. MOLONY B. & D. ELLIS. 1989. Monograph for Clinical Investigation of Ticlopidine hydrochloride (RS-99847-XX-07-0). A Platelet Aggregation Inhibitor. Property of Syntex Research, Palo Alto, California 94304.

9. HASS, W., J. D. EASTON, H. P. ADAMS, W. PRYZE-PHILLIPS, B. A. MOLONY, S. ANDERSON & B. KAMM, FOR THE TICLOPODINE ASPIRIN STROKE STUDY GROUP. 1989. A randomized trial comparing ticlopidine hydrochloride with aspirin for the prevention of stroke in high-risk patients. N. Engl. J. Med. **321:** 501–507.

10. GENT, M., J. D. EASTON, V. C. HACHINSKI, E. PANAK, J. SICURELLA, J. A. BLAKELY, D. J. ELLIS, J. W. HARBISON, R. S. ROBERTS, A. G. G. TURPIE, AND THE CATS GROUP. 1989. The Canadian American Ticlopidine Study (CATS) in Thromboembolic Stroke. Lancet **1**(for 1989): 1215–1221.

11. WEISS, H. J. & L. M. ALEDORT. 1967. Impaired platelet/connective tissue reaction after aspirin ingestion. Lancet **2:** 495–497.

12. ANTIPLATELET TRIALISTS' COLLABORATION. 1988. Secondary prevention of vascular disease by prolonged antiplatelet treatment. Br. Med. J. **296:** 320–331.
13. SHERMAN, D.G., M.L. DYKEN, M. FISCHER, M. J. G. HARRISON, & R. G. HART. 1989. Antithrombotic therapy for cerebrovascular disorders. Chest **95**(Suppl. 2): 140S–155S.
14. UK-TIA STUDY GROUP. 1988. United Kingdom transient ischemic attack (UK-TIA) aspirin trial: interim results. 1988. Br. Med. J. **296:** 316–320.
15. A SWEDISH COOPERATIVE STUDY. 1987. High-dose acetylsalicylic acid after cerebral infarction. Stroke **18:** 325–334.
16. GENT, M., J. A. BLAKELY, V. HACHINSKI, R. S. ROBERTS, H. J. M. BARNETT, N. H. BAYER, S. G. CARRUTHERS, S. M. COLLINS, M. G. GAWEL, M. HOPKINS, P. JAIN, M. LAMY, J. P. MELOCHE, E. SAERENS, J. SICURELLA & A. G. G. TURPIE. 1985. A secondary prevention, randomized trial of suloctidil in patients with a recent history of thromboembolic stroke. Stroke **16:** 416–424.
17. THE STEERING COMMITTEE OF THE PHYSICIANS' HEALTH RESEARCH GROUP. 1988. Preliminary report: findings from the aspirin component of the Ongoing Physicians' Health Study. N. Engl. J. Med. **318**(4): 262–264.
18. PETO, R., R. GRAY, R. COLLINS, K. WHEATLEY, C. HENNEKENS, K. JAMROZIK, C. WARLOW, B. HAFNER, E. THOMPSON, S. NORTON, J. GILLILAND & R. DOLL. 1988. Randomized trial of prophylactic daily aspirin in British male doctors. Br. Med. J. **296:** 313–316.
19. ORME, M. 1988. Aspirin all round? Br. Med. J. (Editorial) **298:** 307–308.

Dietary Recommendations to Prevent Coronary Heart Disease

W. VIRGIL BROWN

Medlantic Research Foundation
108 Irving St., NE
Washington, DC 20010

There is now widespread agreement that the habitual dietary pattern of a population has major influence on the prevalence and incidence of arteriosclerotic vascular disease. This is particularly manifest in the coronary heart disease (CHD) rates in geographical groupings. Studies of many societal groups around the world have provided strong evidence that a few specific components of the total nutrient intake define the diets with atherogenic potential. Three of these: high intake of saturated fats, cholesterol and calories (in excess of need leading to obesity) are uniformly associated with a higher blood cholesterol and higher frequency of myocardial infarction and death from CHD. Animal studies and carefully controlled human trials confirm the relationships of dietary saturated fat and cholesterol intake to both blood cholesterol and coronary heart disease.

Health policy leading to recommendations for a population as a whole have emanated from governmental and voluntary health agencies after considering the evidence. More recently very specific guidelines have been issued for health professionals to aid in the dietary management of high blood cholesterol levels in patients.

From time to time it is valuable to reexamine our recommendations to determine if they remain optimal for the present, asking if they are compatible with the most recent scientifically gathered information. It is also useful to review the reasoning process that led to the recommendation regarding a specific nutrient. Are there gaps in the data that need filling? Would fundamental knowledge relating nutrition to physiological or biochemical changes be helpful in refining the recommendation? Finally, are new recommendations needed based on the knowledge gained about other dietary components such as omega-3 fatty acids, soluble fiber or alcohol?

This paper will briefly examine the current dietary guidelines as put forward by the American Heart Association[1] and the United States National Cholesterol Education Program[2] by attempting to answer such questions where they seem relevant.

Health Objectives of Dietary Change

Before considering the dietary changes one must determine the specific objectives to be achieved. Prevention of clinically manifest coronary heart disease and an increase in healthful longevity are the ultimate goals, but other measures such as blood plasma cholesterol, blood pressure and excess body weight are useful as guideposts. Given the strong causal links drawn with disease, changes in these parameters for the individual or for groups of individuals are quite acceptable endpoints of dietary therapy.

Reduction of low density lipoprotein (LDL) cholesterol is universally recommended. LDL is the best documented factor inducing arteriosclerosis in both human and animal studies. Clinical trials of cholesterol lowering which show efficacy in reducing coronary heart disease have (when measured) been associated with LDL reduction.[3-5] An LDL cholesterol below 130 mg/dl is considered desirable, below 100 is probably ideal. Al-

376

though higher levels of high density lipoprotein (HDL) are correlated with reduced risk, changes in HDL as a result of dietary changes have not been linked to change in the incidence of coronary heart disease. Similarly, reductions in triglycerides with diet (or drug) interventions have not been associated by modern statistical analyses with reduced coronary heart disease rates. The absence of adequate studies in certain subgroups leaves open the question of whether benefit may accrue from altering triglycerides and HDL with diet. At this time, the evidence is not sufficient to develop specific dietary guidelines for these objectives.

Excess body fat, particularly that located in the abdominal and chest regions is an independent risk factor for coronary heart disease.[6,7] In addition, it is associated with higher LDL and HDL cholesterol. Higher blood pressure and increased risk of diabetes mellitus also frequently accompany obesity. Losing weight to achieve those ranges given in the Metropolitan Life Insurance table of 1959 is recommended by the American Heart Association.

Lowering blood pressure to values below 140/90 mm Hg is a widely accepted recommendation for adults.[8] Values even lower are associated with reduced risk of stroke and clinical disease in other arterial systems.[9] Dietary factors can play an important roll in this effort and will be discussed later. Chief among these is reducing excess body weight and alcohol consumption. Restriction of dietary sodium and possibly increasing potassium are also potentially beneficial in reducing the incidence of high blood pressure.

Reducing LDL cholesterol, reducing excess body fat and controlling blood pressure can be achieved wholly or in part by appropriate dietary changes. The effects of changing eating patterns are determined by the genetic makeup of the individual, the baseline diet composition and the adherence to the prescribed eating behavior. The rationale for changing specific nutrients is given in order of the potential benefit to the largest number of people (author's opinion).

Saturated Fats

The fully saturated fatty acids: lauric (C 12), myristic (C 14) and palmitic (C 16) have sizable effects on raising blood cholesterol,[10] parimarily through raising the level of the atherogenic LDL cholesterol.[11] Although this effect has been observed in comparisons of populations and confirmed by animal and human intervention studies, the actual mechanisms of action of saturated fats in raising LDL cholesterol is still not well understood. The most frequently observed measurable physiologic change is a slowing in the clearance of LDL from the blood stream,[12] but there is some evidence that LDL synthesis may also be reduced in some individuals.[13] Since most LDL is normally removed from the plasma space by the liver through specific cell surface receptor mechanisms,[14] the number or the rate of functioning of this receptor has been the subject of investigation.[15] The incorporation of these saturated fatty acids into cell membranes and into the LDL molecules provides an opportunity for several potential mechanisms to be operative. The LDL receptor binds to a specific region of apolipoprotein B (apo B), the major protein component of the lipoprotein.[16] It is possible that saturated fats may alter the configuration of apo B and reduce the affinity for the receptor. To date this has not been investigated. Once bound LDL is taken into the cell and ultimately into a lysosome where it is released from the receptor and degraded.[15] The receptor returns to the cell surface to begin the process anew. The increased content of saturated fats could reduce the mobility of the receptor in its movement and thereby increase the time for the cycling of the receptor between cell surface and the lysosomal compartment. This would reduce the apparent number of LDL receptors and thereby slow the clearance of LDL from the plasma compartment. Replacement with monounsaturated and polyunsaturated fats would tend to increase the fluidity of the cell membranes and facilitate receptor function. At the moment these concepts remain theoretical and need much experimental investigation.[16]

Saturated fatty acids of less than 12 carbon units do not raise blood cholesterol.[17] Stearic acid (C 18) also does not increase plasma LDL in human or animal studies.[18] There is strong experimental evidence that this fatty acid is rapidly desaturated between the ninth and tenth carbons as counted from the terminal methyl carbon at the "Omega" end of the molecule.[19] The product of this reaction is oleic acid (C 18:6, Ø-9) the most common monounsaturated fatty acid. Oleic acid has no significant effect in changing LDL cholesterol.[20] Saturated animal fats containing stearic acid would be expected to have less impact on LDL levels due to this effect.

In choosing an appropriate target for saturated fat intake the most reliable guide is the morbidity experience of groups with differing habitual consumptions. This was exactly the data Ancel Keys gathered in his "Seven Countries Study."[21] Finnish, Dutch and American communities were consuming approximately 20% of total calories as saturated fat when this study was done thirty years ago. Populations around the Mediterranean, on Crete and Corfu were eating 10% or less of calories from saturated fat and some Japanese fishing villages were consuming even less, 3 to 4% of calories from this source. The coronary heart disease mortality and the serum cholesterol were closely correlated with the saturated fat intake. Further guidance has been provided by a large number of experiments with human volunteers eating controlled diets, both inside institutions[22] and in free living groups in the community. The Diet Heart Feasibility Study done in this country in the 1960s also gave very useful information about changes in serum cholesterol when saturated fat content was altered.[23]

The current goal for the general population is to reduce saturated fats to less than 10% of calories. If this does not achieve a sufficient reduction in LDL cholesterol in the individual patient, the physician is advised to reduce further, to less than 7% of calories. A diet containing 10% of calories from saturated fat is easily achieved with very few changes in eating patterns for Americans. To reduce the intake to below 7% requires more careful planning and is best achieved with professional advice, preferably from a Registered Dietitian:

Dietary Cholesterol

Much controversy about the efficacy of diet has turned about the issue of dietary cholesterol and its specific effects on blood cholesterol. Studies in which additional dietary cholesterol was given to young persons eating a "normal American diet" often show little resulting change in serum cholesterol. Only when you examine the composite results of several studies does the reason become apparent.[24] The serum response is not linear. Most changes are observed as dietary cholesterol is increased from 0 to 200 mg of cholesterol intake per 1000 Kcal. per day. Since the "average American" consumes almost 200 mg per 1000 Kcal/day, it is not surprising that only modest change occurs in studies where additional cholesterol is added to the existing diet. When one removes the cholesterol from the diet and then adds it back in a controlled manner, a very consistent rise of about 12 mg/dl occurs for each 100 mg of dietary cholesterol added per 1000 Kcal.[25] In animal studies, this rise is primarily in the LDL fraction. The magnitude of the increase in serum cholesterol is also affected by the saturated fat content of the diet, the higher the baseline saturated fat intake the greater the rise in response to dietary cholesterol.[26]

Another sobering consideration is that dietary cholesterol has been associated with coronary heart disease mortality in at least three major studies.[27–29] This effect was independent of other risk factors including serum cholesterol levels. These observations and a series of animal experiments have increased the speculation that the cholesterol carrying chylomicrons formed during a fatty meal would be atherogenic before they were cleared by the liver as suggested by Zilversmit.[30]

Vegetarians eat virtually no cholesterol and enjoy considerably lower LDL cholesterol than age matched meat eaters.[31] There seems to be no requirement whatever for dietary cholesterol; the body synthesizes more than it needs each day. In choosing a daily limitation, the major consideration is dietary palatability. Having meat and dairy products in the diet does make reaching certain Recommended Dietary Allowances easier, *e.g.*, Vitamin B-12 and iron. The American Heart Association and after it, the National Cholesterol Education Program have suggested that we limit our intake to less than 300 mg/day. If a more restrictive diet (Step 2 Diet) is needed, the consumption should be less than 200 mg/day. Both are quite easily achieved with moderate changes in eating patterns for most Americans.

One consideration these simple recommendations do not make is that cholesterol intake when measured in free living communities is closely tied to dietary calories. Over 200 milligrams of cholesterol per 1000 calories were consumed by adult men and women across most age groups in the Nationwide Food Consumption Survey of 1977–1978 conducted by the United States Department of Agriculture.[32] Other studies have confirmed this finding. The recommendation of limiting the intake to less than 300 mg/day (Step 1) or 200 mg/day (Step 2) applies to normally active adult males but is an overestimate of the cholesterol needed to achieve the same degree of serum cholesterol reduction in a woman or a small inactive man. The "average American woman" is consuming approximately 300 mg of cholesterol per day at the present time.[33]

Calorie Balance

The prevention of obesity is no simple matter in the great majority of people. The physicians's advice that "if you eat it, you must use it or it accumulates as fat on your body" is one of those simple truths which simply does not address the problem in most patients. Inspiring the patient to eat less and to increase the exercise level is the only long-term course to weight control that is likely to be successful and healthful. However, we must recognize that we do not understand how weight is maintained within a relatively narrow range in most people and we certainly do not understand why others are driven to eat excessively or to remain inactive. Finally, our knowledge about the factors that control where fat is deposited (omental and truncal as opposed to buttocks and extremities) is very limited.

The between-population comparisons and the studies of large groups of individuals within populations have repeatedly confirmed that obesity (particularly abdominal obesity) is strongly related to higher blood cholesterol, higher triglycerides, lower HDL cholesterol, higher blood pressure, higher incidence of diabetes mellitus and increased rates of heart attack and mortality due to heart disease.[34] Unfortunately, virtually no long-term studies have been completed to demonstrate the efficacy of weight reduction on these cardiovascular endpoints.

In considering what can be done to reduce the excess fat storage on American bodies, comparisons to societies where the problem is less frequent usually reveal the major difference to be our reduced caloric expenditure rather than excess consumption.[35] Increasing exercise is therefore the intervention which most clearly mimics successful control occurring spontaneously in other socieites.

Total Fat Intake

Much emphasis has been placed on reduction of total fat intake. The standard recommendation has been to lower dietary fat to less than 30% of calories. Until recently, the recommendation for more effective dietary control was to further reduce the fat intake to 20% of calories. From other quarters have come calls for diets as low as 10% of calories from dietary fat. The argument for severe fat restriction has stemmed from the observation that peoples eating 10 to 20% of calories as fat have very little coronary heart disease.[21] What was forgotten is that they are uniformly eating very little animal fat (saturated fat) and cholesterol. The argument for lower fat is bolstered by the fact that very low fat diets tend to be low in caloric density and quite high in bulky low calorie fruits and vegetables with more fiber and rich in minerals and certain vitamins. Finally, there is no actual biochemical need for fat intake beyond a very few grams of polyunsaturated fats of the omega-6 and probably the omega-3 varieties.

Many questions have not been answered about the true value of restricting all fats. Will persons lose weight and maintain a more desirable adipose tissue mass on a diet containing 10 to 20% of calories as fat when compared to one of 30 to 35%? Does planning a 20% fat diet make eating patterns for reducing saturated fat and cholesterol easier? Is it more likely that the person attempting to reduce total fat will achieve the saturated fat and dietary cholesterol goals? Certainly, many observations have confirmed that the most important issues for blood cholesterol and coronary heart disease are the saturated fat and cholesterol content, not the total fat in the diet. Vegetarians eating 35% of calories as fat have cholesterol levels and LDL levels approaching those of the Tarahumara Indians of central Mexico who eat less than 20% fat.[31,37] In controlled dietary trials, replacing saturated fat with monounsaturated or polyunsaturated fat achieved equal reduction of LDL cholesterol as with carbohydrate replacement.[38] Vegetarians are thinner and have lower blood pressure even though their total fat intake is almost as high as other Americans.

The recommendation to restrict of total dietary fat should be built on a better scientific base than currently exists. Otherwise, we may be limiting the variety of foods in a healthful diet with no true benefit. This is more than an esthetic issue since the pleasure of the diet may play a crucial roll in determining the long-term adherence.

Monounsatured Fats

If one recognizes the importance of controlling calories and limits all fats accordingly, monounsaturates appear relatively benign as a dietary component. They occur abundantly in nuts, olives and meats. Beef contains almost equal amounts of oleic and palmitic acid esters. In fact, when saturated animal fats are restricted, monounsaturates tend to fall commensurately. There seems little reason not to allow those to be replaced in the form of vegetables oils. Diets containing 15 to 20% of calories from monounsaturates seem quite healthful on Crete and Corfu where coronary disease is relatively infrequent.[21]

There has been much recent interest in the observation that HDL cholesterol remains higher when monounsaturated fats replace saturates as opposed to the reduction in HDL values observed when either carbohydrates or omega-6 polyunsaturated fats are used as replacements.[20] However, it should be noted that most studies of lipoprotein levels in populations eating low saturated fats have lower HDL levels and very low incidence of coronary heart disease.[31,37] The highest HDL levels are often seen in countries with high saturated fat intakes and high rates of vascular disease. We simply do not know the implications of an HDL change induced by diet. When omega-6 polyunsaturates are increased by diet HDL might fall because of more rapid transport of cholesterol into the liver for excretion in the bile. On the other hand, monounsaturates might promote the uptake of cholesterol by HDL in peripheral tissues—presumably a very positive effect. Until we understand the benefit of these changes to arteriosclerosis and the related clinical complications, it seems premature to recommend monounsaturates over polyunsaturates, particularly when the LDL reduction is equivalent if either is used to replace saturated fats. The appropriate issue is not one or the other but determining the upper limit of consumption for each at a level with documented safety. Fifteen to twenty percent of calories could be consumed as monounsaturates with reasonable certainty of no ill effects. However, fat restriction to less than thirty percent of calories will require very severe restrictions in saturates or a reduction of polyunsaturates below average intake in America if such high consumption of monounsaturates is desired.

Polyunsaturated Fats

Polyunsaturated fats are those containing fatty acids with two or more double bonds between the carbon atoms. From a dietary standpoint, polyunsaturated fatty acids fall into major groups, classified by whether the first double-bonded carbon atom is at the third or the sixth position from the terminal (omega) methyl group—thus the designation omega-3 or omega-6 fatty acids.

Omega-6 fatty acids are not synthesized in the body but play essential roles in cell structure and prostaglandin synthesis.[39] This need is met if the intake is sufficient to supply 1 to 2% of calories. At the beginning of this century, American dietary intake was only slightly above this requirement but with the rising availability of vegetable oil, the consumption of linoleic acid (the predominant omega-6 fatty acid) has risen from approximately 2% to 7% of total calories.[40]

Over the years there has been considerable debate as to whether this increase in omega-6 fatty acids was beneficial to health and might be expected to help reduce heart disease rates. Total plasma cholesterol falls more when polyunsaturates replace saturated fatty acids than when either monounsaturated fatty acids or carbohydrates are substituted.[41] Diets high in polyunsaturated fats do not cause arteriosclerosis in animal models.[42] In large community-based studies higher polyunsaturated fat intake and higher content of linoleic acid in adipose biopsies have been associated with lower rates of vascular disease.[28] Only a few years ago therapeutic diets were based more on a desirable ratio of the mass of polyunsaturated to saturated fat than on the total content of any particular type of fat. Many persons with hypercholesterolemia were advised to aggressively increase intake of oils rich in linoleic acid to gain greater reduction of blood cholesterol.

More recently the promotion of omega-6 polyunsaturates has been tempered by animal studies showing potentiation of chemical carcinogens producing a variety of tumors in rodent species.[43,44] In one major study by Dayton et al.[22] it appeared that cancers had increased in the human subjects after eight years of a diet containing increased linoleic acid. In other investigations immunologic mechanisms were found to be compromised by in vitro testing.[45] Epidemiologists noted that no large groups were known to have eaten omega-6 polyunsaturated fats in excess of 10% of calories as a habitual diet and therefore we had no long-term experience to be able to judge the consequences of diets using 15% or more as was frequent.

More recently lipoprotein levels have been monitored in various dietary trials and it seems clear that much of the excess cholesterol reduction of polyunsaturates (linoleic acid) versus monounsaturates (oleic acid) resulted from reductions in HDL cholesterol. LDL cholesterol declines about equally when either type of fat is substituted for saturated fats.

Many of the positive attributes of polyunsaturates seemed to fade and considerable caution about their overuse came into vogue. However, further analysis tends to reduce the fear of moderate increases in consumption of oils rich in linoleic acid. The concern about cancer potentiation is mitigated when one recognizes that the increased response to chemical carcinogens by rodents occurred when polyunsaturates were added at only 2 to 5% of the calories, with little or no further increase at higher intake.[44] Furthermore, these rates were compared to very artificial diets containing virtually all fats as saturated fatty acids. This is of questionable relevance to whether one eats 2% or 10% of calories from this source. In the one human trial where total cancer incidence was increased, the numbers were not statistically significant and many of the individuals affected were found not to be adhering to the prescribed diet. Finally, and most reassuring, the North Karelians in Eastern Finland have increased linoleic acid intake as a part of a public health effort to lower their very high rates of heart disease for the past two decades. In this population total cancer rates seem to be declining.[46] During this same period the United States has shown a dramatic fall in cardiovascular mortality with no rise in overall cancer death rates (age adjusted) as polyunsaturated fat intake has increased from 2% to 7% of total calories.[47] The current recommendation is to not exceed 10% of calories from this source. Countries such as Israel and Norway, where consumption is already 9 to 10% of calories, will be important to monitor for any clues to either positive or negative outcomes.

Omega-3 polyunsaturated fats are most probably essential components of the diet, for they are quite selectively concentrated in certain tissues such as the testis, retina and the central nervous system.[48] The daily requirement is not known but is probably quite small since deficiency states are not described in the medical literature. Much attention has been given to the potential benefit of omega-3 fatty acids due to observations that groups eating diets relatively high in marine oils have very low rates of coronary heart disease.[49,50] Further impetus to study these effects has come from the reduced platelet aggregation in patients and animals given oily fish or extracts of their fats.[51] The more recent demonstration of significant triglyceride reduction in hypertriglyceridemic patients with similar treatment has further heightened interest.[52]

Dietary sources of omega-3 fatty acids include green leafy vegetables (linolenic acid, C-18:2, Ø-3) and all marine life which participates in the food chain beginning with the plankton where eicosapentaenoic acid (C-20:5, Ø-3) and docosahexaenoic acid (C-22:6, Ø-3) are synthesized. Certain fish such as salmon and mackerel are particularly rich in these fats.

Recent studies of Western communities in which fish consumption was correlated with significantly less coronary heart disease has added interest to the potential benefits of fish oil consumption. In Zutphen (Netherlands), the Western Electric Study (Illinois, USA) and the Boston Irish Study, fish consumption of only one to two meals a week seemed beneficial.[27-29] However, much of the fish eaten in these studies was from fresh waters. This is not totally consistent with the operative nutrient being the omega-3 fatty acids, since the latter are enriched only in ocean fish. Perhaps other components of fish are protective or alternatively moderate fish eaters also have other healthful habits.

Using fish oil supplements to lower triglycerides has proven effective at doses of 6 to 12 grams per day.[53] The major effect is to reduce hepatic synthesis of triglycerides. This is expensive treatment, but it may be the preferred therapy for certain patients with extremely high triglyceride levels, i.e., over 1000 mg/dl. Unfortunately, carefully controlled trials have found little benefit in attempts to lower LDL or raise HDL cholesterol in patients with hypercholesterolemia.[54] Diabetics have shown worsening of glucose control when treated with fish oils. On the other hand, animal studies indicate some protection from the atherogenic effects of a high cholesterol diet.[5] Whether this might be a result of alterations in platelet function or immune cell function by the omega-3 polyunsaturated fatty acids is not yet clear.

At present the dietary recommendation to consume fish as a natural part of the diet on at least two or three occasions each week is consistent with the long-term studies of human populations. Supplements of several grams of fish oils each day should be considered medical treatment and taken only with the advice of a physician. Many fascinating scientific questions remain regarding the effects of each omega-3 fatty acid on prostaglandin metabolism and the potential impact of this biochemistry on physiology of platelets, immune mechanisms and the function of other cells of the arterial wall. Some relevance to arteriosclerosis or the thrombotic consequences seems highly probable.

Dietary Protein

Americans consume approximately 15% of their calories as protein. This does not appear to differ significantly from other industrialized nations. Much speculation has existed about the potential value of reducing animal protein and increasing vegetable sources. Animal products currently supply about two thirds of our protein intake.[56] The lower blood cholesterol and lower blood pressure in vegetarians have been attributed to lack of animal protein by some. However, it is difficult to separate this from the many other differences between those who eat meat and true vegetarians including lower saturated fat intake, lower body weight, less smoking, etc. Animal studies have suggested that diets exclusively containing protein from animal sources are much more prone to raise blood cholesterol and are atheroslcerosis producing when compared to those containing only vegetable proteins.[57] The experiments demonstrating marked differences have most often used very high protein diets. However, mixing animal and vegetable sources seems to ameliorate these differences over a wide range of relative contributions from the two sources. Thus it is difficult to relate these studies to recommendations for healthful human diets.

With a primary dietary recommendation to lower saturated fat calories, one possible replacement could be additional protein. However, this seems unwise for several reasons. Firstly, the majority of our population is already exceeding the Recommended Dietary Allowance (0.8 g/kg) and additional protein is not likely to be beneficial. Some concern has been expressed about high protein diets as a potentiator of carcinogenesis,[58] osteoporosis[59] and renal disease.[60] In animal studies, certain carcinogens are enhanced by protein intake of 2 to 3 times the usual requirement. High protein intake can accelerate renal calcium loss but the data in humans over the range normally consumed has not yet provided convincing evidence for a causal relationship with bony loss. Both animal and human studies suggest that function in the compromised kidney may deteriorate more rapidly with high protein diets. Much is yet to be learned about this before specific recommendations can be made.

The quality of the protein is best guaranteed by eating a wide variety of foods but at present the amount of dietary protein should be increased.

Dietary Carbohydrate

The contribution by carbohydrate to the Western diet has been declining for most of the twentieth century and is small compared to developing countries. However it remains greater than any other nutrient with approximately 45% of calories consumed by Americans as carbohydrate.[61] Of this almost half (20% of calories) is from simple sugars; sucrose, fructose and other corn syrup sugars. The remainder (approximately 25%) is in the form of complex carbohydrates such as starch which are derived mainly from grains, vegetables and fruits.

In considering the most appropriate replacement of saturated fat, increasing carbohydrate has many appealing features. The low prevalence of vascular disease in societies where high consumption of complex carbohydrates has been evident for centuries is reassuring. The concerns that dietary carbohydrate specifically contributes to the etiology of diabetes mellitus and obesity has been largely dispelled by noting the confounding factors as well as the weakness and inconsistency of the associations in epidemiological studies. Animal studies have also failed to consistently support these concepts. Increasing plant sources of carbohydrates provides dietary enhancement of most micronutrients (vitamins and minerals) and of soluble and insoluble fiber adding to the attractiveness of the recommendation.

One might also consider additional sugars instead of saturated fats. There is little evidence that the sugar content of the diet has a direct impact on cardiovascular disease. Convincing evidence exists only for dental caries being increased by diets high in sucrose in particular.[62] However, these tend to be calories empty of the other nutritional attributes of grains, fruits and vegetables and therefore complex carbohydrates from these sources seem a far better choice.

An increase in our complex carbohydrate calories from an average intake of 25% to 35% or more with a concomitant reduction in saturated fats and simple sugars would be consistent with current dietary recommendations.

Alcohol as a Nutrient

Ethanol is a significant source of calories in many countries. In the United States it is estimated to make up 5% of total calories and 10% of calories when considering only that segment of population which drinks alcoholic beverages.[32] This does not include other calories (sugar, etc.) inherent in the formulation of beer, wine and other alcoholic drinks.

Population-based studies have noted that the coronary heart disease rates are often less in moderate drinkers than in those who do not use alcohol at all.[62] HDL cholesterol (HDL_2 and HDL_3) is well documented to be higher in relation to alcohol consumption.[63] These facts have led some to consider advising moderate alcohol intake as a preventative measure. This seems unwise when one considers the prevalence of alcohol addiction and its social and health consequences. Alcohol has not been shown to prevent vascular disease in animal experiments or in clinical trials in humans. Finally, some aspects of cardiovascular disease are strongly associated with drinking alcohol. High blood pressure and stroke are more frequent in persons who drink more than one ounce of ethanol each day,[64] and myocardiopathy is caused or made worse by this agent in a small but important group. The recommendation to limit all alcohol to less than one ounce daily seems well founded.

Dietary Fiber

Plants contain a large number of polymeric substances, primarily carbohydrate in structure, which are not digestible by the human intestinal enzymes and are therefore not absorbed. They are passed into the large intestine where bacterial enzymes are often able to degrade these substance partially or completely. A distinction has been made between those polymers which dissolve in water, often forming gels (soluble fiber) and those which rapidly settle to the bottom of aqueous mixtures (insoluble fiber). The soluble fibers include pectins, gums, mucilages and some hemicelluloses. Lignin, celluloses and most hemicelluloses are insoluble. Most plants are composed of both types of fiber but the relative amounts vary markedly; wheat bran is rich in insoluble fiber with virtually no soluble fiber whereas the fiber in psyllium seeds is approximately 80% soluble.

Clinical and laboratory methodological problems have made difficult an accurate estimate of fiber content in American diets. Estimates range from 10 to 18 grams per day for average intake in adults.[65] Of this, only 3 to 6 grams are estimated to be soluble fiber.

A variety of studies in animals and humans have found that the soluble fiber lowers LDL cholesterol with no significant effect on other lipoprotein levels. Insoluble fiber has no measurable effect on lipoproteins. Controlled clinical trials with soluble fiber at doses of 10 to 20 grams per day have shown reductions in LDL of 20% or more.[66] The largest effects seem to occur when the diet is not changed. After instituting the dietary recommendations of the American Heart Association and establishing a stable baseline of lipoprotein observations on this diet, LDL cholesterol is usually observed to decline 5 to 10% with 10 grams of soluble fiber divided into two or three doses daily.[67] It is of note that the American Heart Association diet as often instructed would result in an intake of approximately 6 grams of soluble fiber each day. Currently there is insufficient data to recommend the optimum dose of soluble fiber but it is probably less than 20 grams per day.

The mechanism by which soluble fiber lowers plasma cholesterol is not known. We do not know whether less LDL is made and secreted into human plasma or if it is taken up more rapidly by the liver. Some evidence suggests bile acid excretion in the stool is increased but other studies have failed to confirm these findings.[68] Bile appears to become less lithogenic and gall stones are reduced in guinea pigs.[69]

No serious side effects are currently associated with increased intake of soluble fiber. However, some concern has been expressed that a large increase in insoluble fiber may be associated with decreased absorption of minerals, particularly iron and zinc. Most of the experiments in which mineral absorption appeared compromised was done with wheat bran. This effect seems associated with phytates and similar compounds which may bind to iron and zinc in the intestine. However clinical studies with mixtures of fibers suggest this is unlikely to be a health concern at the levels consumed by humans.[70]

SUMMARY

The evidence that limiting dietary saturated fat and cholesterol will lower LDL cholesterol and contribute to the reduction in risk of cardiovascular disease is adequate for sound dietary recommendations to patients and to the public at large. Reduction of intake of all saturated fats to less than 10% of calories is a practical and achievable goal for Western man. Further reduction to less than 7% of calories is possible with a motivated and well instructed patient. The mechanism by which saturated fatty acids, particularly palmitate and laurate raise LDL cholesterol need detailed biochemical and physiologic study.

Dietary cholesterol is unnecessary and clearly contributes to vascular disease in Western man. This vascular effect appears to be only partially explained by its effect on LDL cholesterol. Reduction to less than 300 mg per day for men of average size is achievable. Women and those eating fewer calories should strive for even less.

Monounsaturated fats (oleic acid) can be consumed at levels of 20% of calories without significant concern if total calories are within limits to maintain desirable weight.

Omega-6 polyunsaturated fats do not offer a significant health concern and need not be limited below the current intake of 7% of calories in the United States. Populations eating higher levels should be monitored to determine if such intakes are associated with either improved health or long-term ill effects since this level of intake has not been a long-standing tradition in any known culture.

Omega-3 fatty acids might be increased to 2 or 3% of calories with potential benefit. Eating fish and marine animals is the most clearly documented safe method for achieving this. Larger intakes and particularly the use of fish oil supplements is unproven therapy for vascular disease prevention and needs much further study as a medical treatment for a variety of disorders.

Protein intake is more than adequate in the USA and further increases could have negative effects on the prevalence of renal disease and osteoporosis. Although these issues are of hypothetical interest at the moment, they are worthy of considerable investigation.

Complex carbohydrates consumed as components of vegetables, fruits and grains should be considered proven safe and healthful. Increasing calories from these sources at the expense of saturated fats and simple sugars should prove highly beneficial to Western populations. Fiber from these sources may have beneficial effects on blood cholesterol and intestinal function. Soluble fiber is documented to lower LDL cholesterol but the mechanism of this effect is not established and is worthy of considerable study. At present sufficient information is not available to give a quantitative recommendation for fiber intake.

Alcohol increases HDL cholesterol and has been associated with decreased incidence of coronary heart disease in community studies. However, the negative effects of alcohol use including addiction, stroke and high blood pressure justify the current recommendation to limit intake to less than one ounce per day.

Alterations in the Western diet along the lines currently recommended by a variety of health agencies in many countries could lead to a very large reduction in coronary heart disease without significant increases in other chronic diseases. The current efforts should be devoted to: (1) understanding mechanisms of dietary effects so that these can be enhanced; (2) providing healthful foods in more attractive forms; (3) improving food labeling so that consumers can make healthful choices at the point of purchase; and (4) providing our educational institutions and health professionals with improved teaching tools for their students and patients. Fostering a continuing change toward the dietary goals outlined above will require a consistent effort by all segments of our society including government, food manufacturers, food retailers, restauranteurs, health professionals and the consumer.

REFERENCES

1. NUTRITION COMMITTEE, AMERICAN HEART ASSOCIATION. 1986. Circulation 74: 1465A–1468A.
2. NATIONAL CHOLESTEROL EDUCATION PROGRAM. 1988. Arch. Intern. Med. 148: 36–69.
3. LIPID RESEARCH CLINICS PROGRAM. 1984b. J. Am. Med. Assoc. 251: 365–374.
4. FRICK, M. H., O. ELO, K. HAAPA, et al. 1987. N. Engl. J. Med. 317: 1237–1245.
5. ARNTZENIUS, A. C., D. KROMHOUT, J. D. BARTH et al. 1985. N. Engl. J. Med. 312: 805–811.
6. ASHLEY, F. W., JR & W. B. KANNEL. 1974. J. Chronic Dis. 27: 103–114.
7. LARSON, B., K. SVARDSUDD & L WELIN. 1984. Br. Med. J. 288: 1401–1404.
8. WORLD HEALTH ORGANIZATION. 1978. TECHNICAL REP. SER. 628. WHO. GENEVA. 58 pp.
9. POOLING PROJECT RESEARCH GROUP. 1978. J. Chronic Dis. 31: 201–306.
10. AHRENS, E. H., JR., P. H. BLANKENHORN & T.T. TSALTAS. 1954. Proc. Soc. Exp. Biol. Med. 86: 872–878.
11. GRUNDY, S. M. & G. L. VEGA. 1988. Am. J. Clin. Nutr. 47: 822–824.
12. SHEPHERD, J., C. J. PACKARD, J. R. PATSCH et al. 1978. J. Clin. Invest. 61: 1582–1592.
13. TURNER, J. D., N.-A. LE & W. V. BROWN. 1981. Am. J. Physiol. 241: E57–E63.
14. BROWN, M. S. & J. L. GOLDSTEIN. 1986. Science 232: 34–47.
15. SPADY, D. K. & J. M. DIETSCHY. 1985. Proc. Natl. Acad. Sci. USA 82: 4526–4530.
16. SORIA, L. F., E. H. LUDWIG, H. R. G. CLARKE, et al. 1989. Proc. Natl. Acad. Sci. USA 86: 587–591.
17. GRANDE, F., J. T. ANDERSON & A. KEYS. 1970. Am. J. Clin. Nutr. 23: 1184–1193.
18. BONANOME, A. & S. M. GRUNDY. 1988. N. Engl. J. Med. 318: 1244–1248.
19. KEYS, A. 1970. Circulation (Suppl.) 41:I 1–1211.
20. AMERICAN HEART ASSOCIATION. 1970. Circulation 41: 1–195.

21. DAYTON, S., M. L. PEARCE, S. HASHIMOTO. *et al.* 1969. Circulation **39**: Suppl. II.
22. HAGSTED, D. M., R. B. McGANDY, M. L. MYERS *et al.* 1965. Am. J. Clin. Nutr. **17**:281–295.
23. KEYS, A. 1984. Am. J. Clin. Nutr. **40**: 351–359.
24. MATTSON, F. H., B. A. ERICKSON, & A.M. KLIGMON. 1972. Am. J. Clin. Nutr. **25**: 589–594.
25. SCHONFELD, G., W. PATSCH, L. L. RUDEL *et al.* 1982. J. Clin. Invest. **69**: 1072–1080.
26. KROMHOUT, D. & C. DELEZENNE CULANDER. 1984. Am. J. Epidemiol. **119**: 733–741.
27. SHEKELLE, R. B., A. M. SHRYOCK, O. PAUL *et al.* 1981. N. Engl. J. Med. **304**: 65–70.
28. KUSHI, L. H., R. A. LEW, F. J. STARE *et al.* 1985. N. Engl. J. Med. **312**: 811–818.
29. ZILVERSMIT, D. B. 1979. Circulation **60**: 473–485.
30. BURSLEM, J., G. SCHONFELD & M. A. HOWALD. 1978. Metabolism **27**: 711–719.
31. U.S. DEPARTMENT OF AGRICULTURE. 1984. Report No. I-2. Consumer Nutrition Division, Human Nutrition Information Service. Hyattsville, MD. 439 pp.
32. U.S. DEPARTMENT OF AGRICULTURE. 1985. Report No. 85-1. Nutrition Monitoring Division, Human Nutrition Information Service. Hyattsville, MD. 102 pp.
33. HUBERT, H. B., M. FEINLEIB, P. M. McNAMARA *et al.* 1983. Circulation **67**: 968–977.
34. DEBOER, J. O., A. J. VANES, L. C. ROOVERS *et al.* 1986. Am. J. Clin. Nutr. **44**: 585–595.
35. KEYS, A. 1975. Atherosclerosis. **22**: 149–192.
36. CONNOR, W. E., M. T. CERGUEIVA & R. W. CONNOR. 1978. Am. J. Clin. Nutr. **31**: 1131–1142.
37. GRUNDY, S. M., L. FLORENTIN, D. NIX *et al.* 1988. Am. J. Clin. Nutr. **47**: 965–969.
38. VONSCHACKY, C. 1987. Ann. Intern. Med. **107**: 890–899.
39. U.S. DEPARTMENT OF AGRICULTURE. 1986. Report NO. 85-3. Nutrition Monitoring Division, Human Nutrition Information Service. Hyattsville, MD. 94 pp.
40. KEYS, A., J. T. ANDERSON & F. GRANDE. 1965. Metabolism. **14**: 776–787.
41. MENDELSOHN, D., L. MENDELSOHN & D. G. HAMILTON. 1980. S. Afr. J. Sci. **76**: 225–228.
42. BULL, A. W., J. C. BRONSTEIN & N. D. NIGRO. 1988. Proc. Am. Assoc. Cancer Res. **29**: 149.
43. IP, C., C. A. CARTER & M. M. IP. 1985. Cancer Res. **45**: 1997–2001.
44. ERICKSON, K. L. 1986. Prog. Clin. Biol. Res. **222**: 555–586.
45. REDDY, B. S. & L. A. COHEN. 1986. *In* Macronutrients and Cancer. Vol. 1: 175. CRC Press. Boca Raton, FL.
46. DEVESA, S. S., D. T. SILVERMAN & J. L. YOUNG, JR. 1987. J. Natl. Cancer Inst. **79**:701–770.
47. VONSCHACKY, C., S. FISHER & P. C. WEBER. 1985. J. Clin. Invest. **76**: 1626–1631.
48. KEYS, A., N. KIMURA, B. KUSUKAWA *et al.* 1985. Ann. Intern. Med. **48**: 83–94.
49. LEAF, A. & P. C. WEBER. 1988. N. Engl. J. Med. **318**: 549–557.
50. MARCUS, A. J. 1987. Platelet eicosanoid metabolism. *In* Homostasis and Thrombosis: Basic Principles and Clinical Practice, 2nd edit. R. W. Coleman, J. Hirsch, V. J. Maarden & E. W. Salzman, Eds. 676–688. J.B. Lippincott. Philadelphia, PA.
51. ILLINGWORTH, D. R., W. S. HARRIS & W. E. CONNOR. 1984. Arteriosclerosis **4**: 270–275.
52. NESTEL, P. J., W. E. CONNOR, M. F. REARDON *et al.* 1984. J. Clin. Invest. **74**: 82–89.
53. CONNOR, W. E. 1986. *In* Health Effects of Polyunsaturated Fatty Acids in Seafoods. A. P. Simopoulos, R. R. Kifer & R. E. Martin, Eds. Academic Press. New York, NY.
54. VONSCHACKY, C. 1987. Ann. Intern. Med. **107**: 890–899.
55. MARSTON, R. & N. ROPER. 1987. Natl. Food Rev. **36**: 182.
56. CARROLL, K. K. 1978. Nutr. Rev. **36**: 1–5.
57. NATIONAL RESEARCH COUNCIL. 1982. Report of the Committee on Diet Nutrition and Cancer. Assembly of Life Sciences. National Academy Press. Washington, DC. 478 pp.
58. SHUETTE, S. A. & H. M. LINKSWILER. 1982. J. Nutr. **112**: 338–349.
59. BRENNER, B. M., T. W. MEYER & T. H. HOSTETTER. 1982. N. Engl. J. Med. **307**: 652–659.
60. GLINSMAN, W. H., H. IRAUSQUIN & Y. K. PARK. 1986. J. Nutr. **116**: 51–5216.
61. FRIEDMAN, L. A. & A. W. KIMBALL. 1986. Am. J. Epidemiol. **124**: 481–489.
62. BARRETT-CONNOR, E. & L. SUAREZ. 1982. Am. J. Epidemiol. **115**: 888–893.
63. GILL, J. S., A. V. ZUZULKA, M. J. SHIPLEY *et al.* 1986. N. Engl. J. Med. **315**: 1041–1046.
64. LANZA, E., D. Y. JONES, G. BLOCK *et al.* 1987. Am. J. Clin. Nutr. **46**: 790–797.
65. LIFE SCIENCES RESEARCH OFFICE. 1987. Physiological Effects and Health Consequences of Dietary Fiber. Federation of American Societies for Experimental Biology. Bethesda, MD. 236 pp.

66. BELL, L.P., K. HECTORNE, H. B. REYNOLDS, T. K. BALM & D. HUNNINGHAKE. 1989. J. Am. Med. Assoc. **261:** 3419–3423.
67. STORY, J.A. 1986. In Dietary Fiber: Basic and Clinical Aspects. C. V. Vahouny & D. Kritchevsky, Eds. Plenum Press, Newly.
68. KRITCHEVSKY, D., S. A. TEPPER & D. M. KLUNFELD. 1984. Experientia **40:** 350–351.
69. WALKER, A. 1985. Mineral metabolism. *In* Dietary Fibre, Fibre-Depleted Foods and Disease. H. Trowell, D. Burkitt & K. Heaton, Eds. 361–375. Academic Press. New York, NY.

Clinical Studies on Atherosclerosis in Diabetics

YOSHIO GOTO, KEN-ICHI YAMADA, TAKESHI OHYAMA,
AND KEI SATO

*Department of Medicine
and
Department of Neurology
Tohoku Kousei-Nenkin Hospital
Miyaginoku, Sendai 983, Japan*

INTRODUCTION

Diabetes is a risk factor of atherosclerosis, and vascular complications, especially ischemic heart disease are the first ranking cause of death among diabetics in the United States and some European countries. In Japan, myocardial infarction was very rare even in diabetics until 1960, as reported by Rudnick and Anderson who stayed in Hiroshima and published an article on the complications of diabetes in Japan. Since 1960, the prevalence of diabetes in Japan has been increasing year by year, and the average fasting blood glucose of the Japanese population over 40 years old has been increasing by 0.3–0.8 mg/dl every year. These facts indicate that Japanese people have been exposed to diabetogenic environmental factors. The nutrient intake has changed from the traditional high-carbohydrate, low-fat diet to the relatively high-fat Western diet, although the total energy intake has remained steady. The average body mass index (BMI) of Japanese people over 40 years old has been increasing during the last 30 years and is thought to be due to less physical activity of the people. The increase in BMI and the increase in the elderly population may be the main reasons for the increase in the diabetic population.

FREQUENCY OF ATHEROSCLEROTIC FINDINGS IN DIABETICS

Macroangiopathy in Diabetic Autopsy Cases

The Japanese Society of Pathology has published the Annual Report of Pathological Autopsy Cases since 1958. The cases recorded in the Annual Report were registered from more than two hundred hospitals all over the country. We have collected the cases of diabetes mellitus from the reports of 1958–1985. The chronological change in frequency of arteriosclerotic diseases in diabetic autopsy cases is shown in TABLE 1. The figures of the nondiabetic cases are shown in the last column. The freqencies of the diseases are higher in diabetics than nondiabetics; myocardial infarction has been increasing over the last 30 years, though cerebral infarction and hemorrhage have not.

Calcification of the Arterial Wall

There are several clinical methods of quantitative assessment of atherosclerosis. Measurement of the calcified area of the aorta on X-ray CT film is a simple and reliable one. We measured the calcified area of the abdominal aorta in each CT slice and gave points

TABLE 1. Chronological Change in Frequency of Cardiovascular Disease in 60–69-Year-Old Diabetic Autopsy Cases (%)

Autopsy Finding		Diabetic						Nondiabetic
Autopsy Finding	Year (No)	1958–65 (288)	66–70 (724)	71–75 (927)	76–80 (1190)	81–82 (582)	83–85 (1134)	1978 (7011)
Myocardial infarction		13.2	15.2	18.1	22.2	25.6	26.6	4.1
Cerebral infarction		15.3	17.1	15.9	14.5	14.8	11.6	3.2
Cerebral hemorrhage		2.1	5.4	6.9	7.7	6.2	4.6	4.2

as follows: if the calcified area was one quarter, then one point was given, if two quarters, two points, if three quarter, three points, and if all of the aortic wall was calcified, four points. The calcification index was calculated as the mean of the slices. The calcification index of the abdominal aorta was significantly higher in patients treated with oral hypoglycemic agents than those treated with insulin or diet alone. By classification of the duration of diabetes, the calcification index was higher in patients with more than 10 years than in those with 10 years or less. When they were compared by serum total cholesterol and triglyceride levels, however, there was no significant difference between the cases of hyperlipidemic and normolipedemic cases. In this study, serum lipids were the means of the values obtained at every clinical visit. The index was higher in hypertensive cases than normotensive cases, and higher in patients with proteinuria. However, there was no significant difference between the patients with and without retinopathy or neuropathy.

Pulse Wave Conduction Velocity

Measurement of pulse wave conduction velocity (PWV) of the aorta is a simple noninvasive method to assess sclerosis of the aorta. It was demonstrated clearly that there was a very close correlation between the pulse wave conduction velocity and sclerotic change of the aorta at autopsy. There was no significant difference in PWV between 30–39-year-old diabetics and 30–39-year-old healthy subjects. However, the difference between the two groups was significant after the age of 40. In other words, the aorta of diabetic patients gets older by 10 years or more than healthy subjects after the age of 40. PWV was significantly faster in hypertensive diabetics than normotensive diabetics, but it was not significantly different between diabetics with and without calcification of tibial arteries. It was not significantly different among the groups classified by diabetes-treatment methods, duration of diabetes, or condition of glycemic control. PWV was significantly greater in the cases of diabetic proliferative retinopathy and in those of persistent proteinuria compared with the cases without retinopathy or without proteinuria. These results suggest that sclerosis of the aorta may progress in parallel with diabetic microangiopathy.

Carotid Artery Blood Flow and Circulatory Resistance

Volume and velocity of carotid arterial blood flow and presence of plaque formation and calcification of the arteries were measured and observed by doppler imaging technique and B-mode real time ultrasound using ultrasonographic equipment (SSD-980, Aloka Co., Tokyo) in diabetic and nondiabetic patients. The blood flow volume was significantly reduced and circulatory resistance was significantly greater in diabetic patients than in nondiabetic patients (TABLE 2). Elasticity of the carotid arterial wall was reduced in diabetics, and calcification and plaque formation were not infrequently observed in diabetics.

COMMENTS: ATHEROGENETIC FACTORS IN DIABETICS

Hyperlipidemia is common in diabetic patients. Mean cholesterol was 215 ± 43 mg/dl (mean $\pm$ SD, n = 294) and triglyceride was 138 ± 121 mg/dl. These figures are very low when compared with those of diabetics in the United States and European countries. This may be one of the reasons for the lower frequency of ischemic heart disease among Japanese diabetics. The serum lipids decreased significantly after 5 years of diabetic treatment. The most frequent phenotype of lipidemia was type IIa of the World Health Organization (WHO) classification (14%) and type IV (12%), then followed by type IIb (10%) and V (0.3%) in 323 diabetics with diabetes treatment history of more than five years.

Why is diabetes a risk factor of atherosclerosis? It was demonstrated that low density lipoprotein (LDL) is glucosylated in the hyperglycemic condition. Goto and co-workers confirmed that the LDL and HDL of diabetic patients was glucosylated more than those of nondiabetic patients, and that the LDL of diabetic patients was more negatively charged than that of nondiabetics when electrophoretic mobility was estimated by the Laser Zee System 3000 (Pen Ken, Inc., New York). They also found that glucosylated LDL stimulated DNA synthesis of the cultured human arterial smooth muscle cells, and noted a significantly higher sorbital content of the erythrocytes in the diabetics with aortic sclerosis estimated by PWV measurement than those without aortic sclerosis. This suggests a possible role of the polyol pathway for the development of atherosclerosis in diabetics. A decrease in prostacyclin production from alloxan diabetic rabbit aorta was also confirmed. This impaired prostacyclin production may accelerate atherosclerosis in diabetics. Platelet sensitivity to ADP and prostacyclin *in vitro* was measured in connection with pulse wave velocity. Diabetic patients with hypersensitivity to ADP showed greater frequency of abnormal PWV values and those with hyposensitivity to prostacyclin also showed greater frequency of PWV abnormality than those with normal sensitivity of platelets. This result suggests that abnormal platelet function is closely related to the development of atherosclerosis. They also confirmed a higher plasma content of von Willebrand factor in diabetics with increased PWV than those with normal PWV.

CONCLUSION

Our studies on diabetics showed a high prevalence of atherosclerotic changes estimated by fluorscopic and functional examinations. The reasons for this high prevalence

TABLE 2. Carotid Blood Flow Volume and Circulatory Resistance in Diabetics and Nondiabetics

Age	Blood Flow Volume (ml/sec)			Circulatory Resistance (mmHg/ml/sec)		
	Nondiabetic	Diabetic	p	Nondiabetic	Diabetic	p
<50	10.02 ± 1.04 (8)*	8.23 ± 2.60 (5)	<0.01	9.36 ± 0.59 (8)	13.74 ± 2.48 (5)	<0.01
50–59	8.88 ± 1.37 (13)	7.00 ± 2.17 (13)	<0.01	12.26 ± 2.59 (13)	16.61 ± 7.00 (13)	<0.01
60–69	6.37 ± 1.49 (13)	6.39 ± 2.03 (10)	ns	17.74 ± 4.78 (13)	19.73 ± 2.48 (10)	ns
≥70	6.28 ± 1.87 (8)	5.96 ± 1.28 (8)	ns	20.14 ± 6.78 (8)	19.86 ± 5.23 (8)	ns

*M $\pm$ S D (no).

TABLE 3. Factors Accelerating Atherosclerosis in Diabetics

1. Hypertension
2. Hyperlipidemia
3. Obesity
4. Hyperinsulinemia
5. Hyperaggregability of platelets
6. Decrease in PGI_2 production in arterial wall
7. Increase in von Willebrand factor release from vessel wall
8. Glycation of arterial tissue protein and LDL
9. Activation of polyol pathway in arterial wall
10. Diabetic autonomic neuropathy

of atherosclerosis in diabetic patients may be as follows (TABLE 3). Hypertension is common among diabetic patients because of their hyperinsulinemic state and hypersensitive state to norepinephrine and angiotensin II. Hyperlipdemia is also common and many epidemiological studies suggest that an increase in triglyceride is more closely associated with diabetic macroangiopathy than cholesterol, although the mechanism is as yet unknown. Obesity is common among diabetics. Hyperinsulinemia is usually observed among obese diabetic patients. Abnormality of platelet function is frequently observed among diabetics and this abnormality does not become normal by glycemic control. Decrease in prostacyclin production and increase in von Willebrand factor release from the vessel wall may also be a cause of the high prevalence of atherosclerosis in diabetics. Glycation of vessel wall tissue protein and lipoproteins, and activation of the polyol pathway may be a cause of atherosclerosis, and if so, glycemic control may be important for the prevention of atherosclerosis in diabetics. Autonomic neuropathy, which may cause abnormalities in the metabolism of the arterial wall, may also be a cause of atherosclerosis. Integration of these factors will accelerate atherosclerosis in diabetic patients and, conversely, control of these factors may be essential for the prevention of atherosclerosis in diabetic patients.

REFERENCES

1. RUDNICK, P. A. & P. S. ANDERSON. 1962. Diabetes mellitus in Hiroshima, Japan. Diabetes **11:** 533–543.
2. OIKAWA, S, R. ABE, & Y. GOTO. 1982. Calcification of leg arteries in diabetics. J. Jpn. Atheroscler. Soc. **9:** 1035–1039.
3. GOTO, Y. 1986. Diabetes and atherosclerosis. J. Jpn. Atheroscler. Soc. **14:** 247–258.
4. GOTO, Y., R. ABE, S. OIKAWA, R. SANO & Y FUJII. 1985. Serum lipids in diabetic patients. J. Jpn. Atheroscler. Soc. **12:** 1351–1357.

Mutations in the Low Density Lipoprotein Receptor Gene in Japanese Patients with Familial Hypercholesterolemia

HIROSHI MABUCHI, KOUJI KAJINAMI, HAJIME FUJITA,
JUNJI KOIZUMI, AND RYOYU TAKEDA

Second Department of Internal Medicine
Kanazawa University School of Medicine
Kanazawa 920, Japan

Familial hypercholesterolemia (FH) is a common autosomal dominant disorder produced by mutations in the LDL receptor gene.[1] The chromosomal location of the human LDL receptor gene was shown to be in the short arm of chromosome 19. The normal LDL receptor gene is about 45.5 kb, and includes 18 exons and 17 introns.[2,3] More than 35 mutants of the LDL receptor gene have been reported.[4] The locations of these mutations are shown above the schema of the gene in FIGURE 1. We have found four new variants of the LDL receptor gene: FH-Tonami-1,[5] FH-Tonami-2,[6] FH-Kanazawa,[7] and FH-Okayama,[7] through analysis with Southern blotting of DNA samples from the members of 200 unrelated Japanese families.

FH-Tonami-1[5]

A typical family with FH-Tonami-1 is shown in FIGURE 2.[5] DNA samples were digested with Bam HI, and hybridized by labeled pLDLR-2HHI. Subjects with 16.0 kb band only showed normocholesterolemia. Thus, hypercholesterolemia and the 10.0-kb abnormal fragment completely cosegregated in all studied members.[5]

The location of this 6-kb deletion was between the Kpn I site in intron 14 and the Xba I site in intron 15. As mRNA splicing intron 14 to exon 15 should not change the reading frame, this mutant gene product might delete the O-linked sugar domain (FIG. 3).

We studied the biosynthesis of this mutant LDL receptor protein. The cultured skin fibroblasts from a heterozygote were pulse-labeled with ^{35}S-methionine following precipitation with IgG-C7 and SDS-PAGE. In this heterozygote of FH-Tonami-1, normal LDL receptor protein precursors of 120 KDal are processed to their mature form of 160 KDal. However, the mutant precursor of about 100 KDal disappeared rapidly after chase without processing to mature forms.[8] Thus, the O-linked sugar domain is thought to be a critical portion for processing of the LDL receptor protein.

FH-Tonami-2[6]

The normal LDL receptor gene shows one hybridized fragment of about 26 kb after Eco RV digestion. Case H.Y. showed a single 16-kb fragment, while patient K.H. showed two fragments; one was 26 kb and the other 16 kb. By digestion with several other

393

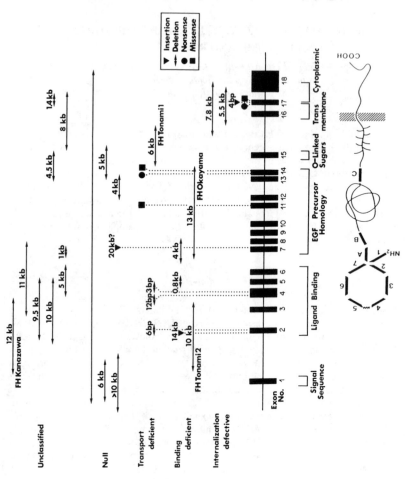

FIGURE 1. Location of familial hypercholesterolemia mutations in the low density lipoprotein (LDL) receptor gene. Biochemical classes of mutations are shown on the *left side*.[4]

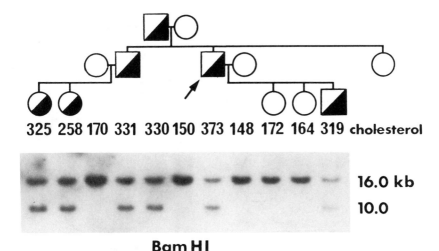

325 258 170 331 330 150 373 148 172 164 319 **cholesterol**

16.0 kb
10.0

Bam HI

FIGURE 2. Analysis of the LDL receptor gene in a family of FH-Tonami-1 (K.Y.). In all patients with heterozygous FH (◨,◑), the abnormal fragments (10.0 kb) are found after digestion by BamHI. Non-FH members do not show this abnormal fragment.[6]

restriction enzymes, this mutant gene has been proved to have approximately a 10-kb deletion which eliminated exons 2 and 3. By the intensity of the hybridyzed fragments, H.Y. was considered to be a "true homozygote" and K.H. a heterozygote with this mutant gene. The deletion in this mutant gene eliminated exons 2 and 3, and mRNA splicing of exons 1 to 4 should not change the reading frame. Thus, the first two repeats of the ligand binding domain are thought to be deleted (FIG. 3).

To characterize the biosynthesis of this mutant receptor, the cultured skin fibroblasts were pulse-labeled with ^{35}S-methionine following precipitation with IgG-C7 and SDS-PAGE. No cross reactive material could be detected on the lane of H.Y. As IgG-C7 recognizes the first repeat of the ligand binding domain, this mutant cannot be detected by this receptor protein antibody. This mutant LDL receptor activity of the true homozygote (H.Y.) was approximately 40% of normal internalization and degradation. And in the heterozygotes, the receptor activity was about 70%. In Scatchard analysis, this mutant receptor affinity for LDL particles was lower and its number was relatively higher than normal values.[8]

Clinical characteristics of patients with FH-Tonami-2 are unique. All 4 true homozygotes were born to consanguineous parents. Their serum cholesterol levels (587 ± 38 mg/dl) were lower than those of Japanese classical homozygotes. All these homozygotes are presently still alive at ages 62, 51, 48, and 33 years.

Previously we reported case H.Y. under the title of "Normalization of LDL levels and disappearance of xanthomas during pregnancy in a woman with heterozygous familial hypercholesterolemia".[9] At that time we thought this to be a case of heterozygote, because the LDL receptor activity of her cultured skin fibroblasts showed 40% of normal, and her father's cholesterol level was normal, 168 mg/dl. However, by LDL receptor gene analysis she has been proved to be a true homozygote, and her father an obligate heterozygote. She showed dramatic reductions of LDL-cholesterol during her two pregnancies, and also by estradiol she showed a definite reduction of LDL-cholesterol levels. At the same time her skin xanthomas almost disappeared during pregnancy. Also in WHHL

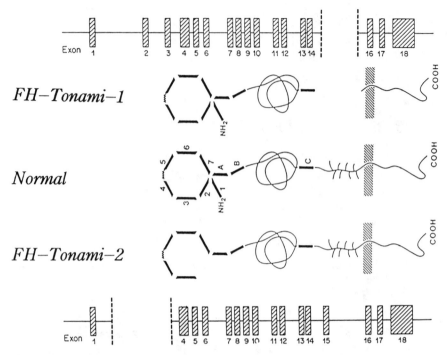

FIGURE 3. Deletions of LDL receptor gene and their corresponding mutant LDL receptor proteins. The 6-kb deletion in the LDL receptor gene of FH-Tonami-1 eliminates exon 15. This mutant gene might delete the O-linked sugar domain of the LDL receptor protein. The 10-kb deletion in the LDL receptor gene of FH-Tonami-2 eliminates exons 2 and 3, and might delete the first two repeats of the ligand binding domain of the LDL receptor protein.

rabbits, similar reductions of serum cholesterol levels were observed during pregnancies.[10] Thus, estrogens induce the biosynthesis of LDL receptor protein in this mutant gene as well as in normal genes.

In summary, in FH-Tonami-1 the LDL receptor precursor protein cannot be processed into mature form. However, in FH-Tonami-2, the partially abnormal receptor can be synthesized and processed, and FH-Tonami-2, caused by a partially impaired LDL receptor with small deletion in its ligand binding domain, produces a mild type of FH.

REFERENCES

1. GOLDSTEIN, J. L. & M. S. BROWN. 1989. Familial hypercholesterolemia. *In* The Metabolic Basis of Inherited Disease. C. R. Scriver, A. L. Beaudet, W. S. Sly & D. Valle. Eds. 6th edit. 1215–1250. McGraw-Hill Company. New York, NY.
2. YAMAMOTO, T., C. G. DAVIS, M. S. BROWN, M. L. CASEY, J. L. GOLDSTEIN & D. W. RUSSELL. 1984. The human LDL receptor: A cysteine-rich protein with multiple Alu sequences in its mRNA. Cell **39:** 27–38.
3. SÜDHOF, T. C., J. L. GOLDSTEIN, M. S. BROWN, & D. W. RUSSELL. 1985. The LDL receptor gene: A mosaic of exon shared with different proteins. Science **228:** 815–822.
4. RUSSELL, D. W., V. ESSER & H. H. HOBBS. 1989. Molecular basis of familial hypercholesterolemia. Arteriosclerosis 9(Suppl. I):I-8–I-13.

5. KAJINAMI, K., H. MABUCHI, H. ITOH, I. MICHISHITA, M. TAKEDA, T. WAKASUGI, J. KOI-
   ZUMI & R. TAKEDA. 1988. New variant of low density lipoprotein receptor gene. FH-Tonami.
   Arteriosclerosis **8:** 187–192.
6. KAJINAMI, K., H. FUJITA, J. KOIZUMI, H. MABUCHI, R. TAKEDA & M. OHTA. 1989. Genetically determined mild type of familial hypercholesterolemia including normocholesterolemic patients: FH-Tonami-2. Circulation **80:** II-278.
7. KAJINAMI, K., H. MABUCHI, A. INAZU, H. FUJITA, J. KOIZUMI, R. TAKEDA, T. MATSUE &
   M. KIBATA. Novel gene mutations at the low density lipoprotein receptor locus: FH-
   Kanazawa and FH-Okayama. J. Intern. Med. In press.
8. FUJITA, H. Manuscript in preparation.
9. MABUCHI, H., Y. SAKAI, A. WATANABE, T. HABA, J. KOIZUMI & R. TAKEDA. 1985. Normalization of low-density lipoprotein levels and disappearance of xanthomas during pregnancy in a woman with heterozygous familial hypercholesterolemia. Metabolism **34:** 309–
   315.
10. SHIOMI, M., T. ITO & Y. WATANABE. 1987. Increase in hepatic low-density lipoprotein
   receptor activity during pregnancy in Watanabe heritable hyperlipidemic rabbits; an animal
   model for familial hypercholesterolemia. Biochim. Biophys. Acta **917:** 92–100.

Lessons in Prevention of Atherosclerosis Learned from Recent Studies of Japanese Youth

KENZO TANAKA

Department of Pathology
Faculty of Medicine
Kyushu University
3-1-1, Maidashi, Higashi-ku
Fukuoka 812, Japan

Atherosclerotic disease is one of the most significant causes of death in many countries. It is important to learn the natural history of atherosclerosis, particularly its geographico-pathological differences in different areas of the world, and to study its etiology and how to prevent it.

In this report, the incidence of myocardial infarction in consecutive autopsy cases from 1940 to 1987 at Kyushu University, as an example demonstrating a recent trend of the ischemic heart disease in Japan[1-5] and the recent status of the extent and severity of atherosclerosis and its risk factors in Japanese youth[5-8] are presented.

In addition, the role of fibrinogen-fibrin metabolism in the arterial wall in atherogenesis[9-12] is reported.

Incidence of Myocardial Infarction in Autopsy Cases in Japan

The incidence of myocardial infarction, pulmonary thromboembolism, and thrombosis in consecutive autopsy cases over 40 years old at Kyushu University during the period between 1940 and 1987 is shown in FIGURE 1.[1-3,5]

The incidence of myocardial infarction has been increasing during the last 48 years, and was 12.2% among the 539 autopsy cases over 40 years old during the recent three years, 1985 to 1987. The incidence of thromboembolism at any site has been increasing and was 38.1% in the autopsy cases from 1985 to 1987.

Total calories uptake shows no significant changes in this observation period, but fat intake is 16 g in 1946, 27.8 g in 1961, and 56.8 g in 1985, showing about a twofold increase in the last 25 years.

TABLE 1 shows the incidence of myocardial infarction and thromboembolism in the autopsy cases at Kyushu University during the periods 1951–1956, 1961–1963, and 1985–1987.[3-5] There is an increase in the incidence of myocardial infarction from 3.4% to 12.2%.

The incidence of myocardial infarction in autopsy cases over 40 years old in Boston, USA during the period 1959–1962 is shown in TABLE 1.[1,2,4] There was a marked difference, namely, a 10-fold difference, in the incidence of myocardial infarction in these two nations during the same period, as shown in TABLE 1.

It is interesting that the incidence of myocardial infarction in the Japanese autopsy cases has increased recently, but its incidence in 1985–1987 is still almost half of that in the American autopsy cases in 1960–1962.

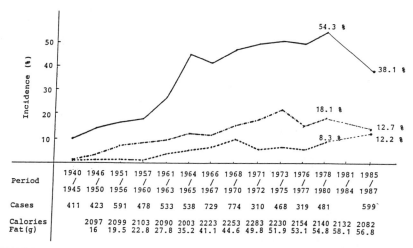

FIGURE 1. Incidence of thrombosis, pulmonary thromboembolism, and myocardial infarction: autopsy cases over 40 years old at Kyushu University, 1940–1987. *Solid line,* thromboembolism at any site; *dashed and dotted line,* pulmonary thromboembolism; *dashed line,* myocardial infarction. (From Tanaka.[5] Reprinted by permission from the *Journal of the Japanese Atherosclerosis Society.)*

Extent and Severity of Atherosclerosis and Its Risk Factors in Japanese Youth

Atherosclerotic changes begin to develop in childhood. It was recently proposed that primary prevention of atherosclerosis should be initiated in pediatric age groups. A nationwide cooperative study of atherosclerosis in Japanese infants, children, and young adults was carried out, the objective being to observe the history of atherosclerosis and its risk factors during the first 39 years of life in the present day Japanese population.[8]

Pathologists of 8 major laboratories in Japan collected 2320 aortas, 1620 coronary arteries, and 344 cerebral arteries from 2856 autopsied patients who ranged in age from

TABLE 1. Incidence of Myocardial Infarction and Thromboembolism in Autopsy Cases in Fukuoka and Boston[a]

	Fukuoka 1951–56	Fukuoka 1961–63	Boston 1959–62	Fukuoka 1985–87
No. of Cases	591	533	600	599
	%	%	%	%
Thromboembolism, any site, gross & micro	16.4	27.2	47.6	38.1
Myocardial infarction				
Fresh	0.5	0.4	11.8	6.0
Old	2.9	2.1	12.8	6.2
Total	3.4	2.4	24.6	12.2
Pulmonary embolism (or infarction)	1.5	3.4	23.8	12.7
Venous thrombi	3.9	4.7	3.0	15.0

[a]From Tanaka.[5] Reprinted by permission from the *Journal of the Japanese Atherosclerosis Society.*

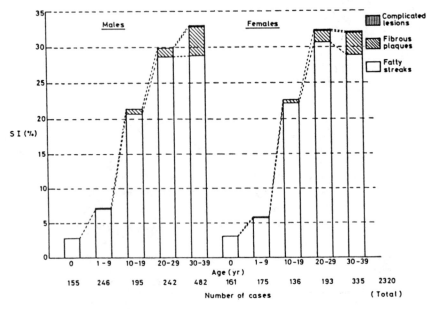

FIGURE 2. Mean of surface involvement of various types of atherosclerotic lesions in aortas. (From Tanaka *et al.*[8] Reprinted by permission from *Atherosclerosis.*)

1 month to 39 years. All autopsies were performed between January 1978 and December 1982.

As the causes of death of the examined autopsy cases, malignancy including leukemia and lymphoma accounted for 46% of the total.

The collected arteries were opened longitudinally and fixed in 10% formalin, and the adventitial adipose tissue was removed. The intimal surface was stained with Sudan IV and the grade of atherosclerosis determined.

Quantitative assessment of the atherosclerotic lesions of the arteries was performed by the point counting method. A transparent plastic sheet with dots at 5-mm intervals was applied to the aorta, and those at 3-mm intervals to the coronary and cerebral arteries.

They evaluated each point of the arteries indicated by a dot on the plastic sheet, as having no atherosclerotic lesions (N) or three different types of atherosclerotic lesions: fatty streaks (F), fibrous plaques (P), and complicated lesions (C) including ulceration, mural thrombus, and calcification.

Several scores such as surface involvement (SI) and atherosclerotic index (AI) were calculated as below, and utilized as indexes of extent and severity of atherosclerosis of each artery.

$$Surface\ involvement\ SI\ =\ \frac{F+P+C}{N+F+P+C}\ \times 100$$

$$Atherosclerotic\ index\ AI\ =\ \frac{F+P\ \times\ 10+C\ \times\ 100}{N+F+P+C}$$

The mean values of SI in males, as shown in FIGURE 2, were lower in the 3rd decade than those in females, but higher in the 4th decade than those in females. However, differences were not statistically significant.

Fatty streaks predominated and occupied most of the lesions in those under 1 year of age, and approximately 90% of the lesions in the 4th decade in both sexes, and it increased with age, compared to the preceding decade except for that in the 4th decade. In the 4th decade, fibrous plaques rather than fatty streak showed a rapid increase. Complicated lesions showed an increase with age, but the extent was slight compared with other lesions.

Means of the surface involvement of three different types of the lesions of coronary arteries with sex and age are shown in FIGURE 3. The mean of SI in the 4th decade was higher in males than in females because SI in males showed a rapid increase from the 3rd decade to the 4th decade. Fatty streaks were predominant as was also noted in the aortas. However, fibrous plaques and complicated lesions occupied 28% of the lesions in the 4th decade in males, that is larger proportion than observed in the aortas.

Likewise, SI of each type of atherosclerotic lesion in the cerebral arteries increased with age, as shown in FIGURE 4. However, the atherosclerotic changes were found in only a small percentage of patients and were markedly less extensive compared with findings in the aortas and coronary arteries. SI in the 4th decade was significantly higher in males than in females.

In contrast to aortas and coronary arteries, fibrous plaques predominated over fatty streaks in the cerebral arteries.

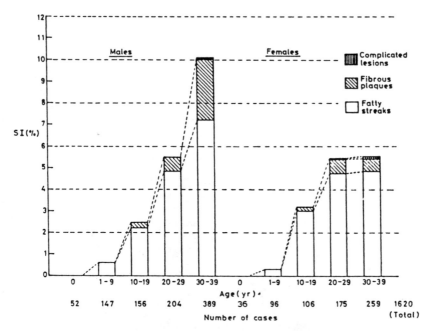

FIGURE 3. Mean of surface involvement of various types of atherosclerotic lesions in coronary arteries. (From Tanaka et al.[8] Reprinted by permission from *Atherosclerosis.*)

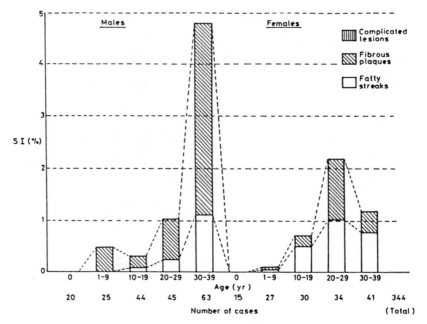

FIGURE 4. Mean of surface involvement of various types of atherosclerotic lesions in cerebral arteries. (From Tanaka *et al.*[8] Reprinted by permission from *Atherosclerosis.*)

Simple correlation coefficients between various scores of atherosclerosis and the risk factors are summarized in TABLE 2. Age, systolic and diastolic blood pressure, and serum cholesterol significantly correlated with each value of SI of aorta, coronary arteries, and cerebral arteries.

On the other hand, triglyceride, uric acid, and platelet counts showed no significant correlation.

From the viewpoint of the difference of the arteries, serum cholesterol was more

TABLE 2. Simple Correlation Coefficients between Selected Measures of Risk Factors and Indexes of Atherosclerosis of Various Arteries[a]

Aorta				Coronary Arteries				Cerebral Arteries			
SI		AI		SI		AI		SI		AI	
AGE	0.58412*	AGE	0.28733*	AGE	0.31050*	CHOL	0.21279*	SBP	0.53595*	SBP	0.56569*
SBP	0.27518*	SBP	0.21450*	SBP	0.21227*	SBP	0.18559*	DBP	0.44034*	DBP	0.43410*
DBP	0.22662*	DBP	0.17905*	CHOL	0.18854*	DBP	0.14414*	AGE	0.21307*	CHOL	0.21850*
CHOL	0.19221*	CHOL	0.11273*	DBP	0.18328*	TRIG	0.12787	CHOL	0.20588*	AGE	0.18673*
TRIG	0.02236	UA	0.02564	TRIG	0.07564	AGE	0.11771*	UA	0.17353	UA	0.12187
UA	0.01089	TRIG	0.00084	UA	0.05192	UA	0.05436*	TRIG	0.09832	TRIG	0.10819
PLT	−0.05407	PLT	−0.01128	PLT	0.02909	PLT	0.02560	PLT	0.00715	PLT	0.02242

[a]Abbreviations: SBP, systolic blood pressure (mm Hg): DBP, diastolic blood pressure (mm Hg); CHOL, serum cholesterol (mg/dl); TRIG, triglyceride (mg/dl); UA, uric acid (mg/dl); PLT, platelet count (per mm³). (From Tanaka *et al.*[8] Reprinted by permission from *Atherosclerosis.*)
    *Significant correlation ($p < 0.05$).

highly correlated with SI and AI of the coronary arteries, and systolic and diastolic blood pressure was more highly correlated with that of the cerebral arteries.

Multivariate analysis was employed to estimate the relative importance of one factor after taking the effect of other related factors into account, because there was a correlation among the antemortem data. The results of the analysis are summarized in TABLE 3.

Atherosclerosis of the aorta significantly correlated with age, mean blood pressure, and serum cholesterol. Age was the strongest factor for both SI and AI. Serum cholesterol rather than mean blood pressure was the stronger factor in SI, and vice versa in AI. This result was explained by the observations that serum cholesterol was a stronger factor for progression of fatty streaks (surface involvement by fatty streak, SIF) and that mean blood pressure was a stronger factor for progression of fibrous plaques (surface involvement by

TABLE 3. Specified Risk Factors Contributing to Variability of Atherosclerosis: Stepwise Multiple Regression Analysis[a]

SIF		SIP		SIC		SI		AI	
Aorta									
AGE	14.16*	AGE	6.43*	AGE	0.47	AGE	19.01*	AGE	4.08*
CHOL	2.08*	MBP	2.50*	MBP	0.26	CHOL	3.23*	MBP	1.25*
MBP	0.14	CHOL	1.25*	SEX	0.15	MBP	0.68*	CHOL	0.81*
SEX	0.00	SEX	0.03	CHOL	0.10	SEX	0.01	SEX	0.13
Sum of $r^2 \times 100 =$	16.18		10.21		0.99		22.93		6.27
Coronary arteries									
AGE	4.14*	MBP	1.88*	CHOL	4.78*	AGE	5.27*	CHOL	5.30*
CHOL	0.89*	AGE	1.08*	MBP	0.89*	CHOL	2.66*	MBP	1.43*
SEX	0.89	CHOL	1.00*	SEX	0.15	SEX	1.24*	AGE	0.08*
MBP	0.21	SEX	0.64	AGE	0.00	MBP	0.94*	SEX	0.01
Sum of $r^2 \times 100 =$	6.13		4.60		5.82		10.11		6.82
Cerebral arteries									
MBP	11.76*	MBP	13.94*	AGE	0.00	MBP	16.66*	MBP	14.63*
CHOL	0.60	AGE	0.57	SEX	0.00	AGE	0.64	AGE	0.59
AGE	0.41	SEX	0.36	MBP	0.00	SEX	0.11	SEX	0.32
SEX	0.02	CHOL	0.09	CHOL	0.00	CHOL	0.03	CHOL	0.05
Sum of $r^2 \times 100 =$	12.79		14.96		0.00		17.44		15.59

[a]r^2 = coefficient of determination. Each numeric value indicates the percent of variation accounted for $r^2 \times 100$. Abbreviations: MBP: mean blood pressure (mm HG); CHOL: serum cholesterol (mg/dl). (From Tanka et al.[8] Reprinted by permission from *Atherosclerosis*.)
*Significant correlation ($p < 0.05$).

fibrous plaque, SIP) because AI values are much more influenced by the extent of fibrous plaques.

In coronary arteries, age, serum cholesterol, and mean blood pressure were significant factors for SI and AI. Sex was also a significant factor for SI, and this can possibly be ascribed to the finding that SI in the 4th decade was significantly higher in males than in females. Surface involvement by fatty streak (SIF) was more highly affected by serum cholesterol than by mean blood pressure, and vice versa for surface involvement by fibrous plaque (SIP). A similar result was noted in the aortas.

In cerebral arteries, mean blood pressure was the only significant factor for SI and AI of cerebral arteries. In comparison to the findings in the aortas and coronary arteries, the most characteristic feature of the cerebral arteries was a strong link to mean blood pressure.

The present study confirms that susceptibility to risk factors varies with the sites of arteries in early lesions of atherosclerosis observed in the young subjects.[6-8]

It was also clarified that the extent of fatty streaks was strongly dependent on serum cholesterol levels and that the extent of fibrous plaques was also strongly dependent on blood pressure levels.[6-8]

The Role of Fibrin in Atherosclerosis

Proliferation of smooth muscle cells is the key process in the development and progression of atherosclerosis. Several factors such as platelet derived growth factor (PDGF), macrophage derived growth factor (MDGF), endothelial cell derived growth factor (EDGF), growth factor derived from smooth muscle cells, low density lipoprotein (LDL) especially of the hyperlipidemia, interleukin I, and hormones were reported as the growth factors. Our hypothesis is, in addition to them, fibrin is important in the proliferation of smooth muscle cells.[9-10]

The localization of fibrin in the arterial wall was observed by immunofluorescence technique in the specimens of human cerebral arteries obtained from 65 subjects ranging in age from a fetus of 38 weeks of gestation to 87 years.[10] Main bifurcations were used from the middle cerebral, internal carotid, and basilar arteries. The sections were incubated with the FITC-conjugated anti-human fibrinogen rabbit/antiserum or FITC-conjugated anti-human-low-density-lipoprotein rabbit/antiserum.

The inner surface and edges of the fibrous plaque gave a bright specific fluorescence for fibrinogen. Specific fluorescence was demonstrated in the inner layer of the advanced plaques, where musculoelastic hyperplasia was seen in the thickened intima.

Early plaques showed some streaks or spots of specific fluorescence for fibrinogen in the interstices of the intima and also between the layers of the reduplicated internal elastic lamina.

Specific fluorescence was frequently seen in the subendothelial region of the uninvolved intima at the bifurcations of the cerebral arteries.

The earliest intimal thickening in a boy of 4 years showed a small amount of fibrinogen deposition.

Specific fluorescence for LDL was first observed in the endothelial cell cytoplasm in a small intimal cushion located in the outer wall of the bifurcation of the middle cerebral artery in an 8-year-old male. In small intimal cushions, fluorescence was located in the inner part of the thickened intima. With advance in intimal thickening, LDL tended to be distributed extracellulary in a wavy manner along elastic fibers and collagen bundles.

The incidence of fibrinogen and LDL deposition in the cerebral arterial wall is summerized in TABLE 4. The deposition of both plasma proteins was most marked in the bifurcation of the middle cerebral arteries and least obvious in the basilar arteries in all age groups. In general, deposition of LDL was associated with deposition of fibrinogen. Lone deposition of LDL in the absence of fibrinogen was only rarely seen. Deposition of these proteins was more frequent with advancing age and increase in intimal thickening.

These observations suggest that deposition of fibrinogen in the intima might precede LDL deposition and possibly play a more important role than LDL in the development of atherosclerotic lesions in the cerebral arteries, especially in their early stage.[10,13,14] Severe atherosclerosis at the bifurcations may in part be due to increased permeation of these plasma proteins and other growth factors, possibly as a result of hemodynamic stress.

Duguid and Astrup suggested that the balance between the deposition of fibrin on the vessel wall and fibrinilytic activity of the vascular intima may play a role in the formation of atheroma.[9]

The effects of fibrin, free from or rich in plasminogen, on the growth of smooth muscle cells in culture obtained from bovine aortas were compared with the effects of agar alone.

The cells began to proliferate on the agar plate containing 5 mg/ml of fibrin, free from plasminogen, at 6 h and continued to proliferate at 48 h.

Incorporation of [^{3}H] thymidine by the cells seemed to be dose-dependent for fibrin, free from plasminogen, during the experimental period, as shown in FIGURE 5.

The cells began to proliferate on the agar plate containing 5 mg/ml of fibrin, rich in

TABLE 4. Deposition of Fibrin and LDL in Intima and Media of the Cerebral Arteries Shown by Immunofluorescence Antibody Technique[a]

Age (Yr)	No. of Cases		MCA	ICA	BA
Fibrin					
−9	14	intima	4 (28.6)	1 (7.1)	1 (7.1)
		media	0	0	0
−29	9	intima	6 (66.7)	7 (77.8)	3 (33.3)
		media	0	0	0
−59	18	intima	14 (77.8)	13 (72.2)	10 (55.6)
		media	4 (22.2)	0	0
60−	24	intima	19 (79.2)	18 (75.0)	14 (58.3)
		media	7 (29.2)	4 (16.7)	3 (12.5)
Total	65	intima	43 (66.2)	39 (60.0)	28 (43.0)
		media	11 (16.9)	4 (6.2)	3 (4.6)
LDL					
−9	14	intima	1 (7.1)	0	1 (7.1)
		media	0	0	0
−29	9	intima	3 (33.3)	0	0
		media	0	0	0
−59	18	intima	3 (16.7)	2 (11.1)	1 (5.6)
		media	0	1 (5.6)	0
60−	24	intima	8 (33.3)	6 (25.0)	4 (16.7)
		media	2 (8.3)	1 (4.2)	0
Total	65	intima	15 (23.1)	8 (12.3)	6 (9.2)
		media	2 (3.1)	2 (3.1)	0

[a]MCA = bifurcation of middle cerebral artery, ICA = bifurcation of internal carotid artery, BA = basilar artery. Figures in brackets: %. (From Sadoshima and Tanaka.[10] Reprinted by permission from *Atherosclerosis*.)

plasminogen, at 6 h. Prominent proliferation of the cells was noted at 24 h, but the cells degenerated and detached from the agar plate at 48 h. The lysed area of the fibrin agar plates was obscure under the phase-contrast microscope, but fibrin degradation products (FDP) were detected in the culture medium.

Incorporation of [^{3}H] thymidine by the cells proliferating in the fibrin agar plate containing plasminogen, as shown in FIGURE 6, became increasingly dose dependent at 24 h, but decreased at 48 h. The growth pattern of the cells on agar alone is shown by closed circles.

A fibrinolysis autograph of smooth muscle cells cultured on a microslide showed lysed areas of fibrin film, corresponding to the proliferating multilayered smooth muscle

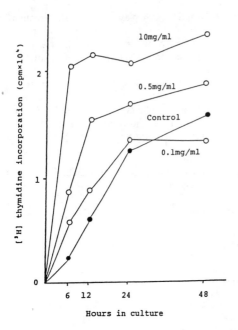

FIGURE 5. Effect of fibrin (plasminogen free) on the incorporation of [³H]thymidine into aortic smooth muscle cells in culture. (From Ishida and Tanaka.⁹ Reprinted by permission from *Atherosclerosis.*)

cells, but there was no lysis on the plasminogen-free fibrin films. Smooth muscle cells cultured in triplicated bottles were extracted with potassium isocyanate. The fibrinolytic activity of the samples was $0.027 + 0.011$ IU of urokinase/mg of protein in the extract. Fibrinolytic activity on the plasminogen-free fibrin plate was nil.

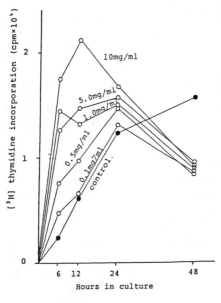

FIGURE 6. Effect of fibrin (plasminogen rich) on the incorporation of [³H]thymidine into aortic smooth muscle cells in culture. (From Ishida and Tanaka.⁹ Reprinted by permission from *Atherosclerosis.*)

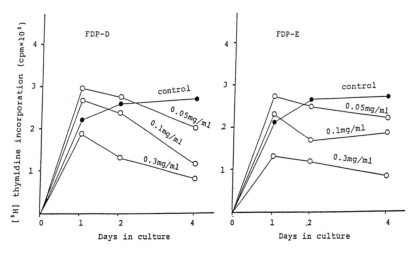

FIGURE 7. Effects of fibrinogen-degradation products on the incorporation of [³H] thymidine by aortic smooth muscle cells in culture. (From Ishida and Tanaka.[9] Reprinted by permission from *Atherosclerosis*.)

The effects of FDP-D and -E (0.05, 0.1, 0.3 mg/ml) added to serum-free culture media were compared with those of serum-free culture media alone. Increasing concentration of FDP-D and -E in the medium resulted in a greater inhibition of the incorporation of [³H] thymidine, as shown in FIGURE 7.

The effects of thrombin or urokinase added to the serum-free culture media were compared with the findings with serum-free culture media alone. There was no smooth muscle cell proliferation. It is interesting that thrombin enhances the production and release of tissue plasminogen activator from the endothelial cells.[15]

These results support the hypothesis that the proliferation of smooth muscle cells is stimulated by fibrin and later inhibited by FDP, as produced by the fibrinolytic activity of smooth muscle cells and endothelial cells. In our previous studies, degradation products of fibrinogen demonstrated a permeability enhancing and chemotactic activities,[16] induced degeneration of endothelial cells,[11] and inhibited PGI₂ synthesis by endothelial and smooth muscle cells.[12] It is proposed that the metabolism of fibrin in the arterial wall, as shown in FIGURE 8, may be of importance in the regulation of smooth muscle cell proliferation.[9]

Advanced age, smoking, obesity, hyperlipidemia, diabetes mellitus, and hypertension are all associated with reduced fibrinolysis. If fibrinolysis is indeed inadequate in such patients, the deposited fibrin would remain in the arterial wall and promote smooth muscle cell proliferation.

SUMMARY

1) The incidence of myocardial infarction, as well as thrombosis, has been increasing recently in the consecutive autopsy cases over 40 years old in Kyushu University, but is still less frequent than those in the autopsy cases in Boston around 1960. Increased fat

intake might play a significant role in the increasing frequency of myocardial infarction in Japanese.

2) In a nationwide cooperative study of atherosclerosis in young Japanese, atherosclerotic changes were observed to begin developing in childhood. Primary prevention of atherosclerosis should be initiated in the pediatric age group. We should pay more attention to subclinical atherosclerosis.

Age, serum cholesterol, and blood pressure were significantly and positively correlated with SI and AI of aortas and coronary arteries.

Serum cholesterol was more strongly correlated with the extent of fatty streaks than was mean blood pressure and vice versa with that of fibrous plaques.

Atherosclerosis of cerebral arteries, however, showed a significant correlation only with the factor of mean blood pressure.

Therefore the susceptibility to risk factors varies with the artery in the case of early lesions of atherosclerosis in young people.

More attention should be paid to the fact that atherosclerosis is a multifactoral disease.

3) Deposition of fibrinogen in the intima might precede LDL deposition and possibly play a more important role than LDL in the development of atherosclerotic lesions in the cerebral arteries, especially in their early stage.

4) The proliferation of smooth muscle cells is stimulated by fibrin and later inhibited by FDP, as produced by fibrinolytic activity of smooth muscle cells.

The metabolism of fibrin in the arterial wall may be of importance in the regulation of smooth muscle cell proliferation, and the coagulation-fibrinolysis system may play a significant role in atherosclerosis with the effect of other risk factors such as cholesterol and hypertension.

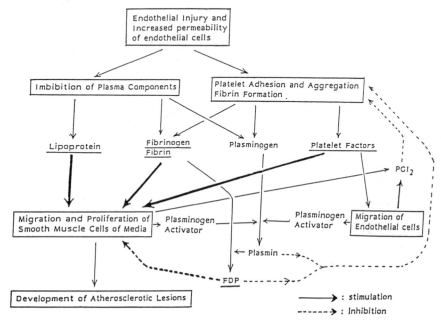

FIGURE 8. Possible role of the coagulation-fibrinolysis system in atherosclerosis. (From Ishida and Tanaka.[9] Reprinted by permission from *Atherosclerosis.*)

REFERENCES

1. GORE, I., A. E. HIRST & K. TANAKA. 1964. Myocardial infarction and thromboembolism. Arch. Intern. Med. **113:** 323–330.

2. HIRST, A. E., I. GORE, K. TANAKA, I. SAMUEL & I. KRISTHTMUKIT. 1965. Myocardial infarction and pulmonary embolism. Arch. Pathol. **80:** 365–370.

3. IMAMURA, T., T. WATANABE & K. TANAKA. 1978. Incidence of thrombosis and myocardial infarction. Statistical analysis of autopsy cases in Fukuoka, Japan. J. Jpn. Coll. Angiol. **18:** 345–348.

4. SUMIYOSHI, A., K. TANAKA, I. GORE & A. E. HIRST, JR. 1965. The incidence of theombolism and myocardial infarction at autopsy in Fukuoka, Japan. Fukuoka Acta Med. **56:** 571–580.

5. TANAKA, K. 1989. Recent trends in the incidence of atherosclerotic diseases in Japan from the pathological point of view (in Japanese). J. Jpn. Atheroscler. Soc. **16.** In press.

6. ARIHIRO, H., A. SUMIYOSHI & K. TANAKA. 1970. A study of Sudanophilia in the coronary artery of infants, children, and young adults. Fukuoka Acta Med. **61:** 481–492.

7. DOKI, K. 1970. Fat deposition in aorta of infants and young adults and its significance in atherosclerosis. Fukuoka Acta Med. **61:** 414–430.

8. TANAKA, K., J. MASUDA, T. IMAMURA, K. SUEISHI, T. NAKASHIMA, I. SAKURAI, T. SHOZAWA, Y. HOSODA, Y. YOSHIDA, Y. NISHIYAMA, C. YUTANI & S. HATANO. 1988. A nation-wide study of atherosclerosis in infants, children and young adults in Japan. Atherosclerosis **72:** 143–156.

9. ISHIDA, T. & K. TANAKA. 1982. Effects of fibrin and fibrinogen-degradation products on the growth of rabbit aortic smooth muscle cells in culture. Atherosclerosis **44:** 161–174.

10. SADOSHIMA, S. & K. TANAKA. 1979. Fibrinogen and low density lipoprotein in the development of cerebral atherosclerosis. Atherosclerosis **34:** 93–103.

11. WATANABE, K. & K. TANAKA. 1983. Influence of fibrin, fibrinogen and fibrinogen degradation products on cultured endothelial cells. Atherosclerosis **48:** 57–70.

12. WATANABE, K., T. ISHIDA, F. YOSHITOMI & K. TANAKA. 1984. Fibrinogen degradation products influence PGI_2 synthesis by cultured porcine aortic endothelial and smooth muscle cells. Atherosclerosis **51:** 151–161.

13. KUROZUMI, T., T. IMAMURA, K. TANAKA, Y. YAE & S. KOGA. 1983. Effects of hypertension and hypercholesteremia on the permeability of fibrinogen and low density lipoprotein in the coronary artery of rabbits. Immunoelectronmicroscopic study. Atherosclerosis **49:** 269–276.

14. KUROZUMI, T., T. IMAMURA, K. TANAKA, Y. YAE & S. KOGA. 1984. Permeation and deposition of fibrinogen and low density lipoprotein in the aorta and cerebral artery of rabbits. Immunoelectron microscopic study. Br. J. Exp. Pathol. **65:** 355–364.

15. NAKASHIMA, Y., K. SHEISHI & K. TANAKA. 1988. Thrombin enhances production and release of tissue plasminogen activator from bovine venous endothelial cells. Fibrinolysis **2:** 227–234.

16. SUEISHI, K., S. NANNO & K. TANAKA. 1981. Permeability enhancing and chemotactic activities of lower molecular weight degradation products of human fibrinogen. Thromb. Haemostasis **45:** 90–94.

Atherosclerosis in Japanese Youth with Reference to Differences between Each Artery[a]

ISAMU SAKURAI, KAORI MIYAKAWA, AKIO KOMATSU, AND
TATSUO SAWADA

Department of Pathology
Nihon University School of Medicine
30-1 Ohyaguchi-kami-machi, Itabashi-ku
Tokyo 173, Japan

INTRODUCTION

Various diseases caused by arterial atherosclerosis are generally considered to be clinically geriatric diseases, but arterial lesions recognizable as early changes of atherosclerosis, such as fatty streaks, may often be seen in the arteries of young people. If one thinks that such arterial changes in youth may be early lesions, which may be expected to progress to more advanced atherosclerosis decades later, a clinically latent period should be very long.[1] Thus, precise investigations of arteries in youth seem to be very important in order to make clear what the initial factors in atherosclerosis are and how early lesions progress to more advanced ones in humans, playing an important role later in developing ischemic diseases in various organs in people past middle age.

As part of a multiinstitutional cooperative study of atherosclerosis in infants, children, and young adults in Japan (group director: Dr. Kenzo Tanaka, Kyushu University, Fukuoka),[2] the present study pays special attention to the differences between each artery, particularly between aortae and coronary arteries.

Atherosclerotic Index

As shown in FIGURE 1, the studied cases, composed of 418 aortae and 326 coronary arteries from Japanese youth aged from zero to 40 years, were divided into 5 groups by age; the youngest group below the age of 1 year, a group aged 1 to 10, a group aged 11 to 20, a group aged 21 to 30, and the eldest group aged 31 to 40. The atherosclerotic indices (AI), according to modified Gore's index, were also grouped in five categories by severity. Group A meant an AI of 0.000, indicating no sclerotic lesions or lipid deposition at all. Group B was categorized by an AI between 0.001 and 0.039, group C was that between 0.040 and 0.099, group D was that between 0.100 and 0.499, and group E, the most severely affected one, was over 0.500.

Atherosclerotic indices tend to rise as age increases in both aortae and coronary arteries, but differences between both arteries are significant by obviously higher values of the indices in the aortae in each age group.

Namely, in the case of aortae, of 48 newborn babies 58.4% were in group A, 10.4% in group B, 20.8% in group C, and 10.4% in group D. Of 72 children between 1 and 10

[a]Supported by a grant from the Ministry of Health and Welfare, Japan.

years, only 8.3% were categorized in group A, 31.9% in group B, 27.9% in group C, and 31.9% in group D. Of 48 cases of the third decade, all had more or less sclerotic lesions. 4.2% were in group B, 20.8% in group C, 70.8% in group D, and 4.2% in group E. Of 84 subjects between 21 and 30, only 1.2% were in group B, 10.7% in group C, 76.2% in group D, and 11.9% in the most severe group E. Of 166 aged between 31 and 40, 1.8% were in group B, 6.6% in group C, 51.2% in group D, and 40.4% in group E.

On the other hand, in the coronary arteries, all of 22 subjects of newborn babies were in group A. That meant that none of the newborn babies had sclerotic lesions in the coronary arteries. Also of 40 children under the age of 10, 95.0% had no sclerotic lesions, and only 5.0% had group C sclerosis. Of 39 subjects of the third decade, 77.0% still had no lesions, and 5.1% were in group B, 5.1% in group C, and 12.8% in group D. Of 84 subjects aged between 21 and 30, 63.2% were categorized with no lesions, 9.5% in group

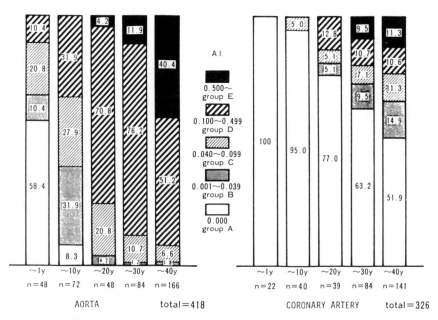

FIGURE 1. Atherosclerotic index by aging in children and young adults.

B, 7.1% in group C, 10.7% in group D, and 9.5% in group E. Of 141 cases aged between 31 and 40, 51.9% had yet no lesions. 14.9% were in group B, 11.3% in group C, 10.6% in group D, and 11.3% in group E.

Thus, the differences in arterial changes in youth and by aging between the aortae and coronary arteries are obviously significant.[6] Among the newborn babies, there was no trace of lipid deposition encountered as only 58.4% in the aortae, whilst on the contrary, 100% in the coronary arteries. In other words, about 40% of new born babies had morphologically detectable lipid deposits of various severity ranging from 0.001 to 0.499 of AI in the aortic intima, while none of the age-matched objectives did so in the coronary arteries. Over 11 years of age, all Japanese youth showed lipid deposits of various degrees in the aortae in this series, but approximately half the subjects (51.9%) of rather aged people between 31 and 40 still had no trace of lipid in the intima of the coronary arteries.

Fat deposits and early lesions of sclerosis obviously begin to appear earlier in the aortic
intima than in the coronary arteries.

The atherosclerotic index is one of the indicators for an evaluation of atherosclerosis
expressed by a combination of both lesion extent and its severity. It is evaluated and
calculated by naked-eye observations on the intimal surface by measuring how widely and
severely the arteries are involved by atherosclerotic lesions of various qualities. In other
words, AI does not express how thick the arterial intima or each sclerotic lesion is.

Intimal Thickness

We have tried, therefore, to investigate how much the intimas of each artery are
thickened on the sections taken from the locations of each artery indicated by the study
group.

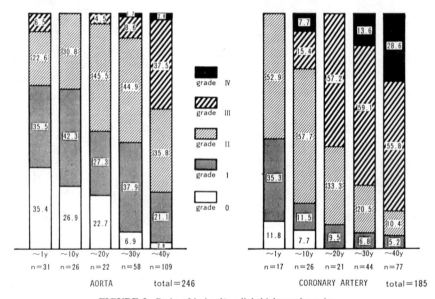

FIGURE 2. Ratio of intimal/medial thickness by aging.

FIGURE 2 shows the age distribution of intimal thickness in the aortae and coronary
arteries, which was histometrically measured at the thickest point on every histology
section of each case by the ratio of the intima/media thickness graded from 0 (intima not
thickened) to IV (ratio of intima/media, 3/1 and over) according to Sakurai.[7]

In the aortae of infants under the age of 1 year, 35.4% were of grade 0, 35.5% of
grade I, 22.6% of grade II, and 6.5% of grade III. In those of children aged between 1
and 10 years, 26.9% were grade I, 42.3% of grade I, and 30.8% of grade II. At ages
between 11 and 20 years, 22.7% were of grade 0, 27.3% of grade I, 45.5% of grade II,
and 4.5% of grade III. At ages between 21 and 30 years, 6.9% were of grade I, 37.9%
of grade I, 44.9% of grade II, 8.6% of grade III, and 1.7% of grade IV. At ages between
31 and 40 years, 2.8% were of grade 0, 21.1% of grade I, 35.8% of grade II, 37.5% of
grade III, and 2.8% of grade IV.

TABLE 1. Frequency of Each Lesion: Aorta (418 Cases)

Age	Total	Fatty Streak (%)	Fibrous Plaque (%)	Complicated Lesion (%)
0–1	48	20 (41.7)	0	0
1–10	72	66 (91.7)	0	0
11–20	48	47 (97.9)	7 (14.6)	0
21–30	84	84 (100.0)	20 (23.8)	0
31–40	166	166 (100.0)	89 (53.6)	2 (1.2)

On the contrary, in the coronary arteries of infants under the age of 1 year, 11.8% were of grade 0, 35.3% of grade I, and 52.9% of grade II. At ages between 1 and 10 years, 7.7% were of grade 0, 11.5% of grade I, 57.7% of grade II, 15.4% of grade III, and 7.7% of grade IV. At ages between 11 and 20 years, none of them was of grade 0, 9.5% were of grade I, 33.3% of grade II, and 57.2% of grade III. At ages between 21 and 30 years, 6.8% were of grade I, 20.5% of grade II, 59.1% of grade III, and 13.6% of grade IV. At ages over 31 years, 5.2% were of grade I, 10.4% of grade II, 55.8% of grade III, and 28.6% of grade IV.

These results of the intimal thickness in both arteries indicate that the intimal thickening of the vessels tend to be significantly stronger in the coronary arteries than in the aortae, although the atherosclerotic index was remarkably higher in the aortae than in the coronary arteries. Microscopically, the intimal thickening seen in the coronary arteries was characteristically based upon significant and diffuse fibrocellular proliferation with proteoglycan accumulation and lesser lipid depostion, but such intimal changes were obviously weaker in the aortae than in the coronary arteries. In the aortae of youth, generally its intima was not so thickened, but it tended to be insudated and loaded by lipid substances at young ages.[6]

Frequency of Each Lesion of Atherosclerosis

As to the frequency of each lesion recognized on the intimas of both aortae and coronary arteries in each age group, TABLES 1 and 2 summarize the results.

On the aortic intimas 41.7% of the infants already had fatty streaks, and most of the objectives aged between 1 and 10, and between between 1 and 10 years, and between 11 and 20 years of age had fatty streaks with frequencies of 91.7% and 97.9%, respectively. All cases over 21 years of age had fatty streaks at certain point(s) in the vessels. Fibrous plaques began to be discovered in the aortae during ages of 11 to 20 years with 14.6% frequency. At ages between 21 and 30 years, fibrous plaques were found in 20 subjects among 84 with 23.8% frequency. Over 31 years of age, over half the people had fibrous plaques with 53.6% occurrence. Complicated lesions were demonstrable at ages over 31

TABLE 2. Frequency of Each Lesion: Coronary Artery (326 Cases)

Age	Total	Fatty Streak	Fibrous Plaque (%)	Complicated Lesion (%)
0–1	22	0	0	0
1–10	40	2 (5.0)	0	0
11–20	39	6 (15.4)	4 (10.3)	0
21–30	84	23 (27.9)	13 (15.5)	0
31–40	141	60 (42.5)	22 (15.6)	2 (1.4)

years in 2 cases out of 166 (1.2%). On the other hand, the coronary arteries revealed that none of cases had any lesions of atherosclerosis in infants below 1 year of age. Only 2 cases (5.0%) among 40 aged between 1 and 10 years demonstrated fatty streaks. Six subjects (15.4%) of 39 aged between 11 and 20 years, 23 subjects (27.9%) of 84 aged between 21 and 30 years, and 60 cases (42.5%) of 141 cases aged over 31 had fatty streaks on the coronary arterial intimas. Fibrous plaques could be observed in none of them aged below 10 years, 4 cases (10.3%) of 39 aged between 11 and 20 years, 13 subjects (15.5%) of 84 aged between 21 and 30 years, and 22 cases (15.6%) of 141 over age of 31 years. Complicated lesions were found in only 2 cases (1/4%) aged over 31 years.

The Youngest Age at Which Each Lesion Is First Recognizable

As shown in TABLE 3, a fatty streak was found in an aorta obtained from a case at the age of 1 month, while at the age of 5 years in the coronary arteries. As to fibrous plaques and complicated lesions, there was not much difference in the youngest age, at which each lesion was first recognized, between the aortae and coronary arteries. The data concerning the youngest age disclosed fibrous plaque at age of 15 years in the aortae and at age of 11 years in the coronary arteries, and complicated lesion at age of 36 years in the aortae and at age of 35 years in the coronary arteries.

TABLE 3. Lesion-Recognizable Youngest Age

	Aorta	Coronary
Fatty streak	1 m	5 y
Fibrous plaque	15 y	11 y
Complicated lesion	36 y	35 y

Immunohistochemistry of Apo B

An immunohistochemical approach was attempted on both arteries, though the studied arteries were in small numbers. TABLE 4 summarizes the immunohistochemical results for Apo B infiltration to the intimas. Apo B often proved to be intra- or extracellularly present in the intimas of both aortae and coronary arteries at any ages.

Cerebral Arteries

Although the number of the cerebral arteries was limited to a total of 38 cases aged between 0 and 30 years because of the low autopsy rate for brain examinations, the study was done by histopathological observations on serial sections of the middle cerebral arteries and strio-thalamic arteries.[8] None of the cases at any age, however, demonstrated any lipid deposits indicating fatty streaks and atheromatous plaques, as shown in TABLE 5. Intimal thickening of the vessels was occasionally demonstrated, particularly with a predominance of the middle cerebral arteries, as shown in TABLE 6. In particular, grade 2 thickening was found in the middle cerebral arteries in one of 3 cases aged between 11 and 20 years, and in 3 subjects out of 4 aged between 21 and 30. The cerebral arteries

TABLE 4. Immunohistochemistry of Apo B in Aortic and Coronary Intima

	Aorta		Coronary	
Age	Intra-cellular	Extra-cellular	Intra-cellular	Extra-cellular
0–1	0/2	2/2	1/3	3/3
1–10	2/4	2/4	2/5	4/5
11–20	1/3	2/3	1/3	2/3
21–30	1/1	0/1	2/2	0/2
31–40	3/4	2/4	3/4	4/4

obtained from seven newborn infants were studied immunohistochemically for identification of infiltrations of fibrinogen, low-density lipoproteins, and albumin in the vessel walls, but obvious positive reactions were not obtained for any of those serum-derived substances.

DISCUSSION AND CONCLUSIONS

All the cases of the present study were hospital deaths with various diseases. Accidental deaths would reflect a natural history of atherosclerosis in Japanese, but it seems difficult to obtain enough numbers of cases for study.

In summary, differences between the aortae and coronary arteries seem to be significantly evident. Also in Japanese youth fatty streaks in the aortae are frequently encountered with 41.7% occurrence even in infants aged below 1 year, and increase rapidly with age to the plateau in the second decade. However, the coronary arteries are different. The subjects under 10 years of age never had any trace of lipid deposits with frequencies of atherosclerotic lesions of 0% in subjects below the age of 1 year, and 5.0% in cases aged between 1 and 10 years. Even in the elder group aged over 31 years, about half the cases are free from fatty streaks. Histological studies on cross sections of the vessels generally indicate that the coronary arteries of young people are characterized by diffuse intimal thickening with fibrocellular proliferation, migration of medial smooth muscle cells to the intimas through widened pores in internal elastic laminae, proteoglycan accumulation,

TABLE 5. Fatty Streaks and Atheromatous Plaques in Cerebral Arteries by Aging

Age	Site	Fatty Streak	Athero-matous Plaques
Below I m	MCA[a]	0	0
(n: 18)	Striothalamic	0	0
1 m—1 yr	MCA	0	0
(n: 7)	Striothalamic	0	0
1 yr—4 yrs	MCA	0	0
(n: 2)	Striothalamic	0	0
5 yrs—10 yrs	MCA	0	0
(n: 4)	Striothalamic	0	0
11 yrs—20 yrs	MCA	0	0
(n: 3)	Striothalamic	0	0
21 yrs—30 yrs	MCA	0	0
(n: 4)	Striothalamic	0	0

[a]MCA = proximal portion of middle cerebral artery.

and less lipid deposition, while the youth aortae start to be loaded with fat in thinner intimas during the very early period of life. The reasons why such differences exist in the progress of atherosclerosis between the two arteries are unknown. The differences of wall structure between the two arteries seem to indicate that each artery may have its own biological activities, which may be characteristic or specific to each of the arteries. Experimental studies on the pathogenesis of atherosclerosis have been widely and generally done on the aortae, particularly on rabbit's aortae, but changes seen in the aortae do not always express qualitatively and quantitatively those of other arteries. Therefore, further studies on atherosclerosis should be done on the basis of each artery with the use of *in vivo* and *in vitro* means. Even though a single lesion is severe enough to obliterate vascular lumens, the Atherosclerotic Index would be still low, though a clinically manifested ischemic disease might occur. This is particularly important in the coronary and cerebral arteries. Further studies and preventive procedures against atherosclerosis should be planned and performed with special attention to the biological specificity of and differences between each artery.

As a part of the study, we made an analysis of relations between total cholesterol

TABLE 6. Intimal Thickness by Aging (Cerebral Arteries)

Age	Site	Grade			
		0	1	2	3
Below 1 m	MCA[a]	16	2	0	0
(n: 18)	Striothalamic	17	1	0	0
1 m—1 yr	MCA	5	2	0	0
(n: 7)	Striothalamic	7	0	0	0
1 yr—4 yrs	MCA	0	2	0	0
(n: 2)	Striothalamic	2	0	0	0
5 yrs—10 yrs	MCA	2	2	0	0
(n: 4)	Striothalamic	4	0	0	0
11 yrs—20 yrs	MCA	2	0	1	0
(n: 3)	Striothalamic	3	0	0	0
21 yrs—30 yrs	MCA	0	1	3	0
(n: 4)	Striothalamic	3	1	0	0

[a]MCA = proximal portion of middle cerebral artery.

values in the sera and the severity of atherosclerosis by dividing into three groups: low cholesterol group (under 120 mg/dl), normal cholesterol group (120 to 200 mg/dl), and high cholesterol group (over 200 mg/dl). We were not able to get significantly positive interrelations between serum cholesterol and the severity of atherosclerosis in the series of the present study. For recent years, however, the dietary habit of Japanese people has rapidly become Westernized by an intake of more fat and proteins of animal sources, as was indicated by Yamamoto[9] who observed that the average value of total cholesterol in children in primary schools nearby the large cities in Japan was a steady 150–160 mg/dl tested before 1970, but thereafter rose to 170–180 mg/dl in a recent study. It is strongly urged that preventive plans against progress of atherosclerosis should be started early in childhood.

REFERENCES

1. DARIA HAUST, M. 1978. Atherosclerosis in childhood. *In* Perspectives in Pediatric Pathology. H. S. Rosenberg & R. P. Bolande, Eds. Vol. 4: 155–126. Year Book Med. Pub., Inc. Chicago, IL.

2. TANAKA, K., J. MASUDA, T., IMAMURA, *et al.* 1988. A nationwide study of atherosclerosis in infants, children and young adults in Japan. Atherosclerosis **72**(2,3): 143–156.
3. GORE, I. & C. TEJADA. 1957. The quantitative appraisal of atherosclerosis. Am. J. Pathol. **33**(5): 875–885.
4. MITCHELL, J. R. A. & W. I. CROSTON. 1965. A simple method for the quantitative assessment of aortic disease. J. Atheroscler. Res. **5**: 135–144.
5. MAE, A. 1971. A comparative study of atherosclerosis of the aorta, coronary artery and large arteries of the circle of Willis in man. J. Kurume Med. Assoc. **34**(12): 1261–1307 (in Japanese with English abstract).
6. MIYAKAWA, K. 1985. Arteriosclerosis in children and young adults among Japanese. Nihon Univ. Med. J. **27**(5): 317–336.
7. SAKURAI, I. 1978. Childhood coronary sclerosis. Acta Pathol. Jpn. **28**(1): 41–52.
8. SAWADA, T. 1982. Morphological study on the structure of cerebral arterial wall in childhood and adult. Nihon Univ. Med. Bull. **41**(9): 889–899 (in Japanese with English abstract).
9. YAMAMOTO, A. 1988. Preface. *In* Serum Lipids—For Establishment of Standards. A. Yamamoto, H. Nakamura & T. Yasugi, Eds. Kyowa Kikaku Tsushin. Tokyo. In Japanese.

The Contribution of Studies of Atherosclerotic Lesions in Young People to Future Research[a]

ROBERT W. WISSLER, DRAGOSLAVA VESSELINOVITCH, AND
AKIO KOMATSU[b]

Department of Pathology
University of Chicago Medical Center
5841 South Maryland Avenue, Box 414
Chicago, Illinois 60637
and
Second Department of Pathology
Nihon University School of Medicine
Itabashi, Tokyo, Japan

INTRODUCTION

This paper has three main messages. The first part of the report is designed to acquaint the reader with the structure and function of the study which benefits from the participation of a very active, talented, and experienced steering committee (TABLE 1) and for which Dr. Wissler has the responsibility to serve as Program Director. It is called the Multicenter Cooperative Study of the Pathobiological Determinants of Atherosclerosis in Youth (PDAY-USA) (FIG. 1). The second part of this report outlines the most evident valuable contributions which this study is designed to make. The third component considers the future research which these PDAY discoveries are likely to stimulate.

The Structure and Function of PDAY

This study is a logical outgrowth of the outstanding multicenter studies supported by the National Heart, Lung and Blood Institute in the late 1950s and the 1960s.[1–3] It also offers the opportunity to extend observations made in the International Atherosclerosis Project and to provide additional quantitative cell biological, ultrastructural, and microchemical (including immunohistochemical and enzymological) data over and above those provided by the community pathological studies,[4–7] and to add a genetic component to the risk factors considered previously. This data is focused on the age span between 15 and 34 years, an age period in which the atherosclerotic process is likely to become manifest and to progress substantially in individuals most at risk.

In addition to its emphasis on modern technology to achieve quantitative morphometric and cell biological results as well as its focus on a critical period in plaque development in the youth of the USA, the study has a number of important features which make it likely to be especially valuable.

[a]Supported by National Institutes of Health Grant HL 33740.
[b]Present address: First Department of Pathology, Kyorin University School of Medicine, 6-20-2 Shinkawa, Mitaka-Shi, Tokyo 181, Japan.

TABLE 1. "PDAY" Steering Committee

THE PATHOBIOLOGICAL DETERMINANTS OF ATHEROSCLEROSIS IN YOUTH
Robert W. Wissler, Ph.D., M.D., Program Director
The University of Chicago School of Medicine

Henry McGill	University of Texas Medical School at San Antonio, and the Southwest Foundation for Biomedical Research
Jack Strong	Louisiana State University Medical School, New Orleans
Abel Robertson	University of Illinois College of Medicine at Chicago
Fred Cornhill	The Ohio State University College of Medicine, Columbus
Alex McMahan	Health Science Center at San Antonio, University of Texas

1. Its multicenter structure (TABLE 2) makes it possible to study disease developing in widely separated parts of the USA and to provide sufficient numbers of cases in a relatively short time so that adequate numbers of samples in each of the age and race "cells" can be reached and significant results can be achieved in virtually all measurements. The plan also calls for the ultimate collection of sufficient cases in order to demonstrate the finer details and the cellular pathobiological features of the important sex differences in disease development.
2. The exclusive use of samples from sudden unexpected death cases decreases the

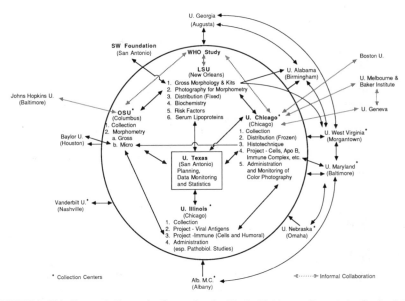

FIGURE 1. This diagram indicates the Centers involved in the Multicenter Cooperative Study of the Pathobiological Determinants of Atherosclerosis in Youth (PDAY). Those Centers in the *inner circle* are involved in all cases collected and take part in the core protocol studies which are mainly concerned with the effects that age, sex, race, the major risk factors (serum lipids, cigarette smoking, hypertension), and diabetes as well as certain additional factors altering endothelial integrity (viruses, immune complexes) have on atherogenesis. The *outer circle* depicts the Centers which are involved primarily in special studies of selected cohorts of cases or in the collection of cases or both. A few Centers (*dotted lines*) are involved informally in studying PDAY cases utilizing approaches not readily available elsewhere.

TABLE 2. Institutions Participating in the PDAY Multicenter Cooperative Study

University of Alabama School of Medicine, Birmingham	Medical College of Georgia, Augusta
Albany Medical College, Albany	University of Nebraska Medical Center, Omaha
Baylor College of Medicine, Houston	The Ohio State University College of Medicine, Columbus
The University of Chicago School of Medicine, Chicago	Southwest Foundation of Biomedical Research, San Antonio
Louisiana State University Medical Center, New Orleans	Vanderbilt University School of Medicine, Nashville
University of Maryland School of Medicine, Baltimore	West Virginia University School of Medicine, Morgantown
University of Illinois College of Medicine at Chicago	University of Texas Medical School at San Antonio

potential effects which might be expected from chronic disease and therapeutic manipulation which are likely to complicate many cases autopsied in community hospitals and medical centers.

3. The use of a number of well established and some relatively new methods to assess the risk factors of hyperlipidemia, diabetes, smoking, hyperglycemia (TABLE 3), as well as circulating immune complexes, DNA polymorphisms in candidate genes for atherosclerosis, etc., make it possible to quantitate reliably a number of risk factors in large numbers of cases.

4. The carefully constructed protocol and the manual of procedures accompanied by multiple training sessions help to achieve carefully collected, standardized samples for analysis, as well as high quality processing, preservation, and distribution of study samples.

5. The relatively short postmortem intervals in most cases between death and refrigeration of the corpse (average 2 hours) as well as between death and autopsy (average ca. 17 hours) help to insure the use of reliable samples. The samples are collected with special precautions to avoid mechanical damage to the aortic intima during the autopsy and the sampling procedures.

6. The sampling strategy developed and adopted for Phase 2[8] makes it possible to compare:

   a. the areas of high prevalence of aortic lesion with low prevalence of lesions in each aortic sample;

TABLE 3. Risk Factors Measured in Autopsied Persons

Risk Factor	Initiating Centers	Marker
Blood lipids	LSU	total cholesterol, HDL cholesterol and apolipoprotein concentrations including Lp(a) in postmortem serum
Smoking	LSU	thiocyanate concentrations in postmortem serum
Blood pressure	LSU	wall thickness of renal arteries and arterioles, and heart weight/BW
Diabetes mellitus	LSU	glycosylated hemoglobin concentrations in postmortem red blood cells
Obesity	all collection centers*	panniculus adiposus thickness; BW/BL and torso indexes
Genetic factors	SWF	DNA polymorphisms in liver

*OSU, Chicago, Nebraska, Illinois, Georgia, Maryland, West Virginia, Vanderbilt, Albany.

    b. the thoracic aortic with the abdominal aortic samples;

    c. the microscopic features of the left anterior descending coronary artery samples with those of the aortic samples;

    d. the right coronary artery gross topographic features with the gross morphometric results of the aortic lesion study;

    e. some of the chemical results obtained from analysis of the left circumflex coronary artery with the aortic chemistry; and

    f. the results obtained on the same or adjacent samples for many of the special study determinations and some of the core chemistry determinations.

7. The computer-assisted gross and microscopic morphometric methods utilizing image processing developed at the Ohio State University and Louisiana State University facilitate gathering accurate quantitative data realtively quickly on large numbers of samples.[9] For some of the special studies, computer-assisted digitized results for cells, lipoproteins, and other quantitatively determined lesion components are measured on specified samples from a limited number of carefully selected cases at the University of Illinois and at the University of Chicago.

8. Frequent consultations by conference calls among the steering committee members along with the convenor of the "Protocol and Manual of Procedures Committee" are aiding the progress of the study.

9. The reviews by a Data Review Board and the constant involvement of the NHLBI scientific staff (especially Drs. Momtaz Wassef and Gardner McMillan), as well as the important input from the Scientific Advisory Committee, are of great value.

10. Quality control is strengthened by means of tutorial instruction sessions with all workers at all centers involved in collection procedures and in quantitative microscopy.

11. There is constant monitoring and input from the University of Texas statistical center, the Louisiana State University processing, distribution, morphology, tissue lipid chemistry, and risk factor center, and the University of Chicago collection, preservation, processing, distribution, macrophotography, histotechnique and study center.

12. The Annual Scientific Days where results are reported and problems are discussed and solved are of great value.

Data Being Gathered on All Cases and on the Special Study Cases

In addition to the risk factor data which are gathered as indicated in TABLE 3, other important information is obtained on almost all cases. This is listed in TABLE 4, along with the various special analyses being carried out on age- and race-balanced groups of carefully selected cases in which all the conditions of quality of samples, postmortem intervals, and complete relevant information are available.

As can be appreciated from TABLES 3 and 4, the data from these analyses offer remarkable opportunities to evaluate in quantitative terms many of the important components of developing lesions and to relate these results to age, to the differences between disease progression in the thoracic and abdominal aortas, to the differences between areas of high prevalence and areas of low prevalence of lesions of the aortas and the right coronary arteries, and to several of the classical risk factors. These results also make it possible to relate the quantitative data from the gross and microscopic analyses of the lesions to results reflecting some newly established or newly suspected risk factors.

Although many of the results from the more than 1200 Phase 2 cases which we have now collected are not yet available for analysis, some of the core data results from 343 Phase 1 (feasibility study) cases have been analysed.

A few of the trends from core data indicate that even with relatively small numbers of cases, the study can be expected to yield significant correlations of certain risk factors such as age, race, sex, serum cholesterol values, and the lipoprotein levels (both low and high density classes) with lesion severity. Evidence of smoking is being evaluated and correlated with the extent of lesions of the abdominal aorta and the right coronary artery. Furthermore, it is clear that both the feasibility study (Phase 1) and the more definitive Phase 2 studies are yielding abundant data which, in general, agree and which open new areas for further study of the cellular and biochemical details of progression of atherogenesis in young people.

TABLE 4. The Major Measurements Being Made on Each Case at the Core Centers and Trends Being Evaluated

Correlates	Preliminary Results (Study Status)
Age and size of lesion	age (5 year groups) and extent of gross lesions are associated; what are the age-race-sex-lesion type relationships?
Race, size and type of lesion	black and white males—interesting differences in atheromatous involvement
Serum cholesterol, HDL-C, LDL-C, VLDL and size of lesions	cholesterol and calculated serum LDL-C cholesterol and gross lesion—how strongly correlated?
Tobacco use (thiocyanate) and size of lesion	thiocyanate blood levels and gross lesions; clear-cut results being obtained
HDL-C and size of lesion	need more cases to improve the power of the test
Hyperglycemia and size of lesion	glycosylated hemoglobin with gross lesions (developing data base)
Hypertension and size of lesion	arterioles and small vessels with gross lesions (developing data base)
DNA apolipoprotein polymorphisms with size of lesion	genetic deviations of apolipoproteins B and E appear likely to be correlated with arterial lesion involvement
Adipose tissue fatty acids with chemical and cellular markers and severity of lesion	with special emphasis on the reflections of dietary fat containing tropical oils, marine oils, saturated, mono- and polyunsaturated fatty acids, on the type and extent of arterial lesions—need more cases studied
Obesity	obesity and body build as related to severity of lesions in young males and females.

A number of important relationships among risk factors and lesion components—both cellular and chemical—are becoming available for systematic studies, particularly for these age-race-sex groups. Among these are the data on DNA lipoprotein phenotypes, a number of which are revealing new relationships to lesion extent and severity. Similarly, the data on apolipoproteins in the sera and in the lesions as well as the immunological assessments being made on the serum and on the lesions are definitely pioneering efforts.

Although it is not the purpose of this report to present any data or conclusions, several of the most productive investigations yielding important data from both the core study and the specialized studies are given in TABLES 4 and 5. Here the most obvious impending relationships of lesions to quantitative results of risk factors and other corollary measurements are given. Much of the quantitation of lesions has been carried out by a time-

TABLE 5. The Measurements Made in Special Studies Centers and Trends Being Evaluated

Correlates	Initiating Center	Study Status
Microthrombi in standard samples by SEM as related to blood lipids, characteristics of lesions, use of tobacco (thiocyanate), t-lymphocytes, macrophages, etc.	Georgia (Chandler)	many cases studied; correlations with smoking and definitive paper being prepared for publication
Phenotypic modulation (shift to synthetic cell type in the intima); being evaluated and quantitated to help to determine onset of progressive atherogenesis	Georgia (Rao)	numerous cases evaluated; correlations with lesion lipid staining, other cells in lesions, CT pattern, etc., being pursued
Collagen types I–V as determined by immunohistochemistry correlated with position in plaque and with newly discovered CT patterns	Alabama (Gay)	determinations have covered most of special study cases distributed
T-lymphocytes in developing lesions as an indicator of immune interactions to alter the histogenesis of atherosclerosis	Illinois (Emeson, Robertson)	to document, quantitate, and correlate with the pathogenetic mechanisms which involve cellular immune reactions
Viral antigens and viral genomes in early lesions correlated with size and the cells of plaques	Illinois (Yamashiroya, Robertson)	progressing well and capable of numerous correlations
Mast cells, histamine, and other vasoactive amines and their contribution to lesion severity and artery vasospasm	Vanderbilt (Virmani, Atkinson)	leading to a better understanding of the factors involved in arterial reaction to catecholamines and the contribution of spasm to atherosclerosis
Quantitative data on cellular populations in lesions correlatedwith "lesion prone" and "lesion resistant" areas, various parts of the aorta, and coronary arteries	Chicago (Wissler, Vesselinovitch, Komatsu, Kusumi)	yielding quantitative data and being related to data from several other determinations, (*i.e.,* apolipoproteins, lesion size, and lipid localization)
Quantitation of apolipoproteins B, E, Lp(a), etc. in standard core samples correlated with lesion severity, etc.	Chicago (Wissler, Vesselinovitch, Komatsu)	excellent progress with all case samples; results correlated with "lesion prone," "lesion resistant" areas, etc.
Immune complexes in serum correlated with lesion architecture and cellular makeup of the developing plaque, immunocomplexes in lesions, etc.	Chicago (Wissler, Vesselinovitch, Ko)	progressing, with preliminary results presented and published
Three-dimensional quantitation of lesion components including lipid deposits, SMC, macrophages, foam cells, etc., to correlate with risk factors, transfer of lipid, etc. using confocal laser light scope	Baylor (Smith)	new technology offers promise; reported in preliminary results
Trans-cis fatty acids and lesion characteristics	West Virginia (Jagannathan)	useful data being generated which should be valuable when related to the other lesion components, especially lesion progression and fatty acids in triglycerides

continued

TABLE 5. *Continued.*

Correlates	Initiating Center	Study Status
Quantitation of proteoglycans in lesion samples and their changes with risk factors and progression	West Virginia (Jagannathan)	may be especially important in diabetes and hypertension; too early to evaluate
Quantitation of collagen in standard samples using microchemical approaches to relate to location of sample, risk factors, type of artery, blood and tissue lipid, etc.	Alabama (Miller)	excellent progress in obtaining data and utilizing it for comparing coronary and aortic analyses
Tissue lipid chemistry to correlate with types of lesions known to result from consumption of various food fats (coconut oil, peanut oil, fish oil, olive oil, etc.)	LSU (Strong, (Malcom)	abundant data being generated which can be correlated with many lesion components being measured

honored system of grading gross extent of atheromatous lesions which was developed at Louisiana State University,[10] which recently has been found to agree with the computer-assisted quantitative method of evaluating the extent of atheromatous plaques developed /at the Ohio State University. The latter system is being utilized for numerous studies involving PDAY and other cases. It makes it possible to quantitate overall disease and to give a quantitative and topographical rendition of the extent of disease in any given sample being used for specialized studies in this research program.

A number of other determinations are being made on very large numbers of cases and can, for all practical purposes, be thought of as core data. These include the extensive fatty acid analyses on adipose tissue being carried out at Louisiana State University, hepatic DNA analyses which are being performed at the Southwest Foundation for Biomedical Research, and the quantitative gross and microscopic morphometric analyses being performed at the Ohio State University. The latter make it possible to compare the disease at five-year age intervals in the right coronary artery versus the thoracic aorta versus the abdominal aorta. Furthermore, lesion thickness, both grossly and microscopically, as well as certain other state of the art quantitative measurements of the developing intimal arterial disease are proving to be of great value as correlates of risk factors. They hold promise as correlates of the development of certain cellular and immunohistochemical aspects of the ahterosclerotic plaque.

Several of the results being obtained from the specialized study centers also appear to be making important original contributions to our understanding of the development and the progression of atherosclerosis in young people (TABLE 5).

The detailed studies being carried out at the Medical College of Georgia are focused on the intimal surface of both the aorta and the anterior descending coronary arteries at standardized sites. The scanning electronmicroscopic data derived from these autopsies with less than twelve hour postmortem intervals utilize sufficiently large artery samples to make it possible to scan areas of the intimal arterial surface so that sampling bias can be diminished.[11] The results indicate that microthrombi can be found in some cases and not in others, thus making it possible to relate the findings to some of the prevalent risk factors.

The second specialized study being conducted at the Medical College of Georgia Center is aimed at quantitating the relative distribution of smooth muscle cell phenotypes expressing vimentin, desmin, myosin, and two different forms of actin at the light microscopic level, using immunohistochemical reagents to identify the presence of these cytoskeletal proteins as a measure of differentiation of the cell population and as an indicator of lesion activity. Ultimately these studies should be able to differentiate relatively quiescent intimal thickening of the "diffuse fibrous" type from the active, developing, frequently lipid laden, and progressing atheromatous lesions.

Another specialized study of note is that being carried out at the University of Alabama School of Medicine at Birmingham. Advanced techniques in collagen biochemistry and collagen immunohistochemistry are applied to the samples from young individuals. Specific antibodies for human collagen types I, II, III, IV, and V are being utilized to identify, quantitate, and map the pattern of collagen deposition in various parts of the plaque. Over 250 cases have now been studied using the indirect immunofluorescence technique and polyclonal as well as monoclonal antibodies which have been fully characterized for their titer and specificity. The determinations are performed on unfixed cryostat sections and are revealing collagen patterns in the paracellular and interstitial matrix of the various defined parts of the artery (endothelial, subendothelial, and medial) for each sample. These results are being correlated with new collagen and elastin patterns which have been discovered to be quite frequent in the small raised lesions in both core and special study samples being examined at the University of Chicago Center. It is evident that some of the unusual collagen patterns in the developing lesions may be of considerable importance relative to the risk factor stimuli which are involved and in limiting the aterial medial involvement by lesions.

Other aspects of the pathobiology of these atheromatous lesions in young people being studied at the University of Illinois are relating the T-lymphocyte population of these early atherosclerotic lesions to risk factors and to a number of morphometric observations being made both at Ohio State University and at the University of Illinois.[12] Furthermore, these data can be meaningfully related to the quantitative observations being made at the University of Chicago Center, where the monocyte-derived macrophages of these lesions in young people are being quantitated in the core samples from both the left anterior descending arteries and the standard samples of the aorta. The University of Illinois researchers are now collecting this kind of quantitative data on the formalin fixed samples and are collecting data on the presence of herpes simplex virus (HSV) and cytomegalovirus (CMV) DNA by in situ hybridization and viral antigen by immunocytochemical methods in cells of atherosclerotic plaques.[13] These data are being quantitatively correlated with a number of characteristics of the atheromatous lesions and with the risk factors which are being measured. Viral DNA and viral antigen data are also being obtained in liver and spleen samples of these same cases.

At the Vanderbilt University School of Medicine Center, the histamine, serotonin, and the total catecholamines in standard arterial samples and their relationships to the extent and type of atherosclerosis and to known risk factors are being examined. This study also involves a measure of vascular spasm in selected samples as a possible mechanism of endothelial injury and quantitation of mast cells in relation to these developing atheromatous lesions. These cellular and chemical responses of the arteries during this period of atherosclerotic lesion development can be related not only to risk factors, but also to the cellular phenomena being quantitated at the other specialized Centers of research, notably at the Medical College of Georgia, the University of Illinois, and the University of Chicago, all of which are studying adjacent samples from identical cases which have been carefully selected and balanced to offer the best opportunity to obtain significant results.

At the University of Chicago Study Center, major emphasis is being placed on the quantitation of the monocyte-derived macrophages and the quantitation, both morphometrically and microchemically, of several of the apolipoproteins in the lesions, especially apo B and E, and Lp(a). Furthermore, progress is being made in quantitating immune complexes in the serum of patients and in the atheromatous artery.

The data from all of these special studies will be related to many of the risk factors being studied, as well as to the cellular, biochemical, and the connective tissue phenomena being observed at other special study centers as soon as suffieicnt numbers of observations are available to make this a worthwhile undertaking.

As part of the intensive investigation of the cells of the developing plaque and their relationship to connective tissue and lipoprotein elements in the plaque, Baylor College of Medicine in Houston has been exploring the three-dimensional study of microscopic elements of the plaque utilizing the laser scanning confocal microscope. A recent report by this group at the International Conference on Atherosclerosis and Cardiovascular Disease in Bologna has indicated considerable promise for this improved methodology.

The other major components of these specialized studies are those being performed on the core biochemical samples of thoracic aorta, abdominal aorta, and left circumflex coronary arteries. The most intensive and extensive studies of these arterial specimens are being carried out at Louisiana State University, where not only total cholesterol, free cholesterol, esterified cholesterol, cholesteryl ester fatty acids and phospholipid analyses are performed, but samples of lipid-free arterial residue are prepared and distributed to the Medical School of West Virginia and the University of Alabama School of Medicine in Birmingham. These residues are analyzed for proteoglycans at West Virginia and for certain types of collagens at Alabama. The LSU Core Center also helps to process and distribute suitable processed frozen samples of liver and spleen to both the University of Illinois Center and the Southwest Foundation Center for the analyses involving viral genome (University of Illinois) and DNA probes (Southwest Foundation). The Louisiana State University Center also performs fatty acid analyses on adipose tissue and contributes lipid-containing samples which can be used for trans- and cis-fatty acid analyses at the West Virginia Center.

The utilization of common chemical samples of arteries for several of these determinations makes it possible to interpret the results in relation to the total lesion and in turn to relate the chemical results to the cellular and histochemical results. These studies are greatly facilitated by the adjacent anatomical location of chemical and core histological samples.

Contributions to the Future That the PDAY Study is Likely to Foster

The space limitations of this paper and the relatively early stages of the study make it impossible to evaluate completely the contributions which its results may make to the research carried out on human and experimental atherosclerosis in the next decade or two.

Nevertheless, it is clear that results are likely to provide in quantitative terms the clearest, the least biased, and the most accurate information to date on how the various components and the several measurable dimensions of the atherosclerotic lesions develop during a period of life, *i.e.*, from 25 through 34 years of age, when the plaques are beginning to become raised and progressive in those who are most at risk. As these data are correlated with risk factors and with the detailed data on the cellular and chemical makeup of the lesions, it seems likely that new insights and new relationships will be found so that one will be able to design enlightened intervention trials to interrupt the progression of atherogenesis.

Furthermore, it seems likely that some of the more conspicuous paradoxes of lesion formation and progression as related to race and sex should be resolved by the increased knowledge of what is happening to the cellular and chemical constitutents of these lesions. The more conspicuous fatty streaks in the aortas of young females and in particular in the aortas from young black females, and the definite tendency for raised lesion progression to occur in the male aorta, are examples of paradoxes[6,14] which are being confirmed in this study but which remain to be explained. When sufficient female cases are obtained, it should be possible to design studies to explain these phenomena in relation to some of the risk factors being analyzed—especially those in the lipid/lipoprotein/DNA and hypertension areas.

The results of studies being carried out at the Medical College of Georgia should, as they are related to risk factors and lesion severity, help to:

1. provide some areas needing further study in relation to the sporadic and relative infrequency of the microthrombi;
2. establish the basis for further work to determine the usefulness of a phenotypic classification of "smooth muscle cells" as a way to differentiate more easily the developing plaque from diffuse intimal thickening and/or the "cushion lesion."[15,16]

The interesting connective tissue patterns discovered and described at the University of Chicago in these early lesions, *i.e.*, the condensed collagen often observed under the internal elastic lamina (IEL) and the frequent presence of the condensed elastin near the intimal surface, will serve as a stimulus for further study of the process by which the fiber proteins are produced by the smooth muscle cells. They may offer a prospect of learning more about the form of the collagen and the elastin which is present in these curious patterns. They may help to determine whether collagen in combination with proteoglycans may be of more importance than the IEL in binding the lower density lipoproteins, and in limiting the early lesions to the intima.

The work at the University of Illinois is most promising. Thus far, it appears that viruses and T-lymphocytes are found very commonly in early atheromatous lesions. As the evidence increases that injurious immune phenomena at the cellular level may be important in atherogenesis,[17-20] it seems possible that viral antigens may trigger some of these autoimmune phenomena or even be a part of "immune complex" formation. Furthermore, there is increasing evidence of the correlation of immune complexes, monocyte-derived macrophages, T-lymphocytes, and other components of immunological injury in the lesions with the production of autoimmune reactions by increased amounts of oxidized LDL and/or oxidized VLDL in the lesions. It now appears that we will need several studies of the frequency and severity of the immunological aspect of atherosclerosis in human arteries before we will understand more completely its contribution to the progression of atherosclerosis. At present, our own studies indicate that between 10 and 20% of human cases may have an immunological component to their coronary artery lesions.[21,22] This number may increase substantially as we learn to recognize the more subtle arterial architectural, cellular, and other pathobiological influences of immune complex phenomena. The special studies of the catecholamines, histamine, and serotonin will build on the evidence previously presented by the Vanderbilt group and others[23-25] implicating these substances and the arterial mast cell population of the artery in liberating these substances, coupled with various types of functional studies.

The localization of low density lipoproteins in the lesions of these young people, which differs in areas where the disease progresses as compared to areas where it is likely to remain stationary, can be quantitated both immunohistochemically and by extraction and by microimmunochemical analysis. This is proving to be a very useful quantitative determination. The same is true of the enumeration of monocyte-derived macrophages, whether or not they are loaded with lipid (FIGS. 2 and 3) and the overwhelming predominance of lipid-laden smooth muscle cells (FIGS. 4 and 5). Of almost equal interest is the lack of evidence that Lp(a) localizes in the lesions. So far, most of the positive staining of the sections with antibodies to Lp(a) seems to be localized at the lumenal surface of the artery intima with only a little staining of internal artery wall elements, mostly in or on macrophages.

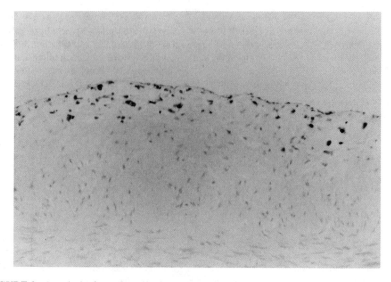

FIGURE 2. A typical "fatty plaque" which may be considered to be the transitional raised lesion between a "fatty streak" and a "fibrous plaque." It is located in the "lesion prone" area of sample #44 of the left anterior descending (LAD) coronary artery. It is prepared using HAM 56 as the primary antibody and the Vector Elite ABC Kit. It is clear that the relatively small numbers of monocytes and monocyte-derived macrophages are located in the superficial part of this rather thick lipid containing lesion.

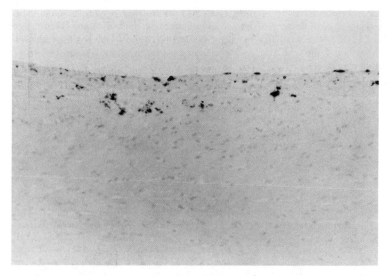

FIGURE 3. A typical "fatty streak" in the "lesion prone" dorsal area of the thoracic aorta (sample #1) of the same case as that shown in FIGURE 2 and prepared in the same way with the same reagents. This rather flat lipid-rich lesion contains only a few HAM 56 positive cells located in all layers of the slightly thickened intima.

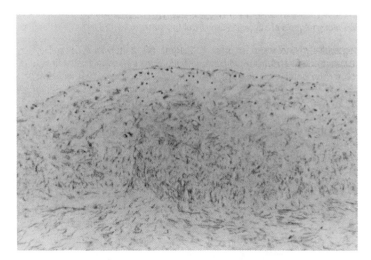

FIGURE 4. This is an adjacent section from the same sample #44 shown in FIGURE 2 and prepared using HHF 35 to identify smooth muscle cells in the lesion using the Vector Elite ABC peroxidase method. The photomicrograph is from the same lesion prone area and shows that the majority of cells in the fatty plaque are positive for the smooth muscle antigen which this reagent specifically identifies. Also note the small dark cells in the superficial area of the lesion. These are probably lymphocytes.

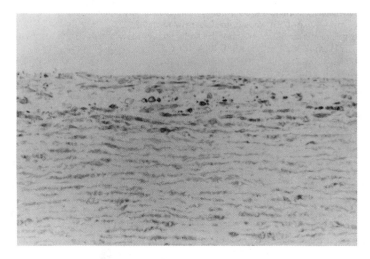

FIGURE 5. This is an adjacent section from the same sample #1 from the thoracic aorta as shown in FIGURE 3. It shows the same area of the same fatty streak. It is prepared using the same HHF 35 antibody used to prepare the section shown in FIGURE 4. Note that most of the cells of the lesion with methyl green positive nucleus stains are also positive for this antigen. The picture shows a number of cells which might be called ''foam cells'' which are strongly positive for the SMC actin antigen.

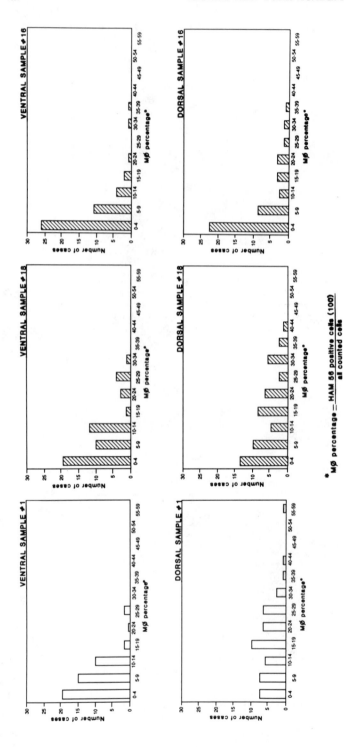

FIGURE 6. Histograms showing that there is a strong trend in the aorta for the dorsal (lesion prone) areas of samples #1 and #18 to have a larger population of monocyte/macrophages than the ventral areas. No such trend is seen in sample #16 where the aortic lesions are likely to progress most rapidly with age. The *bar graphs* give the number of times on the vertical axis that these 50 cases showed the percentage of positive monocyte/macrophages (MØ) cells shown on the horizontal axis.

The quantitation of the cells of sections which have been allowed to react with antibodies to monocyte-derived macrophages has already indicated results which are highly correlated with the presence or absence of lipid-containing lesions (FIG. 6).

It is likely that continuation of these studies will provide many opportunities to correlate these cytological, biochemical, and immunological findings with known risk factors as well as providing a national and international resource for future investigations. These studies are likely to lead to a number of new concepts concerning the pathogenesis and progression of atheromatous lesions in young people.

ACKNOWLEDGMENTS

The authors thank Gertrud Friedman, Cynthia Chamberlain, and Alexander Arguelles for their help in preparing the manuscript.

PATHOBIOLOGICAL DETERMINANTS OF ATHEROSCLEROSIS IN YOUTH

Participating Institutions and Investigators

Program Director
Robert W. Wissler, PhD, MD, University of Chicago; Associate Director: Abel L. Robertson, Jr., MD, PhD, The University of Illinois
Steering Committee
J. Fredrick Cornhill, PhD, The Ohio State University; Henry C. McGill, Jr., MD, and C. Alex McMahan, PhD, The University of Texas Health Science Center at San Antonio; Abel L. Robertson, Jr., MD, PhD, The University of Illinois; Jack P. Strong, MD, Louisiana State University Medical Center; Robert W. Wissler, PhD, MD, University of Chicago
Convener of Protocol and Manual of Operations Committee
Margaret C. Oalmann, Dr. P.H., Louisiana State University Medical Center
Internal Advisory Committee
Jack C. Geer, MD, University of Alabama; James E. Grizzle, PhD, F. Hutchinson Cancer Center, Seattle, WA; Paul E. Lacy, MD, Washington University School of Medicine; Robert W. Prichard, MD, Wake Forest University; Robert Selzer, MS, Jet Propulsion Laboratory, California Institute of Technology
Participating Centers
University of Alabama, Birmingham, AL. UAB Medical Center: Principal Investigator: Steffen Gay, MD; Coinvestigators: Renate E. Gay, MD, Guo-quiang Huang, MD [HL-33733]; UAB Department of Biochemistry: Principal Investigator: Edward J. Miller, PhD; Coinvestigators: Donald K. Furuto, PhD, Margaret S. Vail, Annie J. Narkates [HL-33728]*
Albany Medical College, Albany, NY. Principal Investigator: Assaad Daoud, MD; Coinvestigators: Adriene S. Frank, PhD, Mary A. Hyer, E. Carol McGovem [HL-33765]
Baylor College of Medicine, Houston, TX. Principal Investigator: Louis C. Smith, PhD [HL-33750]
University of Chicago, Chicago, IL. Principal Investigator: Robert W. Wissler, PhD, MD; Coinvestigators: Dragoslava Vesselinovitch, DVM, MS, Akio Komatsu, MD, PhD, R. Timothy Bridenstine, MS, Robert J. Stein, MD, Robert H. Kirschner, MD, PhD,

Manuela Bekermeier, HTL (ASCP), Blanche Berger, HTL (ASCP), Laura Hiltscher, HTL (ASCP) [HL-33740]

The University of Illinois, Chicago, IL. Principal Investigator: Abel L. Robertson, Jr., MD, PhD; Coinvestigators: Robert J. Stein, MD, Eugene E. Emeson, MD, Luna Ghosh, MD, Herbert M. Yamashiroya, PhD, Robert J. Buschmann, PhD; Assistant Investigator: Janes J. Gabrovsek, DDS, Collection: Edmund R. Donoghue, Jr., MD, Robert H. Kirschner, MD, PhD, Tae Lyong An, MD, Michael Chambliss, MD, Eupil Choi, MD, Nancy Jones, MD, Mary I. Jumbelic, MD, Mitra S. Kalelkar, MD, Uuksel Konakci, MD, Barry Lifschultz, MD, Michael I. Schaffer, PhD, Shaku Teas, MD, Margarita Amuza, MD, James Dianovsky, BA, Frances Norris, HTL (ASCP), Donald Waterford, BA, Special Studies: Mei-Ling Shen, PhD, Richard Yang, MS, Frances Norris, HTL (ASCP), Dana Gylys, HT (ASCP) [HL-33758]

Louisiana State University Medical Center, New Orleans, LA. Principal Investigator: Jack P. Strong, MD; Coinvestigators: Gray T. Malcom, PhD, William P. Newman Ill, MD, Margaret C. Oalmann, Dr PH, Paul S. Roheim, MD, Ashim K. Bhattacharyya, PhD, Miguel A. Guzman, PhD, Ali A. Hatem, MD, Conrad A. Hornick, PhD, Carlos D. Restrepo, MD, Richard E. Tracy, MD, PhD [HL-33746]

University of Maryland, Baltimore, MD. Principal Investigator: Wolfgang J. Mergner, MD, PhD; Coinvestigators: Margaret L. Couture, PhD, James H. Resau, PhD, Robert D. Vigorito, MS, PA, Q.-C. Yu, MD, PhD [HL-33752]

Medical College of Georgia, Augusta, GA. Co-Principal Investigators: A. Bleakley Chandler, MD, Raghunatha N. Rao, MD; Coinvestigators: D. Greer Falls, MD, Benjamin O. Spurlock, BA; Associate Investigators: Kalish B. Sharma, MD, Joel S. Sexton, MD; Research Assistants: P.M. Faliman, BS, G.W. Forbes (HL-33772]

University of Nebraska Medical Center, Omaha, NE. Principal Investigator: Bruce M. McManus, MD, PhD; Coinvestigators: Jerry W. Jones, MD, Todd J. Kendall, MS, Jerrold A. Remmenga, BS, William C. Rogler, BS [HL-33778]

The Ohio State University, Columbus, OH. Principal Investigator: J. Fredrick Cornhill, PhD; Coinvestigators: William R. Adrion, MD, Patrick M. Fardel, MD, Brian Gara, MS, Edward Herderick, BS, John Meimer, MS, Larry R. Tate, MD [HL-33760]

Southwest Foundation for Biomedical Research, San Antonio, TX. Principal Investigator: James E. Hixson, PhD [HL-39913]

The University of Texas Health Science Center at San Antonio, San Antonio, TX. Principal Investigator: C. Alex McMahan, PhD; Coinvestigators: George M. Barnwell, PhD, Henry C. McGill, Jr., MD, Yolan N. Marinez, MA, Thomas J. Prihoda, PhD, Herman S. Wigodsky, MD, PhD [HL-33749]

Vanderbilt University, Nashville, TN. Principal Investigator: Renu Virmani, MD; Coinvestigators: James B. Atkinson, MD, PhD, Charles W. Harlan, MD [HL-33770]

West Virginia University Health Sciences Center, Morgantown, WV. Principal Investigator: Singanallur N. Jagannathan, PhD; Coinvestigators: Bruce Caterson, PhD, James L. Frost, MD, K. Murali K. Rao, MD, Nathaniel F. Rodman, MD [HL-33748]

*Brackets [] indicate number of National Heart, Lung, and Blood Institute grant.

REFERENCES

1. McGILL, H. C., JR. 1968. Fatty streaks in the coronary arteries and aorta. Lab. Invest. **18:** 560–564.
2. STRONG, J. P. & H. C. McGILL, JR. 1969. The pediatric aspects of atherosclerosis. J. Atheroscler. Res. **9:** 251–265.
3. STRONG, J.P. 1986. Coronary atherosclerosis in soldiers. A clue to the natural history of atherosclerosis in the young. J. Am. Med. Soc. **256:** 2863–2866.
4. OALMANN, M. C., G. T. MALCOM, V. T. TOCA, M. A. GUZMAN & J. P. STRONG. 1981.

Community pathology of atherosclerosis and coronary heart disease: postmortem serum cholesterol and extent of coronary atherosclerosis. Am. J. Epidemiol. **113:** 396–403.

5. ROCK, W.A., JR., M. C. OALMANN, H. C. STARY, R. E. TRACY, M. T. MCMURRY, R. W. PALMER, R. A. WELSH & J. P. STRONG. 1972. A standardized method for evaluating myocardial and coronary artery lesions. *In* The Pathogenesis of Atherosclerosis. R. W. Wissler & J. C. Geer, Eds. 247–260. The Williams & Wilkins Company. Baltimore, MD.

6. STRONG, J. P., M. C. OALMANN, W. P. NEWMAN III., R. E. TRACY, G. T. MALCOM, W. D. JOHNSON, L. H. MCMAHAN, W. A. ROCK, JR., & M. A. GUZMAN. 1984. Coronary heart disease in young black and white males in New Orleans: Community Pathology Study. Am. Heart J. 108(Part 2): 747–759.

7. SOLBERG, L. A. & J. P. STRONG. 1983. Risk factors and atherosclerotic lesions. A review of autopsy studies. Arteriosclerosis **3:** 187–198.

8. WISSLER, R. W., D. VESSELINOVITCH, A. KOMATSU & R. R. BRIDENSTINE. 1988. The arterial wall and atherosclerosis in youth. *In* Biology of the Arterial Wall. 265–274. CIC Edizioni Internazionali. Rome.

9. CORNHILL, J. F., E. E. HERDERICK & H. C. STARY. 1990. Topography of human aortic sudanophilic lesions. Monogr. Atherosclerosis. 13–19. Karger. Basel.

10. GUZMAN, M. A., C. A. MCMAHAN, H. C. MCGILL, JR., J. P. STRONG, C. TEJADA, C. RESTREPO, D. A. EGGEN, W. B. ROBERTSON & L. A. SOLBERG. 1968. Selected methodologic aspects of the International Atherosclerosis Project. Lab. Invest. **18(5):** 479–497.

11. SPURLOCK, B. O., & A. B. CHANDLER. 1987. Adherent platelets and surface microthrombi of the human aorta and the left (anterior descending) coronary artery: a scanning electron microscopy feasibility study. Scanning Microsc. **1:** 1359–1365.

12. EMESON, E. E. & A. L. ROBERTSON. 1988. T = lymphocytes in aorta and coronary intimas—their potential role in atherogenesis. Am. J. Pathol. **130:** 359–369.

13. YAMASHIROYA, J. H., L. GHOSH, R. YANG & A. L. ROBERTSON, JR. 1988. Herpesviridae in coronary arteries and aorta of young trauma victims. Am. J. Pathol. **130:** 71–79.

14. TEJADA, C., J. P. STRONG, M. R. MONTENEGRO, C. RESTREPO & L. A. SOLBERG. 1968. Distribution of coronary and aortic atherosclerosis by geographic location, race, and sex. Lab. Invest. **18(5):** 509–526.

15. CAMPBELL, G. R. & J. H. CAMPBELL. 1985. Smooth muscle phenotypic changes in arterial wall homeostasis: implications for the pathogenesis of atherosclerosis. Exp. Mol. Pathol. **42:** 139–162.

16. MOSSE, P. R. L., G. R. CAMPBELL, Z. L. WANG & J. H. CAMPBELL 1985. Smooth muscle phenotypic expressions in human carotid arteries. I. Comparison of cells from diffuse intimal thickening adjacent to atheromatous plaques with those of the media. Lab. Invest. **53:** 556–562.

17. STEINBERG, D., S. PARTHASARATHY, T. E. CAREW, J. C. KHOO & J. L. WITZTUM. 1989. Beyond cholesterol: modifications of low-density lipoprotein that increase its atherogenicity. N. Engl. J. Med. **320:** 915–924.

18. JURGENS, G., H. F. HOFF, G. M. CHISOLM III & H. ESTERBAUER. 1987. Modification of human serum low density lipoprotein by oxidation—characterization and pathophysiological implications. Chem. Phys. Lipids **45:** 315–336.

19. JONASSON, L., J. HOLM, O. SKALLI, G. BONDJERS & G. K. HANSSON. 1986. Regional accumulations of T cells, macrophages, and smooth muscle cells in the human atherosclerotic plaque. Arteriosclerosis **6:** 131–138.

20. OREKHOV, A. N., V. V. TERTOV & D. N. MUKHIN. 1989. Atherogenic factors of atherosclerotic patients' blood plasma. I. Modified low density lipoproteins. 29. European Atherosclerosis Society. Linkoping.

21. WISSLER, R. W., D. VESSELINOVITCH, H. R. DAVIS P. H. LAMBERT & M. BEKERMEIER. 1985. A new way to look at atherosclerotic involvment of the artery wall and the functional effects. Ann. N.Y. Acad. Sci. **454:** 9–22.

22. WISSLER, R. W., D. VESSELINOVITCH & C. KO. 1989. The effects of circulating immune complexes on atherosclerotic lesions in experimental animals and in younger and older humans. Transplant Proc. **21:** 3707–3708.

23. ATKINSON, J. B., L. J. ROBERTS, K. A. AULSEBROOK, C. E. HARLAN & R. VIRMANI. 1987. Role of histamine in atherogenesis. Arteriosclerosis **7:** 53a.

24. ATKINSON, J. B., L. J. ROBERTS, K. AULSEBROOK, C. E. HARLAN & R. VIRMANI. 1988. The role of histamine in progression of atherosclerosis in the young. Circulation **78:** II–146
25. ATKINSON, J.B., R. VIRMANI, M. V. TANTENGCO, W. H. MERRILL, W. H. FRIST, & R. M. ROBERTSON. 1989. Influence of age and atherosclerosis on coronary reactivity. Lab. Invest. **60:** 39.

Effects of Preceding Mural Thrombus on the Pathogenesis of Final Obstructive Coronary Thrombosis

TAKESHI SHOZAWA

Second Department of Pathology
Akita University School of Medicine
1-1-1 Hondo
Akita 010, Japan

INTRODUCTION

Occlusive thrombosis of coronary artery in patients with acute myocardial infarction (AMI) is usually considered to be caused by the sudden break of the brittle lining of atherosclerotic lesions. However, the older part of the thrombus that was often seen in the deep zone, at the thrombus-plaque or -ulcer interface was insufficiently studied. In the coronary arteries of patients who died suddenly of ischemic heart disease, recent thrombi often covered over atheromatous plaque fissures, and most coronary thrombi have a layered structure of thrombus material of differing age. Exact knowledge of the relationship between the older part of coronary thrombus and plaque ulcers in patients with AMI is lacking. In fresh thrombosis, the older part of thrombus indicates recent thrombus.

In this study, the early stages of coronary thrombi of AMI were studied histologically in an attempt to clarify the topographical relationship between recent thrombi and plaque ulcers with respect to the pathogenesis of fatal coronary thrombosis.

MATERIALS AND METHODS

In this study, hearts of 37 AMI patients with recent thrombus material in the deep layer of thrombosis in the coronary artery supplying the necrotic myocardium were selected from 64 AMI patients who had died within 4–5 days from onset and were necropsied within 3 hours after death. The patients were from Akita, between 1977 and 1989. All patients had transmural infarction with an area of myocardial destruction of 3 cm or greater in at least one dimension. Twenty-two were male with a mean age 70.6 ± 9.24 years, ranging from 42 to 83. The rest were female with a mean age 71.1 ± 5.37 years, ranging from 60 to 77. Mean heart weight was 419.3 ± 80.94 g, ranging from 300 to 610 g in males and 406.8 ± 65.91 g, ranging from 320 to 580 g in females.

The hearts were cut transversely at the apical third and fixed carefully in formalin. After fixation, three main stems, including epicardial main branches were removed from the heart. After decalcification, they were carefully cut transversely in segments of 3 to 4 mm. The segments were carefully inspected, diagrammatically sketched, and marked on the proximal site of the specimen with india ink. They were then dehydrated, embedded in paraffine and sectioned. When fresh or organizing thrombi or intimal hemorrhage were present, both the diseased segments of the coronary artery and the segments just proximal and distal to them were sectioned transversely and for each, two 5-micron-thick sections were picked up, at a distance of 50 microns apart. One section was stained with elastica Masson's trichrome stain and the other was stained with Hematoxylin-eosin or phosphotangstic acid hematoxylin. The hearts were cut into slices 1 cm thick and at least 2 slices, at 5 cm and at 2 cm from the apex, were embedded in paraffin in order to determine the site, size, and age of the infarcted area.

AMI age was determined by clinical data and histological age using Mallory's criteria modified with Lodge-Patch's and Bouchadry and Majno's findings. The hearts were divided in two groups showing myocardial changes within 24 hours and from 2 to 5 days after onset. AMI at more than 5 days from onset was excluded from this study.

Coronary thrombi were classified into 4 stages—fresh, recent, organizing, and organized. Fresh thrombi consist of tightly packed but discernible platelets, red cells, and white cells entrapped in fibrin, often with Zahn's line present (less than 2 days of age). Recent thrombi appear homogenously compact with small slitlike spaces and sometimes with spindle shaped mesenchymal cells sprouting from the vessel wall (less than 6 days). Organizing thrombi showed a proliferation of small vessels and deposition of collagen fibrils and hemosiderin. Later the number of collagen fibers increased and recanalization progressed gradually (less than 3 weeks). Organized thrombi show the formation of fewer but larger channels of small vessels (over 3 weeks).

TABLE 1. Types of Acute Coronary Lesions Where Recent Thrombi Had Adhered and Number of Cases Who Died of AMI within the First 24 Hours, and between 2 and 5 Days

Type of Acute Coronary Lesion[a]	Age of AMI		Total
	<24 Hours	From 2 to 5 Days	
I = a	10	20	30
I = b		2	2
II = a	1	2	3
II = b	1	1	2
Total	12	25	37

[a]Type I, recent thrombus combined with plaque ulcer: a) with hemorrhage in the atheroma; and b) with no hemorrhage in the atheroma. Type II, recent thrombus adhered to the thick intima: a) with hemorrhage in the atheroma; and b) with no hemorrhage in the atheroma.

RESULTS

Recent thrombi located in the deep layer of the coronary thrombosis were classified into two main groups according to whether they were associated with plaque ulcers or not (TABLE 1.) The first group associated with plaque ulcers of the atheroma was further classified into two subgroups with or without intraatheromatous hemorrhage (Type I-a and I-b). The second group with no ulcers in the thick intima or plaque, was also classified in two subgroups with and without intraatheromatous hemorrhage (Type II-a and II-b). The number of cases in each group with respect to AMI age is shown in TABLE 1. All thrombosis within the coronary artery was occlusive except for 2 cases of between 2 to 5 days of age in Type I-a.

Recent thrombi were usually located in the severely stenosed arterial segment, fixed in eroded intima and usually associated with hemorrhage or edema in the underlying connective tissue. In Type I coronary lesions, recent thrombi were not located only near plaque ulcers, but in the opposite site to the ulcer. Sometimes, they covered plaque ulcers or ragged cloth-like plaque ulcers (FIGS. 1, 2, and 3). In cases 4–5 days of age, spindle

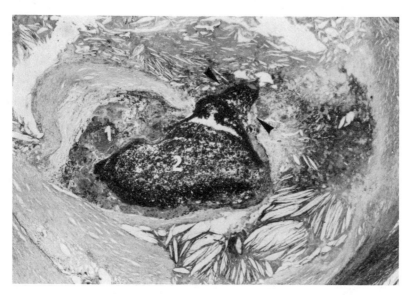

FIGURE 1. Transverse section of a Type I-a coronary lesion in a case of AMI, on the 2nd day from onset. Recent thrombi (1) occupied about half of the area, adhering to the thick atheroma capsule on the opposite site of the plaque rupture in a nodular shape. Fresh coagulation thrombus (2) in the right half of the lumen. Note the ulcer (▶ ◀) extending into the atheroma accompanied by hemorrhage. Stain: elastica and Masson's trichrome. × 10.

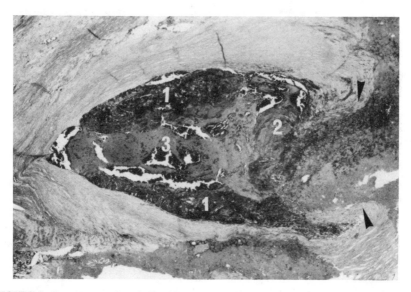

FIGURE 2. Transverse section of a Type I-a coronary lesion in a case of AMI within 24 hours from onset. Recent thrombi (1) are visible in the deep portion, which adhered to the intima near and on the opposite site to the rupture. More recent thrombus (2) sealed the volcano-like plaque rupture (▶ ◀). Fresh thrombus material (3) fills the area between these recent thrombi. Stain: elastica and Masson's trichrome. × 10.

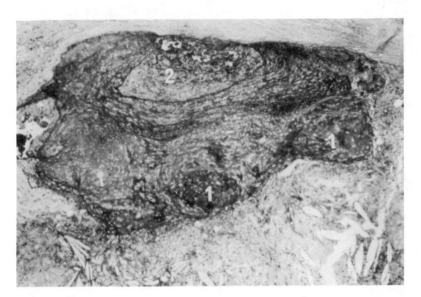

FIGURE 3. Transverse section of a Type I-a occluded artery from a patients who died on the 2nd day. A recent thrombus (1) sealed a ragged cloth-like plaque ulcer. Fresh thrombus (2) is filled in the upper half of the lumen. Stain: elastica and Masson's trichrome. ×20.

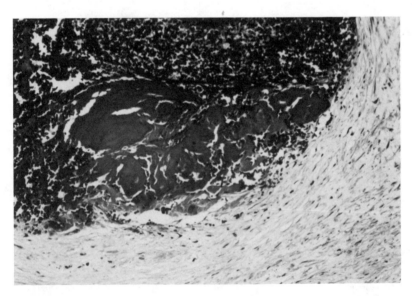

FIGURE 4. Basal portion of an occluded thrombus in a severely stenosed segment of the coronary artery of an AMI case within 24 hours from onset (Type II-b). A recent thrombus has adhered to the bleeding intima and a few spindle mesenchymal cells are sprouting into the basal portion from the underlying connective tissue. Stain: hematoxylin and eosin. × 50.

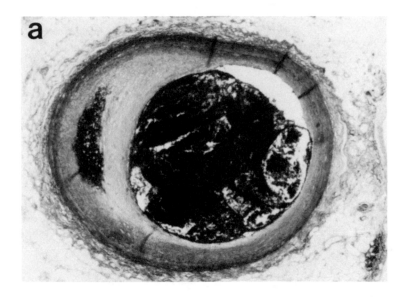

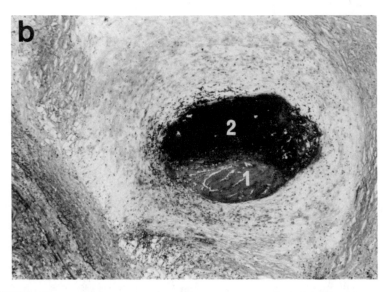

FIGURE 5. Two stepped transverse sections of the coronary artery of a 4–5-day Type II-a case. (**a**) The proximal section which is 4 mm apart from section (b), showed luminal dilatation and was filled by a red thrombus and intraatheromatous hemorrhage. (**b**) In the lower half of the occluded thrombus, a recent thrombus (1) adhered to the eroded thick edematous intima with hemorrhaging in the underlying connective tissue. Fresh thrombus (2) obliterated the rest of the lumen. Stain: elastica and Masson's trichrome. (a) × 5 and (b) × 20.

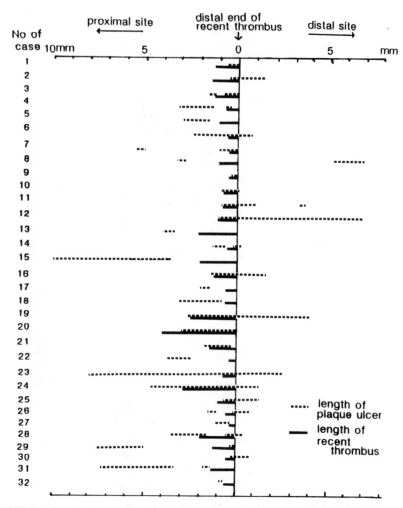

FIGURE 6. Length of recent thrombi and plaque ulcers and the topographical relationship between them in 32 cases of Type I.

mesenchymal cells sprouted into the base of the recent thrombi from the underlying connective tissue (FIGS. 4 and 5). The length of recent thrombi and plaque ulcers and the topographical relationship between them in a Type I coronary lesion is shown in FIG. 6. The length of recent thrombi and plaque ulcers varied from one case to another. In two third of cases, plaque ulcers were mainly located in the segment to which a recent thrombus adhered (FIGS. 1 and 2). Sometimes, they were also extended to the proximal or distal site, but were rarely found apart from the recent thrombus (FIG. 7). In Type I-a, both recent thrombi and plaque ulcers were seen in the height of the middle or distal third portion of the intraatheromatous hemorrhage. A plaque ulcer was sometimes located near the proximal end of the atheroma, causing a large hemorrhage to extend downwards into the atheroma to the level of the recent thrombus (FIG. 7).

The number of plaque ulcers also varied. Two or more plaque ulcers were found in 21 Type I cases. Of more than 53 plaque ulcers in total, 15 showed ulcers sealing with thrombosis, 6 went deep into the atheroma and the rest were ragged-cloth like ulcers.

Most fresh thrombi extending into the proximal site were red, and sometimes reached a few centimeters in length. Most fresh thrombi that covered recent thrombi and plaque ulcers were of varied types, extending in short distances distally, and transformed into red thrombi. In a few cases, white thrombi extended distally from a recent thrombus.

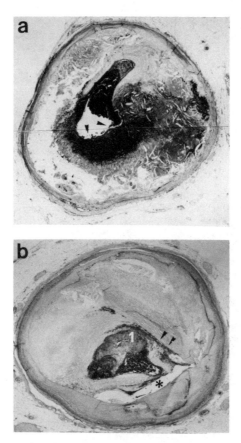

FIGURE 7. Two stepped transverse sections of the coronary artery in AMI on the 2nd day from onset. This case is the 15th case shown in FIGURE 6. (**a**) In the proximal segment 4 mm apart from the recent thrombus shown in (b), a large ulcer (▼ ▼) with intraatheromatous hemorrhage extends downward and communicates with the coronary lumen through rents near section (b). (**b**) Recent thrombus (1) adheres to the thick intima of the severely stenosed segment. In the underlying connective tissue, there is a hemorrhaging (▼ ▼), which is communicated with the atheroma cavity (*). Red cells on the inner surface of the cavity wall indicate that it was filled by fresh hemorrhaging. Stain: elastica and Masson's trichrome. × 5.

DISCUSSION

Organization of coronary thrombosis progresses in the same fashion as thrombosis observed in other arteries. Ridolfi *et al.* pointed out that fresh thrombi are usually formed in the first 48 hours and the subsequent changes which occur from 2 to 14 days after onset were histologically classified into early, middle and late stages. In this study, thrombi that he classified as early stage (from 2 to 5 days after onset) were used as recent thrombi. Thrombi of the other two stages were included in the organizing stage, because proliferation of mesenchymal cells and small vessels is a characteristic finding in granulation tissue. AMI age was divided in two groups; within the first 24 hours and from 2 to 5 days. If recent thrombi were found in the first group, acute lesions had begun earlier at the coronary arterial wall than had the formation of a fresh occluded thrombus within the lumen due to a plaque ulcer.

Crawford pointed out that in 2/3 of the cases he studied, recent thrombi were found in the deep zone of the fresh ones. Ridolfi *et al.* also observed that in 14% of the cases, the focal area of a thrombus that is several days older than the associated myocardial infarction was found in the deep layers covering a plaque ulcer. In patients with ischemic heart disease, recent thrombi which covered plaque ulcers of the atheroma seemed to play an important role in causing unstable angina or sudden death.

In this study, recent thrombi were not only found in 32 cases to be associated with plaque ulcers, but were also found in 5 coronary arterial lesions without plaque ulcers. In both groups, recent thrombi mainly adhered to the eroded thick intima of the coronary artery, showing over 75% luminal stenosis. In the underlying connective tissue, edema, bleeding, or degenerated collagen fibers were usually observed, and in some cases, sprouting of spindle mesenchymal cells into the recent thrombus was also seen. In the thick intima of Type II coronary lesion, modified smooth muscle cells and fine elastic fibers were proliferated. Lumen of the plaque ulcer segment were often wider than stenosed segments where recent thrombi had adhered. Plaque ulcers located in the proximal site away from any recent thrombi, were frequently associated with fresh red thrombosis within the arterial lumen, and hemorrhage into the atheroma.

These findings indicate that recent thrombi were induced at the intima of severely stenosed segments of the coronary artery earlier than or at least in the same stage as the formation of the plaque ulcer. Recent studies of flow patterns in poststenotic segments of the human coronary artery indicate that the volume of coronary flow decreased clearly in the severely stenosed segment. A prominent decrease in coronary flow might induce damage easily on the thick intima or atheromatic plaque of severely stenosed segments. The observation that ragged cloth-like ulcers made up over half of the 53 plaque ulcers in this study, and that layered structures with thrombus material of differing ages are often located at the thick intima of severely stenosed coronary arteries might support our opinion, although the destruction of the atheromatic plaque might also have progressed rapidly by hemorrhage in the atheroma.

SUMMARY

Of sixty-four acute myocardial infarcts showing myocardial necrosis within 5 days after onset, 37 had fresh coronary occlusive thrombi with recent thrombus in the deep layer. The recent thrombi were usually located in the severely stenosed segment of arteriosclerotic coronary arteries. They adhered to the intima not only near but on the opposite site to the plaque ulcers and sometimes covered the ulcer. In two thirds of the cases, both the recent thrombi and plaque ulcers were located in the same segment. In the others, the topographical relationship of plaque ulcers to recent thrombi in the longitudinal direction varied from one case to another. These findings show that the recent thrombus might play an important role in the formation of a fresh occlusive thrombus and plaque ulcer of coronary arteriosclerotic lesions.

REFERENCES

1. CHAPMAN, I. 1965. Arch. Pathol. **80:** 256–261.
2. CONSTANTINIDES, P. 1966. J. Atheroscler. Res. **6:** 1–7.
3. FRIEDMAN, M. & G. J. VAN BOVENKAMP. 1966. Am. J. Pathol. **48:** 19–44.
4. HORIE, T., M. SEKIGUCHI & K. HIROSAWA. 1973. Br. Heart J. **40:** 153–161.
5. CRAWFORD, T. 1977. Pathology of Ischemic Heart Disease Butterworth. London.
6. RIDOLFI, R. & G. HUTCHINS. 1977. Am. Heart J. **93:** 468–486.
7. SHOZAWA, T., M. SAGESHIMA, T. TSUBURAYA, M. KOBAYASHI, M. MIURA, M. ITOH & M. HAYASHI. 1981. J. Jap. Atheroscl. Soc. **9:** 425–426.
8. DAVIES, M. & A. C. THOMAS. 1984. N. Engl. J. Med. **310:** 1137–1140.
9. FALK, E. 1983. Br. Heart J. **50:** 127–134.
10. MALLORY, C. K., P. D. WHITE & SALCEDO-SALGAR. 1939. Am. Heart J. **18:** 647–671.
11. LODGE-PATCH, I. 1951. Br. Heart J. **13:** 37–42.
12. BOUCHADRY, B. & G. MAJNO. 1974. Am. J. Pathol. **74:** 301–330.
13. DUGUID J.B. 1946. J. PATHOL. BACTERIOL. **58:** 207–212.
14. KAJIYA, F., K. TSUJIOKA, Y. OGASAWARA, Y. WADA, S. MATSUOKA, O. HIRAMATSU, S. TADAOKA, M. GOTO & T. FUJIWARA. 1987. Circulation **76:** 1092–1100.

The Role of Calcium and Magnesium in the Development of Atherosclerosis

Experimental and Clinical Evidence[a]

HAJIME ORIMO AND YASUYOSHI OUCHI

Department of Geriatrics
University of Tokyo
7-3-1, Hongo, Bunkyo-ku
Tokyo 113, Japan

INTRODUCTION

Little attention has been paid to the role of calcium (Ca) in the development of atherosclerosis, because pathological studies have revealed that Ca deposition in the arterial wall, found in calcified atherosclerotic plaque and Mönckeberg's type arteriosclerosis, appears in the final stage of atherogenesis. Ca deposition, thus, has been considered to be the result, rather than the cause, of atherosclerosis. Recently, accumulated evidence, however, indicated that Ca might play a crucial role in the development of atherosclerosis. First, Blumenthal et al.[1] reported that Ca deposition was present in the human aorta even in the developing stage of atherosclerosis. Strickberger et al.[2] also reported the increase, by 4.8-fold, of Ca transport across the aortic plasma membrane and the increase of both intracellular and extracellular Ca in cholesterol-fed rabbits. Second, cytosolic calcium has been shown to regulate some important cellular functions such as secretion of biological products, muscle contraction, proliferation and gene expression in various types of cultured cells.[3,4] Although the mechanism of atherogenesis has not been fully elucidated, many biological phenomena in atherogenesis have been found to be Ca dependent. Third, there is evidence that the Ca antagonist may have an antiatherogenic effect. Rosenblum et al.[5] showed that sodium ethane hydroxydiphosphonate, an anticalcifying agent, prevented lipid accumulation in the aorta of cholesterol-fed rabbits. Since then, many experimental studies have suggested that Ca antagonists, including lanthanum,[6] nifedipine,[7,8] nicardipine,[8] verapamil,[9] diltiazem,[10] and nilvadipine,[11] may have an antiatherogenic effect.

Since Ross et al.[12,13] proposed the "response-to-injury" hypothesis, the importance of arterial cells such as endothelial cells (ECs) and smooth muscle cells (SMCs) in the development of atherosclerosis has been emphasized. Therefore, we investigated the function of arterial cells with special reference to intracellular Ca metabolism. We also investigated the effect of dietary magnesium (Mg) on the development of experimental atherosclerosis in rabbits, and the effect of long-term use of nifedipine on the magnitude of coronary artery stenosis in humans.

[a]This study was supported by Grants-in-Aid for Scientific Research (No. 61480247 and No. 01570472) from the Ministry of Education, Science, and Culture of Japan, and a grant from Takeda Medical Foundation.

444

MATERIALS AND METHODS

Experimental Evidence

Experiment 1. Effect of Free Radicals on Cytosolic Free Calcium Concentration and Low-Density Lipoprotein (LDL) Transport in Cultured Endothelial Cells

ECs were obtained from the thoracic aorta of a six-month-old male pig by scraping the luminal surface with a razor blade. Cells were cultured in minimal essential medium (MEM) supplemented with 10% fetal calf serum (FCS) at 37°C in 5% CO_2 and 95% air. Cells at the 3rd to 7th passage were used for the experiment.

Linoleate hydroperoxide (LHO) was prepared according to the procedure described by Thomas and Pryor.[14] Briefly, 0.22 g of linoleate was dissolved in 0.7 ml of ethanol and further dissolved in 100 ml of borate buffer (0.05 M, pH 9). Soybean lipoxidase (4050 units/ml) was added and the mixture was incubated for 10 min at 0°C. The reaction was terminated by adding HCl. LHO was then extracted with 20% ether/hexane 3 times, evaporated at 24°C, and dissolved in 1 ml of ethanol. LHO was subsequently stored at -20°C until the time of the experiment. The LHO activity was assayed employing the method described by Yagi.[15]

Cytosolic free calcium concentration ($[Ca^{++}]i$) in ECs was measured according to the procedure reported by Tsien *et al.*[16] and Capponi *et al.*[17] with minor modification as described elsewhere.[18] The fluorescence of quin 2-loaded cells was measured by a Hitachi 650-10S fluorescence spectrophotometer. LHO or xanthine/xanthine oxidase (X-XO) was added and quickly mixed, and fluorescence was measured once or twice per minute for 10 minutes. ECs were pretreated respectively with nifedipine (3.2 μM) or scavenger enzymes 10 minutes and 1 minute before the addition of LHO or X-XO. At the end of fluorescence measurement, 20 μM of digitonin was added to the cells to measure F_{max}, or the fluorescence intensity of calcium-saturated quin 2. F_{min}, or the fluorescence intensity of calcium-free quin 2 was calculated from the equation; $F_{min} = 0.16 \times (F_{max} -$ background) + background. The background, that is, the autofluorescence of cells and coverslips, was finally measured by adding 0.5 mM of $MnCl_2$. The $[Ca^{++}]i$ was calculated from the equation; $[Ca^{++}]i = Kd \times (F - F_{min})/(F_{max} - F)$. Kd, previously determined by Tsien *et al.*, was 115 nM.[16]

LDL transport across endothelial cells was measured according to the method described by Territo *et al.*[19] ECs from pig aorta were cultured on gelatin-coated polycarbonate filter (pore size; 5 μm) placed in a modified Boyden chamber. LDL fraction was obtained from pig plasma by using ultracentrifugation and was iodinated with the iodine monochloride method. At confluency, ^{125}I-LDL was added to the medium in the upper chamber with and without LHO (3.2 μM) and was incubated at 37°C for 60 min. Radioactivity in the lower chamber was then counted and was considered to be the amount of transported LDL.

The effects of X-XO and LHO on $[Ca^{++}]i$ in ECs and ^{125}I-LDL transport across monolayered ECs were investigated. The effect of pretreatment by nifedipine (Bayer, Leverkusen, FRG) on X-XO-induced and LHO-induced change was also investigated.

Experiment 2. Relationship between Cytosolic Free Calcium Concentration and DNA Synthesis Stimulated by Growth Factors in Cultured Rat Aortic Smooth Muscle Cells

SMCs were isolated from aortic media of 5-week-old male Wistar rats according to the method as described elsewhere.[18] Briefly, small explants were aseptically cut off from the thoracic aorta and were subjected to culture in medium 199 supplemented with 20%

of fetal calf serum (FCS) in 5% CO_2 and 95% air at 37°C until cells migrated from the explants. The explants were removed and culture was continued until cells became confluent. Confluent cells were detached with trypsin (0.125%)/ethylenediamine tetraacetic acid (EDTA: 0.005%) solution, and subcultured in MEM supplemented with 10% of FCS. Cells at 8th to 10th passage were used for the experiments.

DNA synthesis of SMCs was measured as the incorporation of [³H]thymidine. Confluent SMCs were detached with trypsin/EDTA solution, suspended in MEM with 10% FCS and inoculated onto 96-multiwell plates (0.32 cm^2/well). The cells were incubated until they became confluent after approximately two days. Growth of the cells was arrested for 24 hr by substitution of MEM with 0.1% FCS for the previous medium. Nifedipine or vehicle was firstly added and either epidermal growth factor (EGF; Collaborative Research, Lexington, MA), platelet-derived growth factor (PDGF; Collaborative Research, Lexington, MA) or somatomedin-C (Sm-C; Fujisawa Pharmaceutical Co., Osaka, Japan) was then added to the medium. The effect of BAY K 8644 (Bayer), a calcium agonist, was also investigated. [³H]Thymidine was finally added to give the concentration of 1 μCi/ml. After 36 hr of incubation, medium was discarded and cells were washed with ice-cold phosphate buffered saline without containing Ca^{++} and Mg^{++} and subsequently incubated in ice-cold trichloroacetic acid (TCA: 5%) for 20 min. After removal of TCA, cells were lyzed with 50 μl of NaOH (0.5 N) and the cell lysate was titrated with the same volume of HCl (0.5 N). Radioactivity of the mixture was counted with a liquid scintillation counter (Aloka LSC 700, Tokyo, Japan) and was considered to be the amount of DNA synthesis.

$[Ca^{++}]i$ in SMCs was measured by using the same method as that described in Experiment 1.

Experiment 3. Effect of Magnesium on Experimental Atherosclerosis in Rabbits

Male New Zealand white rabbits weighing about 2.5 kg each were kept individually in stainless steel cages in a room where temperature was around 23°C. The rabbits were divided into 5 groups and were put on 5 kinds of diets: (A) regular (n = 6), (B) 1% cholesterol (n = 6), (C) 1% cholesterol plus an additional 0.3% Mg diet (n = 6), (D) 1% cholesterol plus an additional 0.6% Mg (n = 7), (E) 1% cholesterol plus an additional 0.9% Mg (n = 6). Cholesterol and/or Mg sulfate was added to the regular diet (RC4; Oriental Yeast Co., Ltd., Tokyo, Japan). Since the regular diet and 1% cholesterol diet contained 0.4% Mg, the diets (C), (D) and (E) actually contained a total of 700, 1000, and 1300 mg of Mg per 100 g, respectively. Rabbits were allowed free access to tap water containing negligible amounts of Ca and Mg. One hundred grams of the assigned diet were given daily to each rabbit. All rabbits were fed the whole diet every day of the experiment. Diets containing additional Mg were well tolerated throughout the experiment. Systolic blood pressure and body weight were measured once a week. After 10 weeks, 10 ml of blood was collected from the ear vein into a plastic syringe containing 0.13 ml of EDTA (0.5 M). An additional 10 ml of blood was collected into a plastic syringe, which did not contain anticoagulants. These blood samples were centrifuged at 1,500 g for 15 min. at 4°C. Plasma and serum were stored at −20°C until the time of chemical analysis. Rabbits were then bled to death under pentobarbital anesthesia. Total cholesterol and high density lipoprotein (HDL)-cholesterol concentration in the plasma were measured with an enzymatic method and a heparin-Mn^{++} precipitation-enzymatic method, respectively.

Aortas were carefully removed from the aortic root to the bifurcation. Surrounding adventitial tissues were cleaned, and the entire aorta was washed twice with saline. Aortas were longitudinally divided into anterior and posterior halves of approximately the same size. The posterior half of each aorta was affixed to a plastic board, and was fixed by incubating in 3.5% formaldehyde solution for 24 hr. Aortas were then washed with distilled water and stained by incubating in Oil Red O solution for 20 min, as described by Willis et al.[8] After staining, the intimal surface was photographed, and the area of the stained intimal surface was measured with a X-Y digitizer connected to a microcomputer. The ratio of the stained area to the whole intimal surface of the posterior half of the aorta was considered the magnitude of atherosclerosis.

Clinical Evidence

Patients with ischemic heart disease, on whom coronary angiography (CAG) was repeatedly performed, were randomly selected. Sixteen subjects were on nifedipine therapy (40 mg/day; nifedipine group; 14 males and 2 females, age 53 ± 2) and 13 subjects were not on nifedipine therapy (control group; 11 males and 2 females, age 58 ± 3). No significant differences were observed between the two groups in clinical backgrounds including age, sex, cardiac diagnosis, the presence of coronary risk factors, and medication other than nifedipine. The severity of coronary artery stenosis was also similar. The interval between two CAG examinations was 733 ± 237 days for the control group and was 561 ± 103 days for the nifedipine group.

CAG examination was performed using the Judkins method. Right and left coronary angiograms were taken at several positions of the right and left anterior oblique views before and after sublingual administration of 0.3 mg of nitroglycerine. These angiograms were recorded on 35 mm cinefilm and the shots after nitroglycerine administration were analyzed by XR-70 coronary analyzer (Vanguard, Melville). That is, the first CAG was carefully observed, and all lesions with 25 to 75% stenosis were defined as region of interest (ROI). The regions which were judged to have more than 75% stenosis were excluded from this study to avoid the possible influence of vasospasm and thrombus formation. The cinefilm of CAG was loaded into the projector (Vanguard XR-35) and the magnitude of coronary artery stenosis was quantitatively measured by using videodensitometry[20] (XR-70 coronary analyzer), which was connected to the XR-35 projector, for each ROI on the first and second CAG. The magnitude of coronary artery stenosis was measured from a single plane angiogram which provided the details of the stenotic site. The magnitude of stenosis for each ROI on the first CAG was again measured on the same view of the second CAG, and the change in the magnitude was compared between the control group and the nifedipine group.

Statistics

Data were analyzed with one-factor analysis of variance. When the statistically significant effect was found, Newman-Keuls test was performed to isolate differences between groups. Student t test for paired and unpaired data was also performed when appropriate. A p value of less than 0.05 was considered to be significant. All data are presented in the text, tables and figures as means $\pm$ SEM.

RESULTS AND DISCUSSION

Experimental Evidence

Experiment 1

As shown in TABLE 1, $[Ca^{++}]i$ in quiescent ECs was 111.9 ± 11.2 nM. Both X (0.1 mM)-XO (2.5–40 mU/ml) and LHO (0.032–1 µM) increased $[Ca^{++}]i$ in a dose-dependent manner and peak values were obtained at 5 to 7 minutes after the addition of X-XO or LHO. Both superoxide dismutase (SOD) and SOD-catalase significantly suppressed the increase in $[Ca^{++}]i$ provoked by X-XO, suggesting that the response was mediated by generated superoxide. Nifedipine (3.2 µM) also suppressed the increase. The pretreatment by glutathione (GSH)-glutathione peroxidase (GPox), however, was not effective. In contrast, GSH-GPox suppressed the increase in $[Ca^{++}]i$ provoked by LHO (0.32 µM). Nifedipine was again effective. The effect of SOD-catalase was not significant. It has been reported that the generation of superoxide in human leucocytes stimulated by concanavalin A and by chemotactic peptides is mediated by intracellular calcium.[21,22]

TABLE 1. Effects of Xanthine/Xanthine Oxidase (X-XO) and Linoleate Hydroperoxide (LHO) on Cytosolic Free Calcium Concentration (nM) in Cultured Pig Aortic Endothelial Cells[a]

No Treatment			111.9 ± 11.2 (30)	
Agents	X-XO	(n)	LHO	(n)
Vehicle	577.9 ± 118.9 §§	(14)	873.0 ± 199.1 §§	(13)
SOD + catalase	236.8 ± 11.9 **	(12)	594.3 ± 135.1 §§	(8)
SOD	312.4 ± 22.8 §,*	(9)	N.D.	
GSH + GPox	369.2 ± 67.0 §	(6)	480.1 ± 102.8 §,*	(9)
Nifedipine	231.2 ± 11.9 **	(6)	306.4 ± 43.7 **	(8)

[a]The final concentrations of nifedipine, X, XO, and LHO were 3.2 µM, 0.1 mM, 40 mU/ml, and 0.32 µM, respectively. SOD = superoxide dismutase (100 µg/ml), GSH = glutathione (10 µM), GPox = glutathione peroxidase (10 mU/ml), N.D. = not determined. §$p < 0.05$, §§ $p < 0.01$ vs no treatment; *$p < 0.05$, **$p < 0.01$ vs vehicle. Number of experiments is shown in parentheses.

However, the involvement of cytosolic calcium in the action of reactive oxygen has not been reported. The results obtained in this experiment clearly indicate that both LHO and X-XO increase $[Ca^{++}]i$ in cultured endothelial cells.

As shown in FIGURE 1, both X-XO and LHO significantly increased LDL transport across the endothelial cell layer. The importance of intracellular calcium was directly indicated from the observation that calcium ionophore, ionomycin, also increased the transport (FIG. 1). SOD-catalase significantly suppressed the increase in LDL transport provoked by X-XO, suggesting that the response was mediated by generated superoxide. Although the underlying mechanism has not been elucidated, possible mechanisms of the transport could be LDL receptor-mediated transcytosis, nonreceptor-mediated transcytosis, and transport through the cellular junction. Further studies should be performed to elucidate the exact mechanism.

We found that nifedipine suppresses the increase in $[Ca^{++}]i$ provoked by reactive oxygen together with the inhibition of increase in LDL transport (TABLE 1, FIG. 2). Since it has been reported that voltage-dependent calcium channels do not exist in cultured endothelial cells, the effect of nifedipine might result not from the inhibition of voltage-

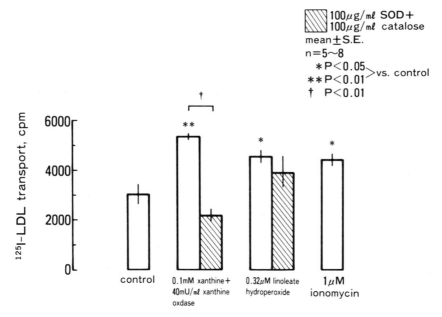

FIGURE 1. Effects of xanthine (X; 0.1 mM)/xanthine oxidase (XO; 40 mU/ml), linoleate hydroperoxide (LHO; 0.32 μM), and ionomycin (1 μM) on ^{125}I-low density lipoprotein (LDL) transport across cultured pig aortic endothelial cell layer. Effects of superoxide dismutase (SOD)/catalase on X-XO- and LHO-induced changes in LDL transport are also shown.

dependent calcium channels, but possibly from another action such as membrane stabilizing action.

Reactive oxygen species are known to be a risk factor for the development of atherosclerosis. These molecules provoke many adverse biological effects on endothelial cells such as morphological alteration,[23–25] impairment of prostacyclin production,[26] and the increase of vascular permeability,[27,28] all of which could promote the atherosclerotic

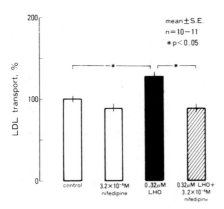

FIGURE 2. Effects of linoleate hydroperoxide (LHO; 0.32 μM) and nifedipine (3.2 μM) on ^{125}I-low density lipoprotein (LDL) transport across cultured pig aortic endothelial cell layer. Nifedipine alone did not affect the transport; however, nifedipine significantly inhibited the increase in LDL transport provoked by LHO.

process. The results obtained in this experiment suggest a new mechanism by which calcium antagonists foster the antiatherogenic action.

Experiment 2

As shown in FIGURE 3, EGF enhanced DNA synthesis and increased $[Ca^{++}]i$ in cultured vascular SMCs. The results indicate that cytosolic calcium might be involved in the proliferation of vascular SMCs provoked by EGF, because pretreatment by nifedipine suppressed both the enhancement of DNA synthesis and the increase in $[Ca^{++}]i$ provoked by EGF (FIG. 4). As shown in FIGURE 5, PDGF provoked similar effects on DNA synthesis and $[Ca^{++}]i$ in cultured vascular SMCs. The effect of nifedipine on the PDGF-

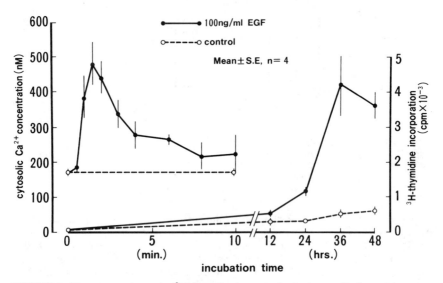

FIGURE 3. Time course change in [³H]thymidine incorporation and cytosolic free calcium concentration (*inset*) in cultured rat aortic smooth muscle cells treated with epidermal growth factor (EGF; 100 ng/ml).

induced increase in DNA synthesis was, however, somewhat different from that produced by EGF. Although the increase in $[Ca^{++}]i$ was suppressed by nifedipine, the increase in DNA synthesis was not suppressed (FIG. 4). To explain the discrepant result, two possibilities must be considered. First, there might be another mechanism independent of cytosolic free calcium for the promotion of DNA synthesis by PDGF. A possible mechanism is an activation of protein kinase C through the generation of diacylglyceride.[29,30] Protein kinase C has been reported also to be a promoter for DNA synthesis in cultured fibroblasts.[31,32] Therefore, the lack of an inhibitory effect of nifedipine on the PDGF-induced increase in DNA synthesis might be explained by the hypothesis that an activation of protein kinase C caused by PDGF is enough to promote DNA synthesis in SMCs. In contrast to PGDF, Hesketh *et al.*[33] showed that EGF increases $[Ca^{++}]i$ in 3T3 fibroblasts without accompanying inositol phospholipid breakdown or activation of protein kinase C. Second, the possibility must be considered that calcium release from intracellular stores,

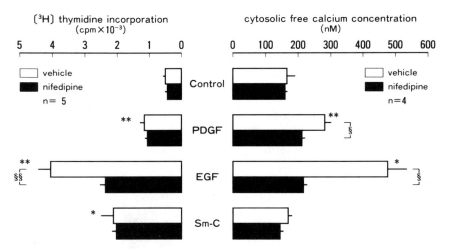

FIGURE 4. Effects of platelet-derived growth factor (PDGF; 1 U/ml), epidermal growth factor (EGF; 100 ng/ml) and somatomedin-C (Sm-C; 100 ng/ml) on [³H]thymidine incorporation (*left panel*) and cytosolic free calcium concentration (*right panel*) in cultured vascular smooth muscle cells. Effects of nifedipine (3.2 μM) on growth factor-induced changes are also shown. *p <0.05, **p <0.01 vs control (vehicle), §p <0.05, §§p <0.01.

which might have been masked because of the calcium chelating effect of quin 2,[34] might contribute to DNA synthesis provoked by PDGF. It has been shown that PDGF binds to the receptors in 3T3 fibroblasts, leads to inositol phospholipid breakdown in the cell membrane, and generates inositol trisphosphate which releases calcium from the intracellular stores.[35,36] Nifedipine is known to act on calcium channels in cell membrane and

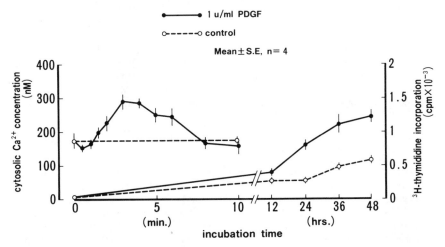

FIGURE 5. Time course change in [³H]thymidine incorporation and cytosolic free calcium concentration (*inset*) in cultured rat aortic smooth muscle cells treated with platelet-derived growth factor (PDGF; 1 U/ml).

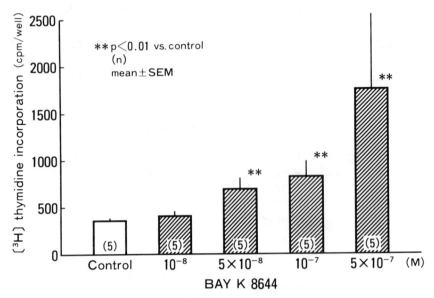

FIGURE 6. Effect of BAY K 8644 on [³H]thymidine incorporation in cultured rat aortic smooth muscle cells. **p <0.01 vs control.

to have no effect on the calcium release from the intracellular stores. Thus, nifedipine might not be effective on the action of PDGF. On the other hand, the calcium agonist BAY K 8644 increased DNA synthesis in a dose-dependent manner (FIG. 6). The result provides direct evidence of the contribution of cytosolic free calcium to DNA synthesis.

On the other hand, Sm-C was found to increase DNA synthesis without accompanying the increase in [Ca⁺⁺]i (FIG. 7). Moreover, nifedipine did not affect the enhancement of DNA synthesis induced by Sm-C (FIG. 4). These results indicate that calcium mobilization is not involved in the mechanism of action of Sm-C on DNA synthesis.

As demonstrated in this experiment, the transient rise in [Ca⁺⁺]i, thus, might play an important role in the proliferation of SMCs stimulated by EGF. In contrast, the rise in [Ca⁺⁺]i might not be involved in the mechanism of proliferation of SMCs provoked by Sm-C. The role of cytosolic free calcium in the proliferation of SMCs provoked by PDGF was not definitive and another factor might participate in the mechanism.

Experiment 3

The administration of 1% cholesterol diet significantly increased the Oil Red O-positive atherosclerotic area which covered the aortic intimal surface (3.2 ± 1.4% vs 37.3 ± 1.3%, p <0.01). Supplementation of 0.3% Mg did not affect the area of atherosclerotic plaque. However, supplementation of 0.6% and 0.9% Mg significantly suppressed the area to 11.7 ± 0.9% and 9.2 ± 1.5%, respectively (p <0.01 vs 1% cholesterol group). These results indicate that dietary Mg has an antiatherogenic effect. This would support the epidemiological observations that suggest that high Mg intake decreases mortality from atherosclerotic diseases.[37-39] Antiatherogenic action did not result from the effect of Mg on blood pressure or body weight, because these parameters were similar in the five groups of rabbits throughout the experiment. Dietary Mg significantly decreased cholesterol content in the aorta without reducing total cholesterol concentration in plasma. Moreover, Mg supplements did not further affect plasma HDL-cholesterol concentration which was reduced when an 1% cholesterol diet was administered. These findings suggest that Mg might prevent the development of atherosclerosis by decreasing cholesterol accumulation in the aortic wall.

The pharmacological basis of the inhibitory effect of Mg on the development of atherosclerosis has not been elucidated. However, Mg has been shown to modulate Ca influx in vascular smooth muscles. Altura *et al.* found that acute reduction in extracellular Mg concentration increased Ca content in vascular smooth muscles, and acute elevation had the opposite effect.[40] Furthermore, the increase in extracellular Mg concentration has been reported to decrease the influx of ^{45}Ca into the aorta and portal veins of rats[41] and also into cultured rat aortic smooth muscle cells.[42] The effect of extracellular Mg is considered to result from the competition with Ca^{++} at binding sites in vascular smooth muscle cell membranes.[43] Extracellular Mg, thus, could be considered to have Ca entry blocking action. Calcium entry blocking action of Mg may contribute, at least in part, to the suppression of the development of atherosclerotic lesions, because lanthanum, which is known to block Ca entry by occupying Ca binding sites[44] in various types of cell membranes, has been reported to suppress the development of atherosclerosis in cholesterol-fed rabbits.[6]

Clinical Evidence

As shown in TABLE 2, the magnitude of stenosis showed a small and statistically insignificant increase for the 37 ROIs in the control group. In contrast, it showed a significant decrease for 33 ROIs in the nifedipine group. These results suggest the possibility that the long-term use of calcium antagonist nifedipine might be effective against the progression of coronary atherosclerosis in humans. The effect of nifedipine was more

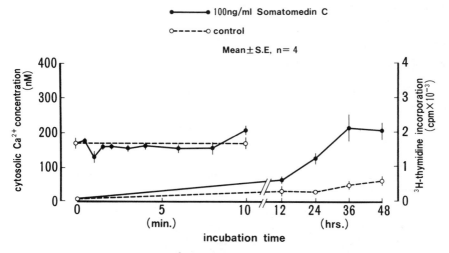

FIGURE 7. Time course change in [^{3}H]thymidine incorporation and cytosolic free calcium concentration (*inset*) in cultured rat aortic smooth muscle cells treated with somatomedin-C (Sm-C; 100 ng/ml).

TABLE 2. Effect of Long-Term Use of Nifedipine on the Magnitude of Coronary Artery Stenosis Measured by Videodensitometric Analysis of Coronary Angiogram (CAG)[a]

	Control Group % Stenosis		Nifedipine Group % Stenosis	
	1st CAG	2nd CAG	1st CAG	2nd CAG
Total ROIs	54.1 ± 2.6	58.6 ± 3.3 (37)	52.5 ± 3.8	46.2 ± 4.3 *,§ (33)
ROIs in RCA	45.4 ± 3.6	50.9 ± 5.9 (11)	47.9 ± 4.7	45.3 ± 6.1 (14)
ROIs in LCA	57.8 ± 3.2	61.8 ± 3.9 (26)	55.8 ± 5.7	46.9 ± 6.0 *,§ (19)

[a]ROIs = regions of interest, RCA = right coronary artery, LCA = left coronary artery. Number of ROIs is shown in parentheses. *$p < 0.05$ vs 1st CAG in nifedipine group; §$p < 0.05$ vs 2nd CAG in control group.

apparent on the lesions of the left coronary artery than on those of the right coronary artery. The reason for this is not clear. It is unlikely that nifedipine is more effective on the lesions of the left coronary artery. Moreover, the location of coronary artery stenosis was not found to affect the progression and regression rate.[45] The possible cause might be the difference in the magnitude of stenosis between the right and left coronary arteries on the first CAG.

Many experimental studies have been done to elucidate the effect of calcium antagonists on atherogenesis by using animal models such as cholesterol-fed rabbits[5-8] and Watanabe heritable hyperlipidemic rabbits.[46] Although the results from these experimental studies are still controversial, the focus has been placed on a clinical trial to determine the effect of calcium antagonist on the development or progression of coronary atherosclerosis. Klein et al.[47] analyzed the repeated CAG in patients on and not on nifedipine or diltiazem therapy, and they reported that the incidence of the regression of coronary artery stenosis was higher in patients on diltiazem therapy. Yabe[48] also reported that the incidence of progression of coronary artery stenosis was lower and that of regression was higher in patients on nifedipine therapy for approximately one year. Although these studies were performed by using semiquantitative analysis of CAG, the results were compatible with those demonstrated in this study. A large-scale clinical trial named the International Nifedipine Trial on Antiatherosclerotic Therapy (INTACT) is presently under way.[49] The final results, however, have not been published.

Although this study was retrospectively done, the results obtained were encouraging. A prospective and multicentric double-blind study should be performed to obtain a final conclusion regarding the antiatherogenic action of calcium antagonist in humans.

SUMMARY AND CONCLUSION

Based on the findings presented in this study, we propose the hypothesis that calcium could be a mediator for the development of atherosclerosis. FIGURE 8 shows a schematic illustration of the hypothesis. The presence of risk factors such as hypertension, hyperlipidemia, and smoking may increase the influx of calcium into vascular ECs. We have shown that reactive oxygen species, which are considered to be a risk factor for the development of atherosclerosis, actually increase $[Ca^{++}]i$ in vascular ECs. Increased intracellular calcium may damage the function of ECs, resulting in platelet aggregation at the damaged site. Increased intracellular calcium may also increase uptake of macromolecules in plasma such as fibrinogen and LDL, eventually forming atherosclerotic plaque. We have also shown that the influx of calcium into vascular ECs is associated with LDL transport across vascular ECs. The pretreatment by nifedipine inhibited both the increase in $[Ca^{++}]i$ and the increase in LDL transport, suggesting that intracellular calcium modulates LDL transport across ECs. Growth factors released from platelets may provoke migration and proliferation of medial SMCs in the aterial intima. It has been reported that migration of SMCs from arterial media to intima is enhanced by the presence of calcium, and can be inhibited by the pretreatment of calcium antagonist.[50] As demonstrated in this study, calcium also plays an important role in the proliferation of SMCs provoked by some kinds of growth factors such as EGF.

On the other hand, we found that an increased amount of dietary Mg suppressed the development of atherosclerotic lesions in the aorta of cholesterol-fed rabbits without affecting plasma total cholesterol and HDL-cholesterol concentrations. The mechanism of action might also be related to the calcium entry blocking action. The clinical and nutritional implications of these phenomena should be investigated further.

The evidences presented in this study, however, would not be sufficient to fully explain the etiological role of calcium in atherogenesis. Further studies are required to elucidate the mechanism of the contribution of calcium to atherogenesis. The efficacy of calcium antagonist for the prevention of atherosclerosis in humans should also be investigated further.

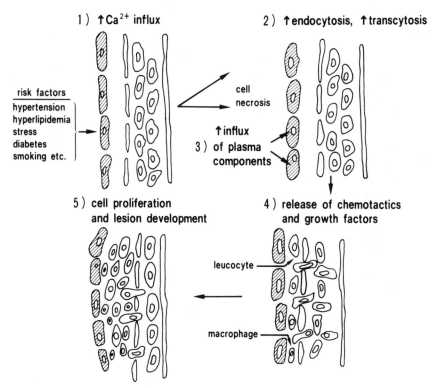

FIGURE 8. Schematic illustration showing the hypothetical role of calcium in the process of atherogenesis. *Hatched cells* indicate arterial endothelial cells, and *open cells* indicate smooth muscle cells in the arterial media.

REFERENCES

1. BLUMENTHAL, H. T., A. I. LANSING & P. A. WHEELER. 1950. Am. J. Pathol. **26:** 989–1009.
2. STRICKBERGER, S. A., L. N. RUSSEK & R. D. PHAIR. 1988. Circ. Res. **62:** 75–80.
3. CAMPBELL, A. K. 1983. *In* Intracellular Calcium: Its Universal Role as Regulator. H. Gutfreund, Ed. John Wiley & Sons. Chichester.
4. HESKETH, T. R., G. A. SMITH, J. P. MOORE, M. V. TAYLOR & J. C. METCALFE. 1983. J. Biol. Chem. **258:** 4876–4882.
5. ROSENBLUM, I. Y., L. FLORA & R. EISENSTEIN. 1975. Atherosclerosis **22:** 411–424.
6. KRAMSCH, D. M., A. J. ASPEN & C. S. APSTEIN. 1980. J. Clin. Invest. **65:** 967–981.
7. HENRY, P. D. & K. I. BENTLEY. 1981. J. Clin. Invest. **68:** 1366–1369.
8. WILLIS, A. L., B. NAGEL, V. CHURCHILL, M. A. WHYTE, D. L. SMITH, I. MAHMUD & D. L. PUPPIONE. 1985. Arteriosclerosis **5:** 250–255.
9. BLUMLEIN, S. L., R. SIEVERS, P. KIDD & W. W. PARMLEY. 1984. Am. J. Cardiol. **54:** 884–889.
10. GINSBURG, R., K. DAVIS, M. R. BRISTOW, K. MCKENNET, S. R. KODSI, M. E. BILLINGHAM & J. S. SCHROEDER. 1983. Lab. Invest. **49:** 154–158.
11. KOIBUCHI, Y., S. SAKAI, S. MIURA, T. ONO, F. SHIBAYAMA & M. OHTSUKA. 1989. Atherosclerosis **79:** 147–155.
12. ROSS, R. & J. A. GLOMSET. 1976. N. Engl. J. Med. **295:** 420–425.
13. ROSS, R. 1986. N. Engl. J. Med. **314:** 488–500.
14. THOMAS, M. J. & W. A. PRYOR. 1980. Lipids **15:** 544–548.
15. YAGI, K. 1976. Biochem. Med. **15:** 212–216.
16. TSIEN, R. Y., T. POZZAN & T. J. RINK. 1982. J. Cell Biol. **94:** 325–344.
17. CAPPONI, A. M., P. P. LEW & M. B. BALLOTON. 1985. J. Biol. Chem. **260:** 7836–7842.
18. ORIMO, H., M. WATANABE & Y. OUCHI. 1988. Biochem. Biophys. Res. Commun. **150:** 1282–1286.
19. TERRITO, M., J. A. BERLINER & A. M. FOGELMAN. 1984. J. Clin. Invest. **74:** 2279–2284.
20. NICHOLS, A. B., F. O. CHRISTOPHER, B. A. GABRIELI, J. J. FENOGLIO & P. D. ESSER. 1984. Circulation **69:** 512–522.
21. SCULLY, S. P., G. B. SEGEL & M. A. LICHTMAN. 1986. J. Clin. Invest. **77:** 1349–1356.
22. NAKAGAWARA, M., K. TAKESHIGE, H. SUMIMOTO, J. YOSHITAKE & S. MINAKAMI. 1984. Biochim. Biophys. Acta **805:** 97–103.
23. WEISS, S. J., J. YOUNG, A. F. LOBUGLIO, A. SLIVKA & N. F. NIMEH. 1981. J. Clin. Invest. **68:** 714–721.
24. YAGI, K., H. OHKAWA, N. OHISHI, M. YAMASHITA & T. NAKASHIMA. 1981. J. Appl. Biochem. **3:** 58–65.
25. SASAGURI, Y., T. NAKASHIMA, M. MORIMATSU & K. YAGI. 1984. J. Appl. Biochem, **6:** 144–150.
26. SASAGURI, Y., M. MORIMATSU, T. NAKASHIMA, O. TOKUNAGA & K. YAGI. 1985. Biochem. Int. **11:** 517–521.
27. SHASBY, D. M., S. E. LIND, S. S. SHASBY, J. C. GOLDSMITH & G. W. HANNINGHAKE. 1985. Blood **65:** 605–614.
28. SHASBY, D. M., S. S. SHABY & M. J. PEACH. 1983. Am. Rev. Respir. Dis. **127:** 72–76.
29. TAKAI, Y., A. KISHIMOTO, U. KIKKAWA, T. MORI & Y. NISHIZUKA. 1979. Biochem. Biophys. Res. Commun. **91:** 1218–1224.
30. NISHIZUKA, Y. 1984. Nature **328:** 693–698.
31. TUPPER, J. T., L. KAUFMAN & P. V. BODINE. 1980. J. Cell. Physiol. **104:** 97–103.
32. ROZENGURT, E., A. RODRIGUEZ-PENA, M. COOMBS & J. SINNET-SMITH. 1984. Proc. Natl. Acad. Sci. USA **81:** 5748–5752.
33. HESKETH, T. R., J. P. MOORE, J. D. H. MORRIS, M. V. TAYLOR, J. RONGERS, G. A. SMITH & J. C. METCALFE. 1985. Nature **313:** 481–484.
34. TSIEN, R. Y. 1980. Biochemistry **19:** 2396–2404.
35. BERRIGDE, M. J. & R. F. IRVINE. 1984. Nature **312:** 315–321.
36. BERRIDGE, M. J., J. P. HESLOP, R. F. IRVINE & K. D. BROWN. 1984. Biochem. J. **222:** 195–201.
37. KOBAYASHI, J. 1957. Berichte Ohara Inst. **11:** 12–21.
38. SCHROEDER, H. A. & W. BRATTLEBORO. 1960. J. Chron. Dis. **12:** 586–591.

39. Morris, J. N., M. D. Crawford & J. A. Heady. 1961. Lancet **1:** 860–862.
40. Altura, B. M. & B. T. Altura. 1971. Am. J. Physiol. **220:** 938–944.
41. Turlapaty, P. D. M. V. & B. M. Altura. 1978. Eur. J. Pharmacol. **52:** 421–423.
42. Smith, J. B., E. J. Cragoe, Jr. & L. Smith. 1987. J. Biol. Chem. **262:** 11988–11994.
43. Altura, B. M. & B. T. Altura. 1981. Fed. Proc. **40:** 2672–2679.
44. Weiss, G. B. 1974. *In* Annual Review of Pharmacology. H. W. Elliot, R. Okun & R. George, Eds. Annual Reviews, Inc. Palo Alto, CA.
45. Bruschke, A. V. G., T. S. Wijers, W. Kolsters & J. Landmann. 1981. Circulation **63:** 527–536.
46. Watanabe, N., Y. Ishikawa, R. Okamoto, Y. Watanabe & H. Fukuzaki. 1987. Artery **14:** 283–294.
47. Klein, W., A. Lutfy & H. Schreyer. 1983. *In* New Calcium Antagonists: Recent Developments and Prospects. A. Fleckenstein, Ed. Gustav Fischer Verlag. Stuttgart, F.R.G.
48. Yabe, Y. 1985. J. Jpn. Atheroscler. Soc. **13:** 793–807.
49. Lichtlen, P. R., U. Nellessen, W. Rafflenbeul, S. Jost & H. Hecker. 1987. Cardiovasc. Drugs Ther. **1:** 71–80.
50. Nakao, J., H. Itoh, T. Ohyama, W-C. Chang & S. Murota. 1983. Atherosclerosis **46:** 309–319.

Clinical and Experimental Approaches to the Prevention of Atherosclerosis by Immunological Regulations

FUMIO KUZUYA, MASAFUMI KUZUYA, MASAHIRO YASUE,
MICHITAKA NAITO, CHIAKI FUNAKI, TOSHIO HAYASHI,
AND KANICHI ASAI

Department of Geriatrics
Nagoya University School of Medicine
65, Tsuruma-cho, Showa-ku
Nagoya 466, Japan

INTRODUCTION

It has been supposed that a variety of factors affects the initiation and development of atherosclerosis. Immunity and inflammation may also be involved in the atherosclerotic process. Recent studies have shown that immunoglobulins,[1] complement components,[2] and C5b-9 terminal complexes[3] have been observed in human or experimental atherosclerotic lesions. The detection of C5b-9 indicates that complement activation has occurred *in situ*. It is known that crystalline cholesterol[4] and cholesterol oxidation derivatives[5] activate the human complement system to completion *in vitro*, causing cleavage of C5, generation of C5a, and formation of terminal C5b-9 complexes. Recently Seifert *et al.*[6] reported that in cholesterol-induced atherosclerosis in rabbits C5b-9 complexes were observed to colocalize with extracellular lipid in the subendothelial space, and these depositions preceded monocyte infiltration and foam cell development. They hypothesize that early cholesterol accumulation in the aortic intima results in complement activation and that complement activation products may provide a mechanism by which monocytes are attracted to arterial regions of lipid accumulation. The complement activation in the vascular wall may induce not only the recruitment of inflammatory cells due to the release of chemoattractants but also the complement-mediated cell lysis with subsequent tissue injury. These events would be relevant to atherogenesis.

Recently it has been reported that dextrans exhibit anticomplementary properties as well as anticoagulant activities.[7] Dextrans inhibit the formation of C3 convertases and the anticomplementary activity is dependent on the molecular weight.[8] In Japan sodium dextran sulfate (DS) prepared by hydrolysis of polymer dextran (molecular weight approximately 400,000) to a preparation comprising molecules of molecular weight 7,000–8,000 has been used clinically for hyperlipidemia. Recently a primary prevention study for arteriosclerotic diseases in Japan proved that the long-term administration of DS was useful for the primary prevention of ischemic heart diseases.[9] We hypothesize that if DS inhibits activation of the complement system, its effectiveness for the prevention of arteriosclerotic diseases is possibly due in part to its anticomplementary property.

In the present study we investigated the effect of DS on the activation of the complement pathway *in vitro*. We also monitored the changes in the complement system of the subjects following the administration of DS.

In addition, we investigated the effect of another agent, camostat mesilate (CM), which has anticomplementary activity[10] on cholesterol-induced atherosclerosis in rabbits.

MATERIALS AND METHODS

Materials

DS (molecular weight 7000) was kindly supplied by Meito Co. (Japan) and CM by Ono Pharmaceutical Co. (Japan).

Effect of DS on Complement Activation in Whole Serum

Normal human serum was obtained from healthy donors. DS was dissolved in saline and 0.1 ml of solution was added to 0.9 ml of whole serum. Then classical pathway (CH_{50}) and alternative pathway activity ($APCH_{50}$) were determined in the serum. CH_{50} was assessed according to the method of Mayer[11] with slight modification and $APCH_{50}$ was assessed by the hemolytic activity of human serum with Mg-EGTA against unsensitized rabbit erythrocytes.

Effect of Administration of DS on the Complement System

DS (900 mg/day) was administered to 10 subjects, aged 63 ~ 81 years (male: 3, female: 7; no immune-mediated diseases were present in their past history), in order to study its effect on the complement system. CH_{50}, C3, C4 and C3a were measured at 2-week intervals. CH_{50} was assessed according to the method of Mayer[11] with slight modification, C3 and C4 were assessed by single radical immunodiffusion method and C3a by using radioimmunoassay kits (Upjohn Co.).

Effect of CM on Cholesterol-Induced Atherosclerosis in Rabbits

White Japanese male rabbits (n = 23) were fed a 1% cholesterol diet for 2 weeks, and then divided into two groups so as not to make a statistical difference in the serum total cholesterol levels between the two groups. One group (n = 12) was continued on a 1% cholesterol diet as a control. The other group (n = 11) was fed a 1% cholesterol diet plus camostat mesilate (CM) (300 mg/day). At the end of the 14-week period, all animals were killed and autopsied. The aortas were removed and measured by planimetry of the areas containing the atheromatous lesion. The lesioned areas were presented as a percentage of the total surface area of aorta. Serum lipids and body weight were determined every 4 weeks. Serum total cholesterol and phospholipid were measured by the enzymatic method, triglyceride by the acetyl acetone method, and high density lipoprotein (HDL)-cholesterol by the heparin-Ca method.

RESULTS

Effect of DS on CH_{50} and $APCH_{50}$

As shown in FIGURE 1, DS was able to inhibit the total classical as well as the alternative pathway activities in whole serum as assessed by its dose-dependent capacity to inhibit lysis of sensitized sheep erythrocytes and lysis of rabbit erythrocytes in Mg-EGTA. To be more precise, more than 10^{-4} M of DS, and 10^{-5} M of DS significantly inhibit classical and alternative pathway activities, respectively.

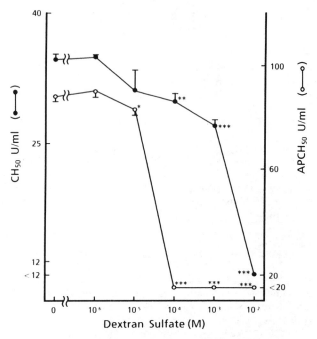

Mean ± SD (n = 3), *P<0.05, **P<0.01, ***P<0.001

FIGURE 1. Effect of dextran sulfate on CH_{50} and $APCH_{50}$. Dextran sulfate in 0.1 ml saline was added to 0.9 ml human serum. Then CH_{50} and $APCH_{50}$ were determined. Statistical significance was compared to control (dextran sulfate 0 M).

Effect of Administration of DS on the Complement System

During the administration of DS for 4 weeks, there were no significant changes in CH_{50}, C3, and C4 levels in the serum of subjects (TABLE 1). The level of C3a in the plasma in the 4th week was significantly reduced as compared with that before the administration (TABLE 1, FIGURE 2).

Effect of CM on Cholesterol-Induced Atherosclerosis

No significant difference was observed between the two groups in serum total cholesterol level and body weight throughout the experiment (TABLE 2). The percentage of

TABLE 1. Effect of Administration of Dextran Sulfate on Serum Complement Levels[a]

	CH_{50} (U/ml)	C_3 (mg/ml)	C_4 (mg/ml)	C_{3a} (ng/ml)
Before	29.9 ± 2.3	91.9 ± 8.9	42.2 ± 9.2	423.4 ± 123.6
2 wk	28.0 ± 2.9	86.2 ± 6.6*	38.2 ± 9.7	333.8 ± 137.5
4 wk	32.2 ± 4.1	87.3 ± 9.9	40.8 ± 9.4	283.9 ± 35.4**

[a]Mean ± SD (n = 3); *$p < 0.05$, **$p < 0.01$ vs before.

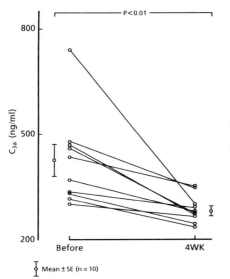

FIGURE 2. Effect of administration of dextran sulfate on the C3a level. The level of C3a in the plasma of 10 subjects was determined before and after the administration of dextran sulfate (900 mg/day).

intimal surface area of aorta involved in atheromatous lesion revealed $33.34 \pm 7.18\%$ (mean $\pm$ SE) in the control group, and it tended to be inhibited in the CM-treated group, being $17.32 \pm 4.99\%$ (FIGURE 3), but this difference was not statistically significant. Total complement activity (CH_{50}) was reduced significantly in the CM-treated group as compared with the control group (TABLE 3).

DISCUSSION

A number of immunohistochemical investigations demonstrated that the immune-related proteins present high levels in the atherosclerotic lesion.[1-3] However, it is not clear that the deposition of complement components and complexes in atherosclerotic lesions is a consequence of the formation of atherosclerotic lesion or a cause of it. To demonstrate the involvement of the complement system in the formation of atherosclerosis, it is necessary either to use animal models that are complement-deficient animal strains or to use agents that specifically inhibit the complement system. It has been

TABLE 2. Changes in Serum Lipids and Body Weight on 1% Cholesterol Diet[a]

	2 Weeks		14 Weeks	
	Control (N = 12)	Treated (N = 12)	Control (N = 12)	Treated (N = 11)
Total cholesterol (mg/dl)	699.3 ± 328.4	697.6 ± 353.7	934.2 ± 311.6	1290.5 ± 613.4
Triglyceride (mg/dl)	143.3 ± 96.6	128.2 ± 112.5	259.6 ± 136.0	487.0 ± 380.8
Phospholipid (mg/dl)	470.0 ± 214.6	501.5 ± 216.3	496.9 ± 125.8	708.8 ± 295.0
HDL-cholesterol (mg/dl)	31.9 ± 9.6	37.4 ± 12.2	36.9 ± 11.0	$27.9 \pm 7.2*$
Body weight (g)	2967.5 ± 168.1	2876.4 ± 188.1	3307.5 ± 191.8	3136.4 ± 369.1

[a]Mean $\pm$ SD; $*p < 0.05$ vs control.

1% cholesterol diet

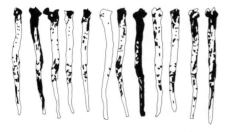

FIGURE 3. Tracing of aortic surface area involvement with atherosclerotic lesions.

1% cholesterol diet + camostat mesilate

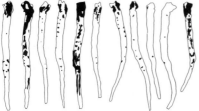

reported that congenital C6-deficient rabbits exhibit a reduced incidence and severity in aortic lesion formation compared with control rabbits when fed a cholesterol-supplemented diet.[12] However, the use of agents to study the involvement of the complement system in atherogenesis has not yet been investigated, since at present there are no available agents that specifically inhibit the complement system. Furthermore, even if we could use the agent that specifically depletes the complement system such as cobra venom factor, we could not ignore a propensity towards infection and thrombotic disorders. Therefore, it is difficult to study a functional role for the complement system in the formation of atherosclerotic lesions.

There have been a number of reports that suggest DS is effective not only in inhibiting cholesterol-induced atherosclerosis in experimental animals[13] but in preventing ischemic heart disease in the primary prevention study.[9] These reports came to the conclusion that the effectiveness of DS on inhibition of atherosclerosis or prevention of atherosclerotic disease was ascribed to its usefulness in improving serum lipid levels. Recently it has been reported that dextran derivatives of various molecular weights exhibit anticomplementary activities.[7,8] In the present study we demonstrate that DS (molecular weight 7000), which has been clinically used in Japan, inhibits both classical and alternative complement pathways *in vitro*. Therefore, it is possible that the antiatherogenic effect of DS is ascribed at least in part to its anticomplementary activity. We could not find any significant changes in CH_{50}, C3, and C4 levels in subjects following the administration of DS (900

TABLE 3. Effect of Administration of Camostat Mesilate on CH_{50} in Rabbits[a]

	4 Weeks	6 Weeks
Control group (n = 5)	9.38 ± 0.55	10.30 ± 1.65
CM-treated group (n = 5)	$8.32 \pm 0.37*$	9.34 ± 1.07

[a]Mean ± SD; *$p < 0.05$ vs control.

mg/day). However, C3a levels were reduced after the administration of DS. Though it is not clear what this reduction of C3a levels implies exactly, it is possible that the administration of DS would inhibit C3 cleavage *in vivo.*

CM is one of p-guanidinobenzoate derivatives, and it is a strong and reversible inhibitor of $C\overline{1}r$ and C1 esterase.[10] As shown in our results, CM prevented cholesterol-induced atherosclerosis in rabbits without any apparent effect on suppressing the increased serum cholesterol level. And also CM suppressed CH_{50} in rabbits. These observations may indicate that the anticomplementary activity of CM inhibits the formation of atherosclerotic lesion induced by cholesterol feeding. However, whether only the anticomplementary activity is important to the action of CM in the prevention of cholesterol-induced atherosclerosis in rabbits remains to be established, since CM also has the inhibitory effect of thrombin.[10]

The above results may suggest but unfortunately do not prove satisfactorily the possibility of the complement system being relevant to atherogenesis. It is hoped at some future time to test experimentally and clinically whether a new agent which specifically inhibits complement activity could prevent atherosclerosis.

SUMMARY

To evaluate the involvement of the complement system in atherogenesis, we investigated the effect of camostat mesilate (CM), $C\overline{1}r$, and C1 esterase inhibitor on cholesterol-induced atherosclerosis in rabbits. We also examined the effect of sodium dextran sulfate (DS, molecular weight: 7000), which is reported to be effective in preventing arteriosclerotic diseases and in inhibiting cholesterol-induced atherosclerosis in experimental animals, on complement activation *in vitro* and *in vivo.* The administration of CM reduced the formation of atherosclerotic lesions in cholesterol-fed rabbits. DS inhibited complement pathway *in vitro,* and the administration of DS reduced the C3a level in subjects. These results suggest that complement activation may possibly be involved in the atherosclerotic process.

REFERENCES

1. VLAICU, R., H. G. RUS, F. NICULESCU & A. CRISTEA. 1985. Atherosclerosis **55:** 35–50.
2. PANG, A. S. D., A. KATZ & J. O. MINTA. 1979. J. Immunol. **123:** 1117–1122.
3. VLAICU, R., F. NICULESCU, H. G. RUS & A. CRISTEA. 1985. Atherosclerosis **57:** 163–177.
4. HASSELBACHER, P. & J. L. HAHN. 1980. Atherosclerosis **37:** 239–245.
5. SEIFERT, P. S. & M. D. KAZATCHKINE. 1987. Mol. Immunol. **24:** 1303–1308.
6. SEIFERT, P. S., F. HUGO, G. K. HANSSON & S. BHAKDI. 1989. Lab. Invest. **60:** 747–754.
7. MAUZAC, M., F. MAILLET, J. JOZEFONVICZ & M. D. KAZATCHKINE. 1985. Biomaterials **6:** 61–64.
8. CREPON, B., F. MAILLET, M. D. KAZATCHKINE & J. JOZEFONVICZ. 1987. Biomaterials **8:** 248–253.
9. GOTO, Y., A. KUMAGAI, F. KUZUYA, N. YOSHIMINE, S. YOSHIDA, T. IRITANI, H. IIDA, Y. UMETADA, H. OKABE, Y. EHATA, Y. SATO, H. FUKUI, N. MATSUOKA, M. KURITA, Y. SAITO, Y. MIZUNO, M. MORISE & T. TANAKA. 1987. J. Clin. Biochem. Nutr. **2:** 55–70.
10. FUJII, S. & Y. HITOMI. 1981. Biochim. Biophys. Acta **661:** 342–345.
11. MAYER, M. M. 1961. *In* Experimental Immunochemistry. E. A. Kabat & M. M. Mayer, Eds. 133–240. Charles C. Thomas. Springfield, IL.
12. GEERTINGER, P. & H. SORENSEN. 1975. Artery **1:** 177–184.
13. YAMADA, K., F. KUZUYA & M. NODA. 1961. Jpn Circ. J. **25:** 570–578.

Possible Role of Dietary Proteins and Amino Acids in Atherosclerosis[a]

HERSCHEL SIDRANSKY

Department of Pathology
The George Washington University
Medical Center
Washington, DC 20037

INTRODUCTION

At the onset of this century, in 1909, a pathologist, Ignatowski,[1] was the first to provide a clear demonstration that diet affected the course of atherosclerosis. He observed that rabbits fed animal products, such as eggs, meat and milk, showed atheromas of the aorta which he attributed to the protein component of these foods. However, all of his dietary components contained cholesterol.

In 1913, Anitschkow and Chalatow[2] reported that diets containing cholesterol in vegetable oil could produce atherosclerosis. This shifted research emphasis towards cholesterol and other lipids and away from proteins. Nonetheless, epidemiologic data[3,4] relating diet to heart disease in 1957 revealed that the incidence of ischemic heart disease could be correlated with intake of animal protein as easily as with intake of fat.

Since this review will focus predominantly on proteins and amino acids as possible influential factors in atherosclerosis, I plan to cover selected studies dealing with these dietary components. However, from the outset it is necessary to stress that whenever one dietary component is altered, it influences the effects or actions of other dietary components. Thus, an imbalanced state may be induced which then has diverse implications on the pathogenesis of disease states, especially one such as atherosclerosis. Thus, one simple alteration or rearrangement of amino acids in proteins can have considerable impact on the overall metabolism relating to many dietary components, which then can manifest itself with pathological lesions.

Nutritional imbalances are induced by altering the quality and/or quantity of diet intake. Poor quality of essential foodstuffs induces a variety of pathological states, which in the past have mainly been considered under specific deficiency states. It has also been established that the quantity of intake will influence the pathological picture induced by the poor quality diet. In relation to amino acid deficient diets, the quantity of dietary intake influences the pathological responses in a variety of organs.[5] A human counterpart is the contrasting pathological findings in infants with marasmus versus those with kwashiorkor, where the amount of diet intake plays a major role.

It might be worthwhile in this introduction to stress the importance of nutritional imbalance in relation to the quality as well as quantity of diet as influenced by dietary amino acids and proteins by citing some of our own earlier experimental studies dealing with amino acid deficient diets.[5] We were concerned with the induction of experimental models of marasmus and kwashiorkor. From our experimental studies, we learned early

[a]This work was supported by United States Public Health Service Research Grants DK-27339 from the National Institute of Arthritis, Diabetes, and Digestive and Kidney Diseases and CA-41832 from the National Cancer Institute.

TABLE 1. Influence of the Amounts of Intake of Balanced or Unbalanced Diet on the Induction of Experimental Models of Marasmus and Kwashiorkor

	Intake of Diet			
	Balanced		Unbalanced	
Condition	Adequate	Inadequate	Adequate	Inadequate
Marasmus		X	X	X
Kwashiorkor			X	

that the amount of intake and the degree or state of the dietary balance or imbalance were of great importance. TABLE 1 demonstrates that while the marasmus model could be induced by a decreased intake of a balanced diet or by an adequate or decreased intake of certain unbalanced diets, the kwashiorkor model could only be induced by an adequate intake of an unbalanced diet. TABLE 2 cites experimental conditions whereby the two models could be induced. The results stress the importance of amounts and/or quality of diet intake in the induction of the two different disease entities. Thus, manipulation of several variables can influence the overall pathological picture. It is essential to have a clear understanding of these possibilities before formulating concepts regarding the pathogenesis of these two specific nutritional diseases as well as of other diseases, which are considered to be diet induced or related.

For many years, it has been known that animals, rabbits and rats, show a hypercholesterolemic response when fed animal protein in comparison to vegetable protein. Usually, this is demonstrated by feeding casein and soy protein, but the metabolic response also occurs with a number of animal proteins when compared to vegetable proteins (FIG. 1).[6] Since there is much experimental and epidemiological evidence linking elevated serum cholesterol levels with a higher risk of atherogenesis,[7] it is important to assess whether dietary protein or amino acids may play a role in the induction and maintenance of atherosclerosis in animals as well as in man. A number of reviews have considered this important problem.[8-10]

In this presentation, I plan to review data collected by numerous researchers for many years pertaining to findings dealing with the effects of proteins and/or amino acids on the pathogenesis of atherosclerosis (mainly in relation to the development of hypercholester-

TABLE 2. Requirements for Induction of Pathologic Changes in Experimental Models of Marasmus and Kwashiorkor[a]

Marasmus
  Decreased intake of diet
    Balanced—complete diet
    Unbalanced—single essential amino acid devoid diet
                —poor quality protein diet
  Adequate intake of diet
    Unbalanced—low carbohydrate, single essential amino acid devoid diet
                —amino acids devoid diet
Kwashiorkor
  Adequate intake of unbalanced diet
    Essential amino acid devoid diet
      Need for other amino acids
      Adequate quantity of carbohydrate
    Poor quality protein diet

[a]Data derived from experimental studies described in review article.[5]

olemia). I shall emphasize points which I feel are of importance and/or may need further explanation in order to help clarify how proteins and amino acids may act in influencing serum cholesterol levels. These selections are biased in view of my own past experience with the role that dietary amino acids and proteins play in other nutritionally related conditions. Nonetheless, I feel that much basic information needs to be collected about nutritional imbalances as induced by proteins and amino acids before an understanding of how they are involved in nutritionally induced or related diseases such as atherosclerosis is fully and rationally accomplished. Such an approach should receive high priority and offers a promising area for future research. Should this presentation stimulate further investigation into the basic aspects of the consequences of specific nutritional imbalances (how they occur, act, and may be alleviated), I feel that my review will have been of value.

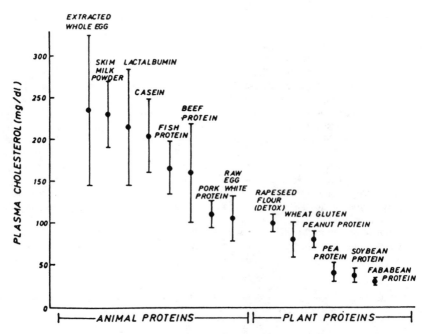

FIGURE 1. Effect of different dietary proteins on serum cholesterol levels in rabbits. Four to six animals were fed a low fat, cholesterol-free semisynthetic diet for 28 days. Means ± SEM are given (according to Carroll and Hamilton[6]).

Role of the Quality of Dietary Protein

Shortly after Ignatowski[1] reported that rabbits fed animal protein developed arterial lesions, a number of other investigators reported interesting findings in regard to the type of dietary proteins used. Rabbits fed high dietary casein (30 g/day) developed arterial lesions, but those fed soybeans did not.[11,12] Also, lean beef muscle in the diet induced atherosclerosis.[13] Studies with other species have likewise produced different effects depending upon the type of proteins used. These reports have been described in a number of review articles.[8-10] In general, the plasma cholesterol levels have become higher in some animals fed animal proteins and lower in some animals fed plant proteins.

Although it is still not clear whether animal proteins contain something that produces a hypercholesterolemic response, especially in rabbits, or whether plant proteins contain some hypocholesterolemic component, it has been considered that the differences in the amino acid compositions of the two types of proteins are responsible for their different responses. Feeding mixtures of L-amino acids as present in casein or egg yolk protein induced hypercholesterolemic responses similar to those obtained with the intact proteins. Feeding mixtures of L-amino acids as present in soy protein isolate or sunflower seed protein induced lower levels of plasma cholesterol but not as low as those obtained with the intact proteins.[14,15] It is conceivable that part of the difference in the response to protein in contrast to L-amino acids may be related to the different rates of intestinal absorption of the amino acids under the two feeding conditions. Likewise, the tonicity of the blood following intestinal absorption may become altered with the more rapid influx of the L-amino acids. In earlier studies from our laboratory, we demonstrated that anisotonicity is of importance in affecting protein synthesis in the liver.[16]

The above and other feeding experiments provided evidence that dietary amino acids could influence the level of plasma cholesterol, especially in rabbits, but in spite of many studies, it is still not clear which amino acids alone or combinations of amino acids are mainly responsible for the effects.[15] Since higher levels of essential amino acids are present in animal than in plant proteins, this consideration was evaluated. Supplementation of isolated soybean protein with seven essential amino acids to levels comparable to those found in animal proteins failed to produce a hypercholesterolemic response.[8]

Further experimental studies have revealed that the hypercholesterolemic response due to animal protein can be modified by other dietary constituents. High levels of polyunsaturated fat in the diet can prevent the effect[17,18] while dietary carbohydrate and dietary fiber, as well as dietary fat, have been found to modify the response.[19-22] These observations stress aspects pertaining to nutritional alterations or imbalances which can radically affect the overall response.

In searching for clues as to how different dietary proteins may influence serum lipid levels in susceptible species of animals, many investigators have reported on differences, gastrointestinal and metabolic, observed in animals consuming casein or soy proteins.[10] Under gastrointestinal effects, soy protein induces a lowering of intestinal steroid absorption and a rise of fecal steroid excretion[23] probably by reducing the bioavailability of bile acids due to the fiber content of soy preparations.[24] Under metabolic effects, the differences in amino acid composition of the different types of proteins have already been mentioned. Also, differences in endocrine response have recently been described, particularly in view of the knowledge that some endocrine disorders give rise to abnormal serum cholesterol levels.[10] Soy protein isolate fed to pigs caused significant increases in total thyroxine concentrations over that in pigs fed casein.[10] In rats, Cree and Schalch[25] observed higher thyroxine levels in animals eating a gluten diet as compared to casein. Thus, it is conceivable that effects of vegetable protein, particularly soy protein, in inducing hypocholesterolemia may be attributable to elevated plasma thyroxine levels.[10] Others have attributed the hypercholesterolemia due to casein to elevated serum insulin levels.[26]

In consideration of the mechanisms by which dietary proteins influence serum cholesterol levels in experimental animals, Carroll et al.[23,27] have been concerned with the effects on cholesterol metabolism and on the turnover of plasma cholesterol and lipoproteins. They found that the mass of cholesterol in the plasma (present within 2 pools) was greater in casein-fed rabbits than in the plasma of the soy protein-fed rabbits, whereas the plasma cholesterol of the latter group turned over much more rapidly than that of the casein-fed rabbits.[23] Also, the intestinal absorption of cholesterol of the casein-fed rabbits

occurred more readily than those of soy protein-fed rabbits.[23] Analysis of plasma lipoproteins revealed that the excess serum cholesterol of casein-fed rabbits was carried in the
low-density lipoprotein (LDL) fraction with little change in the high-density lipoproteins
(HDL).[28] Using radiolabeled intermediate density lipoproteins (IDL), Carroll and co-
workers found that the protein component of the lipoprotein, like the cholesterol, turned
over more rapidly in soy protein-fed rabbits.[23] However, the results of experiments with
very low-density lipoproteins (VLDL) labeled with radioiodine were different in that the
level of radioactivity in plasma decreased at much the same rate overall in both casein-
and soy protein-fed rabbits, although there was a more rapid decrease during the first hour
with lipoproteins derived from soy protein-fed compared with those from casein-fed
rabbits. In the rat, it has been reported that casein induces higher rates of VLDL secretion
by liver *in vivo*.[29] The label was transferred from VLDL to HDL more rapidly when the
labeled lipoprotein was derived from the soy protein-fed doners.[27] In studies of the
composition of the apoproteins of the different lipoprotein fractions,[30] the concentration
of apo E was markedly increased in the VLDL and IDL of casein-fed rabbits compared
with those fed soy protein. Also, apo C in the VLDL of casein-fed rabbits showed an
increase.[27] Others have reported different apo B,E receptor activities between casein and
soy-fed rats.[31] It is of interest that the concentration of apo E is influenced by cholesterol
feeding and thyroid function.[32] A recent study[33] reported that casein-fed rats had higher
proportions of apo Cs and lower proportions of apo A-1 than soy-fed rats and suggested
that dietary proteins may affect plasma cholesterol by altering its distribution among
plasma lipoproteins as well as through modifications in the soluble apolipoprotein composition of lipoproteins.

Role of the Quantity of Dietary Protein

Beginning with an early study by Newburgh and Clarkson[13] and subsequently by
many other studies (TABLE 3), it has been demonstrated that not only the quality of the
dietary protein, but also the quantity consumed was important in altering the serum
cholesterol levels in experimental animals. As indicated in TABLE 3, in most cases, the
higher the intake of a specific dietary protein, the greater its effect, be it hypercholesterolemia or hypocholesterolemia, depending on the specific dietary protein (animal or
vegetable). Thus, the nutritional imbalance induced by alterations in the quantity of
dietary protein consumed played an important role in influencing the levels of serum
cholesterol.

Summarized in TABLE 3 are the results obtained by feeding different dietary levels of
proteins (animal or vegetable) to a number of species. In rabbits, the data clearly indicate
that the hypercholesterolemic effect of a protein is enchanced by increasing the proportion
of the protein in the diet. However, no effect occurs when the proportion of a protein
without hypercholesterolemic properties is altered. In rats, the results are somewhat
inconsistent. Although an explanation for the differences in the rats is not available,
variability among the experiments may be responsible since there were major differences
in duration, strain and age, quantity of diets consumed, and other factors. In birds, a
species difference between pigeons and chickens appears to be present, but again the
experimental conditions were variable. In other species, the experimental results are
limited.

In review of the experimental studies with many species, in most cases the levels of
dietary proteins used in the diets were described without much information concerning the
actual amounts of total diet consumed. Thus, the influence of actual total diet eaten of
each test diet is not clear, and this in itself could be an important variable which may only
be carefully controlled by measuring daily diet intake and using pair-feeding or by force-

feeding of all diets. Although a number of studies use body weight changes as an indication of diet consumption, it is fallacious to assume that this always correlates with similar intake of diet even when the control and experimental diets might be isocaloric in composition. Of course, age and sex are important variables which have usually been adequately controlled. As indicated in TABLE 3, the results clearly show a specific trend that high levels of specific proteins show greater effects (up and down) on serum cholesterol. Nonetheless, some experimental studies are not in agreement. The discrepencies might be attributed to variable experimental conditions.

Other neglected or uncontrolled variables in experimental studies are the amounts of

TABLE 3. Evidence for Influence of Quantity of Dietary Protein on Serum Cholesterol Levels in Different Species

Species	Hypercholesterolemia	Hypocholesterolemia	No Change
Rabbits	lean beef muscle (36 > 27%)[13a] casein (54 > 27%)[14] casein (40 > 20 > 10%)[35]		vegetable proteins (38,22,&13%)[34] soybean (54&27%)[14] casein (30&8%)[36]
Rats	casein (16 > 10 > 4%)[37] casein (30 > 15 > 7.5%)[44] casein (10&69% > 30%)[45] casein (40 > 7.5 > 12–18%)[46] casein (5,40,60 > 10,20%)[47a]	casein (high vs low)[38–42] soybean (60 > 40 > 10%)[41] soybean (40 > 10%)[45] fibrin (40 > 10%)[45] pork (40 > 10%)[45] wheat gluten (68.5 > 40> 30 > 20 > 10%)[45]	casein (27&12%)[43]
Birds	*pigeons* casein + cholesterol (30 > 15 > 5%)[48a,49] casein + cholesterol (20,40 > 10%)[64,65]	*chickens* soybean or sesame (high vs low)[50–63] casein (high vs low)[55,56,66–68]	
Pigs	soybean (18 > 12%)[69]	soybean (16 > 9%)[70]	soybean (13.7&4.9%)[71]
Dogs	casein (0 > 4.4g/day/kg)[72]		
Calves	soybean (9 > 25%)[73] soybean (low > high)[74]		
Monkeys	casein (25 > 10%)[75] commercial + casein (25,4 > 8%)[76,77]		commercial diet (25&9%)[78]

[a]Findings based upon morphologic observations.

diet eaten at each feeding as well as the times of feedings. Changes in these factors or conditions can conceivably alter metabolic responses. A number of reports have stressed the differences in the effects of nibbling versus meal eating of diets which may influence the outcome or consequences of the intake of a specific diet.[79–83] Jenkins et al.[84] recently reported that humans consuming a nibbling diet had reduced fasting serum cholesterol levels in comparison with those fed a three-meal diet. Normal eating habits of different species are quite different. For example, rats eat continuously during the night, while man eats three meals during the day.

The preceding information casts light on important issues, which are frequently ignored or given less emphasis than they merit. Dietary levels of nutrients as well as dietary intake are important variables in all types of experimentation dealing with nutrition or nutritionally-related diseases or syndromes. In general, animals appear to be more sensitive to minor nutritional impairments (deficiencies, excesses, imbalances) than are humans. Their instinctive adaptive response to a bad diet is usually a rapid diminished intake of diet. Thus, control of diet intake is vital in comparing results of experimental animals with those of control animals (consuming a good, balanced diet). Many experimental studies dealing with proteins and amino acids in relation to the induction of hypercholesterolemia have failed to adequately control for this variable—comparable intake of diets.

Species Differences

It has clearly been established that different dietary proteins determine different serum cholesterol levels if fed in a semisynthetic diet to some, but not all, animal species. In the rabbit, hypercholesterolemia can be induced without adding high cholesterol or sucrose supplements that need to be added to diets of rats or pigs to cause a similar response. In normal man, most studies have demonstrated that animal (casein) or vegetable (soy) proteins do not induce different serum cholesterol levels.[10] Fortunately, the rabbit was used as the earliest experimental animal, and it proved to be the most sensitive species when animal (casein) and vegetable (soybean) proteins were compared. The rat has also been used in many experimental studies but is less sensitive than the rabbit, and a number of other nutritional factors (carbohydrate,[85] cholesterol,[85,86] and triglyceride[86]) enhance the hypercholesterolemic effect of animal (casein) protein. Also, female and growing rats appear to be more sensitive to changes in dietary protein than male and adult rats.[87,88] The pig has demonstrated a hypercholesterolemic response due to casein provided that elevated dietary cholesterol and fiber were included in the diet.[89] In monkeys, the results are mixed. One study described hypocholesterolemia due to soy isolate,[90] but another study reported no change in serum cholesterol when changing soy protein isolate for casein.[6] In man, Barth and Pfeuffer[10] have reviewed a number of "tightly controlled studies" and reported that in 11 of 13 studies animal and vegetable proteins did not appreciably change serum cholesterol levels. Van Raaij et al.[91,92] fed humans and rabbits the same semisynthetic diets and found that soy protein caused a marked effect in the rabbit but none in man. Thus, Barth and Pfeuffer[10] conclude that overall experimental evidence does not support that soy protein causes a hypocholesterolemic effect in normal man. Even in hyperlipidemic humans, the effect of soy protein on serum cholesterol levels is questionable in that a hypocholesterolemic response was found in only 5 of 15 studies.[10] Nonetheless, others do not agree with the interpretation by Barth and Pfeuffer.[10] Erdman and Fordyce in a recent review article[93] conclude that the prevailing interpretation of the literature suggests that in controlled studies soy protein depresses serum cholesterol in hypercholesterolemic human subjects. Differing dietary protocols from different laboratories may account for a great deal of variability in the results.

Role of Amino Acids

As described above, different proteins were influential in altering the serum cholesterol levels and atherogenesis. Therefore, it was natural that investigators began to explore the amino acid composition of proteins in hopes of gaining some insight into the possible importance of the amino acids. A number of earlier studies dealt with the role of particular amino acids in rabbits,[94] rats[40,44,95,96] and chickens.[55,97,98] I shall review data based upon experimentation with specific amino acids.

TABLE 4 summarizes experimental data from many experimental studies in which investigators studied the effects of eight specific amino acids (histidine, glutamic acid, methionine, taurine, glycine, tyrosine, leucine and cystine) on serum cholesterol levels of different species of animals.

This paper will focus attention on five animo acids which merit review. Two amino acids, lysine and arginine, gained much recognition in regard to the induction of hyper-cholesterolemia as advocated by Kritchevsky.[130] He suggested that the lysine to arginine ratio may be of significance, but experimental studies by others[131] failed to show much correlation between the level of plasma cholesterol and the ratio of lysine to arginine. The concept that a change in the ratio of two amino acids, such as the ratio of lysine to arginine, as proposed by Kritchevsky,[130] in influencing cholesterolemia, is an interesting

TABLE 4. Effects of Single Amino Acids on Serum Cholesterol Levels in Different Species

Species	Hypocholesterolemia	Hypercholesterolemia	No Change
Rabbits		histidine[99]	glutamic acid[100]
		methionine[101]	methionine[102]
Rats	cystine[42,103,104]	glutamic acid[100]	methionine[105]
	taurine[42,106]	histidine[107–109]	
	methionine[42,95,110–113]	methionine[37,114]	
	glycine[115]	tyrosine[116]	
Mice	cystine[104]		
	methionine[104]		
Chicks	glutamic acid[100]		
	methionine[54,117]		
Pigs			methionine[118]
Monkey	cystine[119,120]	histidine[121]	
	taurine[120]		
	methionine[119,120]		
Man	glutamic acid[122–124]		histidine[125]
			cystine[126]
			taurine[127]
			methionine[126,128]
			leucine[129]

one and stresses the possible consequences of amino acids imbalances. Even though there is disagreement as to the importance of these two specific amino acids, it is possible that other amino acid imbalances may indeed prove to be influential. Two other essential amino acids, threonine and tryptophan, have been under investigation in our laboratory and may indirectly have some relationship to heart disease and/or atherosclerosis. The fifth amino acid, homocysteine, has recently been implicated in a specific type of vascular disease.

Lysine and Arginine

In regard to the recent interest in lysine and arginine and particularly the ratio of arginine to lysine,[130] I have decided to review some of the earlier experimental studies dealing with lysine deficiency. Our own early study[132] with rats force-fed or fed ad libitum a purified diet devoid of lysine revealed a number of morphologic and biochemical changes in different organs in rats tube-fed but not in those fed ad libitum in comparison to controls consuming the complete diet. The differences in the results between the force-feeding (adequate intake) and ad libitum (ate less) regimens were explained in terms of differences in the quantity of the deficient diet consumed. In light of our own findings, it was important to review the data of some of the others who investigated the effects of lysine on cholesterolemia in rats and rabbits and carefully consider the amounts of diet consumption in each study.

In 1964 Weigensberg et al.[133] reported that, when rabbits were fed a diet composed of zein, rice and barley containing 1% cholesterol and deficient in lysine, they had lower serum lipid (including cholesterol) levels together with less aortic atherosclerosis than those fed a diet with sufficient lysine. Diet consumption was not measured, but the rabbits fed the deficient diet lost significant body weight suggesting less consumption. In 1971, McGregor[134] reported that rats consuming a wheat gluten diet (limiting in lysine) but supplemented with lysine did not alter the serum cholesterol level. The rats on the deficient diet gained much less (25%) though they ate relatively more than the supplement diet fed rats. Likewise, when lysine was added to a casein diet, no significant changes in serum lipids (including cholesterol) were observed.[44,96] Added 5% lysine reduced food intake by 5–11% with minor decreases in body weight changes. On the other hand, addition of lysine to a commercial diet resulted in a decrease in the serum cholesterol after 30 days in rats.[135] Diet consumption and body weight changes were not given, but the authors implied that supplementation would cause increased growth. Kritchevsky[130] reported that the supplementation of soybean protein with lysine resulted in an increase of serum cholesterol levels. The experimental conditions of the above studies were quite different, and the quantity of diet consumption and the weight changes using different diets were difficult to assess. Therefore, one must be cautious in attempting to conclude what effect lysine itself may have on serum cholesterol levels. Could the changes be due to the effect on diet intake and little more? An answer is as yet not clear.

Threonine

Although there are no specific data available that suggest this essential amino acid acts to influence the process of atherosclerosis, it might be appropriate to mention that deficiency of dietary threonine has been reported to induce cardiac hypertrophy.[136] In this study, young rats were force-fed a complete or threonine-devoid diet for 3 days. The findings with heart muscle of the experimental animals (hypertrophy and increased protein synthesis) contrasted with those dealing with skeletal muscle where atrophy and decreased protein synthesis was observed.[136] Whether and how smooth muscle (such as in vessels) may be effected under such experimental conditions needs to be explored.

Tryptophan

In 1975, Raja and Jarowski[137] discovered that the administration of capsules containing L-tryptophan (69 mg) and L-lysine monohydrochloride (205 mg) three times daily after meals resulted in a significant drop in plasma cholesterol and triglyceride levels in six human cases.

Another interesting finding attributed to increased dietary tryptophan in rats was by Fregly et al.[138] who found that chronic dietary tryptophan (25 and 50 g/kg) given to DOCA-treated rats provided significant protection against the development of DOCAinduced hypertension, polydipsia, polyuria and cardiac hypertrophy in rats. Other workers[139–143] have reported that tryptophan (50 mg/kg) administered acutely to spontaneously hypertensive rats rapidly reduces blood pressure. Also, Feltkamp et al.[144] reported a modest reduction in the blood pressure of 14 humans with essential hypertension when tryptophan was administered orally (50 mg/kg). Most investigators speculated that the effect was mediated through increased synthesis and release of brain serotonin. However, some workers questioned this assumption.[143] Also, our laboratory has demonstrated that tryptophan itself has a rapid and important direct effect on protein synthesis in the rat liver,[145] while others have described such effects on lung,[146] kidney,[147] stomach,[148] and brain[147] which are independent of the effect through serotonin. Thus, other actions of tryptophan (other than via serotonin) may be implicated in its effect in reducing blood pressure in the hypertensive animal.

Choline Deficiency and Tryptophan

Many years ago, several laboratories[149–151] reported that rats fed a choline deficient diet developed aortic atherosclerosis in addition to fatty liver due to choline deficiency. Much experimental work has been conducted in an attempt to elucidate the pathogenesis of the liver lesion due to choline deficiency.[152] However, only a limited number of experimental studies have been concerned with the cardiovascular lesions, including atherosclerosis, which occur with choline deficiency.[149–151]

In our own laboratory, we have been concerned with the effects of elevated dietary tryptophan and of a choline-deficient diet on the promotion of γ-glutamyltranspeptidase positive foci in rat livers.[153] These foci have been considered as precursor lesions in the development of hepatocarcinomas. In one recent study,[154] we observed that elevated (2%) dietary tryptophan affected the serum lipid levels of rats fed a choline-deficient diet for 1 week. The added dietary tryptophan to the choline-deficient diet caused within 1 week a return in serum cholesterol, HDL cholesterol and triglyceride values to levels present in rats fed the choline supplemented diet. The significance of the alterations in serum lipids due to added dietary tryptophan is unknown. Yet it stresses how a specific amino acid excess creates a further nutritional imbalance, which can influence altered circulating serum lipids due to choline deficiency. The alterations in serum lipid due to choline deficiency may influence the development of atherosclerosis in the rat and possibly added dietary tryptophan may prevent the effect. Further experimental studies are needed to determine whether this indeed may occur.

Homocysteine

Accumulation of excessive quantities of homocysteine accompanies inborn errors of metabolism that decrease the conversion of homocysteine to cystathionine. The homocysteinemia and homocystinuria resulting from these inherited defects are associated with precocious vascular disease and with arterial and venous thrombosis.[155] Thus, a role for homocysteine in the pathogenesis of arteriosclerotic disease has been postulated. Recently, a number of clinical studies have indicated that homocysteine accumulates in both cobalamin and folate deficiencies.[156] Folic acid administration has been demonstrated to reduce plasma homocysteine levels.[157] The relationship between the homocysteinemia of inherited cystathionine synthetase deficiency and vascular disease is well established. However, this association cannot be extrapolated to the overall population. Yet it is possible that homocysteine might constitute a risk factor for the development of premature vascular disease. If this is indeed true, then the imbalance induced by cobalamin and folate deficiencies may be of importance in the pathogenesis of this type of vascular disease.

Amino Acid Effects

From the diverse effects described for various single amino acids, it is at present difficult to assess what role or roles they may play in influencing cholesterolemia or atherosclerosis. It has been suggested that a role for amino acids or peptides liberated during protein digestion may be as stimulators of hormone secretion. Indeed, many single amino acids stimulate hormonal responses.[145,158-160] Several hormones, such as insulin, glucagon, thyroxine and catecholamines, can mediate the activity of enzymes, which are involved in cholesterol metabolism, such as β-hydroxy-β-methyl glutaryl CoA reductase.[159,160] Further studies are needed before conclusions regarding any single amino acid are drawn.

CONCLUDING COMMENTS

This presentation has attempted to be a concise review of previous experimental studies dealing with aspects pertaining to the possible influence of dietary protein and amino acids on the development of hypercholesterolemia, which is considered to be intimately associated with atherosclerosis. Review of the extensive data collected over many years from numerous experimental studies reveals unfortunately that our understanding as to how dietary components, particularly proteins and amino acids, may act in the pathogenesis of this process is not clear. One is forced to conclude that the process is a complex one, whereby a number of variables, such as quality and quantity of protein, amino acid composition and proportions, relationships with other dietary components, susceptibility and resistance, and other factors are influential under specific experimental circumstances. Thus, at the present time, one may speculate that the dietary-induced alterations in serum cholesterol levels by proteins and amino acids are related to nutritional imbalances induced by unbalanced dietary intake and/or internal derangements. The complexity of the problem is further emphasized by the species variability in experimental studies. In general, man appears to be more resistant to alterations due to changes in dietary proteins and amino acids than do other species. Nonetheless, in-depth studies of the process in susceptible species under carefully controlled experimental conditions may still offer the best approach to a better overall understanding of the problem. Future experiments may benefit from greater consideration of the concept of nutritional imbalances which can be induced in a variety of ways, each of which may be important as well as vital. Results using experimental models, whereby numerous variables (as many as possible) are simultaneously controlled should offer more definitive and conclusive answers than are currently available. Utilization of the newly developed approaches of molecular biology in conjunction with classical nutritional experimental studies should offer basic information toward a better understanding of the consequences of nutritional imbalances including those induced by dietary proteins and amino acids in relationship to the pathogenesis of cholesterolemia (atherosclerosis).

REFERENCES

1. IGNATOWSKI, A. 1909. Uber die Wirkung des tierischen Einweisses auf die Aorta und die parenchymatosen Organe der Kaninchen. Virchows Arch. A **198:** 248–270.

2. ANITSCHKOW, N. & S. CHALATOW. 1913. Uber experimentelle Cholesterinsteatose und ihre Bedeutung fur die Entstehung einiger pathologischer Prozesse. Zentralbl. Allg. Pathol. Anat. **24:** 1–9.

3. YUDKIN, J. 1957. Diet and coronary thombosis: hypothesis and fact. Lancet **1:** 155–162.

4. YERUSHALMY, J. & H. E. HILLEBOE. 1957. Fat and diet and mortality from heart disease: a methodologic note. N.Y. State J. Med **57:** 2343–2354.

5. SIDRANSKY, H. 1976. Nutritional disturbances of protein metabolism in the liver. Am. J. Pathol. **84:** 649–667.

6. CARROLL, K. K. & R. M. G. HAMILTON. 1975. Effects of dietary protein and carbohydrate on plasma cholesterol levels in relation to atherosclerosis. J. Food Sci. **40:** 18–23.

7. KANNEL, W. B., W. P. CASTELLI & T. GORDON. 1979. Cholesterol in the prediction of atherosclerosis disease. New Perspectives based on the Framingham study. Ann. Intern. Med. **90:** 85–91.

8. CARROLL, K. K. 1982. Hypercholesterolemia and atherosclerosis: effects of dietary protein. Fed. Proc. **41:** 2792–2796.

9. TERPSTRA, A. H. M., R. J. J. HERMUS & C. E. WEST. 1983. The role of dietary protein in cholesterol metabolism. World Rev. Nutr. Diet **42:** 1–55.

10. BARTH. C. A. & M. PFEUFFER. 1988. Dietary protein and atherogenesis. Klin. Wochenschr. **66:** 135–143.

11. NEWBURGH, L. H. 1919. The production of Brights' disease by feeding high protein diets. Arch. Intern. Med. **24:** 359–377.

12. NEWBURGH, L. H. & T. L. SQUIER. 1923. High protein diets and arteriosclerosis in rabbits. Arch. Intern. Med. **26:** 38–40.

13. NEWBURGH, L. H. & S. CLARKSON. 1923. The production of atherosclerosis in rabbits by feeding diets rich in meat. Arch. Intern. Med. **31:** 653–676.

14. HUFF, M. W., R. M. G. HAMILTON & K. K. CARROLL. 1977. Plasma cholesterol levels in rabbits fed low fat, cholesterol-free, semipurified diets: effects of dietary proteins, protein hydrolysates and amino acid mixtures. Atherosclerosis **28:** 187–195.

15. HUFF, M. W. & K. K. CARROLL. 1980. Effects of dietary proteins and amino acid mixtures on plasma cholesterol levels in rabbits. J. Nutr. **110:** 1676–1685.

16. LYNN, J. K. & H. SIDRANSKY. 1974. Effect of changes of osmotic pressure of portal blood on hepatic protein synthesis. Lab. Invest. **31:** 332–339.

17. LAMBERT, G. F., J. F. MILLER, R. T. OLSEN & D. V. FROST, 1958. Hypercholesterolemia and atherosclerosis induced in rabbits by purified high fat rations devoid of cholesterol. Proc. Soc. Exp. Biol. Med. **97:** 544–549.

18. MALMROS, H. & G. WIGAND. 1959. Atherosclerosis and deficiency of essential fatty acids. Lancet **2:** 749–751.

19. BAUER, J. E. & S. J. COVERT. 1984. The influence of protein and carbohydrate type on serum and liver lipids and lipoprotein cholesterol in rabbits. Lipids **19:** 844–850.

20. CARROLL, K. K., R. M. G. HAMILTON, M. W. HUFF & A. D. FALCONER. 1978. Dietary fiber and cholesterol metabolism in rabbits and rats. Am. J. Clin. Nutr. **31:** 5203–5207.

21. HAMILTON, R. M. G. & K. K. CARROLL. 1976. Plasma cholesterol levels in rabbits fed low fat, low cholesterol diets. Effects of dietary proteins, carbohydrates and fibre from different sources. Atherosclerosis **24:** 47–62.

22. KRITCHEVSKY, D., S. A. TEPPER, D. E. WILLIAMS & J. A. STORY. 1977. Experimental atherosclerosis in rabbits fed cholesterol-free diets. Part. 7. Interaction of animal or vegetable protein with fiber. Atherosclerosis **26:** 397–403.

23. HUFF, M. W. & K. K. CARROLL. 1980. Effects of dietary proteins in turnover, oxidation and absorption of cholesterol and on steroid excretion in rabbits. J. Lipid Res. **21:** 546–558.

24. CHO, B. H. S., P. O. EGWIN & C. G. FAHEY. 1985. Plasma lipid and lipoprotein cholesterol levels in swine. Modification of protein-induced response by added cholesterol and soy fiber. Atherosclerosis **56:** 39–49.

25. CREE, T. C. & D. S. SCHALCH. 1985. Protein utilization in growth: effect of lysine deficiency on serum growth hormone, somatomedins, insulin, total thyroxine (T_4) and triiodothyronine, free T_4 index, and total corticosterone. Endocrinology **117:** 667–673.

26. HUBBARD, R., C. L. KOSCH. A. SANCHEZ, J. SABATE, L. BERK & G. SHAVLIK. 1989. Effect

of dietary protein on serum insulin and glucagon levels in hyper- and normocholesterolemic men. Atherosclerosis **76:** 55–61.

27. ROBERTS, D. C. K., M. E. STALMACH, M. W. KHALIL, J. C. HUTCHINSON & K. K. CARROLL. 1981. Effects of dietary protein on composition and turnover of apoproteins in plasma lipoproteins of rabbits. Can. J. Biochem. **59:** 642–647.

28. CARROLL K. K., M. W. HUFF & D. C. K. ROBERTS. 1979. Vegatable protein and lipid metabolism. *In* Soy Protein and Human Nutrition. H. L. Wilcke, D. T. Hopkins & D. H. Waggle, Eds. 261–280. Academic Press. New York, NY.

29. PFEUFFER, M. & C. A. BARTH. 1986. Modulation of very low density lipoprotein secretion by dietary protein is age-dependent in rats. Ann. Nutr. Metab. **30:** 281–288.

30. CATAPANO, A. L., R. L. JACKSON, E. B. GILLIAM, A. M. GOTLO, JR., & L. C. SMITH. 1978. Quantification of apo C-II and apo C-III of human very low density lipoprotein by analytical isoelectric focusing. J. Lipid Res. **19:** 1047–1052.

31. COHN, J. S. & P. J. NESTEL. 1985. Hepatic lipoprotein receptor activity in rats fed casein and soy protein. Atherosclerosis **56:** 247–250.

32. DELAMATRE, J. G. & P. S. ROHEIM. 1981. Effect of cholesterol feeding on apoB and apoE concentrations and distributions in euthyroid and hypothyroid rats. J. Lipid Res. **22:** 297–306.

33. JACQUES, H., Y. DESHAIES, K. K. CARROLL, J. M. HRABEK-SMITH & L. SAVOIE. 1988. Effects of dietary proteins on the cholesterol and soluble apolipoprotein composition of plasma lipoproteins in the rat. Nutrition **4:** 439–445.

34. FREYBERG, R. H. 1937. Relation of experimental atherosclerosis to diets rich in vegetable proteins. Arch. Intern. Med. **59:** 660–666.

35. TERPSTRA, A. H. M., L. HARKES & F. H. VAN DER VEEN. 1981. The effect of different proportions of casein in semi-purified diets on the concentration of serum cholesterol and the lipoprotein composition in rabbits. Lipids **16:** 114–119.

36. MUNRO, H. N., M. H. STEELE & W. FORBES. 1965. Effect of dietary protein level on deposition of cholesterol in the tissues of the cholesterol-fed rabbit. Br. J. Exp. Pathol. **49:** 489–496.

37. BAGCHI, K., R. RAY & R. DATTA. 1963. The influence of dietary protein and methionine on serum cholesterol level. Am. J. Clin. Nutr. **13:** 232–237.

38. CHEN, L. H., S. LIAO & L. V. PACKETT. 1972. Interaction of dietary vitamin E and protein level or lipid source with serum cholesterol level in rats. J. Nutr. **102:** 729–732.

39. FILLIOS, L. C., S. B. ANDRUS, G. V. MANN & F. J. STARE. 1956. Experimental production of gross atherosclerosis in the rat. J. Exp. Med. **104:** 539–554.

40. GROOT, A. P. DE. 1958. The influence of dietary protein on the serum cholesterol level in rats. Voeding **19:** 715–718.

41. MOYER, A. W., D. KRITCHEVSKY. J. B. LOGAN & H. R. COX. 1956. Dietary protein and serum cholesterol in rats. Proc. Soc. Exp. Biol. Med. **92:** 736–737.

42. SEIDEL, J. C., N. NATH & A. E. HARPER. 1960. Diet and cholesterolemia. V. Effects of sulfur-containing amino acids and protein. J. Lipid Res. **1:** 474–481.

43. CHANG, M. L. W. & M. A. JOHNSON. 1980. Effect of pectin and protein levels on cholesterol-4-^{14}C metabolism in rats. Nutr. Rep. Int. **22:** 91–99.

44. HEVIA, P., F. W. KARI, E. A. ULMAN & W. J. VISEK. 1980. Serum and liver lipids in growing rats fed casein with L-lysine. J. Nutr. **40:** 1224–1230.

45. NATH, N., A. E. HARPER & C. A. ELVEHJEM. 1959. Diet and cholesteremia. III. Effect of dietary proteins with particular reference to the lipids in wheat gluten. Can. J. Biochem. Physiol. **37:** 1375–1384.

46. JONES, R. J. & S. HUFFMAN. 1956. Chronic effect of dietary protein on hypercholesteremia in the rat. Proc. Soc. Exp. Biol. Med. **93:** 519–522.

47. FILLIOS, L. C., C. NAITO, S. B. ANDRUS, O. W. PORTMAN & R. S. MARTIN. 1958. Variations in cardiovascular sudanophilia with changes in the dietary level of protein. Am. J. Physiol. **194:** 275–279.

48. CLARKSON, T. B., R. W. PRICHARD, H. B. LOFLAND & H. O. GOODMAN. 1962. Interactions among dietary fat, protein, and cholesterol in atherosclerosis-susceptible pigeons. Circ. Res. **11:** 400–404.

49. LOFLAND, H. B., T. B. CLARKSON & H. O. GOODMAN. 1961. Interactions among dietary fat,

protein and cholesterol in atherosclerosis-susceptible pigeons. Effect on serum cholesterol and aortic atherosclerosis. Circ. Res. **9:** 919–924.

50. LEVEILLE, G. A., A. S. FEIGENBAUM & H. FISHER. 1960. The effect of dietary protein, fat and cholesterol on plasma cholesterol and serum protein components of the growing chick. Arch. Biochem. Biophys. **86:** 67–70.

51. LEVEILLE, G. A. & H. FISHER. 1958. Plasma cholesterol in growing chicken as influenced by dietary protein and fat. Proc. Soc. Exp. Biol. Med. **98:** 630–632.

52. LEVEILLE, G. A. & H. E. SAUBERLICH. 1961. Influence of dietary protein level on serum protein components and cholesterol in the growing chick. J. Nutr. **74:** 500–504.

53. LEVEILLE, G. A., J. W. SHOCKLEY & H. E. SAUBERLICH. 1961. Influence of dietary factors on plasma lipid relationships in the growing chick. Proc. Soc. Exp. Biol. Med. **108:** 313–315.

54. LEVEILLE, G. A., J. W. SHOCKLEY & H. E. SAUBERLICH. 1962. Influence of dietary protein level and amino acids on plasma cholesterol of the growing chick. J. Nutr. **76:** 321–324.

55. JOHNSON, D., G. A. LEVEILLE & H. FISHER. 1958. Influence of amino acid deficiencies and protein level on the plasma cholesterol of the chick. J. Nutr. **66:** 367–376.

56. KENNEY, J. J. & H. FISHER. 1973. Effect of medium chain triglycerides and dietary protein on cholesterol absorption and deposition in the chicken. J. Nutr. **103:** 923–928.

57. KOKATNUR, M. G. & F. A. KUMMEROW. 1959. The relationship of corn oil and animal fats to serum cholesterol values at various dietary protein levels. J. Am. Oil Chem. Soc. **36:** 248–250.

58. KOKATNUR, M., N. T. RAND, F. A. KUMMEROW & H. M. SCOTT. 1958. Effect of dietary protein and fat on changes of serum cholesterol in mature birds. J. Nutr. **64:** 177–184.

59. MARCH, B. E., J. BEILY, J. TOTHILL & S. A. HAQQ. 1959. Dietary modification of serum cholesterol in the chick. J. Nutr. **69:** 105–110.

60. NISHIDA, T., F. TAKENAKE & F. A. KUMMEROW. 1958. Effect of dietary protein and heated fat on serum cholesterol and beta-lipoprotein levels, and on the incidence of experimental atherosclerosis in chicks. Circ. Res. **6:** 194–202.

61. ROSE, R. J. & S. L. BALOUN. 1969. Effect of restricted energy and protein intake on atherosclerosis and associated physiological factors in cockerels. J. Nutr. **98:** 335–343.

62. STAMLER, J., R. PICK & L. N. KATZ. 1958. Effects of dietary proteins, methionine and vitamins on plasma lipids and atherogenesis in cholesterol-fed cockerels. Circ. Res. **6:** 442–446.

63. STAMLER, J., R. PICK & L. N. KATZ. 1958. Effects of dietary protein and carbohydrate level on cholesterolemia and atherogenesis in cockerels on a high-fat, high-cholesterol mash. Circ. Res. **6:** 447–451.

64. LITTLE, J. M. & E. A. ANGELL. 1977. Dietary protein level and experimental aortic atherosclerosis. Atherosclerosis **26:** 173–179.

65. SUBBIAH, M. T. V. 1977. Early dietary and medical intervention and the development of atherosclerosis. I. Effect of low protein diet on the age-related accumulation of sterols and steryl-esters in aorta during spontaneous atherogenesis in the white carneau pigeon. Nutr. Rep. Int. **15:** 223–229.

66. FISHER, H., A. FEIGENBAUM, G. A. LEVEILLE, H. S. WEISS & P. GRIMINGER. 1959. Biochemical observations on aortas of chickens. Effect of different fats and varying levels of protein, fat and cholesterol. J. Nutr. **69:** 163–171.

67. KOKATNUR, M., N. T. RAND & F. A. KUMMEROW. 1958. Effect of the energy to protein ratio on serum and carcass cholesterol levels in chicks. Circ. Res. **6:** 424–431.

68. STAMLER, J., R. PICK & L. N. KATZ. 1958. Action of casein, egg albumin and corn germ on cholesterolemia and atherogenesis in cockerels. Fed. Proc. **17:** 155.

69. GREER, S. A. N., V. W. HAYS, V. C. SPEER & J. T. MCCALL. 1966. Effect of dietary fat protein and cholesterol on atherosclerosis in swine. J. Nutr. **90:** 183–190.

70. BARNES, R. H., E. KWONG, W. POND, R. LOWRY & J. K. LOOSLI. 1959. Dietary fat and protein and serum cholesterol. II. Young swine. J. Nutr. **69:** 269–273.

71. BARNES, R. H., E. KWONG, G. FIALA, M. RECHCIGL, R. N. LUTZ & J. K. LOOSLI. 1959. Dietary fat and protein and serum cholesterol. I. Adult Swine. J. Nutr. **69:** 261–268.

72. LI, T. W. & L. FREEMAN. 1946. Experimental lipemia and hypercholesterolemia by protein depletion and by cholesterol feeding. Am. J. Physiol. **145:** 660–666.

73. COCCODRILLI, G. D., P. T. CHANDLER & C. E. POLAN. 1970. Effects of dietary protein on blood lipids of the calf with special reference to cholesterol. J. Dairy Sci. **53:** 1627–1631.
74. CHANDLER, P. T., R. D. MCCARTHY & E. M. KESLER. 1968. Effect of dietary lipids and protein on serum proteins, lipids and glucose in the blood of dairy calves. J. Nutr. **95:** 461–468.
75. STRONG, J. P. & H. C. MCGILL. 1967. Diet and experimental atherosclerosis in baboons. Am. J. Pathol. **50:** 669–690.
76. SRINIVASAN, S. R., B. RADHAKRISHNAMURTHY, E. R. DALFERES & G. S. BERENSON. 1979. Serum α-lipoprotein responses to variations in dietary cholesterol, protein and carbohydrate in different nonhuman primate species. Lipids **44:** 559–565.
77. SRINIVASAN, S. R., B. RADHAKRISHNAMURTHY, E. R. DALFERES, L. S. WEBBER & G. S. BERENSON. 1977. Serum lipoprotein responses to exogenous cholesterol in spider monkeys: effect of levels of dietary protein. Proc. Soc. Exp. Biol. Med. **154:** 102–106.
78. MIDDLETON, C. C., T. B. CLARKSON, H. B. LOFLAND & R. W. PRICHARD. 1967. Diet and atherosclerosis of squirrel monkeys. Arch. Pathol. **83:** 145–153.
79. COHN, C. & D. JOSEPH. 1960. Effects on metabolism produced by the rate of ingestion of the diet. 'Meal-eating' versus 'nibbling.' Am. J. Clin. Nutr. **8:** 682–690.
80. COHN, C., D. JOSEPH, L. BELL & A. OLER. 1963. Feeding frequency and protein metabolism. Am. J. Physiol. **205:** 71–78.
81. HOLLIFIELD, G. & W. PARSON. 1962. Metabolic adaptations to a 'stuff and starve' feeding program. I. Studies of adipose tissue and liver glycogen in rats limited to a short daily feeding period. J. Clin. Invest. **41:** 245–249.
82. FABRY, P. & J. TEPPERMAN. 1970. Meal frequency. A possible factor in human pathology. Am. J. Clin. Nutr. **23:** 1059–1068.
83. WILEY, J. H. & G. A. LEVEILLE. 1970. Influence of periodicity of eating on the activity of adipose tissue and muscle glycogen synthesizing enzymes in the rat. J. Nutr. **100:** 85–93.
84. JENKINS, D. J. A., T. M. S. WOLEVER, V. VUKSAN, et al. 1989. Nibbling versus gorging: metabolic advantages of increased meal frequency. N. Engl. J. Med. **324:** 929–934.
85. HEVIA, P., R. A. CLARY & W. J. VISEK. 1979. Serum and liver lipids in rats fed casein or soybean protein with sucrose or dextrin or sucrose and cholesterol. Nutr. Rep. Int. **20:** 539–548.
86. NAGATA, Y., K. IMAIJUMI & M. SUGANO. 1980. Effects of soy bean protein and casein on serum cholesterol levels in rats. Br. J. Nutr. **44:** 113–121.
87. TERPSTRA, A. H. M., G. VAN TINTELEN & C. E. WEST. 1982. The effect of semipurified diets containing different proportions of cholesterol in whole serum, serum lipoproteins and liver in male and female rats. Atherosclerosis **42:** 85–95.
88. WEST, C. E., K. DEURING, J. B. SCHUTLE & A. H. M. TERPSTRA. 1982. The effect of age in the development of hypercholesterolemia in rabbits fed semipurified diets containing casein. J. Nutr. **112:** 1287–1295.
89. CHO, B. H. S., P. O. EGWIM & G. C. FAHEY. 1985. Plasma lipid and lipoprotein cholesterol levels in swine. Modification of protein-induced response by added cholesterol and soy fiber. Atherosclerosis **56:** 39–49.
90. TERPSTRA, A. H. M., C. E. WEST & J. T. C. M. FENNIS. 1984. Hypercholesterolemic effect of dietary soy protein versus casein in rhesus monkeys (Macaca mulatta). Am. J. Clin. Nutr. **39:** 1–7.
91. RAAIJ, J. M. A. VAN, M. B. KATON & J. G. A. J. HAUTVAST. 1979. Casein, soy protein, serum cholesterol. Lancet **2:** 958.
92. RAAIJ, J. M. A. VAN, M. B. KATAN, J. G. A. J. HAUTVAST, et al. 1981. Effect of casein versus soy protein diets on serum cholesterol and lipoproteins in young healthy volunteers. Am. J. Clin. Nutr. **34:** 1261–1271.
93. ERDMAN, J. W., JR. & E. J. FORDYCE. 1989. Soy products and the human diet. Am. J. Clin. Nutr. **49:** 725–737.
94. HUFF, M. W. & K. K. CARROLL. 1980. Effects of dietary proteins and amino acid mixtures on plasma cholesterol levels in rabbits. J. Nutr. **110:** 1676–1685.
95. GROOT, A. P. DE. 1960. De invloed van eiwitten en andere nutrienten op de cholesterolspiegel van het bloed. Voeding **21:** 374–386.

96. HEVIA, P., E. A. ULMAN, F. W. KARI & W. J. VISEK. 1980. Serum lipids of rats fed excess L-lysine and different carbohydrates. J. Nutr. **110:** 1231–1239.

97. KOKATNUR, M. G. KLAIN, D. SNETSINGER, F. A. KUMMEROW & H. M. SCOTT. 1959. Effect of various amino acids on serum cholesterol levels in chicks. Fed. Proc. **18:** 532.

98. KOKATNUR, M. G. & F. A. KUMMEROW. 1961. Amino acid imbalance and cholesterol levels in chicks. J. Nutr. **75:** 319–329.

99. GEISON, R. L. & H. A. WAISMAN. 1970. Plasma and tissue cholesterol and lipid levels in rabbits on L-histidine-supplemented diets. Proc. Soc. Exp. Biol. Med. **133:** 234–237.

100. BAZZANO, G. 1969. Hypocholesterolemic effect of glutamic acid in the mongolian gerbil. Proc. Soc. Exp. Biol. Med. **131:** 1463–1465.

101. HERMUS, R. J. J. & G. M. DALLINGA-THIE. 1979. Soya, saponins, and plasma-cholesterol. Lancet **1:** 48.

102. HAMILTON, R. M. G. & K. K. CARROLL. 1976. Plasma cholesterol levels in rabbits fed low fat, low cholesterol diets: effects of dietary proteins, carbohydrates and fibre from different sources. Atherosclerosis **24:** 47–62.

103. YOSHIDA K., M. YAHIRO & K. AHIKO. 1989. Effects of addition of arginine cystine, and glycine to the bovine milk-simulated amino acid mixture on the level of plasma and liver cholesterol in rats. J. Nutr. Sci. Vitaminol. **34:** 567–576.

104. FILLIOS, L. C. & G. V. MANN. 1954. Influence of sulfur amino acid deficiency on cholesterol metabolism. Metabolism **3:** 16–26.

105. JONES, R. J., R. W. WISSLER & S. HUFFMAN. 1957. Certain dietary effects on the serum cholesterol and atherogenesis in the rat. Arch. Pathol. **63:** 593–601.

106. HERRMAN, R. G. 1959. Effect of taurine, glycine and -sitosterols on serum and tissue cholesterol in the rat and rabbit. Circ. Res. **8:** 224–227.

107. QURESHI, A. A., J. A. SOLOMON & B. EICHELMAN. 1978. L-Histidine-induced facilitation of cholesterol biosynthesis in rats. Proc. Soc. Exp. Biol. Med. **159:** 57–60.

108. SOLOMON, J. K. & R. L. GEISON. 1978. Effect of excess dietary L-histidine on plasma cholesterol levels in weanling rats. J. Nutr. **108:** 936–943.

109. SOLOMON, J. K. & R. L. GEISON. 1978. L-Histidine-induced hypercholesterolemia: characteristics of cholesterol biosynthesis in rat livers. Proc. Soc. Exp. Biol. Med. **159:** 44–47.

110. PASSANANTI, G. T., N. B. GUERRANT & R. Q. THOMPSON. 1958. Effects of supplementary methionine and choline on tissue lipids and on the vascular structure of cholesterol-fed growing rats. J. Nutr. **66:** 55–74.

111. NATH, N., J. C. SEIDEL & A. E. HARPER. 1961. Diet and cholesterolemia. VI. Comparative effects of wheat gluten lipids and some other lipids in presence of adequate and inadequate dietary protein. J. Nutr. **74:** 389–396.

112. SEIDEL, J. C. & A. E. HARPER. 1962. Effects of ethionine and methionine on serum lipids and lipoproteins. Proc. Soc. Exp. Biol. Med. **111:** 579–582.

113. SHAPIRO, S. L. & L. FREEDMAN. 1955. Effect of essential unsaturated fatty acids and methionine on hypercholesteremia. Am. J. Physiol. **181:** 441–445.

114. ROTH, J. S. & S. W. MILSTEIN. 1957. Some effects of excess methionine on lipid metabolism in the rat. Arch. Biochem. Biophys. **70:** 392–400.

115. KATAN, M. B., L. H. M. VROOMEN & R. J. J. HERMUS. 1981. Reduction of casein-induced hypercholesterolemia and atherosclerosis in rabbits and rats by dietary glycine, arginine and alanine. Atherosclerosis **43:** 381–391.

116. NAGHOKA, S., Y. AOYAMA & A. YOSHIDA. 1985. Effect of tyrosine and some other amino acids on serum level of cholesterol in rats. Nutr. Rep. Int. **31:** 1137–1148.

117. HILL, E. G. 1966. Effects of methionine, menhaden oil and ethoxyquin on serum cholesterol of chicks. J. Nutr. **89:** 143–148.

118. KIM, D. N., K. T. LEE, J. M. REINER & W. A. THOMAS. 1978. Effects of a soy protein product on serum and tissue cholesterol concentrations in swine fed high-fat, high-cholesterol diets. Exp. Mol. Pathol. **29:** 385–399.

119. MANN, G. V., S. B. ANDRUS, A. MCNALLY & F. J. STARE. 1953. Experimental atherosclerosis in cebus monkeys. J. Exp. Med. **98:** 195–217.

120. MANN, G. V., A. MCNALLY & C. PRUDHOMME. 1960. Experimental atherosclerosis. Effects of sulfur compounds on hypercholesteremia and growth in cysteine-deficient monkeys. Am. J. Clin. Nutr. **8:** 491–498.

121. KERR, G. R., R. C. WOLF & H. A. WAISMAN. 1965. Hyperlipemia in infant monkeys fed excess L-histidine. Proc. Soc. Exp. Biol. Med. **119:** 561–562.

122. OLSON, R. E., G. BAZZANO & J. A. D'ELIA. 1970. The effects of large amounts of glutamic acid upon serum lipids and sterol metabolism in man. Trans. Assoc. Am. Physicians **83:** 196–210.

123. OLSON, R. E., M. Z. NICHAMAN, J. NITTKA & J. A. EAGLES. 1970. Effect of amino acid diets upon serum lipids in man. Am. J. Clin. Nutr. **23:** 1614–1625.

124. GARLICH, J. D., G. BAZZANO & R. E. OLSON. 1970. Changes in plasma free amino acid concentrations in human subjects on hypocholesteremic diets. Am. J. Clin. Nutr. **23:** 1626–1638.

125. GERBER, D. A., J. E. SKLAR & J. NIEDWIADOWIEZ. 1971. Lack of an effect of oral L-histidine on the serum cholesterol in human subjects. Am. J. Clin. Nutr. **24:** 1382–1383.

126. MORSE, E. H., S. B. MERROW, M. A. PARKER, E. P. LEWIS & C. A. NEWHALL. 1966. Lipid metabolism and the sulfur-containing amino acids. J. Am. Diet. Assoc. **48:** 496–500.

127. TRUSWELL, A. S., S. MCVEIGH, W. D. MITCHELL & B. BRONTE-STEWART. 1965. Effect in man of feeding taurine on bile acid conjugation and serum cholesterol levels. J. Atheroscler. Res. **5:** 526–532.

128. MANN, G. V., D. L. FARNSWORTH & F. J. STARE. 1953. An evaluation of the influence of dl-methionine treatment on the serum lipids of adult American males. N. Engl. J. Med. **249:** 1018–1019.

129. TRUSWELL, A. S. 1964. Effect of surplus leucine intake on serum cholesterol in man. Proc. Nutr. Soc. **23:** xlvi.

130. KRITCHEVSKY, D. 1979. Vegetable protein and atherosclerosis. J. Am. Oil Chem. Soc. **56:** 135–140.

131. CARROLL, K. K. 1981. Soya protein and atherosclerosis. J. Am. Oil Chem. Soc. **58:** 416–419.

132. SIDRANSKY, H. & T. BABA. 1960. Chemical pathology of acute amino acid deficiencies. III. Morphologic and biochemical changes in young rats fed valine- or lysine-devoid diets. J. Nutr. **70:** 463–483.

133. WEIGENSBERG, B. I., H. C. STARY & G. C. MCMILLAN. 1964. Effect of lysine deficiency on cholesterol atherosclerosis in rabbits. Exp. Mol. Pathol. **3:** 444–454.

134. MCGREGOR, D. 1971. The effects of some dietary changes upon the concentrations of serum lipids in rats. Br. J. Nutr. **25:** 213–224.

135. JAROWSKI, C. I. & R. PYTELEWSKI. 1975. Utility of fasting essential amino acid plasma levels in formulation of nutritionally adequate diets. III. Lowering of rat serum cholesterol levels by lysine supplementation. J. Pharm. Sci. **64:** 690–691.

136. VERNEY, E. & H. SIDRANSKY. 1974. Alterations in cardiac protein metabolism in rats force-fed a threonine-devoid diet. J. Nutr. **104:** 463–472.

137. RAJA, P. K. & C. I. JAROWSKI. 1975. Utility of fasting essential amino acid plasma levels in formulation of nutritionally adequate diets. IV. Lowering of human plasma cholesterol and triglyceride levels by lysine and tryptophan supplementation. J. Pharm. Sci. **64:** 691–692.

138. FREGLY, M. J., O. E. LOCKLEY, J. VAN DER VOORT, C. SUMNERS & W. N. HENLEY. 1987. Chronic dietary administration of tryptophan prevents the development of deoxycorticosterone acetate salt induced hypertension in rats. Can. J. Physiol. Pharmacol. **65:** 753–764.

139. JARROTT, B., A. MCQUEEN, L. GRAF & W. J. LOUIS. 1975. Serotonin levels in vascular tissue and the effects of a serotonin synthesis inhibitor on blood pressure of hypertensive rats. Clin. Exp. Pharmacol. Physiol. Suppl. **2:** 201–205.

140. FULLER, R. W., D. R. HOLLAND, T. T. YEN, K. G. BEMIS & N. B. STAMM. 1979. Antihypertensive effects of fluoxitine and L-5-hydroxytryptophan in rats. Life Sci. **25:** 1237–1242.

141. SVED, A. F., C. M. VAN ITALLIE & J. D. FERNSTROM. 1982. Studies on the antihypertensive action of L-tryptophan. J. Pharmacol. Exp. Ther. **221:** 329–333.

142. WOLF, W. A. & D. M. KUHN. 1984a. Effects of L-tryptophan on blood pressure in normotensive and hypertensive rats. J. Pharmacol. Exp. Ther. **230:** 324–329.

143. WOLF, W. A. & D. M. KUHN. 1984b. Antihypertensive effects of tryptophan are not mediated by brain serotonin. Brain Res. **295:** 356–359.

144. FELTKAMP, H., K. A. MEUER & E. GODCHARDT. 1984. Tryptophan-induced lowering of

blood pressure and changes in serotonin uptake by platelets in patients with essential hypertension. Klin. Wochenschr. **62:** 1115–1119.

145. SIDRANSKY, H. 1985. Tryptophan: unique action by an essential amino acid. *In* Nutritional Pathology. Pathobiochemistry of Dietary Imbalances. H. Sidransky, Ed. Vol. **10:** 1–62. The Biochemistry of Disease. Marcel Dekker, Inc. New York, NY.

146. GACAD, G., K. DICKIE & D. MASSARO. 1972. Protein synthesis in lung: influence of starvation on amino acid incorporation into protein. J. Appl. Physiol. **33:** 381–384.

147. JORGENSEN, A. J. F. & A. P. N. MAJUMDAR. 1976. Bilateral adrenalectomy: effect of tryptophan force-feeding on amino acid incorporation into ferritin, transferrin, and mixed proteins of liver, brain and kidneys *in vivo*. Biochem. Med. **16:** 37–46.

148. MAJUMDAR, A. P. N. 1979. Bilateral adrenalectomy: effect of tryptophan on protein synthesis and pepsin activity in the stomach of rats. Scand. J. Gastroenterol. **14:** 949–954.

149. HARTROFT, W. S., J. H. RIDOUT, E. A. SELLERS & C. H. BEST. 1952. Atheromatous changes in aorta, carotid and coronary arteries of choline-deficient rats. Proc. Soc. Exp. Biol. Med. **81:** 384–393.

150. WILGRAM, G. F., C. H. BEST & J. BLUMENSTEIN. 1955. Aggravating effect of cholesterol on cardiovascular changes in choline-deficient rats. Proc. Soc. Exp. Biol. Med. **89:** 476–479.

151. SALMAN, W. D. & P. M. NEWBERNE. 1962. Cardiovascular disease in choline-deficient rats. J. Nutr. **73:** 26–45.

152. SHINOZUKA, H. & S. L. KATYAL. 1985. Pathology of choline deficiency. *In* Nutritional Pathology. Pathobiochemistry of Dietary Imbalances. H. Sidransky, Ed. Vol. **10:** 279–320. The Biochemistry of Disease. Marcel Dekker, Inc. New York, NY.

153. SIDRANSKY, H., C. T. GARRETT, C. N. MURTY, E. VERNEY & E. S. ROBINSON. 1985. Influence of dietary tryptophan on the induction of γ-glutamyltranspeptidase-positive foci in the livers of rats treated with hepatocarcinogen. Cancer Res. **45:** 4844–4847.

154. SIDRANSKY, H., E. VERNEY & R. N. KURL. 1989. Effect of feeding a choline deficient diet on the hepatic nuclear response to tryptophan in the rat. Exp. Mol. Pathol. **51:** 68–79.

155. MUDD, S. H. & H. L. LEVY. 1983. Disorders of transsulfuration. *In* The Metabolic Basis of Inherited Disease. J. B. Stanbury, J. B. Wyngarden & D. S. Frederickson, Eds. 522–559. McGraw-Hill. New York, NY.

156. Homocysteine, folic acid, and the prevention of vascular disease. 1989. Nutr. Rev. **47:** 247–249.

157. BRATTSTROM, L. E., B. ISRAELSSON, J. O. JEPPSSON & B. L. HULTBERG. 1988. Folic acid—an innocuous means to reduce plasma homocysteine. Scand. J. Clin. Lab. Invest. **48:** 215–221.

158. SUGANO, M., N. ISHIWAKI, Y. NAGATA & K. IMAIZUMI. 1982. Effects of arginine and lysine addition to casein and soybean protein, on serum lipids, apolipoproteins, insulin and glucagon in rats. Br. J. Nutr. **48:** 211–221.

159. FAJANS, S. S., J. C. FLOYD, R. F. KNOPF & J. W. CONN. 1967. Effect of amino acids and protein on insulin secretions in man. Recent Prog. Horm. Res. **23:** 617–656.

160. PALMER, J. P., R. M. WALTER & J. W. ENSINK. 1975. Arginine-stimulated acute phase of insulin and glucagon secretion. I. In normal man. Diabetes **24:** 735–740.

161. EDWARDS, P. A. 1973. Effect of adrenalectomy and hypophysectomy on the circacian rhythm of β-hydroxy-β-methyl-glutamyl coenzyme A reductase activity in rat liver. J. Biol. Chem. **248:** 2912–2917.

162. DUGAN, R. E., G. C. NESS, M. R. LAKSHAMON, C. M. NEPOKROEFF & J. W. PORTER. 1974. Regulation of hepatic β-hydroxy-β-methylglutamyl coenzyme A reductase by the interplay of hormones. Arch. Biochem. Biophys. **161:** 499–504.

The Effect of Milk Intake on Serum Cholesterol in Healthy Young Females

Randomized Controlled Studies[a]

CHIKAYUKI NAITO[b]

Tokyo Teishin Hospital
Department of Internal Medicine
2-14-23, Fujimi, Chiyoda-ku
Tokyo, Japan

INTRODUCTION

Milk intake is regarded as one of the dietary factors causing hypercholesterolemia in spite of its low cholesterol content. To the contrary, quite a few papers have reported that there were some ingredients to lower plasma cholesterol in milk or milk products.[1-4] Moreover, recently in this country, as patients suffering from osteoporosis have been increasing, the Ministry of Welfare recommends taking more milk. Therefore, to see any effect of excess milk intake on plasma lipid levels and also to see whether adaptation would take place when excess milk is given for a longer period of time, we performed randomized, controlled studies.

SUBJECTS AND METHODS

As shown in FIGURE 1, we performed three experiments. Subjects enrolled in these studies were all healthy student nurses (female) 19 years of age, living in the same dormitory. In each experiment a different group of students was used. Those three experiments were performed in different seasons to avoid possible misinterpretation of seasonal variation of cholesterol level. Only normolipidemic persons were selected.

In experiment 1, fourteen subjects were randomly divided in two groups, one of which was given 400 ml regular whole milk everyday for 4 weeks in addition to regular daily food, and the other served as the control, to whom drinking milk and taking milk products were prohibited.

In experiment 2, twenty-seven subjects were enrolled and divided randomly in two groups. Half of them were given 400 ml regular whole milk daily for twelve weeks and the rest served as the control.

In experiment 3, thirty subjects were randomly allocated to three groups. 400 ml of regular whole milk, skim milk and skim milk with added dextrose to match the calorie count of the regular whole milk were given daily for 12 weeks to each person of the first, the second and the third group, respectively.

Blood was obtained from the antecubital vein early in the morning after an overnight fast. At the points marked with arrows in FIGURE 1, body weight, blood pressure, and

[a]Supported by a grant from the National Milk Promotion Association, Japan.

[b]Address for correspondence: Dr. Chikayuki Naito, 35-7, Ootsuka 5, Bunkyo-ku, Tokyo 112, Japan.

blood chemical constituents were measured in these three experiments. The average of the values at one week before and at the starting day of the experiment was regarded as the basal value at 0 time.

The concentrations of serum cholesterol, triglyceride, and phospholipid were determined by enzymatic methods with the aid of an autoanalyzer, in which we used "Determiner" kits for cholesterol, triglyceride and phospholipid, respectively.[5] HDL-cholesterol in serum was measured enzymatically in the supernatant fluid after precipitation of LDL and VLDL with dextran sulfate-Mg^{++}. Concentrations of apolipoproteins in serum were determined immunochemically, basing on the principle of rate nephelometry,[6] by use of "Apo-Auto·2[Daiichi]" kits and a Behring Nephelometer Analyzer. Serum total protein, albumin, calcium and inorganic phosphorus were measured by the routine methods with the aid of an autoanalyzer in the central laboratory in our hospital.

1) Experiment 1

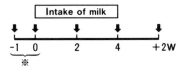

2) Experiment 2

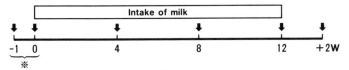

3) Experiment 3

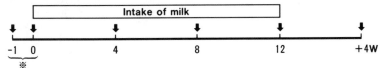

FIGURE 1. Schedule of the experiments. *The average of two values determined at these points was regarded as the basal value at 0 time.

For statistical analysis we used paired sample t test within a group, and analysis of variance for comparison between or among groups.[7]

RESULTS

Blody weight and blood pressure did not change significantly in any groups during the experimental period. Furthermore, no consistent changes were observed in serum calcium, inorganic phosphorus, total protein and albumin concentrations in any groups during the experimental period.

In experiment 1, as shown in FIGURE 2, serum cholesterol concentration increased

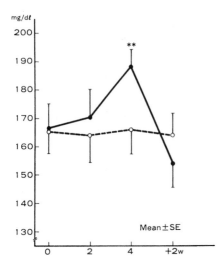

FIGURE 2. Changes in serum total cholesterol concentration by 400 ml daily intake of regular whole milk for 4 weeks. *Black circle and solid line:* milk intake group; *white circle and dashed line:* control group. The value at each check point was compared with that of the basal value; **p <0.02. The difference between the two groups was not statistically significant.

significantly in the regular milk intake group at 4 weeks and the concentration returned to the basal level at 2 weeks after the cessation of milk intake, while the concentration in the control group did not show any significant change. This result suggested that daily intake of 400 ml regular whole milk might increase the serum cholesterol level. Then, to check the reproducibility of the result and to see whether adaptation may occur if we drink it for a longer period of time, we performed experiment 2.

As shown in FIGURE 3, also in experiment 2, serum cholesterol concentration increased at 4 weeks, although it was not statistically significant. Moreover, in this experiment, the concentration maintained that high level at 8 weeks but returned to the basal level at 12 weeks in spite of continuing milk intake, and the basal level was maintained at 2 weeks after stopping milk intake. Serum triglyceride concentration varied inconsis-

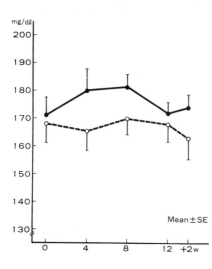

FIGURE 3. Changes in serum total cholesterol concentration by 400 ml daily intake of regular whole milk for 12 weeks. *Black circle and solid line:* milk intake group; *white circle and dashed line:* control group. The value at each check point was not statistically different from that of the basal value. The difference between the two groups was not statistically significant.

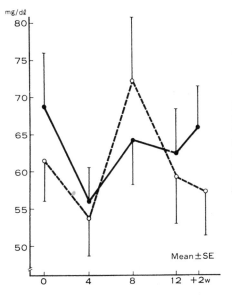

FIGURE 4. Changes in serum triglyceride concentration by 400 ml daily intake of regular whole milk for 12 weeks. *Black circle and solid line:* milk intake group; *white circle and dashed line:* control group. The value at each check point was not statisitcally different from that of the basal value. The difference between the two groups was not statistically significant.

tently (FIG. 4), and HDL-cholesterol tended to increase during the experimental period in both groups (FIG. 5). Serum phospholipid concentration changed almost in parallel with the change in cholesterol concentration.

The increase in cholesterol concentration after daily intake of 400 ml regular whole milk seemed consistent in these two experiments, although the concentration returned to the basal level after a longer period of time in spite of the continuity of milk intake as shown in experiment 2. Therefore, to confirm the phenomenon and to examine whether the phenomenon was caused by fat content in milk or excess calorie intake, we performed experiment 3.

As shown in FIGURE 6, the changes in total cholesterol concentration in the serum or the regular whole milk intake group were very similar to those observed in experiment 2.

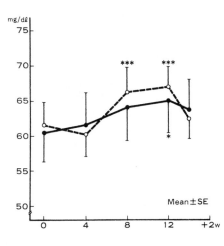

FIGURE 5. Changes in HDL-cholesterol concentration by 400 ml daily intake of regular whole milk for 12 weeks. *Black circle and solid line:* milk intake group; *white circle and dashed line:* control group. The value at each check point was compared with that of the basal value: *$p < 0.05$; ***$p < 0.01$. The difference between the two groups was not statistically significant.

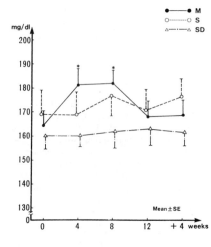

FIGURE 6. Changes in serum total cholesterol concentration in the regular whole milk intake group (M), the skim milk intake group (S) and the skim milk with added dextrose intake group (SD) during 12 weeks. The value at each check point was compared with that of the basal value: *p <0.05. No statistically significant difference was found among the three groups.

However, the cholesterol concentration did not change in the skim milk group and in the skim milk with added dextrose group to make its calorie count equivalent to that of regular whole milk. Changes in phospholipid concentrations were variable, but in general the changes were almost parallel with those in the cholesterol level (FIG. 7). Changes in triglyceride concentration were also variable in these three groups (FIG. 8).

Interestingly, as shown in FIGURE 9, HDL-cholesterol increased significantly during the milk intake period in the regular whole milk intake group, while the concentrations of the skim milk intake group and of the skim milk with added dextrose intake group were kept almost constant. However, the result was not consistent with the result in experiment 2. Further studies will be needed to confirm this point. As for apolipoprotein concentrations, no fractions changed clearly and distinctly (TABLE 1). However, it may be said that apo B appeared to increase slightly at 4 and 8 weeks in the regular whole milk intake

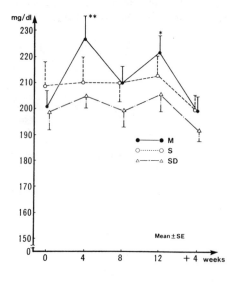

FIGURE 7. Changes in serum phospholipid concentration in the regular whole milk intake group (M), the skim milk intake group (S) and the skim milk with added dextrose intake group (SD) during 12 weeks. The value at each check point was compared with that of the basal value: *p <0.05; **p <0.01. No statistically significant difference was found among the three groups.

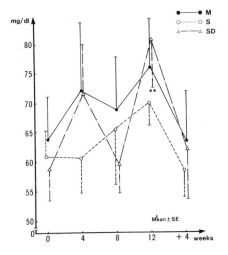

FIGURE 8. Changes in serum triglyceride concentration in the regular whole milk intake group (M), the skim milk intake group (S) and the skim milk with added dextrose intake group (SD) during 12 weeks. The value at each check point was compared with that of the basal value: **p <0.01. No statistically significant difference was found among the three groups.

group, and that apo A-I, A-II, C-II and C-III tended to increase during the experimental period in all three groups. Apo E concentration was almost constant during the experimental period in all three groups.

DISCUSSION

Excess intake of milk is alleged to be a cause of hypercholesterolemia and coronary heart disease in developed countries. From a viewpoint of causing hypercholesterolemia, milk contains a tiny amount of cholesterol (about 10 mg per 100 ml of milk) and about 3.5% fat, which is mostly saturated. Therefore, these saturated fats have been regarded as the cause of hypercholesterolemia due to an ingestion of milk. Nevertheless, several papers[1-4] reported the existence of some factors in milk which lowers the serum cholesterol level. Mann and Spoerry[1] reported a significant decrease in serum cholesterol in

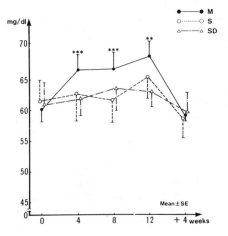

FIGURE 9. Changes in HDL-cholesterol concentration in the regular whole milk intake group (M), the skim milk intake group (S) and the skim milk with added dextrose intake group (SD) during 12 weeks. The value at each check point was compared with that of the basal value: **p <0.01; ***p <0.001. No statistically significant difference was found among the three groups.

spite of a daily intake of more than 4 liters of milk and a gaining in body weight in members of the Maasai tribe aged 16 to 23 years. However, Rossouw et al.[8] reported that skim milk decreased serum cholesterol level, though yoghurt and full cream milk temporarily increased serum cholesterol in adolescent schoolboys aged 16 to 18 years during 4 weeks' experimental period. They ingested 2 liters excess of milk. Rossouw et al.[8] concluded that they could not find convincing evidence of a milk factor, and that a cholesterol-lowering effect of skim milk appeared at least partly due to its low lipid content.

In these previous reports, subjects were given a large amount of milk, which caused some disturbance to regular diet habit, a considerable increase in calorie intake and a gain in body weight.

TABLE 1. Changes in Apolipoproteins in the Regular Whole Milk Intake Group (M), the Skim Milk Intake Group (S) and the Skim Milk with Added Dextrose Intake Group (SD)[a]

Appolipo-protein Group		Duration (Weeks)				
		0	4	8	12	+4
A I	M	125.0 ± 3.7	135.0 ± 4.1**	131.5 ± 5.2	133.2 ± 3.2*	121.4 ± 2.5
	S	125.1 ± 5.6	126.4 ± 6.7	123.3 ± 5.7	128.2 ± 4.7	118.6 ± 3.7
	SD	125.5 ± 6.3	126.3 ± 3.7	124.0 ± 4.3	122.6 ± 2.5	121.2 ± 3.2
A II	M	24.1 ± 1.2	24.9 ± 1.3	25.8 ± 1.5	28.0 ± 1.2***	24.7 ± 0.9
	S	23.9 ± 1.1	25.7 ± 1.6	26.7 ± 1.9	30.2 ± 1.4***	24.9 ± 1.2
	SD	24.6 ± 0.8	26.8 ± 1.2*	26.9 ± 1.1**	29.7 ± 1.6**	25.1 ± 0.8
B	M	64.9 ± 3.6	74.4 ± 4.3***	72.9 ± 3.5*	67.2 ± 12.7	68.6 ± 3.7
	S	65.2 ± 4.4	69.1 ± 4.3	71.4 ± 5.4	71.4 ± 4.3**	72.6 ± 3.7*
	SD	53.6 ± 2.8	66.1 ± 3.7**	63.2 ± 4.0	67.2 ± 6.3	64.7 ± 3.4**
C II	M	2.2 ± 0.3	2.8 ± 0.3***	2.2 ± 0.2	2.6 ± 0.3*	2.5 ± 0.3
	S	2.4 ± 0.3	2.8 ± 0.2	2.2 ± 0.2	2.8 ± 0.2*	2.7 ± 0.3*
	SD	2.3 ± 0.2	2.7 ± 0.2*	2.2 ± 0.2	2.7 ± 0.3	2.8 ± 0.3
C III	M	7.7 ± 0.7	9.5 ± 0.7***	8.9 ± 0.8	9.7 ± 0.5***	7.9 ± 0.7
	S	7.7 ± 0.5	9.3 ± 0.5*	8.6 ± 0.5	9.7 ± 0.5**	7.9 ± 0.5
	SD	7.6 ± 0.6	9.0 ± 0.3*	8.5 ± 0.7	9.2 ± 0.5	8.3 ± 0.5
E	M	4.2 ± 0.5	4.3 ± 0.4	3.9 ± 0.3	4.5 ± 0.3**	4.3 ± 0.5**
	S	3.9 ± 0.3	4.0 ± 0.3	4.0 ± 0.3	4.6 ± 0.2*	4.3 ± 0.7
	SD	4.3 ± 0.3	4.2 ± 0.3	4.4 ± 0.4	4.7 ± 0.2	4.5 ± 0.3

[a]The figures represent the mean ± standard error of the mean. The value at each check point was compared with that of the basal value, respectively: *p <0.05; **p <0.01, ***p <0.001. No statistically significant difference was found in each apolipoprotein concentration among the three groups.

In our experiments we daily added 400 ml milk to the regular diet, because people in Japan ordinarily take one bottle of milk (200 ml) a day, if any. Moreover, we hoped to avoid the effects of a large excess calorie intake, a disturbance to regular diet habit and an increase in body weight on lipid metabolism. We asked the subjects to take milk after breakfast and supper, 200 ml each, to avoid reducing the regular diet intake.

As the consistent result in experiments 1 to 3, we found a significant increase in total cholesterol at 4 weeks in the regular whole milk intake group, and the increased level of cholesterol continued for a further 4 weeks. However, the cholesterol concentration returned to the basal level 4 weeks afterwards in spite of continuing the milk intake. An increase in cholesterol concentration after the milk intake was also observed by Thompson et al.[9] and by Rossouw et al.,[8] but not by Mann et al.[1] Mann et al. reported a decrease in cholesterol level from drinking a large amount of milk as mentioned above. No one except Rossouw et al.[8] reported an initial increase and later decrease in cholesterol concentration under continuation of milk intake. However, their experimental periods were all less than 4 weeks.

The initial increase in cholesterol concentration might not be caused by excess calorie intake or by any factors other than fat, because the cholesterol concentration did not change significantly in the skim milk intake group and in the skim milk with added dextrose intake group in our experiment. The increase seems to relate most probably to fat content. However, the decrease in the concentration under continuation of milk intake cannot be explained properly from our experiments. We think that this is a kind of adaptation to a change in food intake. In our experiments, we did not observe any significant changes in body weight in spite of the excess intake of energy corresponding to 400 ml milk, that is, 200 kcal, during our experimental period. We cannot explain the phenomenon so far, but we think that we could avoid the effect of a gain in body weight on lipid metabolism in our experiments. Any changes in body weight would make it difficult to interpret the results.

CONCLUSIONS

We performed three randomized, controlled studies to examine the effects of milk intake on human serum cholesterol level with the cooperation of healthy student nurses 19 years of age, living in the same dormitory. The conclusions of these experiments are as follows.

1. Contrary to some previous reports, neither regular whole milk nor skim milk decreased serum cholesterol concentration, suggesting that cholesterol-lowering factors might not exist in milk.
2. Excess intake of milk might increase the serum cholesterol level during a short initial period, but adaptation might develop gradually to decrease it to the basal level during a longer period of time.
3. The initial increase in cholesterol level by regular whole milk intake might be caused by milk fat itself, but not by excess calorie intake or by some factors other than fat.

ACKNOWLEDGMENTS

The author gratefully acknowledges the support of Drs. S. Oomori and M. Kawamura throughout the experiments. The author also appreciates the participation of Drs. K. Kawasugi, A. Omoto, and S. Miyazaki during the early stages of these studies.

REFERENCES

1. MANN, G.V. & A. SPOERRY. 1974. Studies of a surfactant and cholesteremia in Maasai. Am. J. Clin. Nutr. **27:** 464–469.
2. MALINOW, M. R. & P. McLAUGHLIN. 1975. The effect of skim milk on plasma cholesterol in rats. Experientia **31:** 1012–1013.
3. MANN, G. V. 1977. A factor in yoghurt which lowers cholesteremia in man. Atherosclerosis **26:** 335–340.

4. THAKUR, C. P. & A. N. JHA. 1981. Influence of milk, yoghurt and calcium on cholesterol-induced atherosclerosis in rabbits. Atherosclerosis **39:** 211–215.

5. ITO, H., C. NAITO, H. HAYASHI & M. KAWAMURA. 1988. Activity of low-density lipoprotein receptors as estimated from concentrations of apolipoprotein B and C-II in serum. Clin. Chem. **34:** 2224–2227.

6. KOSTNER, G. M. 1983. Apolipoproteins and lipoproteins of human plasma: Significance in health and in disease. Adv. Lipid Res. **20:** 1–43.

7. SOKAL, R. R. & F. J. ROHLF. 1969. Biometry. The Principles and Practice of Statistics in Biological Research. W. H. Freeman and Company. San Francisco, CA.

8. ROSSOUW, J. E., E.-M. BURGER, P. V. D. VYVER & J. J. FERREIRA. 1981. The effect of skim milk, yoghurt, and full cream milk on human serum lipids. Am. J. Clin. Nutr. **34:** 351–356.

9. THOMPSON, L. U., D. J. A. JENKINS, M. A. VIC AMER, R. REICHERT, A. JENKINS & J. KAMULSKY. 1982. The effect of fermented and unfermented milks on serum cholesterol. Am. J. Clin. Nutr. **36:** 1106–1111.

Effect of Eicosapentaenoic Acid on the Binding and Degradation of Oxidized LDL and the Production of LTB_4, LTC_4, and PGE_2 in Rat Peritoneal Macrophages

KE-JIAN CHANG, HIROYUKI SAITO, YASUSHI TAMURA, AND
SHO YOSHIDA

Second Department of Internal Medicine
Chiba University School of Medicine
Chiba 280, Japan

It has been shown that macrophages invaded into the subendothelial space and phagocytosed deposited cholesterol through the scavenger pathway, leading to the formation of foam cells.[1] It was recently suggested that low density lipoprotein (LDL) was oxidized in the vessel wall.[2] Macrophages were reported to release eicosanoids when exposed to oxidized LDL (O-LDL).[3] Recently, it was revealed that ingestion of fish oil concentrate, rich in eicosapentaenoic acid (EPA), prevented atherosclerotic tissue changes in animal models.[4,5] To analyze the mechanism of the prophylactic effect of EPA, we tried to reveal the effect of EPA-E ingestion on the capability of binding and proteolytic degradation of iodine 125-labeled-O-LDL (^{125}I-O-LDL) between EPA-rich macrophages obtained from Wistar rats fed 100 mg/kg/day of EPA ethyl ester (EPA-E, 99.8% purity) during four weeks (EPA macrophages) and macrophages on a control diet (control macrophages). And we also compared the amount of eicosanoid production between EPA macrophages and control macrophages exposed to O-LDL.

Even though the EPA content in macrophages was significantly increased, the content of arachidonic acid (AA) was not altered by the ingestion of 100 mg/kg/day of EPA-E (data not shown). Nevertheless, the production of AA-derived eicosanoids (LTB_4, LTC_4, and PGE_2) was significantly reduced by the EPA-E ingestion (FIG. 1). We also found that the binding and degradation of ^{125}I-O-LDL was not influenced by the EPA-E ingestion (TABLE 1), indicating that scavenger activity for O-LDL cannot be influenced by the ingestion of this amount of EPA-E.

These eicosanoids, measured in the present study, are considered to be involved in the development of atherosclerosis. PGE_2 increases vascular permeability and edema.[6] LTB_4 is chemotactic for monocytes[7] and promotes smooth muscle cell proliferation.[8] LTC_4 induces smooth muscle cell contraction[9] and fibroblast proliferation.[10] The present result, therefore, may indicate that the prophylactic effect of EPA on atherosclerotic tissue changes might be partly due to the inhibitory effect of EPA on this eicosanoid production. Further study is now in progress to reveal the effect of larger amounts of EPA-E ingestion on the scavenger pathway.

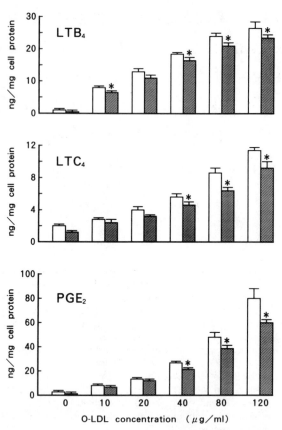

FIGURE 1. Comparison of the production of LTB_4, LTC_4, and PGE_2 between EPA macrophages and control macrophages. Macrophages (10^6 cells) were incubated with O-LDL for 2 h in 5% CO_2–95% air at 37°C. The content of each eicosanoid in the culture medium was determined by using respective specific antibodies. Each experiment was performed in duplicate and each value represents the mean ± SEM of three separate experiments. ☐, control macrophages; ▨, EPA macrophages; *$p < 0.05$.

TABLE 1. Comparison of the Binding and Degradation of ^{125}I-O-LDL between EPA Macrophages and Control Macrophages

O-LDL	Binding[a]		Degradation		Cellular Content	
(μg/ml)	C	E	C	E	C	E
10	0.69 ± 0.15^{b}	0.70 ± 0.05	0.39 ± 0.03	0.35 ± 0.02	0.72 ± 0.20	0.80 ± 0.15
20	1.17 ± 0.09	1.16 ± 0.10	0.67 ± 0.05	0.65 ± 0.04	2.07 ± 0.19	2.22 ± 0.28
40	1.96 ± 0.09	1.93 ± 0.14	1.30 ± 0.06	1.29 ± 0.05	2.57 ± 0.12	2.54 ± 0.17
80	3.11 ± 0.21	$2.78 \pm .016$	2.25 ± 0.09	2.45 ± 0.18	5.34 ± 0.24	5.84 ± 0.62
120	4.18 ± 0.15	3.82 ± 0.14	3.17 ± 0.22	3.26 ± 0.13	7.01 ± 0.28	7.54 ± 1.19

[a]Rat peritoneal macrophages (10^6 cells) were cultured for one day in 5% CO_2–95% air at 37°C before the assay. In the binding study, RPMI-1640 containing 75 μM chloroquine and ^{125}I-O-LDL (100–200 cpm/ng) were added into each culture dish and incubated for 2 h in 5% CO_2–95% air at 37°C. Radioactivities in macrophages were counted in a gamma counter. In the degradation study, after macrophages were cultured for 2 h with ^{125}I-O-LDL, the amount of ^{125}I labeled acid-soluble materials in the culture medium was determined. After the degradation study, radioactivities in macrophages were counted. C, control macrophages; E, EPA macrophages.
[b]Each experiment was performed in duplicate and each value represents the mean ± SEM (μg/mg cell protein) of three separate experiments.

REFERENCES

1. GERRITY, R. G. 1981. Am. J. Pathol. **103:** 181.
2. HEINECKE, J. W., H. ROSEN & A. CHAIT. 1984. J. Clin. Invest. **74:** 1890.
3. YOKODE, M., T. KITA, Y. KIKAWA, T. OGOROCHI, S. NARUMIYA & C. KAWAI. 1988. J. Clin. Invest. **81:** 720.
4. KIM, D. N., H. T. HO, D. A. LAWRENCE, J. SCHMEE & W. A. THOMAS. 1989. Atherosclerosis **76:** 35.
5. DAVIS, H. R. & R. T. BRIDENSTINE. 1987. Arteriosclerosis **7:** 441.
6. WILLIAMS, T. J. & M. J. PECK. 1977. Nature **270:** 530.
7. FORD-HUTCHINSON, A. W. 1985. Fed. Proc. **44:** 25.
8. PALMBERG, L., H. E. CLAESSON & J. THYBERG. 1987. J. Cell Sci. **88:** 151.
9. WARGOVICH, T., J. MEHTA, W. W. NICHOLS, C. J. PEPINE & C. R. CONTI. 1985. J. Am. College Cardiol. **6:** 1047.
10. BAUD, L., J. PEREZ, M. DENIS & R. ARDAILLOU. 1987. J. Immunol. **138:** 1190.

Receptors for Modified Low Density Lipoproteins on Human Umbilical Vein Endothelial Cells in Culture

NORIAKI KUME, HIDENORI ARAI, YUTAKA NAGANO,
HIDEO OTANI, YUKIHIKO UEDA, CHUICHI KAWAI,
KENJI ISHII,[a] AND TORU KITA[a]

Third Division, Department of Internal Medicine
and
[a]Department of Geriatric Medicine
Faculty of Medicine
Kyoto University
54 Kawara-cho, Shogoin
Sakyo-ku, Kyoto 606, Japan

INTRODUCTION

Oxidative modification of low density lipoprotein (LDL) occurs *in vivo* and causes atherosclerosis.[1] We recently showed that mouse peritoneal macrophages have at least three receptors for oxidized LDL and acetylated LDL; one is common to both of the two forms of modified LDL and the others are specific only for either acetylated or oxidized LDL.[2] On the other hand, vascular endothelial cells also have receptors for modified LDL.[3,4] In the present study, we investigated the uptake pathway of acetylated LDL and oxidized LDL in cultured human endothelial cells.

METHODS

Endothelial cells were harvested from human umbilical veins as previously described with a slight modification.[5] We used the first-passaged confluent monolayers in the following experiments. Assays of proteolytic degradation of ^{125}I-labeled lipoproteins by cultured endothelial cells were performed as previously described by Goldstein *et al.*[6] LDL was isolated from human plasma by ultracentrifugation. Acetylated LDL and oxidized LDL were prepared by the previously described method.[7]

RESULTS AND DISCUSSION

Time-course experiments showed linear increase in the degradation of ^{125}I-labeled acetylated or oxidized LDL for up to 24 hours. The dose-response relationship of the specific degradation of ^{125}I-labeled acetylated or oxidized LDL showed saturation kinetics, which suggests that their uptake is receptor-mediated. To investigate the uptake pathway of acetylated LDL and oxidized LDL, we performed the cross-competition study between the two ligands. The degradation of ^{125}I-labeled oxidized LDL in endothelial cells was almost completely inhibited by the 100-fold excess amount of unlabeled acetylated LDL or oxidized LDL. However, the degradation of ^{125}I-labeled acetylated LDL

494

was only partially inhibited by the excess amount of unlabeled oxidized LDL, while unlabeled acetylated LDL inhibited it completely.

These data indicate that cultured human endothelial cells do not have any receptors specific only for oxidized LDL. On the contrary, our data suggest the existence of additional receptors on endothelial cells, as we already indicated on mouse macrophages, which recognize acetylated LDL but not oxidized LDL. However, further studies would be needed to elucidate the pathophysiological significance of the endothelial receptors for modified LDL *in vivo*.

REFERENCES

1. KITA, T. *et al.* 1987. Proc. Natl. Acad. Sci. USA **84:** 5928–5931.
2. ARAI, H. *et al.* 1989. Biochem. Biophys. Res. Commun. **159:** 1375–1382.
3. STEIN, O. *et al.* 1980. Biochim. Biophys. Acta **620:** 631–635.
4. BAKER, D. P. *et al.* 1984. Arteriosclerosis **4:** 248–255.
5. JAFFE, E. A. *et al.* 1973. J. Clin. Invest. **52:** 2745–2756.
6. GOLDSTEIN, J. L. *et al.* 1979. Proc. Natl. Acad. Sci. USA **76:** 333–337.
7. YOKODE, M. *et al.* 1988. J. Clin. Invest. **81:** 720–729.

Characterization of Low Density Lipoprotein Receptors in Normal and Watanabe Heritable Hyperlipidemic Rabbits

KENJI ISHII,[a] NORIAKI KUME,[b] HIDEO OTANI,[b]
CHUICHI KAWAI,[b] HITOSHI SHIMANO,[c]
NOBUHIRO YAMADA,[c] AND TORU KITA[a]

Department of Geriatric Medicine
and
[b]*Third Division, Department of Internal Medicine*
Faculty of Medicine
Kyoto University
Kyoto, Japan
and
[c]*Third Department of Internal Medicine*
The University of Tokyo
Tokyo, Japan

Lipid-laden foam cells are a characteristic in the early stage of atherosclerotic lesions. Many foam cells in these lesions preserve the characteristics of macrophages.[1] Beta-VLDL, which accumulate in the plasma of patients with type III hyperlipoproteinemia and cholesterol-fed animals, is known to transform macrophages into foam cells. Homozygous Watanabe heritable hyperlipidemic (WHHL) rabbits, like their human counterparts with familial hypercholesterolemia, have not only extraordinary high LDL levels, but also a substantially increased concentration of VLDL remnants, which are similar to β-VLDL.[2] In the present study, we investigated the uptake mechanism of β-VLDL by peritoneal macrophages and fibroblasts obtained from normal and WHHl rabbits.

When incubated with peritoneal macrophages from normal and WHHL rabbits, $[^{125}I]\beta$-VLDL was degraded by both macrophages with saturation kinetics. At the saturation, $[^{125}I]\beta$-VLDL degraded by WHHL macrophages was about 30% that by normal rabbit macrophages. Normal rabbit macrophages degraded ^{125}I-LDL with a saturable, high affinity mechanism. However, WHHL rabbit macrophages did little. These results indicated that WHHL rabbit macrophages took up β-VLDL despite the lack of LDL receptor activity. The LDL receptor gene of WHHL rabbits has a small in-flame deletion of 12 nucleotides which results in the loss of four amino acids from the cysteine-rich repeat of the ligand binding domain.[3] Due to its defect, the abnormal LDL receptors of WHHL rabbit fibroblasts do not recognize apo B 100 in LDL particles. However, the precursor of the mutant LDL receptor from WHHL rabbit adrenal gland bind β-VLDL on the nitrocellulose blot.[3] When incubated with fibroblasts from WHHL rabbit, $[^{125}I]\beta$-VLDL was degraded in a saturable, high affinity mechanism. As β-VLDL uptake in fibroblasts is mediated exclusively by the LDL receptors, the result strongly suggested

[a]Correspondence to Kenji Ishii, MD, Department of Geriatric Medicine, Faculty of Medicine, Kyoto University, 54 Shogoin-Kawaracho, Sakyo-ku, Kyoto, 606 Japan.

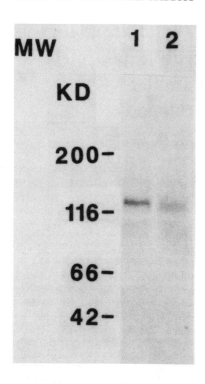

FIGURE 1. Ligand blot of LDL receptors from fibroblasts from normal and WHHL rabbits. Cells were solubilized, electrophoresed, and transferred to nitrocellulose. The nitrocellulose paper was incubated with β-VLDL at the protein concentration of 10 μg/ml. The blots were developed in mouse anti-rabbit apo B 100 monoclonal antibody (20 μg/ml) and horseradish peroxidase conjugated goat anti-mouse IgG. *Lane 1:* fibroblasts from normal rabbits (48 μg/lane); *lane 2:* fibroblasts from WHHL rabbits. The scale gives relative migrations of molecular weight standards.

that the degradation of $[^{125}I]$β-VLDL by WHHL fibroblasts was mediated by mutant LDL receptors. Ligand blotting using β-VLDL detected a single protein in Triton X-100 extracts of WHHL rabbit firboblasts (FIG. 1). The apparent molecular weight of the β-VLDL-binding protein on WHHL rabbit fibroblasts was same as that of normal rabbit fibroblasts. The amount of $[^{125}I]$β-VLDL degraded by fibroblasts from WHHL rabbit at the saturation was about 250 ng/mg cell protein/5 hours, and that by normal rabbit fibroblasts was about 750 ng/mg cell protein/5 hours. The ratio of degraded ^{125}I-β-VLDL by WHHL fibroblasts to that by normal rabbit fibroblasts was almost same as that observed in macrophages. This suggested that degradation of β-VLDL by WHHL cells was mediated by common pathway, *i.e.*, mature mutant LDL receptors. An immunoprecipitation study showed that WHHL rabbit peritoneal macrophages synthesized mature mutant LDL receptors. To verify that the uptake of β-VLDL by WHHL rabbit macrophages is mediated via the mature mutant LDL receptors, we performed the competition study using anti-LDL receptor antibody. One μl/ml of anti-LDL receptor antiserum abolished degradation of $[^{125}]$β-VLDL by WHHL rabbit macrophages. On the other hand, nonimmunized guinea pig serum did not inhibit the degradation of $[^{125}I]$β-VLDL. Our results indicated that mutant LDL receptors of WHHL rabbit peritoneal macrophages recognized β-VLDL despite their inability to recognize LDL, and suggested the implication of the mutant LDL receptor of WHHL macrophages to foam cell formation.

REFERENCES

1. Ross, R. 1986. N. Engl. J. Med. **314:** 488–500.
2. Ishii, K., *et al.* 1989. J. Lipid Res. **30:** 1–7.
3. Yamamoto, T., *et al.* 1986. Science **232:** 1230–1237.

Deletion of the Growth Factor Homology Domain of the Low Density Lipoprotein Receptor in Familial Hypercholesterolemia

TOHRU FUNAHASHI,[a] YASUKO MIYAKE, SHOJI TAJIMA, AND
AKIRA YAMAMOTO

Department of Etiology and Pathophysiology
National Cardiovascular Center Research Institute
553 Fujishirodai, Suita
Osaka, Japan

LDL receptor binds and takes up plasma LDL into the cell. The receptor dissociates the ligand within the cell and recycles back to the cell surface. The mutant receptor produced by expressible cDNA that deletes the gene coding the epidermal growth factor (EGF) homology domain impairs recycling ability.[1] There has been no report of a naturally occurring mutant with impaired recycling ability. The clinical phenotype of this mutation *in vivo* has not been elucidated. We now report a patient with homozygous familial hypercholesterolemia (FH) whose receptor impaired recycling ability.

The patient was a 32-year-old woman. Her plasma level of cholesterol was 517 mg/dl. She had marked xanthomas. Nevertheless, she had no signs of coronary artery disease.

Skin fibroblasts of this patient were sent from Dr. S. Yamashita at Osaka University. Cells of the patient produced a small 115 kD mature receptor. Cell surface binding of anti-LDL receptor antibody indicated a normal amount of receptor protein was present on her cell surface. The mutant receptor could not bind LDL but could bind βVLDL. βVLDL binds to the LDL receptor through its component apo E. When the cells were incubated at 37°C in the presence of βVLDL, βVLDL binding remained at a relatively constant level in normal cells. This is explained by the fact that the normal receptors recycle back and can bind the ligand repeatedly. Surprisingly, in mutant cells βVLDL binding was gradually decreased. Anti-receptor antibody binding also decreased under the presence of ligand. We conclude that the mutant receptor was not efficiently recycled back to the cell surface.

Next we focused on a genetic analysis of the mutant receptor gene. Southern blotting of the genomic DNA from the patient showed a large deletion in the middle portion of the LDL receptor gene. We cloned an abnormal 9.4 kb Eco RI/Xba I fragment in λong C. Mapping analyses revealed that the patient gene had a 12-kb deletion including the exons 7 through 14. Those exons encode an entire region of the EGF homology domain of the receptor. Sequencing analyses of the deletion joint suggested that this mutation arose by recombination of two repetitive Alu sequences in opposite directions in intron 6 and 14. The characteristics of the receptor protein produced by this natural mutation were similar to those of an artificial mutation constructed by Davis *et al.*

From the clinical aspect, the patient showed high levels of cholesterol and xanthomas

---

[a]Address for correspondence: Second Department of Internal Medicine, Osaka University Medical School, 1-1-50 Fukushima, Fukushima-ku, Osaka 553, Japan.

but manifested no signs of coronary artery disease despite being in her 4th decade. The apo E recognizing ability of the receptor may play some role in preventing accumulation of cholesterol in coronary arteries.

(The complete text of this paper has been published.[2])

REFERENCES

1. DAVIS, *et al.* 1987. Nature **326:** 760–765.
2. MIYAKE, Y., *et al.* 1989. J. Biol. Chem. **264:** 16584–16590.

Phosphatidylinositol Turnover in Human Monocyte-Derived Macrophages Was Stimulated by Native and Acetyl LDL

YOSHINORI ASAOKA, YUICHI ISHIKAWA, TAKAHIRO
TANIGUCHI, MASAHIKO TSUNEMITSU, KEN MATSUMOTO,
AND HISASHI FUKUZAKI

First Department of Internal Medicine
Kobe University School of Medicine
7-5-1 Kusunoki-cho, Chuo-ku
Kobe 650, Japan

Monocyte-derived macrophages (MDM) are considered to play a key role in the pathogenesis of atherosclerosis.[1] The process of lipid accumulation in macrophages has been well investigated, though the mechanism of activating the macrophages remains to be clarified. Inositol 1,4,5-triphosphate (IP_3) is well known as a second messenger produced by a receptor-mediated inositol phospholipid hydrolysis and plays a central role in intracellular signal transduction and cell activation. We report the contribution of phosphatidylinositol turnover to native and chemically modified LDL uptake by human MDM.

Human MDM were separated as described by Bøyum.[2] The adherent cells on the dishes were cultured in RPMI 1640 supplemented with 10% autologous serum for 5 days following incubation in serum-free medium for 2 days and used as MDM. After stimulating the cells by various LDL, intracellular IP_3 was assayed using an IP_3 assay kit (Amersham). Native LDL was prepared by the method of Havel *et al*.[3] Acetyl LDL was prepared as described by Basu *et al*.[4] Copper-oxidized LDL was prepared by incubating native LDL with 5 μM $CuSO_4$.[5] Chemically modified LDL showed the anodal migration in agarose gel electrophoresis.

Time course study of IP_3 formation in human MDM stimulated by 30 μg/ml of LDL showed that the maximal effect was observed at 3 min (data not shown). As shown in FIGURE 1, both native and acetyl LDL stimulated IP_3 formation in a dose-dependent manner. The increase of IP_3 in human MDM stimulated by acetyl LDL was 3-fold higher than that by native LDL. TABLE 1 shows the potency of each LDL to produce IP_3 in human MDM. Acetyl, oxidized, and native LDL induced 0.36, 0.33, and 0.12 nmol/mg protein, respectively.

We showed that IP_3 formation stimulated by chemically modified LDL was three times that stimulated by native LDL. Block *et al*. described how native LDL induced the activation of phosphatidylinositol turnover in human platelets, fibroblasts, lymphocytes, and rat smooth muscle cells.[6] The higher IP_3 formation induced by chemically modified LDL than that induced by native LDL may explain the higher potency of chemically modified LDL to activate macrophages. It is likely that the activation of macrophages by LDL results in the metabolic regulation or the release of biologically active substances toward cell proliferation. Especially, macrophages strongly activated by chemically modified LDL could play a central role in the initiation of atherosclerosis.

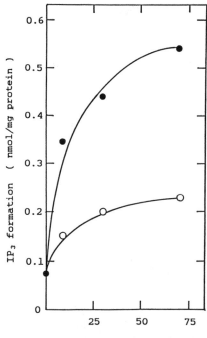

FIGURE 1. IP_3 formation in human MDM stimulated by various concentrations of acetyl and native LDL. Various concentrations of LDL were added to MDM monolayers (20–40 μg cell protein/dish). After 3 min incubation, the reaction was terminated by ice-cold 15% TCA. IP_3 was assayed as described in the text. ●, Acetyl LDL; ○, native LDL.

TABLE 1. IP_3 Formation in Macrophages Stimulated by Various LDL[a]

	IP₃ Formation	
	nmol/mg Protein	Fold
Native LDL	0.12	1.0
Oxidized LDL	0.33	2.7
Acetyl LDL	0.36	3.0

[a]30 μg/ml of various LDL were added to each dish containing human MDM (20–40 μg cell protein/dish), incubated for 3 min. The reaction was terminated by ice-cold 15% TCA. IP_3 was assayed as described in the text.

REFERENCES

1. Ross, R. 1986. N. Engl. J. Med. **314:** 488–500.
2. Bøyum, A. 1968. Scand. J. Clin. Lab. Invest. **21** (Suppl. 97): 77–89.
3. Havel, R. J., H. A. Eder & J. H. Bragdon 1955. J. Clin. Invest. **34:** 1345–1353.
4. Basu, S. K., J. L. Goldstein, R. G. W. Anderson & M. S. Brown. 1976. Proc Natl Acad Sci USA **73:** 3178–3182.
5. Steinbrecher, U. P., S. Parthasarathy, D. S. Leake, J. L. Witztum & D. Steinberg. 1984. Proc Natl Acad Sci USA **81:** 3883–3887.
6. Block, L. H., M. Knorr, E. Vogt, R. Locher, W. Vetter, P. Groscurth, B.-Y. Qiao, D. Pometta, R. James, M. Regenass & A. Pletscher. 1988. Proc Natl Acad Sci USA **85:** 885–889.

Secretory Products of Mouse Peritoneal Macrophages Inhibit the Activity of the Scavenger Receptor on Homogeneous Macrophages

WANG ZONG-LI, ZHANG QING, LI HAO, XIA REN-YI, AND
SHE MING-PENG

Department of Pathology
Institute of Basic Medical Sciences
Chinese Academy of Medical Sciences
Faculty of Basic Medicine
Peking Union Medical College
Beijing 100730, China

Macrophages secret a multitude of products and play an important role in the regulation of cell interactions including macrophages themselves.[1,4]

Recent reports indicate that a secretory product of human monocyte-derived macrophage stimulates LDL receptor activity of both arterial smooth muscle cells and skin fibroblasts.[2] Nevertheless, it is still not clear whether the macrophage's autocrine is required in the process of transformation of macrophage-derived foam cells. In this article, the effect of mouse (BALB/C) peritoneal macrophage conditioned medium on the activity of modified LDL receptor and cholesteryl ester synthesis was studied by using homogeneous macrophages and acetyl-LDL as a model.

Mouse peritoneal cells (2.5×10^6/ml medium) were incubated in M199 containing 5% LPS with con A (10 μg/ml medium) or without con A. After removal of those nonadherent cells, conditioned medium was collected between the 3rd and 6th day and centrifuged at 20,000 for 30 min. In order to determine the effect of macrophage-conditioned medium (MCM) on the binding and degradation of acetyl-LDL in homogeneous macrophages, adherent macrophages preincubated with MCM or control medium for 24 hours were prepared, and ^{125}I-acetyl-LDL (25 μg/ml medium) was added for the measurement of binding and degradation. Results indicated that exposure of macrophages to MCM caused a significant increase of ^{125}I-acetyl-LDL binding and a decrease of degradation of the ^{125}I-acetyl-LDL in macrophages. The ^{125}I-acetyl-LDL binding rate was 165.7% ($p < 0.05$) in MCM from unstimulated macrophages (MCM) and 194.3% ($p < 0.201$) in MCM from stimulated macrophages (MCMS) compared with that of the control medium, which had not been exposed to the macrophage. Inhibition of ^{125}I-acetyl-LDL degradation on average was 38.2% ($p < 0.05$) in MCM and 62.1% ($p < 0.001$) in MCMS, respectively, of that obtained in the control. In addition, a supplement of 5% fresh LDS in the conditioned medium did not affect the binding and degradation rates (TABLE 1.)

The effect of conditioned medium on cholesteryl ester synthesis was tested concurrently. Unlabelled acetyl-LDL and ^{3}H-oleic acid bound to albumin were given over macrophage monolayers which had been exposed to MCM or MCMS for 24 hours beforehand.[3] Both conditioned media also inhibited the incorporation of ^{3}H-oleate (0.1 mM, 7500 cpm/nmol) into cholesteryl ester in the presence of unlabelled acetyl-LDL (25 μg/ml medium) (TABLE 2).

TABLE 1. Effect of Conditioned Medium on the Binding and Degradation of ^{125}I-Acetyl-LDL by Homogeneous Macrophages[a]

	Control	MCM	MCMS	MCM + 1.5% LDS
Binding (μg/mg protein)	1.75 ± 0.23	2.0 ± 0.31	3.4 ± 0.51	3.2 ± 0.2
Degradation (μg/mg protein)	5.87 ± 6.2	3.57 ± 4.9	2.19 ± 3.2	2.79 ± 1.4

[a]Values shown are the mean $\pm$ SD from triplicate wells.

In order to make clear whether the macrophage-conditioned medium exerted cytotoxicity to the homogeneous macrophages, the phagocytosis index on glutaraldehyde-treated sheep red cells (G-SRC) was measured, Nevertheless, no definite effect was involved on the number of G-SRC ingested no matter which medium was selected and which negated the possibility of cytotoxicity.

In conclusion, the data indicated that undialysed conditioned medium from mouse peritoneal macrophages inhibited the activity of the scavenger receptor and the consequent cholesteryl ester synthesis in homogeneous macrophages. Substances produced by macrophages prevent the degradation process of acetyl-LDL in lysosomes, unlike choloquine, which blocks the hydrolysis of acetyl-LDL within lysosomes but does not affect the binding of acetyl-LDL.[6] Here, products from the macrophages also stimulate the binding of acetyl-LDL on macrophages. Many studies have shown that secretory products of macrophages can modulate macrophage function in either a positive or negative feedback manner.[1,4] Current data suggest that such autocrine regulation may be related to synthesis and release of arachidonic metabolites, the interferon of -2-macroglobulin.[1,4,5] Autoregulation of the macrometabolism of modified LDL may be of importance for cholesterol deposition in atherosclerosis.

TABLE 2. Cholesteryl Ester Formation in Mouse Peritoneal Macrophages Incubated with Acetyl-LDL (25 μg/ml Medium for 24 hrs)[a]

Medium	Incorporation of ^{3}H-Oleate into Cholesteryl ^{3}H-Oleate (n mol/mg protein $\pm$ SD)
Control medium (5% LDS in M199)	64.5 ± 3.1
MCM (from unstimulated macrophages)	58.7 ± 6.5
MCMS (from stimulated macrophages)	$*45.2 \pm 3.7$

[a]Values shown are mean $\pm$ SD from triplicate dishes. $*p < 0.01$.

REFERENCES

1. OPPENHEIM, J. J., E. J. KOVACS, K. MATSUSHIMA & S. K. DURUM. 1986. There is more than one interleukin 1. Immunol. Today **11:** 45–55.
2. CHAIT, A. 1982. Monocyte-derived macrophages stimulate LDL receptor activity in arterial smooth muscle cells and skin fibroblasts. Arteriosclerosis **2:** 134–139.
3. CHAIT, A., R. ROSS, J. J. ALBERS & E. L. BLERMAN. 1980. Platelet-derived growth factor stimulates activity of low density lipoprotein receptors. Proc Natl Acad Sci USA **77:** 4084–4088.
4. DEVIES, P., R. J. BONNEY, J. L. HANES & F. A. KUECHI. 1980. The synthesis of arachidonic acid oxidation products by various mononuclear phagocytes. *In* Mononuclear Phagocytes. Functional Aspects. R. Van Furth, Ed. 1317–1345. Martinus Nijhoff. The Hague.
5. EPSTEIN, L. 1981. Interferon as a model lymphokine. Fed. Proc. **40:** 56–61.
6. BROWN, M. & J. L. GOLDSTEIN. 1983. Lipoprotein metabolism in the macrophage: implications for cholesterol deposition in atherosclerosis. Ann. Rev. Biochem. **52:** 223–261.

Role of Plasma Proteins in the Oxidized Low Density Lipoprotein Hypothesis as the Initiating Factor of Atherosclerosis

CHIKAYUKI NAITO,[a] MITSUNOBU KAWAMURA, AND
YUMIKO SUGIMURA

Department of Internal Medicine
Tokyo Teishin Hospital
2-14-23, Fujimi, Chiyoda-ku
Tokyo, Japan

INTRODUCTION

Oxidatively "denatured" human plasma low density lipoprotein (LDL) has recently received increasing attention in atherosclerosis research. The degree of LDL oxidation has been estimated by the thiobarbituric acid (TBA) method, and the values measured (TBARS values) have been shown to correspond well with the amount of "LDL" taken up by macrophages. Macrophages may recognize oxidatively "denatured" LDL through so-called scavenger receptors, suggesting that some modification of the protein moiety of LDL may have taken place by oxidation. The modification of the protein moiety of LDL may be caused by conformation changes of the protein due to lipid peroxidation or by direct oxidative changes in protein moiety. Therefore, although the TBA reaction has been believed to represent lipid peroxides, in order to examine whether TBA reactions also represent such changes in the protein moiety of LDL, we measured TBARS values not only in the whole plasma, LDL, and very low density lipoprotein (VLDL), but also in the lipid fraction of the plasma, lipid moiety of LDL and VLDL, simultaneously, before and during the oxidation by the incubating plasma, LDL or VLDL with cupric ion.

METHODS

TBA reactive substances (TBARS) were determined by the modified Slater's method.[1] The main modification of the method is that we chose a dilute acid instead of a concentrated one. By this means we could reduce the effects of other substances than malondialdehyde (MDA) and make the absorbance at 535 nm wavelength more prominent. Serum lipids were extracted and purified by Folch's method.[2]

RESULTS AND DISCUSSION

The existence of less than 50 μM cupric ion did not so much influence the TBARS value determined directly by the method without removing cupric ion from the samples.

---

[a]Address for correspondence: Dr. Chikayuki Naito, 35-7, Ootsuka 5, Bunkyo-ku, Tokyo 112, Japan.

TABLE 1. Distribution of TBARS in Chloroform-Methanol (2:1) Extract of Serum

Serum Sample	A	B	C
TBARS of whole serum	0.091[a]	0.097[a]	0.157[b]
Chloroform-methanol (2:1) extract			
Water-methanol layer	—[c]	—	0.039
Chloroform layer	0.024	0.025	—
Chloroform + protein layer	—	—	0.131

[a]Absorbance equivalent to 0.25 ml serum.
[b]Absorbance equivalent to 0.5 ml serum.
[c]Not measured.

An addition of a tiny amount of BHT was necessary to prevent the extracted lipids from oxidation during evaporating organic solvent, namely chloroform, even at a lower temperature under N_2 gas stream.

Most of the TBARS were recovered in the "protein fraction" and only small portions of the TBARS in the "lipid fraction" either in plasma, LDL or VLDL (TABLES 1 and 2). Moreover, the increment of TBARS value was much more marked in the "protein fraction" than in the "lipid fraction" in all cases during the incubation with cupric ion. The results suggested that the TBA method might not represent merely lipid peroxides. On the other hand, when the whole heparinized plasma was incubated with cupric ion, the increase in the TBARS value was much less than that in the case in which isolated LDL or VLDL was incubated. Furthermore, as shown in FIGURE 1, as the incubated amount of LDL or VLDL increased, the TBARS value decreased, suggesting some protective effects of the protein moiety of LDL and VLDL against oxidation existed. Because the concentration of LDL and of VLDL used in the experiments was lower than the respective "normal" concentration of LDL and VLDL in the circulation (100 μg/ml of LDL protein correspond to 22 mg/dl of LDL-cholesterol; 100 μg/ml of VLDL protein correspond to 25 mg/dl of VLDL-cholesterol), the results suggested that the occurrence of LDL oxidation in the circulation might be improbable as suggested by Steinberg *et al.*[3] Moreover, the results also suggested that hyper-LDL-emia and/or hyper-VLDL-emia might not accelerate but rather prevent oxidative changes of LDL.

CONCLUSION

1. TBA reaction measured the amount of lipid peroxides as well as protein changes by oxidation.
2. Plasma protein was protective against the oxidation of lipoproteins by cupric ion.

TABLE 2. Distribution of TBARS in LDL and VLDL

	LDL		VLDL	
TBARS (nmole MDA/ml)	Before Incubation	After Incubation[b]	Before Incubation	After Incubation[b]
Total	1.059	12.830	0.353	14.100
Lipid fraction	0.388	0.405	0.088	0.173
Protein fraction[a]	0.971	12.425	0.265	14.027
Protein fraction/total (%)	91.7	96.8	75.1	99.5

[a]Total minus lipid fraction.
[b]Each LDL and VLDL in concentration of 100 μg protein/ml was incubated with 5 μM cupric ion for 24 hours.

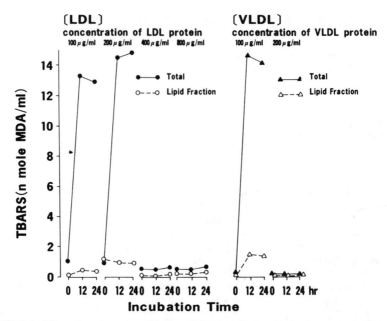

FIGURE 1. Effect of concentration of LDL and VLDL on their oxidation by cupric acid (5 μM).

3. Protein moiety of LDL and VLDL has some protective properties against the oxidation of LDL or VLDL by cupric ion.

REFERENCES

1. NAITO, C. & T. YAMANAKA. 1978. Atherosclerotic diseases and lipoperoxides. Jpn. J. Geriat. **15(3):** 187–191. (In Japanese.)
2. FOLCH, J., M. LEES & G. H. SLOANE STANLEY. 1957. A simple method for the isolation and purification of total lipids from animal tissues. J. Biol. Chem. **226:** 497–509.
3. STEINBERG, D., S. PARTHASARATHY, T. E. CAREW, J. C. KHOO & J. L. WITZTUM. 1989. Modifications of low-density lipoprotein that increase its atherogenicity. N. Engl. J. Med. **320**(14): 915–924.

Arterial Smooth Muscle Cell Response Induced by Loss of Endothelium Continues Even after Apparent Completion of Endothelial Repair

TOYOHIRO TADA, HISASHI TATEYAMA, YUKIO FUJIYOSHI,
AND TADAAKI EIMOTO

Department of Pathology
Nagoya City University Medical School
Mizuho-ku, Nagoya 467, Japan

INTRODUCTION

Previously one of us (T.T.) demonstrated that limited loss of endothelium caused by nylon filament abrasion was associated with a small but significant increase in the ^{3}H-thymidine index of medial smooth muscle cells (SMCs) without intimal thickening.[1] Continuous administration of ^{3}H-thymidine permitted the detection of an elevated rate of cells entering the S phase not observed with standard pulse labeling.[1, 2] The purpose of the present study is to determine precisely when and for how long medial SMCs respond in thoracic aortas of male Sprague Dawley rats which were denuded of a row of endothelial cells approximately 200 μm in width with a fine nylon filament.

MATERIALS AND METHODS

For the 15–20-cell-wide injury, the endothelium was injured by a catheter technique that has been previously described by Reidy and Schwartz.[3] A length of nylon filament (0.35 mm in diameter) was inserted into polyethylene tubing. The top of the nylon filament was bent so that when the filament was extended beyond the polyethylene tubing, it would come into contact with the lumen of the aorta. At various time intervals thereafter, groups of rats received bromodeoxyuridine (BrdU) continuously via an osmotic minipump implanted subcutaneously into the back for three days before sacrifice. Cross sections of each thoracic aorta were processed after perfusion fixation for histological, ultrastructural and immunohistochemical examination, and labeled cells were detected immunohistochemically using monoclonal antibody against BrdU. Cumulative BrdU labeling indices over three days were assessed for animals killed 3 (group 1), 7 (group 2), 10 (group 3), 17 (group 4), and 27 days (group 5) after the initial endothelial injury. The total number of medial SMCs in cross section was obtained by counting the total number of nuclei of medial SMCs in cross section.

RESULTS

It was shown by scanning electron microscopy that a zone of endothelium 15–20 cells wide was removed and the exposed surface was covered with platelets (FIG. 1A). After

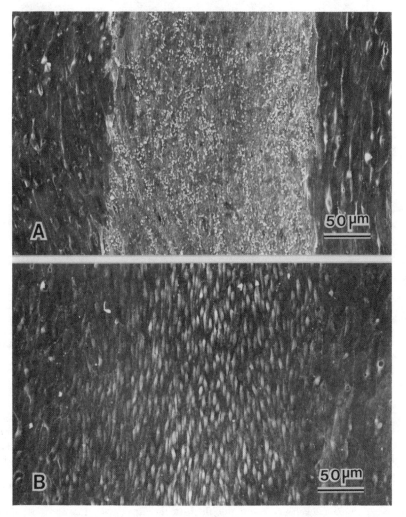

FIGURE 1. Scanning electron micrograph of aorta 2 hours after injury **(A)** shows that a zone of endothelium 15–20 cells wide is removed. Platelets are found adhering to the exposed subendothelium. Injury is completely reendothelialized in approximately 4 days **(B).** The regenerated endothelial cells over the wound were noticeably narrower than the surrounding uninjured cells.

3–4 days, the endothelial layer was fully regenerated (FIG. 1B). The BrdU labeling indices of medial SMCs, however, continued to be significantly increased at least until day 17. The respective values for each group along with the number of medial SMCs are shown in TABLE 1. On the number of medial SMCs, there was no significant difference among groups.

TABLE 1. The BrdU Labeling Indices and Number of Medial SMCs[a]

	Group 1	Group 2	Group 3	Group 4	Group 5	Control
Time after injury (days)	3	7	10	17	27	
BrdU index[b]	3.03 ± 1.56^c	1.65 ± 0.77^c	0.61 ± 0.45^c	0.40 ± 0.23^c	0.24 ± 0.10	0.15 ± 0.17
Number of SMCs[d]	1145 ± 48	1249 ± 173	1079 ± 120	1118 ± 86	1247 ± 141	1361 ± 140

[a]N = 5 for each group.
[b]Mean (%) ± SD.
[c]$p < 0.05$.
[d]Total number of medial SMCs in cross section (mean ± SD).

DISCUSSION

The mechanisms responsible for inducing SMCs to enter the S phase are not known. One hypothesis is that PDGF from platelets adhering to the denuded wall are mitogenic for SMC.[4] Even if this was the case in group 1, however, it could not explain the findings for groups 2, 3, and 4, which showed complete repair of the endothelium. The SMC might, on the other hand, be stimulated by molecules synthesized either by themselves or by regenerated endothelial cells.[5] Of interest is that the total number of medial SMCs in cross sections of injured thoracic aorta from groups 1, 2, 3, 4, and 5 showed no increase compared with the control group values. This suggests that the stimulus produced by endothelial injury induces an increase in polyploid SMCs.

REFERENCES

1. TADA, T. & M. A. REIDY. 1987. Endothelial degeneration: IX. Arterial injury followed by rapid endothelial repair induces smooth muscle cell proliferation but not intimal thickening. Am. J. Pathol. **129:** 429–433.
2. REIDY, M. A. & M. SILVER. 1985. Endothelial degeneration: VII. Lack of intimal proliferation after defined injury to rat aorta. Am. J. Pathol. **118:** 173–177.
3. REIDY, M.A. & S. M. SCHWARTZ. 1981. Endothelial degeneration: III. Time course of intimal changes after small defined injury to rat aortic endothelium. Lab. Invest. **44:** 301–308.
4. ROSS, R., J. GLOMSET & L. HARKER. 1977. Response to injury and atherogenesis. Am. J. Pathol. **86:** 675–684.
5. MUNRO, J. M. & R. S. COTRAN. 1988. The pathogenesis of atherosclerosis: atherogenesis and inflammation. Lab. Invest. **58:** 249–261.

Cytochemical and Immunohistochemical Localization of Superoxide Dismutase (SOD) in the Intima of Swine and Rat Aorta

TAKASHI MAKITA, TETSUYA ISHIDA, MUTSUMI KAWATA,
AND K. T. LEE[a]

Department of Veterinary Anatomy
Yamaguchi University
Yamaguchi 753, Japan
and
[a]Kosin Medical College
Pusan 602-702, Korea

To compare the activity of Cu-Zn-SOD of rat and swine (Tosoh, Tokyo) in the endothelium of the abdominal aorta with that in regenerated endothelial cells, immunocytochemical detection of SOD, using the ABC method at the light microscopic level[1] and the protein A gold method at the electron microscope level, was applied to an intact endothelium and to a regenerated one after one to two weeks of the denudation of it by a ballooning catheter (Fogarty 2F for rat aorta and 8F for swine aorta, Baxter, Tokyo). Exogenous SOD was also detected by either the ABC or the colloidal gold method after perfusion of the swine SOD (0.88 ml, 60,000 unit/kg) or liposomes bearing human SOD (35 mg/kg) to rats (Wister, 250–300g). After one hour, the aorta was dissected, fixed in 4% paraformaldehyde, and embedded in Lowicryl K4M. Polyclonal antibody for the swine and rat SOD, and monoclonal antibody for human SOD were used for immunocytochemistry.[2]

Cu-Zn-SOD was localized both in the cytoplasm and in the nucleus of endothelial cells and in smooth muscle cells in the intima. Endogenous SOD in regenerating cells appeared slightly elevated compared to intact cells. At the electron microscopic level, the distribution of 10 nm colloidal gold in the regenerated cell (FIG. 1) was quite similar to that in the intact endothelial cell. Administered SOD was detected mostly in the perivascular space and also in macrophages (FIG. 2). That was similar to the localization of perfused SOD in Kpffer cells and in the sinusoidal space in liver.[3] These findings suggest that effect of administered SOD may be at the periphery and surface of target cells.

REFERENCES

1. MAKITA, T. & R. LINDBLOM. 1988. Electron microscopic localization of Cu-Zn-SOD of swine in the hepatocyte and parietal cells. Proc. 4th Int. Congress on Cell Biology. K. Charbonneau, Ed. 422. National Research Council of Canada. Ottawa, Canada.
2. MAKITA, T. 1989. Electron microscopic localization of Cu-Zn-SOD in the intima of rat aorta by colloidal gold method. J. Clin. Electron Microsc. **22:** 568–569.
3. MAKITA, T. 1989. Detection of endogenous and exogenous Cu-Zn-SOD by colloidal gold, ABC, and cerium methods in regenerating and tumor cells. Acta Histochem. Cytochem. In press.

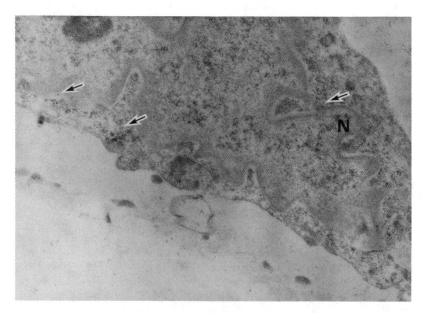

FIGURE 1. After two weeks of ballooning, a regenerated endothelial cell of the rat abdominal aorta contained many colloidal particles *(arrows)* indicating the localization of Cu-Zn-SOD antibodies in the cytoplasm and also, though to a lesser extent, in the nucleus (N).

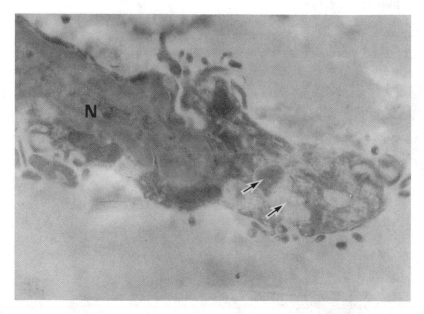

FIGURE 2. Immunocytochemical detection of administered swine Cu-Zn-SOD *(arrows)* in the macrophage in the intima of the rat aorta. Phagocytotic vacuoles contain a number of colloidal gold particles. N: nucleus.

Endothelial Cell Injuries by an Infusion of Various Low Density Lipoproteins into the Rabbit Auricular Vein

TAKEMICHI KANAZAWA, D. H. CHUI, MAKOTO TANAKA,
YUKO FUKUSHI, KOGO ONODERA, HIROBUMI METOKI,[a]
AND YASABURO OIKE[a]

Second Department of Internal Medicine
Hirosaki University School of Medicine
and
[a]*Reimeikyo Rehabilitation Hospital*
5 Zaifu-cho
Hirosaki City, Aomori-Prefecture 036, Japan

To clarify the atherogenicity of LDL, various LDL were infused into the rabbit auricular vein, and histological changes of the basilar artery were compared.

MATERIALS AND METHODS

Three-month-old white rabbits weighing 3 kg were used for the study. LDL was separated by Havel's method.[1] The rabbits were divided into four groups by the kinds of feeding, namely, group 1, standard food; group 2, group 1 + 1% cholesterol; group 3, group 2 + 2% probucol; and group 4, group 2 + 10% soycream (soycream was made from soybeans). LDL which was separated after feeding with each food for 5 weeks, was infused into the rabbit auricular vein. The concentration of the infused LDL was diluted to normal serum cholesterol level, and 400 ml of this diluted LDL were infused into the vein at a rate of 2.2 ml/min for 3 hours. Similarly, LDL separated from the rabbits of the four groups was diluted to the same concentration, and the same amount was infused.

Cerebral basilar arteries were observed by scanning electron microscope and transmission electron microscope,[2] and the findings were compared among the four groups. Platelet aggregability was measured by Born's method.[3]

RESULTS

1) The histological changes of the cerebral basilar arteries by an infusion of saline and LDL of group 1 were not observed. Furthermore, platelet aggregability before and after the infusion did not show a significant difference. 2) Cholesterol-rich LDL was separated from the plasma of group 2. Infusion of the cholesterol-rich LDL, although its infused concentration and amount were the same as the infused LDL of group 1, made the endothelium on the cerebral basilar artery deformed or the mitochondria or the ribosome increased, and the platelet and monocyte adhered to the surface. In addition, platelet aggregability increased. 3) Cholesterol-rich LDL was also obtained from the plasma of group 3. Probucol did not suppress the elevation of LDL-cholesterol. The histological changes after infusion of the LDL treated with probucol was less than those of group 2.

Endocytic vesicles were comparatively numerous, and platelet adhesion was not recognized. The platelet aggregability did not show significant differences before and after the infusion. 4) After the infusion of LDL treated with soycream, histological changes were almost the same as in group 3. However, the development of the endocytic vesicle was less pronounced in this group than in group 3. 5) The changes of tight junction were not observed clearly before or after any of the infusions of LDL.

CONCLUSIONS

1) The endothelial cell injuries of the artery could be made by cholesterol rich LDL infusion in vivo. 2) Even if the same concentration and same amount of cholesterol rich LDL compared to the normal LDL infusion were infused, histological changes were markedly different from each other. 3) Quantitative changes of LDL plays important roles for cell injuries.

REFERENCES

1. HAVEL, R. J., H. A. EDER & J. H. BRAGDON. 1955. The distribution and chemical composition of ultra centrifugally separated lipoproteins in human serum. J. Clin. Invest. **51:** 1486–1494.
2. KANAZAWA, T., C. D. HUA, O. KOMATSU, K. ONODERA & Y. OIKE. 1989. Experimental study on the pathogenesis of cerebral infarction in rabbits by injecting sephandex G-75 (Part I)— Hourly pathological changes of cerebral tissue due to ischemia. Jpn. J. Stroke **11:** 337–346.
3. IZAWA, M., T. KANAZAWA, H. KANEKO, Y. HOSHI, A. MIKUNIYA, K. ONODERA, H. METOKI, Y. SHIMANAKA, R. KAWAHARA, C. NIHEI & Y. OIKE. 1985. Potentiation of platelet aggregation induced by several kinds of aggregating agents. J. Jpn. Atheroscler. Soc. **13:** 89–97.

Detection of Regenerating Cells in Aorta after Ballooning by Immunocytochemical Demonstration of the Thymidine Analogue 5-BromO-2'-Deoxyuridine (BrUdR)

MUTSUMI KAWATA, K. T. LEE,[a] AND TAKASHI MAKITA

Department of Veterinary Anatomy
Yamaguchi University
Yamaguchi City 753, Japan
and
[a]Kosin Medical College
Pusan 602-030, Korea

After denudation of the endothelium of an aorta with a thromboectomy catheter (Fogarty 2F, Baxter, Tokyo), Evans blue was utilized to distinguish blue and nonblue areas in the regenerating surface. The nonblue area, where albumin penetration is blocked by a junctional complex, is regarded as recovered epithelium, while the blue area is supposed to be a slow recovery area. To localize Cu-Zn-SOD, a free radical scavenger, in regenerating cells,[1] as shown in FIGURE 1, another method of identifying the regenerating or proliferating cells by immunocytochemical demonstration of bromodeoxyuridine (BrUdR),[2] a thymidine analogue, was applied for regenerating the endothelium of a rat abdominal aorta (FIG. 2) at the electron microscopic level.

The endothelium was removed by a catheter one to three weeks prior to administration of BrUdR (Takeda, Osaka). During the period of recovery, BrUdR was injected several times at short intervals before dissection of the aorta. Immunocytochemistry of BrUdR was applied by the method of deFazio *et al.*,[2] though sections were not treated with HCl but reacted with 0.1% protease (Sigma, Type VII) in phosphate buffer at pH 7.4. Colloidal gold (10nm) particles were used to localize anti-BrUdR monoclonal antibody. The main site of colloidal gold precipitation was the chromatin area of the nucleus (FIG. 2). We also attempted peroxidase-conjugated Evans blue, but the BrUdr method was more encouraging at the electron microscopic level.

REFERENCES

1. MAKITA, T. 1989. Detection of endogenous and exogenous Cu-Zn-SOD by colloidal gold, ABC, and cerium methods in regenerating and tumor cells. Acta Histochem. Cytochem. In press.
2. DEFAZIO, A., J. A. LEARY, D. W. HEDLEY, & M. H. N. TATTERSALL. 1987. Immunocytochemical detection of proliferating cells *in vivo*. J. Histochem. Cytochem. **35:** 571–577.

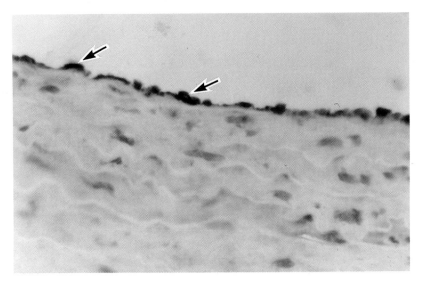

FIGURE 1. Cytochemical localization of Cu-Zn-SOD in the endothelial cells *(arrows)* of rat aorta. Intensive reaction in the endothelium and moderate activity in the smooth muscle were common findings.[1] ABC method with polyclonal antibody of rat SOD.

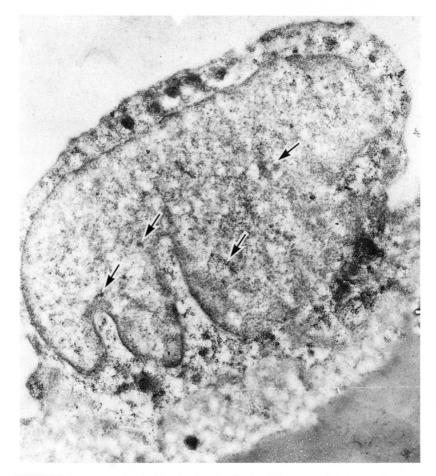

FIGURE 2. Immunocytochemical localization of antibody of BrUdR in the nucleus of a regenerated endothelial cell two weeks after ballooning. Colloidal gold particles *(arrows)* are located in the chromatin substance.

Monoclonal Antibody EMR1a/212D Recognizing the Extracellular Matrix in Atherosclerosis

Purification of Antigenic Material

RYUICHIRO SATO, YASUOMI KOMINE, KEIJI NAKAGAMI,
TSUNEO IMANAKA, AND TATSUYA TAKANO

Department of Microbiology and Molecular Pathology
Faculty of Pharmaceutical Sciences
Teikyo University
Sagamiko, Kanagawa 199-01, Japan

We have developed monoclonal antibodies using a delipidated homogenate of atherosclerotic aorta of Watanabe-heritable hyperlipidemic (WHHL) rabbits as a complex mixture of immunogens. Specific antibodies were selected by indirect immunohistochemical staining of frozen sections of atherosclerotic aorta.[1] One of those antibodies, EMR1a/212D, recognizes extracellular regions of lipid deposits in WHHL rabbit atherosclerotic aorta (FIG. 1a,b). The antigenic material was found in atherosclerotic plaques and serum, and was purified from serum by ion-exchange column chromatography and EMR1a/212D-coupled immunoaffinity column chromatography followed by gel filtration HPLC.[2] The purified antigenic material was a 66-KD glycoprotein with characteristics different from other types of macromolecules known to be found in atherosclerotic plaques. The neuraminidase-treated or trypsin-treated antigenic material lost its antigenic activity, suggesting that sialic acid is one part of the epitope and that the polypeptide backbone around it also participates in it. The amino acid composition of antigenic material was analyzed in a Hitachi Model 835 amino acid analyzer. This glycoprotein was rich in Glx and Asx and poor in Arg and Lys. The amino terminal amino acid sequence of the antigenic material was determined after electroblotting onto polyvinylidene difluoride membrane by a Model 477A Pulse Liquid Phase Sequencer (Applied Biosystems). Twenty amino acid residues in the first 24 amino acid residues of the antigenic material were identical to those of human vitronectin. The purified antigenic material promoted MDCK cell attachment and had a heparin-binding activity. cDNA clones for antigenic material were isolated from a λgt10 library containing cDNA inserts made from Japanese white rabbit liver mRNA. The library was screened with synthetic oligonucleotide probes deduced from the amino terminal amino acid sequence of the antigenic material. Rabbit vitronectin has a 76% amino acid sequence homology with human vitronectin and contains somatomedin B domain, cell attachment domain and glycosaminoglycan binding domain (FIG. 2). Vitronectin is a multifunctional protein promoting attachment and spreading of a variety of cells, and interacting with the C5b-7 complement complex, the thrombin-antithrombin III complex and the plasminogen activator inhibitor. Some of these functions may be involved in the development of atherosclerotic lesions.

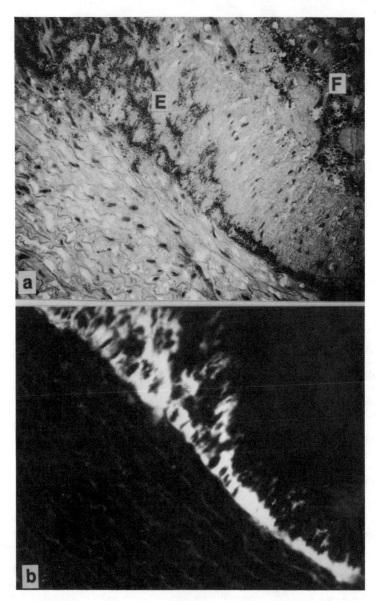

FIGURE 1. Correlation of EMR1a/212D antibody staining and lipid deposits. (a) Two major areas of lipid deposits are observed in atherosclerotic lesions by oil-red O staining. Large droplets stained with oil-red O in contact with nuclei (F) are lipids in the cytoplasm of foam cells, and small scattered droplets near the elastic internal lamina (E) are lipid-deposits in the extracellular matrix. Oil-red O and haematoxylin staining, × 150. (b) Immunofluorescence on EMR1a/212D antibody staining is restricted to extracellular regions with lipid deposits. Indirect immunofluorescent staining of the section adjacent to that for (a), × 150.

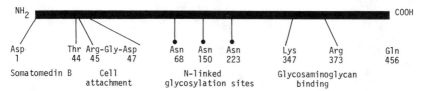

FIGURE 2. Domain structure of rabbit vitronectin. It contains somatomedin B peptide, a cell attachment site, three potential carbohydrate attachment sites, and a glycosaminoglycan binding site.

REFERENCES

1. KIMURA, J., K. NAKAGAMI, K. AMANUMA, S. OHKUMA, Y. YOSHIDA & T. TAKANO. 1986. Virchows Arch. A **410:** 159–164.
2. NAKAGAMI, K., O. SHIMAZAKI, R. SATO, Y. KOMINE, S. OHKUMA & T. TAKANO. 1989. Am. J. Pathol. **135:** 93–100.

Immunohistological Double Labeling of Apolipoprotein E in Different Cell Types of the Human Atherosclerotic Plaque

A. ROESSNER, E. VOLLMER, G. ZWADLO, G. SCHMITZ,
H. ROBENEK, AND C. SORG

Gerhard-Domagk-Institut für Pathologie
Abteilung für Experimentelle Dermatologie der Hautklinik
Institut für Klinische Chemie und Laboratoriumsmedizin
Institut für Arterioskleroseforschung der Westfälischen
Wilhelms-Universität
Münster, Federal Republic of Germany

Although *in vitro* studies of apolipoprotein E secretion by macrophages abound, data about their respective activities in the human atherosclerotic plaque are rather scarce. In recent immunohistochemical investigations, the majority of foam cells in human atherosclerotic plaques were identified as macrophages. In view of the well-known role of apolipoprotein E in what is called "reverse cholesterol transport" it would be most interesting to verify that these macrophage-derived foam cells are actually secreting apolipoprotein E within the atherosclerotic plaque. According to more recent results, even smooth muscle cells are able to secret apolipoprotein E. To find out which cell types in the atherosclerotic plaque are actively involved in apolipoprotein E secretion, we started an immunohistochemical double labeling study with monoclonal antibodies against macrophages, smooth muscle cells, and apolipoprotein E.

Our investigations were performed on samples excised from the ascending aorta of patients undergoing coronary bypass surgery. Macrophages were labeled with the monoclonal antibody 25 F 9 according to Zwadlo *et al.*,[1] and smooth muscle cells were characterized with a monoclonal antibody against desmin. Another monoclonal antibody was available for identification of apolipoprotein E. Immunohistology was performed by indirect peroxidase respectively alkaline phosphatase methods, and for double labeling, a modified so-called APAAP method according to Cordell *et al.*[2] was used, too. The macrophage-derived foam cells showed a strong activity with the antibody against Apo E. The macrophage nature of these secreting foam cells was established in an immunohistochemical double-labeling assay which resulted in a reddish-brown mixed coloring of their cytoplasm, thereby proving that the Apo E-secreting cells are genuine macrophages (FIG. 1). In another immunohistochemical double-labeling assay with monoclonal antibodies against desmin as marker for smooth muscle cells and Apo E, single spindle-shaped cells positive for desmin were also positive for the antibody against Apo E. Obviously, some smooth muscle cells in the atherosclerotic plaque also contain Apo E (FIG. 2).

In conclusion, our *in vitro* investigations of atherosclerotic plaques verify that macrophages transformed to foam cells contain and probably secrete apoprotein E. In addition, there are occasional smooth muscle cells, equally transformed to foam cells and located in the inferior layers of the lesion, the cytoplasm of which obviously contains Apo E. According to Basu *et al.*,[3] the synthesis of Apo E by cholesterol-carrying macrophages is of particular importance for the reverse cholesterol transport towards the liver. The morphologic findings from our study suggest that this metabolic pathway may also play a role in the atherosclerotic plaque.

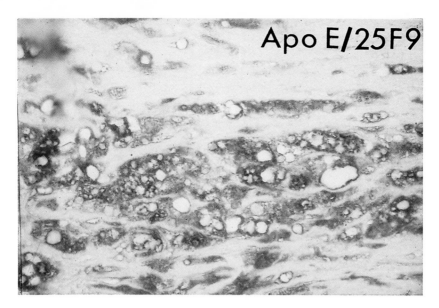

FIGURE 1. Immunohistochemical double labeling: Antibody 25 F 9 against mature tissue macrophages (brown color with the peroxidase method) and antibody against apolipoprotein E (red color with the alkaline phosphatase method). In foam cells we find a mixture of red and brown. ×550.

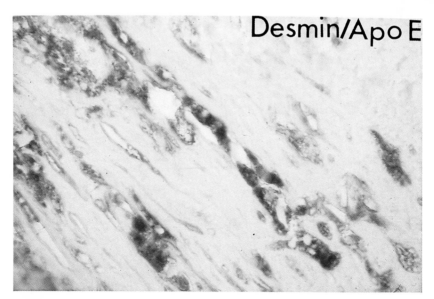

FIGURE 2. Immunohistochemical double labeling with antibodies against desmin (brown color with the peroxidase method) and apolipoprotein E (red color with the alkaline phosphatase method): some spindle-shaped cells are characterized by the brown color as smooth muscle cells which also contain apolipoprotein E. ×550.

REFERENCES

1. G. Zwadlo, E. B. Bröcker, D. B. V. Bassewitz, U. Feige, & C. Sorg. 1985. A monoclonal antibody to a differentiation antigen present on mature human macrophages and absent from monocytes. J. Immunol. **134:** 1487.
2. J. L. Cordell, B. Fallini, W. N. Erber, A. K. Ghosh, Z. Abdulaziz, S. MacDonald, K. A. F. Fulford, H. Stein, & D. Y. Rason. 1984. Immunocytochemical labelling of monoclonal antibodies using immune complexes of alkaline phosphatase and monoclonal anti-alkaline phosphatase. J. Histochem. Cytochem. **22:** 219–229.
3. Basu, S. K., M. S. Brown, Y. K. Ho, R. J. Havel & J. L. Goldstein. 1981. Mouse macrophages synthesize and secrete a protein resembling apolipoprotein E. Proc. Natl. Acad. Sci. USA **78:** 7545–7549.

Fish Oil Depresses the Activity of CTP:Phosphocholine Cytidylyltransferase, Rate-Limiting Enzyme of Phosphatidylcholine Biosynthesis in the Rat

KYOSUKE YAMAMOTO, TERUYOSHI YANAGITA,[a]
NORIYUKI ENOMOTO,[a] AND TAKAHIRO SAKAI

Department of Internal Medicine
Saga Medical School
Saga 849, Japan
and
[a]Department of Applied Biological Sciences
Saga University
Saga 840, Japan

Dietary long-chain fatty acids of fish oils are highly effective in lowering the plasma lipid level in man and in experimental animals. This fall reflects a substantial reduction in hepatic production of very low density lipoprotein (VLDL). Phospholipids (PL), particularly phosphatidylcholine (PC), are prominent components of biological membranes, and recent reports suggest that the active biosynthesis of phosphatidylcholine (PC) is required for the assembly and secretion of VLDL.[1] However, little information is available concerning the effect of fish oil on the PC biosynthesis. We are interested in the possible change in the activity of CTP:phosphocholine cytidylyltransferase (CT), choline kinase (CK) and glycero-3-phosphate acyltransferase by feeding fish oil.[2,3] Male Wistar rats were fed ad libitum by either a beef tallow (BT) or a fish oil (FO) supplemented semipurified diet for one week in experiment 1 and either a corn oil (CO) or a FO-supplemented diet for 3 weeks in experiment 2. The dietary fat level was 10%. Rats were fasted for 8 hr before decapitation.

Weight gain and the relative liver weight were not affected by the dietary treatment in either experiment. As shown in TABLE 1, FO-feeding as compared to BT- or CO-feeding significantly lowered serum triglyceride (TG) and PL levels. The hypocholesterolemic effect of FO-feeding was also evident. Concentration of liver TG was significantly reduced and that of PL was increased in FO-fed rats (TABLE 1). A decrease in VLDL was remarkable in FO-fed rats. FO-feeding as compared to BT- or CO-feeding affects the distribution of PL subclasses in liver microsomes; a decrease in PC and an increase in phosphatidylethanolamine.

The activities of CT, CK and GPAT in liver subcellular fractions are shown in TABLE 2. In experiment 1, the activity of CT in liver microsomes and homogenate decreased remarkably by 50% in FO-fed rats as compared with BT-fed rats. Similarly, the activity of cytosolic CT was significantly lower in the FO-fed rats. The decreased activity of CT in liver microsomes and homogenate by feeding FO was also observed when compared to the CO-fed rats. The activity of cytosolic CK which catalyzes the phosphrylcholine formation was reduced by FO-feeding as compared to BT-feeding. However, there was no change in the CK activity between the FO and CO groups.

TABLE 1. The Concentrations of Plasma and Liver Lipids in Rats Fed Fish Oil (FO) as Compared to Beef Tallow (BT) for One Week (Experiment 1) or FO as Compared to Corn Oil (CO) for 3 Weeks (Experiment 2)[a]

	Experiment 1		Experiment 2	
	BT	FO	CO	FO
Plasma (mg/dl)				
TG	246 ± 32	84 ± 8*	243 ± 64	165 ± 18*
CHOL	125 ± 5	77 ± 5*	143 ± 7	110 ± 9**
PL	230 ± 14	112 ± 12**	256 ± 11	184 ± 17**
Liver (mg/g liver)				
TG	14.4 ± 0.9	5.0 ± 0.2**	18.3 ± 1.2	116 ± 0.6*
CHOL	2.3 ± 0.1	2.1 ± 0.2	2.3 ± 0.2	2.1 ± 0.1
PL	26.3 ± 1.8	30.3 ± 0.6**	26.0 ± 0.9	28.7 ± 0.7**
Microsome				
PC (% PL)	61.3 ± 1.4	56.6 ± 0.3**	60.9 ± 1.1	59.9 ± 0.1
PE (% PL)	14.0 ± 0.4	21.2 ± 0.1*	15.0 ± 0.4	18.8 ± 0.2**
PI + PS (% PL)	13.0 ± 0.4	13.4 ± 0.2	12.5 ± 0.4	13.4 ± 0.2

[a]Each value represents the mean ± SE of 6–7 rats. Abbreviations: TG = triglyceride, CHOL = cholesterol, PL = phospholipids, PC = phosphatidylcholine, PE = phosphatidylethanolamine, PI + PS = phosphatidylinositol + phosphatidylserine. * $p < 0.01$; ** $p < 0.05$.

TABLE 2. The Activities of Liver Phosphatidylcholine Synthetic Enzyme in Rats Fed Fish Oil (FO) as Compared to Beef Tallow (BT) for One Week (Experiment 1) or FO as Compared to Corn Oil (CO) for 3 Weeks (Experiment 2)[a]

	Experiment 1		Experiment 2	
	BT	FO	CO	FO
	(nmol/min/mg protein)			
Cytidylyltransferase				
Homogenate	0.38 ± 0.01	0.25 ± 0.00*	0.45 ± 0.02	0.35 ± 0.01*
Microsome	0.64 ± 0.04	0.36 ± 0.03*	0.56 ± 0.01	0.46 ± 0.01*
Cytosol	1.21 ± 0.04	0.88 ± 0.01*	0.73 ± 0.02	0.81 ± 0.02*
Choline kinase				
Cytosol	3.90 ± 0.10	2.92 ± 0.11*	2.86 ± 0.31	2.63 ± 0.04
Glycero-3-phosphate acyltransferase				
Homogenate	1.29 ± 0.08	1.08 ± 0.07	0.99 ± 0.06	0.72 ± 0.05**
Microsome	2.69 ± 0.10	2.20 ± 0.23	2.61 ± 0.09	2.79 ± 0.07

[a]Each value represents the mean ± SE of 6–7 rats. * $p < 0.01$; ** $p < 0.05$.

These results suggest that the decreased activity of microsomal cytidylyltransferase, the rate-limiting enzyme in PC biosynthesis, in FO-fed rats might suppress the synthesis of PC, which in turn impaired the assembly and secretion of lipoproteins, especially VLDL, in the liver.

REFERENCES

1. YAO, Z. & D. E. VANCE. 1988. J. Biol. Chem. **263:** 2998.
2. YANAGITA, T., K. YAMAMOTO et al. 1989. Jap. Conf. Biochem. Lipids **31:** 259.
3. YANAGITA, T., M. SATOH et al. Biochim. Biophys. Acta **919:** 64.

Cholesterol-Free Diet in Heterozygous Familial Hypercholesterolemia

HIROSHI MOKUNO, NOBUHIRO YAMADA,[a]
TADAO SUGIMOTO,[b] TETSURO KOBAYASHI,[b]
SHUN ISHIBASHI, HITOSHI SHIMANO, TOSHIO MURASE,[b]
AND FUMIMARO TAKAKU

Third Department of Internal Medicine
University of Tokyo
and
[b]*Department of Endocrinology and Metabolism*
Toranomon Hospital
Tokyo, Japan

We have studied the effect of diet therapy on plasma lipoprotein metabolism in heterozygous familial hypercholesterolemia.[1-2]

Seven patients with familial hypercholesterolemia, 5 males and 2 females aged 37 to 66 years, were hospitalized for 2 weeks.[3] A profile of the patients is presented in TABLE 1. Before admission patients had received strict diet therapy; cholesterol less than 300 mg a day and total caloric intake about 30 kcal per kg body weight for more than three months at least. During the period of the ad lib diets, the mean plasma total cholesterol concentration was 337 ± 67 mg/dl. After strict diet therapy in the outpatients, the mean total cholesterol slightly decreased by 4.1%. At the beginning of this study, the mean plasma total cholesterol concentration was 323 ± 67 mg/dl. From the day after admission, the patients received a cholesterol-free diet for 11 days. The content of dietary cholesterol was approximately 1.4 mg a day, and dietary fat, carbohydrate and protein comprised 18.0, 69.2 and 12.8% of calories, respectively. The ratio of polyunsaturated to saturated fatty acids (P/S) was 3:1.

At the end of the study period, plasma cholesterol was lowered by 14.2%, from 323 to 277 mg/dl, as shown in TABLE 2. Among the lipoprotein fractions low density lipoprotein (LDL) cholesterol decreased by 17.5%, from 229 to 189 mg/dl ($p < 0.01$), whereas very low density lipoprotein (VLDL) and intermediate density lipoprotein (IDL) cholesterol levels did not change significantly. High density lipoprotein (HDL) cholesterol decreased by 14.6%, from 41 to 35 mg/dl, a significant change ($p < 0.025$).

Using density gradient ultracentrifugation, we found that the major change in LDL cholesterol was in those fractions with a mean density between 1.034 and 1.042, where cholesterol concentrations decreased from 132 to 87 mg/dl (34%). Cholesterol concentrations in other LDL fractions did not change significantly.[4]

Apolipoprotein B decreased by 16.9%, from 177 to 147 mg/dl. To calculate the cholesterol content in one LDL particle, the plasma LDL cholesterol concentration was divided by the plasma LDL-apolipoprotein B concentration. This ratio, which ranged from 1:59 to 1:71, did not change significantly during the diet therapy.[5]

Our diet decreased the plasma cholesterol concentration significantly, a decrease that

---

[a]Address for correspondence: Nobuhiro Yamada, the Third Department of Internal Medicine, University of Tokyo, Hongo, Bunkyo-ku, Tokyo, Japan 113.

TABLE 1. Profile of Patients (Mean ± SD; N = 7)

Age (years)	51 ± 12
Obesity (%)	1.7 ± 5.6
Cholesterol (mg/dl)	337 ± 67
Family history (+)	6/7
Xanthoma (+)	7/7
Achilles tendon (cm)	
Right	12.1 ± 2.8
Left	13.5 ± 4.5

TABLE 2. The Change of Plasma Lipid (Mean ± SD mg/dl)

	0 Day	4 Day	8 Day	11 Day
Total cholesterol	323 ± 67	303 ± 55	277 ± 57*	277 ± 58*
VLDL-cholesterol	18 ± 11	18 ± 15	19 ± 17	22 ± 27
IDL-cholesterol	34 ± 17	30 ± 13	28 ± 13	27 ± 11
LDL-cholesterol	229 ± 56	213 ± 46	191 ± 53*	189 ± 62*
HDL-cholesterol	41 ± 9	37 ± 8	35 ± 7**	35 ± 10
Triglyceride	106 ± 39	115 ± 67	108 ± 61	132 ± 125
Apolipoprotein B	177 ± 42	156 ± 33	142 ± 28*	147 ± 31*
Ratio of LDL-chol/apo B	1.59	1.71	1.67	1.62

*Significant at $p < 0.01$; ** significant at $p < 0.025$.

was mainly due to a decrease in LDL cholesterol. The concentrations of cholesterol in VLDL, IDL and light fractions of LDL did not change significantly, indicating that the production rate of these lipoproteins did not exceed the rate of removal from the blood circulation. The lack of change in the ratio of LDL cholesterol to LDL apolipoprotein B during diet therapy suggests that the cholesterol-free diet induced a decrease in the number of circulating LDL particles but not in the content of LDL-cholesterol.[6-7]

In our present study, we have demonstrated that diet therapy resulted in a significant reduction in plasma cholesterol, particularly in the LDL fraction. We conclude that diet therapy with free-cholesterol and a high P/S ratio is highly effective in controlling plasma cholesterol levels in heterozygous familial hypercholesterolemia. From the practical point of view, we propose that, prior to the use of medicine for the treatment of hypercholesterolemia, it is necessary to consider whether the patient is on an adequate diet and the activity of LDL receptors are fully activated.

REFERENCES

1. CONNOR, W. E., R. E. HODGES & R. E. BLEILER. 1961. J. Clin. Invest. **40:** 894–901.
2. FERNANDES, J., R. DIJKHUIS-STOFFELSMA, P. H. E. GROOT & J. J. AMBAGTSHEER. 1981. Acta Paediatr. Scand. **70:** 677–682.
3. GOLDSTEIN, J. L. & M. S. BROWN. 1983. The Metabolic Basis of Inherited Disease. 672–712. McGraw-Hill. New York, NY.
4. YAMADA, N., D. M. SHAMES & R. J. HAVEL. 1987. J. Clin. Invest. **80:** 507–515.
5. YAMADA, N. & R. J. HAVEL. 1982. J. Lipid Res. **27:** 910–912.
6. MCNAMARA, D. J., R. KOLB, T. S. PARKER, H. BATWIN, P. SAMUEL, C. D. BROWN & E. H. AHRENS. 1987. J. Clin. Invest. **79:** 1729–1739.
7. MISTRY, P., E. MILLER, M. LAKER, W. R. HAZZARD & B. LEWIS. 1981. J. Clin. Invest. **67:** 493–502.

Long-Term Drinking of MgCl$_2$ Solution and Arterial Lesions in Female SHRSP

NOBORU SAITO,[a] TERUHIKO OKADA,[b] TOSHIAKI MORIKI,[c]
SHOJI NISHIYAMA,[d] AND KOZO MATSUBAYASHI[a]

[a]Department of Geriatrics
[b]Department of Anatomy
[c]Department of Laboratory Medicine
[d]Department of Environmental and Occupational Health
Kochi Medical School
Okohcho, Nankoku,
Kochi 783, Japan

We investigated arteriolar lesions in stroke-prone spontaneously hypertensive rats (SHRSP) and the effects of long-term drinking of MgCl$_2$ solution on these lesions.

METHODS

Two percent MgCl$_2$ solution was administered to 8 female SHRSP aged 2 months for 17 months, and tap water to 9 female age-matched SHRSP, 6 SHRSR (stroke resistant SHR) and 7 WKY (Wistar Kyoto rats) for the same period as controls. Systolic blood pressure was measured by the tail-cuff method (PE-300, Narco). Under anesthesia with urethan, blood sampling was obtained through the abdominal aorta. Magnesium was measured using atomic absorption spectrophotometry (Hitachi 180-80). Rat organs were removed for preparing microscopic specimens with HE-staining. For electronmicroscopy specimens were fixed in 2% glutaraldehyde and in 1% OsO$_4$.

RESULTS

Arterial or Arteriolar Lesions

1. Macroscopically bead-like nodular lesions of the mesenteric artery were most often found in the SHRSP given tap water. 2. Microscopically the bead-like nodular lesions were periarteritis nodosa (FIG. 1). Subendothelial deposits and the damaged internal elastic membrane, enlarged media and adventitia of the mesenteric artery were found in 4 of 5 female SHRSP given tap water (FIG. 1, 1–5), though not in 5 SHRSP given 2% MgCl$_2$ solution (FIG. 1, 6–10). 3. Electronmicroscopically, activated endothelial cells with well developed rough-surface endoplasmic reticulum or Golgi apparatus, subendothelial electron-dense deposits and damaging internal elastic membranes were found in the intima of SHRSP mesenteric arteries (FIG. 2A). The crystal-like electron-dense deposits were fibrin because of 20 to 30 nm stripes in width (FIG. 2B).

The Effect of MgCl$_2$ Solution on Arterial or Arteriolar Lesions

1. Serum magnesium increased in the SHRSP given the MgCl$_2$ solution as compared to the SHRSP given tap water (35.2 ± 4.95 μg/ml (M ± SD) vs 18.23 ± 1.28 μg/ml,

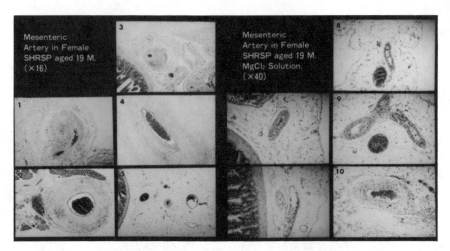

FIGURE 1. Light microscopic figures of the mesenteric artery of female SHRSP aged 19 months (hematoxylin eosin stain). **(1–5)** Mesenteric arteries in female SHRSP given tap water are shown (×16). In 1–4 subendothelial deposits and the enlarged media or adventitia with inflammatory infiltrations are estimated to be periarteritis nodosa, though not in 5. **(6–10)** Mesenteric arteries in female SHRSP given 2% $MgCl_2$ solution are shown (×40). There is no sign of periarteritis nodosa.

p <0.005). 2. Macroscopically the bead-like nodular lesions were found in 89% of 9 SHRSP given tap water, while in 25% of 8 SHRSP given $MgCl_2$ solution and in 0% of 6 SHRSR or 7 WKY given tap water. 3. Microscopically periarteritis nodosa of the mesenteric artery was found in 80% of 5 SHRSP given tap water (FIG. 1, 1–5), though in 0% of 5 SHRSP given $MgCl_2$ solution (FIG. 1, 6–10), and 5 SHRSR or 5 WKY given tap water. The suppressive effects of the $MgCl_2$ solution on arteriolar lesions were also found in SHRSP renal and cerebral tissues. 4. Although serum magnesium increased in the SHRSP given the $MgCl_2$ solution as compared to the SHRSP given tap water, serum cholesterol (73.7 ± 8.3 mg/dl vs 76.6 ± 21.5 mg/dl), fructosamine (1.37 ± 0.14 mM/1 vs 1.33 ± 0.2 mM/1), creatinine (0.52 ± 0.08 mg/dl vs 0.52 ± 0.19 mg/dl) and systolic blood pressure (205 ± 15 mmHg vs 206 ± 27 mmHg) did not differ between them.

DISCUSSION

The occurrence of periarteritis nodosa in the mesenteric artery of old SHR has been observed.[1] We could confirm the frequent occurrence of periarteritis nodosa in SHRSP. In addition to blood pressure the factors such as the increased permeability of the vascular wall or immunological responses may be involved in the occurrence of periarteritis nodosa. Fibrinogen deposits in periarteritis nodosa are reported in SHR.[1] It was very impressive that the supplement of $MgCl_2$ could suppress periarteritis nodosa in SHRSP mesenteric artery.

SUMMARY

1. Macroscopic bead-like nodular lesions were periarteritis nodosa, which were found in SHRSP given tap water. Electronmicroscopically, activated endothelial cells, smooth

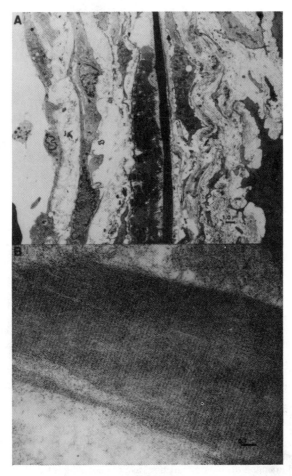

FIGURE 2. Electronmicroscopic figure of the mesenteric artery of female SHRSP aged 19 months (tannic acid stain). **(A)** Endothelial cells are rich in cytoplasm, rough-surface endoplasmic reticulum or Golgi apparatus which show the activated cell states. Subendothelial electron-dense deposits are fibrin. The internal elastic membrane that is very electron dense is stretched. In the intima and the media the activated fibrous or smooth muscle cells are shown. **(B)** Subendothelial crystal-like deposits are fibrin.

muscle cells and fibrous cells were found with well developed rough-surface endoplasmic reticulum or electron-dense particles. 2. The suppressive effects of long-term drinking of MgCl$_2$ solution on arterial or arteriolar lesions, especially on periarteritis nodosa, were observed in this study.

REFERENCES

1. SUZUKI, T., T. MOTOYAMA & R. SATO. 1980. Periarteritis nodosa in spontaneously hypertensive rats—immunohistological study and permeability test. Acta Pathol. Jpn. **30:** 907–915.

Probucol Does Not Act on Lipoprotein Metabolism of WHHL Rabbit Macrophages

YUTAKA NAGANO, NORIAKI KUME, HIDEO OTANI,
HIDENORI ARAI, YUKIHIKO UEDA, CHUICHI KAWAI,
KENJI ISHII,[a] AND TORU KITA[a]

Third Division, Department of Internal Medicine
[a]Department of Geriatric Medicine
Faculty of Medicine
Kyoto University
54 Kawaharacho Shogoin Sakyo-ku
Kyoto 606, Japan

INTRODUCTION

As we have already reported, probucol is very effective for the prevention of atherogenesis in WHHL rabbits, and we also proved that this effect was due to the action of probucol as an antioxidant in preventing the oxidative modification of LDL *in vivo*.[1] However, there might exist other mechanisms of action of this drug concerning the prevention of atherogenesis in WHHL rabbits. Therefore, in this study, its mechanism of action as an antiatherogenic agent other than as an antioxidant was investigated. We paid special attention to the interaction of probucol and WHHL rabbit macrophages, considering that macrophages play important roles in the early stages of atherogenesis.

METHODS

Macrophages of WHHL rabbits were obtained by peritoneal lavage four days after intraperitoneal injection of liquid paraffin oil as previously reported.[2] Macrophages were brought into contact with probucol during 18 hours of preincubation by adding certain amounts of probucol, which were solubilized with ethanol, into the medium. Control macrophages were preincubated in the same medium containing only the same amount of ethanol. In another experiment, macrophages of probucol-fed WHHL rabbits were compared with those of control WHHL rabbits. The effect of probucol on macrophages were estimated by comparing the extent of the uptake of several atherogenic lipoproteins in terms of the intracellular reacylation of [^{14}C]oleate to cholesteryl [^{14}C]oleate following the method of Brown *et al.*[3]

RESULTS AND DISCUSSION

When macrophages pretreated with probucol *in vitro* were incubated with acetyl LDL, β-VLDL or oxidized LDL, they stimulated foam cell transformation of macrophages to the same degree as did control macrophages (Fig. 1). Macrophages obtained from probucol-fed WHHL rabbits also underwent foam cell transformation when incubated with

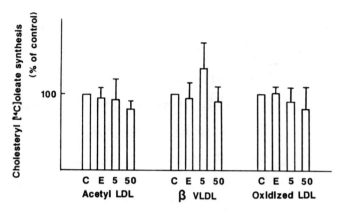

FIGURE 1. Effect of probucol preincubation in vitro on lipoprotein metabolism of WHHL rabbit macrophages. C, probucol (−), ethanol (−); E, probucol (−), ethanol (+); 5, probucol 5 μg/ml in ethanol; 50, probucol 50 μg/ml in ethanol. (Modified from Nagano *et al.*[4])

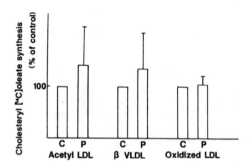

FIGURE 2. Effect of probucol feeding on lipoprotein metabolism of WHHL rabbit macrophages. (Modified from Nagano *et al.*[4])

these lipoproteins, and there were no statistically significant differences between macrophages of probucol-fed rabbits and control rabbits (Fig. 2). We also prepared macrophages that definitely contained probucol using acetyl LDL as a vehicle of probucol,[4] but even in that experiment, no preventive effect of probucol was demonstrated against foam cell transformation of macrophages (data not shown).

The current results give evidence that probucol does not affect lipoprotein metabolism of macrophages, and we confirmed the strong relationship between the antiatherogenic effect of probucol on WHHL rabbits and the action of probucol as an antioxidant.

REFERENCES

1. KITA, T. *et al.* 1987. Proc. Natl. Acad. Sci. USA **84:** 5928–5931.
2. ISHII, K. *et al.* 1988. Biochim. Biophys. Acta **962:** 378–389.
3. BROWN, M.S. *et al.* 1980. J. Biol. Chem. **255:** 9344–9352.
4. NAGANO, Y. *et al.* 1989. Arteriosclerosis **9:** 453–461.

Tissue-Selective Inhibition of Cholesterol Synthesis *In Vitro* and *In Vivo* by Pravastatin Sodium, a 3-Hydroxy-3-Methylglutaryl Coenzyme A Reductase Inhibitor

TEIICHIRO KOGA, YOHKO SHIMADA,[a] MASAO KURODA,[a]
YOSHIO TSUJITA,[a] KAZUO HASEGAWA, AND
MITSUO YAMAZAKI

New Lead Research Laboratories
[a]Fermentation Research Laboratories
Sankyo Co., Ltd.
Hiromachi 1-2-58, Shinagawa-ku
Tokyo 140, Japan

Pravastatin sodium (Pravastatin, CS-514, SQ-31000, Mevalotin®) (FIG. 1) is a competitive inhibitor of 3-hydroxy-3-methylglutaryl coenzyme A (HMG-CoA) reductase, a key enzyme of cholesterol biosynthesis.

In the present study, tissue selectivity of pravastatin in inhibition of cholesterol synthesis was investigated *in vitro* and *in vivo,* and its effect was compared with other HMG-CoA reductase inhibitors, such as lovastatin (MB-530B, Mevinolin, Mevacor®), simvastatin (MK-733, Synvinolin, Zocor®) and ML-236B (Compactin, Mevastatin) (FIG. 1). Inhibition of cholesterol synthesis *in vivo* was measured by incorporation of radioactivity into sterol fraction 1 hr after intraperitoneal injection of [^{14}C]acetate to mice which were orally administered these drugs 2 hr before the acetate injection. When pravastatin was administered to mice at the dose of 20 mg/kg, cholesterol synthesis was inhibited about 90% in the liver and ileum, but the inhibition was less than 10% in the kidney, spleen, adrenal, testis, prostate and brain. This tissue selectivity of pravastatin was also demonstrated even in varying doses (5–40 mg/kg) and time (75–180 min) after drug administration. Other HMG-CoA reductase inhibitors, such as lovastatin and simvastatin in both the lactone and open acid forms, and ML-236B did not show such a tissue-selective inhibition as pravastatin (FIG. 2).

These results were further confirmed by the inhibition of sterol synthesis in various cultured cells and rat lenses (TABLE 1). In freshly isolated rat hepatocytes, pravastatin and other HMG-CoA reductase inhibitors similarly inhibited the sterol synthesis. In the cells from nonhepatic tissues and rat lenses, lovastatin, simvastatin and ML-236B exerted a similar inhibitory activity as observed in rat hepatocytes. In contrast, the inhibitory activity of pravastatin was much less potent in these nonhepatic cells and rat lenses. This tissue selectivity of pravastatin could be explained by lesser cellular uptake of pravastatin into nonhepatic cells.

Thus, pravastatin is shown to be a more distinct tissue-selective inhibitor of sterol synthesis *in vitro* and *in vivo* than other HMG-CoA reductase inhibitors.

REFERENCE

1. TSUJITA, Y. *et al.* 1986. Biochim. Biophys. Acta **877**: 50–60.

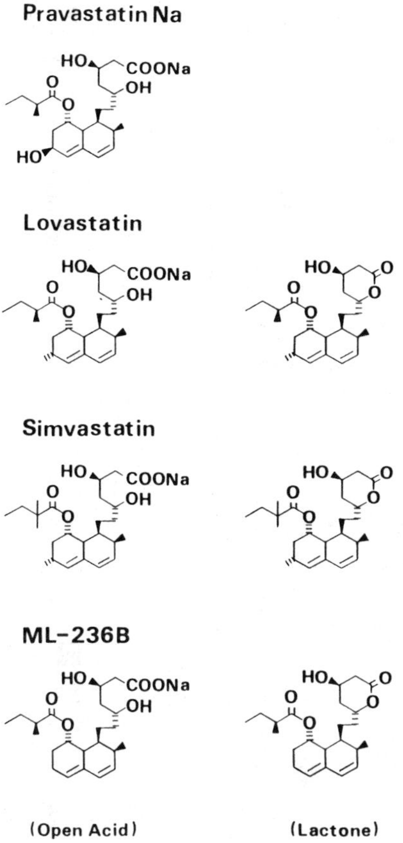

Pravastatin Na

Lovastatin

Simvastatin

FIGURE 1. Chemical structures.

ML-236B

(Open Acid)   (Lactone)

TABLE 1. Effect of Pravastatin, Lovastatin, Simvastatin and ML-236B on the Sterol Synthesis from [^{14}C]Acetate in a Cell-Free Enzyme System, Various Isolated and Cultured Cells and Freshly Isolated Rat Lenses[a]

	Inhibition (IC_{50}, ng/ml)			
	Pravastatin Na	Lovastatin Na	Simvastatin Na	ML-236B Na
Cell-free enzyme system from rat liver	0.8	0.5	0.5	1.7
Rat hepatocytes	2.2	1.9	1.4	7.0
Rat spleen cells	70	1.4	2.2	1.3
Mouse L cells	600	0.8	1.6	2.7
Human skin fibroblasts	200	1.6	1.2	1.6
Rat lenses	185	16.0	9.6	N.D.*

[a]Sterol synthetic activity in cells, rat lenses and a cell-free enzyme system from rat liver was determined[1] by the incorporation of [^{14}C]acetate into digitonin-precipitable sterols and into nonsaponifiable lipids, respectively. The inhibitory activities were expressed by the concentration required for 50% inhibition (IC_{50}). * Not determined.

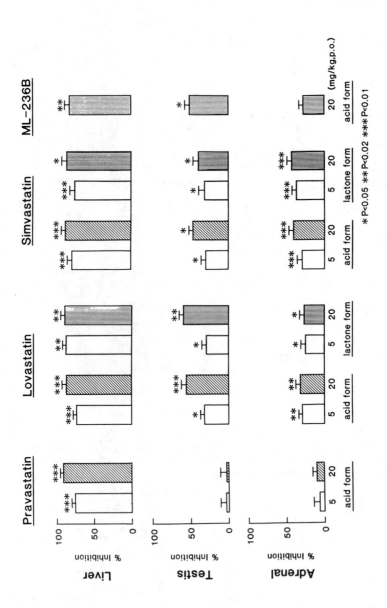

FIGURE 2. The comparative study of tissue selectivity of several HMG-CoA reductase inhibitors in mice *in vivo*. Each drug was orally administered at the doses of 5 and 20 mg/kg to mice 2 hr before the intraperitoneal injection of [^{14}C]acetate. One hr later, each tissue was excised and the incorporation of [^{14}C]acetate into digitonin-precipitable sterols was measured. The data represent the average of values obtained from 4 mice. In adrenal, tissues from 3 mice were pooled and the sterol synthesis was measured. The data indicate the average of values obtained from 4 incubations of 12 mice.

Proliferative Response of Arterial Intimal Smooth Muscle Cells to Epidermal Growth Factor *In Vitro*

MASAKO MITSUMATA,[a] YOJI YOSHIDA,[a] SHINOBU GAMOU,[b]
AND NOBUYOSHI SHIMIZU[b]

*[a]Department of Pathology
Yamanashi Medical College
1110 Tamaho, Nakakoma
Yamanashi 409-38, Japan
and
[b]Department of Molecular Biology
Keio University School of Medicine
35 Shinanomachi, Shinju-ku
Tokyo 160, Japan*

Proliferation of intimal smooth muscle cells is a key event in the pathogenesis of atherosclerosis. Many nuclei of smooth muscle cells (SMCs) were labeled by ^{3}H-thymidine autoradiography in the atherosclerotic intimas of rabbits fed on an atherogenic diet for three months, but few were labeled in the mediae of the aortas. SMCs cultured from atherosclerotic intima (intimal SMCs) proliferated significantly higher in medium containing 10% fetal calf serum on 1, 2, 3 and 5 culture days than the cells from normal aortic media (medial SMCs) (3.6–3.8 times higher in ^{3}H-thymidine uptake). Quiescent intimal SMCs were stimulated to proliferate 6 times more by epidermal growth factor (EGF) at the concentration of 12.5, 25, 100 ng/ml in serum-free medium than the medial SMCs. To disclose the increased growth properties of intimal SMCs, we examined a growth factor signaling pathway that may facilitate the cell proliferation, and also we examined the possibility that additional growth promoting-factors might be secreted by the intimal SMCs under EGF stimulation *in vitro*.

Both intimal and medial SMCs in the serum-free media exhibited high- and low-affinity surface membrane receptors for ^{125}I-labeled EGF. There was no significant difference in the number of specific binding-sites per cell, 1.2×10^5 (intimal) and 1.3×10^5 (medial) receptors/cell, or in the dissociation constant after a four-hour exposure to EGF. There was also no significant difference in the time course of binding and internalization of EGF between the two cells.

C-fos and c-jun mRNA were expressed in both intimal and medial SMCs after incubation with EGF in serum-free medium for one hour by Northern blot analysis. C-myc mRNA also was expressed in both cells after a four-hour incubation (FIG. 1). Minimum contact time for proliferation of intimal SMCs in the serum-free medium with EGF was about eight hours. The addition of lipoprotein-deficient rabbit serum, excluded PDGF (LDS), to the medium with EGF resulted in a significant increase in DNA synthesis of the quiescent medial SMCs. These data suggest the possibility that growth-promoting factors are secreted by intimal SMCs and cooperate with EGF in facilitating cell proliferation. 12.5 and 100 ng/ml EGF stimulated a significant increase in ^{3}H-thymidine incorporation within the medial SMCs in the presence of intimal SMCs compared with that in the culture of medial SMCs alone (FIG. 2). DNA synthesis of medial SMCs, in the conditioned medium from intimal SMCs incubated with serum-free medium, increased significantly (6 times higher) than that from medial SMCs. Additional EGF to conditioned medium accelerated this increased DNA synthesis in medial SMCs. These results suggest that signaling pathways after the expression of c-myc, c-fos, and c-jun mRNA, and possibly growth-promoting factors, which are secreted by the SMC, may regulate the growth properties of intimal SMCs.

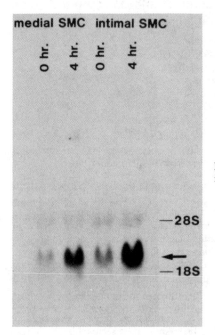

FIGURE 1. C-myc mRNA (*arrow*) in medial and intimal smooth muscle cells stimulated with EGF.

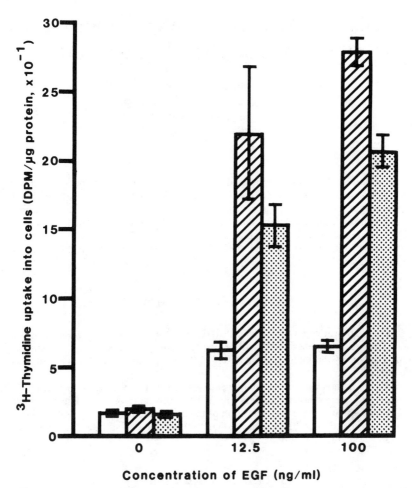

FIGURE 2. Effect of coculture with intimal smooth muscle cells on DNA synthesis in medial smooth muscle cells. *Clear columns,* intimal cell (−); *hatched columns,* intimal cell (+), 3×10^4 cells/well; *stippled columns,* intimal cell (+), 4×10^4 cells/well.

Upregulation of Thrombomodulin on Cultured Endothelial Cells by cAMP

IKURO MARUYAMA AND YASUKO SOEJIMA

Third Department of Internal Medicine
Kagoshima University School of Medicine
1208-1 Usuki-cho
Kagoshima 890, Japan

Thrombomodulin (TM) is an endothelial-cell-associated protein that converts thrombin from a procoagulant protease to an anticoagulant.[1-3] Some factors have an effect on the expression of cell-surface TM. These factors include interleukin 1 (IL-1),[4] tumor necrosis factor (TNF),[4] endotoxin and thrombin.[5] All of these factors downregulate the expression of TM, and no factors which upregulate the expression of TM on the cell surface have been described. This is the first report that endothelial cell-surface TM is upregulated by intracellular cAMP.

MATERIALS AND METHODS

Human umbilical vein endothelial cells (HUVEC) and mouse hemangioma cells were obtained as previously described.[6] All other chemicals were reagent grade products of Sigma. Protein C,[6] thrombin[6] and antithrombin III[6] were of human origin and isolated as indicated.

Confluent monolayer cells in 5-mm wells were washed three times with Medium 199 and incubated with dibutyryl cAMP (dbcAMP), forskolin, or isobutlmethylxanthine (IBMX) for 24 hours. After the incubation of the cells with the above agents, the monolayers were washed three times with Medium 199 and the cell-surface TM activity was measured as previously reported.[6]

RESULTS AND DISCUSSION

Incubation of the monolayers with 2 mM cAMP increased the cell-surface TM by 2–3-fold (FIG. 1). This effect was observed from after 2 hours of incubation and continued up to 24 hours. Northern blotting of mRNA of TM also demonstrated an increase in the time course (date not shown). Treatment of the hemangioma cells with 20 μM of forskolin, 100 μM IBMX or Cilostazol, a newly developed phosphodiesterase inhibitor, also increased the cell-surface TM (FIG. 2). However, the incremental effect was mild and remained up to 2–3-fold of the control level.

These data suggest that expression of TM on HUVEC and hemangioma cells may be regulated by intracellular cAMP. cAMP mediates the hormonal induction of numerous eukaryotic genes through a conserved cAMP responsive element (CRE). However, the mechanism of enhancement of TM expression by cAMP remains to be elucidated at present.

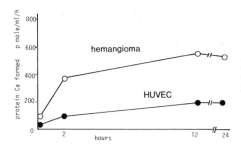

FIGURE 1. Enhancement of TM expression on human umbilical vein endothelial cells and mouse hemangioma cells by 3 mM cAMP.

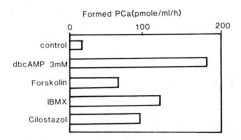

FIGURE 2. Effect of various agents on thrombomodulin activity in mouse hemangioma cells.

REFERENCES

1. ESMON, C. T. & W. G. OWEN. 1981. Indentification of an endothelial cell cofactor for thrombin-catalyzed activation of protein C. Proc. Natl. Acad. Sci. USA **78:** 2249–2250.
2. OWEN, W. G. & C. T. ESMON. 1981. Functional properties of an endothelial cell cofactor for thrombin-catalyzed activation of protein C. J. Biol. Chem. **256:** 5532–5535.
3. ESMON, C. T., N. L. ESMON & K. W. HARRIS. 1982. Complex formation between thrombin and thrombomodulin inhibits both thrombin-catalyzed fibrin formation and factor V activation. J. Biol. Chem. **257:** 7944–7947.
4. COMWAY, E. M. & R. D. ROSENBERG. 1988. Tumor necrosis factor suppresses transcription of the thrombomodulin gene in endothelial cells. Mol. Cell. Biol. **8:** 5588–5592.
5. MARUYAMA, I. & P. W. MAJERUS. 1985. The turnover of thrombin-thrombomodulin complex in cultured human umbilical vein endothelial cells and A549 lung cancer cells. Endocytosis and degradation of thrombin. J. Biol. Chem. **260:** 15432–15438.
6. MARUYAMA, I., H. H. SALEM & P. W. MAJERUS. 1984. Coagulation factor Va binds to human umbilical vein endothelial cells and accelerates protein C activation. J. Clin. Invest. **74:** 224–230.

Genes Expressed during Vascular Smooth Muscle Phenotypic Modulation

GEORGE TACHAS,[a] JULIE H. CAMPBELL,[b] AND
GORDON R. CAMPBELL[a]

[a]Cardiovascular Research Unit
Department of Anatomy
The University of Melbourne
Parkville, Victoria, 3052 Australia
and
[b]Baker Medical Research Institute
Commercial Road
Prahran, Victoria, 3181 Australia

INTRODUCTION

There is a significantly lower volume fraction of myofilaments ($V_V$myo) in smooth muscle cells (SMC) of human diffuse intimal thickenings adjacent to atheromatous plaques compared with cells of the subjacent media or unaffected intima[1] suggesting that changes in SMC phenotype may be important in atherogenesis. Primary cell cultures of arterial medial SMC, under certain conditions, are capable of undergoing a reversible modulation of phenotype from a high $V_V$myo to a low $V_V$myo (in which they are capable of proliferation), then back to a high $V_V$myo following confluency.[2]

The present study investigates changes in mRNA levels of the nuclear protooncogene c-myc, α smooth muscle and $\beta + \gamma$ nonmuscle actin, PDGF A and total poly(A)$^+$ RNA per cell when the SMC are in different phenotypic and proliferative states, in an attempt to gain insight into the genes which may regulate and/or are important in these processes.

RESULTS AND DISCUSSION

Cell Growth and Morphology

Aortic medial SMC from 9-week-old rabbits were dispersed into single SMC and seeded at a density of 1.8×10^6 cells/90-mm dish. The SMC adhered to the culture dish within 24 hours and at 2 days in primary culture the cells were spindle or ribbon shaped and displayed features typical of high $V_V$myo SMC. Day 3 cultures contained cells which had begun to modulate to a low $V_V$myo phenotype and by day 4 the majority of cells were broad and flat, displaying features typical of this phenotype.[3]

Logarithmic growth commenced on day 5 and proliferation continued until confluency (6×10^6 cells/dish) was reached by day 10 (FIG. 1A). A confluent cell monolayer was then maintained up until at least day 16, by which time the SMC cultures had reverted to a high $V_V$myo phenotype.

Changes in α-Actin Isoform mRNA Content as a Percentage of Total Actin and Total Poly(A)$^+$ RNA per Cell

The level of α-actin mRNA expressed as a % of total actin mRNA decreased from 76% in freshly dispersed cells to 42% in day 2 cultured cells and then returned to the

540

original levels by day 10 (81%) in confluent cultures, thereafter remaining high (83%) (FIG. 1B). These data agree with previous studies in our laboratory which have also shown that the changes in α-actin mRNA levels expressed as a % of total actin mRNA, closely resemble the changes in SMC phenotype determined by morphometry ($V_V$myo).[4,5]

The amount of total poly(A)$^+$ RNA per cell increases with time in primary culture to a maximum on day 10. Although dropping slightly as the SMC return to a high $V_V$myo, it does not return to the levels of day 0 (FIG. 1C).

Changes in the Relative Proportions of c-myc, Actin and PDGF A Messages with Time in Culture

A constant amount of mRNA from day 3 to day 16 primary cultures was probed with c-myc,[6] actin[7] and PDGF A[8] cDNA probes and the steady state levels of mRNA per cell determined relative to day 3 (FIG. 2).[9]

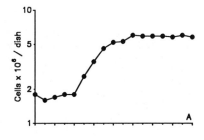

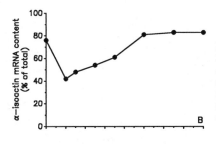

FIGURE 1. **(A)** Growth curve of rabbit aortic SMC grown in primary culture for 16 days. **(B)** α-Isoactin mRNA expression as a percentage of total actin mRNA. **(C)** Total cellular poly(A)$^+$ RNA per cell. These data are for cells seeded at the same seeding density and represent the average of three independent experiments.

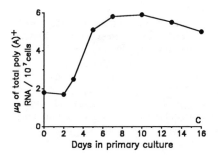

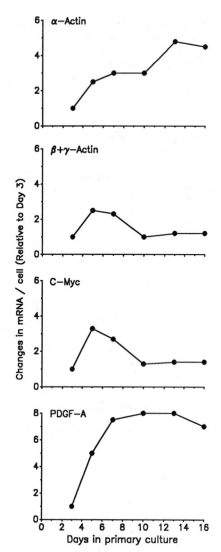

FIGURE 2. Changes in the relative mRNA expressed by rabbit SMC over 16 days in primary culture. The results were determined by multiplying the amount of poly(A)$^+$ RNA per cell (FIG. 1C) by the specific signal obtained using a constant amount of poly(A)$^+$ RNA. Results are given in arbitrary units relative to the signals obtained on day 3.

The β + γ actin mRNA levels increased 2.5-fold from a minimum on day 3 to a maximum on day 5. Near maximal levels were maintained for a further 2 days (while the cells were in logarithmic growth) then returned to the day 3 levels. Similarly, the c-myc mRNA levels increased 3.3-fold from a minimum on day 3 to maximum levels on day 5. These high levels were maintained for a further 2 days (while the cells were in logarithmic growth) and then returned towards the levels expressed in day 3 cultures.

The increase in c-myc and β + γ actin mRNA levels therefore appears to be linked to the onset and maintenance of SMC proliferation and are tightly regulated in a small range of approximately 3-fold. This is consistent with previous findings which have shown c-myc and β actin mRNA are induced in cells that have entered the cell cycle.[10]

In contrast, the α-actin mRNA levels increased 3-fold from day 3 to day 7 and then remained constant until confluency was reached. When cells began to revert to the contractile phenotype by day 13 the α-actin levels increased again and remained high in day 16 cultures. PDGF A levels increased gradually (8-fold) over day 3 to day 10 and then remained constant for a further 3 days before showing a downward trend in day 16 cultures. The PDGF A and α-actin steady state levels are therefore high in both confluent low $V_V$myo and postconfluent high $V_V$myo cells which are not proliferating. The PDGF A levels however show a downward trend in 16 day cultures which have returned to a high $V_V$myo, while the α-actin mRNA levels remain relatively high.

These results indicate that during SMC phenotypic modulation and proliferation, PDGF A and α-smooth muscle actin steady state mRNA levels appear to be controlled independently of c-myc and the nonmuscle $\beta + \gamma$ actin mRNA levels. The increase in c-myc and $\beta + \gamma$ actin expression appears to be linked to SMC proliferation and not phenotypic modulation, while the data for both PDGF A and α-actin are more complex.[5,11,12]

REFERENCES

1. MOSSE, P. R. L., G. R. CAMPBELL & J. H. CAMPBELL. 1986. Arteriosclerosis **6:** 664–669.
2. CHAMLEY-CAMPBELL, J. H., G. R. CAMPBELL & R. ROSS. 1981. J. Cell Biol. **8:** 379–383.
3. CAMPBELL, J. H. & G. R. CAMPBELL. 1987. *In* Vascular Smooth Muscle in Culture. 15–22. CRC Press. Boca Raton, FL.
4. CAMPBELL, G. R., G. TACHAS, G. COCKERILL, J. H. CAMPBELL, J. F. BATEMAN & G. GABBIANI. 1989. Atherosclerosis **8:** 67–71.
5. CAMPBELL, J. H., O. KOCHER, O. SKALLI, G. GABBIANI & G. R. CAMPBELL. 1989. Arteriosclerosis **9:** 633–643.
6. STANTON, L. W., R. WATT & K. B. MARCU. 1983. Nature **303:** 401–406.
7. SHANI, M., U. NUDE, D. ZEVIN-SONKIN, R. ZAKUT, D. GIVOL, D. KATCOFF, Y. CARMON, J. REITER, A. M. FRISCHAUF & D. YAFFE. 1981. Nucleic Acids Res. **9:** 579–589.
8. BETSHOLTZ, C., A. JOHNSSON, C-H. HELDIN, B. WESTERMARK, P. LIND, M. I. S. URDEA, R. EDDY, T. B. SHOWS, K. PHILPOTT, A. L. MELLOR, T. J. KNOTT & J. SCOTT. 1986. Nature **320:** 695–699.
9. ANG, A. H., G. TACHAS, J. H. CAMPBELL, J. F. BATEMAN & G. R. CAMPBELL. 1990. Biochem. J. **265:** 461–469.
10. WOODGETT, J. R. 1989. Br. Med. Bull. **45:** 529–540.
11. CORJAY, M. H., M. M. THOMPSON, K. R. LYNCH & G. K. OWENS. 1989. J. Biol. Chem. **264:** 10501–10506.
12. BLANK, R. S., M. M. THOMPSON & G. K. OWENS. 1988. J. Cell Biol. **107:** 299–306.

Inhibition of Human Vascular Smooth Muscle Cell Proliferation by Interferon Gamma

KENTARO SHIMOKADO AND FUJIO NUMANO

Third Department of Internal Medicine
Tokyo Medical and Dental University
1-5-45 Yushima, Bunkyo-ku
Tokyo 113, Japan

Although T lymphocytes are present in the atherosclerotic lesion, their roles in atherogenesis are still not clear. To elucidate the potential role of the T lymphocyte, we investigated the effects of interferon gamma (INF), a product of activated lymphocytes, on smooth muscle cell proliferation.

METHODS

Human arterial smooth muscle cells (HUA-SMCs) were prepared from human umbilical artery by the method of R. Ross and were maintained in RPMI 1640 medium supplemented with 20% FCS, 10 ng/ml basic FGF. The third passage of HUA-SMCs was seeded in a 24-well tissue culture dish (2 cm^2/well) and cultured in regular medium with or without human recombinant interferon gamma (provided by Takeda Pharmaceutical Co.) for 3–5 days. Cells were trypsinized with 0.25% trypsin/EDTA and the cell number was determined with a Coulter particle counter.

RESULTS AND DISCUSSION

Under our experimental conditions, HUA-SMCs grew logarithmically for 12–15 days and became confluent approximately at 2×10^5 cells/cm^2. When they were cultured in the presence of 0.1–100 u./ml INF, the cell number after 5 days decreased in a dose-dependent fashion with the lowest cell number 40% of that of the control group (FIG. 1). The maximum inhibition was obtained with 100 u./ml INF, and higher concentrations of INF gave no further inhibition of cell proliferation. ED_{50} was 5 u./ml. INF inhibits tumor cell growth either in cytolytic or in cytostatic fashion depending on concentration of INF or cell type. We assessed the mode of the inhibitory effect of INF on HUA-SMCs by measuring LDH release into the culture medium and by dye exclusion with trypan blue. In the presence of 100 u./ml INF, no increase in LDH activity in the culture medium of HUA-SMCs was seen for 3 days. Adherent cells were trypsinized and stained with trypan blue dye. Less than 1% of cells were stained with dye and there was no difference between HUA-SMCs cultured with INF and those without INF. These data suggested that the effect of INF on HUA-SMC growth was cytostatic. Morphological observations substantiated the noncytolytic effect of INF. Under a phase contrast microscope, no morpholog-

544

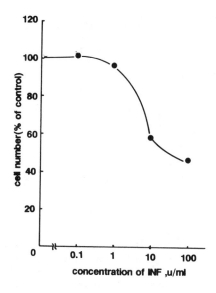

FIGURE 1. Dose-dependent inhibition of HUA-SMC proliferation by INF.

ical difference was detected. Immunocytochemistry using monoclonal antibody HHF35 revealed positive stain both in SMCs treated with INF (FIG. 2) and in untreated cells.

Our results suggest the possibility that lymphocytes in the athrosclerotic lesion are involved in regulation of the growth of SMCs by secreting interferon gamma.

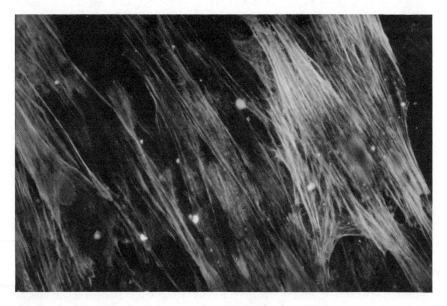

FIGURE 2. HUA-SMCs cultured in the presence of 100 μ/ml INF for 5 days. Stained with monoclonal antibody HHF35.

Transcellular Transport of Angiotensin II through Arterial Endothelial Cells in Monolayer Culture

CHIEKO MINEO, YASUKO YAGYU, TSUNEO IMANAKA, AND
TATSUYA TAKANO

Department of Microbiology and Molecular Pathology
Faculty of Pharmaceutical Sciences
Teikyo University
Sagamiko, Kanagawa 199-01, Japan

Vascular endothelial cells play important roles in the regulation of the transport of macromolecules from blood flow to vascular wall.[1] Angiotensin II (A II) has various actions, related mainly to the vascular smooth muscle contraction and the regulation of blood pressure. We studied the mechanisms of A II transport through cultured porcine arterial endothelial cell monolayer, using the dual chamber method.[2] ^{125}I-A II was added to the upper chamber and the amount of transported ^{125}I-A II to the lower chamber was measured with a gamma counter. When ^{125}I-A II (0.1 nM, 81.4 TBq/mmol) was added in the presence of unlabeled A II (10 μM), the net amount of ^{125}I-A II transport was inhibited 84% (TABLE 1). A II analogue, [Sar^1, Ile^8] A II (50 μm), also inhibited the transport about 70%, while bradykinin (10 μM) had little effect on the transport (data not shown). The transport of ^{14}C-inulin, which was supposed to be transported through cellular junctions, was not affected by unlabeled A II. These results indicated that the transport of ^{125}I-A II through the endothelial cell monolayer was competitively inhibited by the excess amount of unlabeled A II.

We compared the transport of ^{125}I-A II from the apical to basolateral phase, and vice versa, through the endothelial monolayer. As shown in TABLE 1, the transport of ^{125}I-A II from the apical to basolateral phase was inhibited 84% by unlabeled A II (10 μM). On the contrary, the transport of A II from the basolateral to apical phase was not inhibited by the unlabeled A II (about 0%). These results suggest that the transport of A II was unidirectional from the apical to basolateral phase of the endothelial cell monolayer.

^{125}I-A II was transported through the endothelial monolayer in a temperature dependent manner. The amount of ^{125}I-A II transported at 4°C for 2 h was about 44% of that at 37°C (FIG. 1). The transport was inhibited about 96% in the presence of the inhibitors of the ATP generation system, 50 mM 2-deoxyglucose and 10 mM NaN$_3$ (data not shown). The endosomal inhibitor, monensin (50 μM), also inhibited the transport (data not shown). The results suggest that A II transport required an ATP generation system, and endosomal compartment.

We studied the size of the transported A II using Sephadex G-15 column chromatography, and found that A II transported into the lower chamber was not degraded (data not shown). The results demonstrated the ^{125}I-A II was transported through the endothelial cell monolayer without degradation and detected in the intact form.

In this paper, we showed that A II was transported via a specific pathway through the endothelial cell monolayer unidirectionally from the apical to basolateral phase in temperature and energy dependent manner. We suggest that A II is associated with specific binding sites of the endothelial cells, transported through the cells, and released at the basolateral phase to induce contractile responses in smooth muscle cells.

TABLE 1. Competitive Effects of Unlabeled Angiotensin II and Polarity of Transport of ^{125}I-Angiotensin II[a]

Competitive Inhibitors	Transported ^{125}I-AII (fmole/h/dish)	Net Transport (fmole/h/dish)	Inhibition[b] (%)
From apical to basolateral			
None	6.9	3.7	
A II (10 μM)	3.8	0.6	84
From basolateral to apical			
None	6.9	3.7	
A II (10 μM)	7.1	3.9	0

[a]The data shown are the means of 2 or 3 experiments, and in each experiment the transport assay was done in duplicate or triplicate.
[b]Inhibition (%) was calculated as follows:

$$\frac{b-c}{a-c} \times 100 \ (\%)$$

a : ^{125}I-A II transported in the absence of unlabeled A II at 37°C
b : ^{125}I-A II transported in the presence of unlabeled A II at 37°C
c : ^{125}I-A II transported at 4°C.

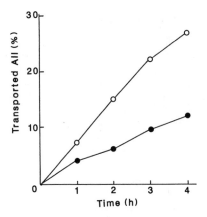

FIGURE 1. Effects of Temperature on Transport of ^{125}I-Angiotensin II. Porcine aortic endothelial cells ($2-5 \times 10^5$ cells/35 mm dish) were seeded and incubated at 37°C in CO_2 incubator to be confluent. After reaching confluent, ^{125}I-A II (18.5 TBq/ml, 10^{-10} M) was added to the upper chamber in 0.1 M Hepes buffer, pH 7.2, containing 120 mM NaCl, 5 mM KCl, 1.2 mM $MgSO_4$, 8 mM glucose, and 0.25% bovine serum albumin, and incubated at 37°C (○) or 4°C (●) for 1, 2, 3, 4, hours.

REFERENCES

1. SIMIONESCU, N., M. SIMIONESCU & G. E. PALADE. 1978. J. Cell Biol. **79:** 27.
2. HASHIDA, R., C. ANAMIZU, Y. YARYU-MIZUNO, S. OHKUMA & T. TATSUYA. 1986. Cell Struct. Funct. **11:** 343–349.

Regulation of Platelet-Derived Growth Factor Gene Expression by Tumor Necrosis Factor and Phorbol Ester in the Human Monocytic Cell Line THP-1

MIKIO NAGASHIMA, YOSHIHIRO FUKUO, AKIRA SAITO,
MINAMI MATSUI,[a] NOBUO NOMURA,[a] RYOTARO ISHIZAKI,[a]
AND AKIRO TERASHI

Second Department of Internal Medicine
[a]Molecular Oncology Laboratory
Nippon Medical School
3-3-5 Iidabashi, Chiyoda-ku
Tokyo 102, Japan

INTRODUCTION

Platelet-derived growth factor (PDGF), which consists of two peptide chains, A and B, is chemotactic and proliferative for mesenchymal cells.[1]

Both A and B chains are transcribed in human atherosclerotic plaque.[2] Thus these can play an important role in the pathogenesis of atherosclerosis.

One of the major sources of PDGF *in vivo* is macrophage. It is not clear what stimulates the expression of PDGF gene in macrophage. Recently tumor necrosis factor (TNF) promoted monocytic differentiation in leukemia cell lines.[3] We study that TNF and/or phorbol 12-myristate 13-acetate (PMA) induce monocytic differentiation and expression of PDGF-A and PDGF-B in a human monoblastic leukemia cell line, THP-1.[4]

METHODS

THP-1 monoblastic cells were grown in RPMI 1640 medium containing 10% fetal calf serum. Recombinant human TNF was added to a final concentration of 10 pM which has been reported to induce monocytic differentiation of these cells.[3] PMA in phosphate buffer was added to a final concentration of 200 ng/ml.

Total RNA was prepared from 10^8 cells by the lysis of NP-40 treatment.

2 μg of polyadenylated RNA, which was selected by chromatography over oligo(dT)-cellulose columns, was subjected to electrophoresis.

PDGF-A, PDGF-B, apo E, and β-actin mRNA were determined by Northern blot analysis.[5]

RESULTS

1. Uninduced THP-1 cells had no detectable PDGF-A and -B mRNA. TNF induced PDGF-A and -B gene expression and the PDGF-A signal was stronger that the

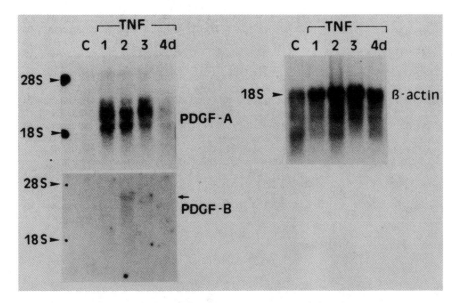

FIGURE 1. PDGF-A and PDGF-B mRNA levels in THP-1 cells treated with TNF. THP-1 cells were cultured for 1, 2, 3, and 4 days without TNF(C), or in the presence of TNF (10 pM).

PDGF-B signal in this stimulation (FIG. 1). The PDGF-A signal was dose-dependently enhanced by TNF (data not shown).

2. PMA-treated cells expressed PDGF-A and -B mRNA about 10-fold stronger than those of the TNF-treated cells. The PDGF-A signal was stronger than the PDGF-B signal in the stimulation of PMA as well as in that of TNF (FIG. 2).

3. The stimulation of the combinations of TNF and PMA strongly enhanced the expression of the PDGF-A and -B gene, especially PDGF-B, as compared with that of PMA alone (FIG. 2).

4. The stimulation of TNF alone was effective in the expression of apo E mRNA in THP-1 cells (FIG. 2).

DISCUSSION

It was suggested that TNF was a differentiating factor and an important inducer of PDGF gene expression in monocytes *in vivo*. TNF enhanced the expression of the PDGF-A and -B gene, especially PDGF-B, in the presence of PMA. It was suggested that the stimulation of TNF in PDGF mRNA expression is more effective after monocytic differentiation by PMA. Because the PDGF-A and -B gene responses by the treatment of TNF and/or PMA were not coordinated, these gene expressions could be regulated by different mechanisms.

TNF is secreted by macrophage, thus macrophage may regulate its PDGF secretion with an autocrine or paracrine system.

TNF also enhanced apo E gene expression in THP-1 cells. This suggested that TNF could be associated with the secretion of apo E in macrophage.

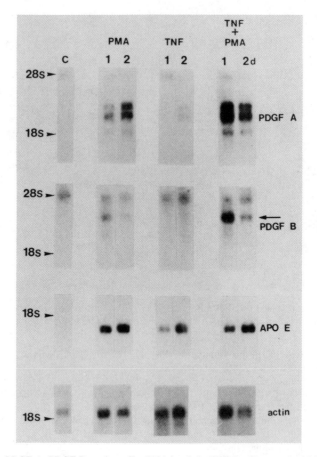

FIGURE 2. PDGF-A, PDGF-B, and apo E mRNA levels in THP-1 cells treated with PMA and/or TNF. These cells were cultured for the indicated times without stimulating agent (C), or in the presence of PMA (200 ng/ml) and/or TNF (10 pM).

REFERENCES

1. Ross, R. 1986. The pathogenesis of atherosclerosis: an update. N. Engl. J. Med. **314:** 488–500.
2. Barrett, T. B. & E. P. Benditt. 1988. Platelet-derived growth factor gene expression in human atherosclerotic plaques and normal artery wall. Proc. Natl. Acad. Sci. USA **85:** 2810–2814.
3. Takeda, K., S. Iwamoto, H. Sugimoto, T. Takuma, N. Kawatani, M. Noda, A. Masaki, H. Morise, H. Arimura & K. Konno. 1986. Nature **323:** 338–340.
4. Tsuchiya, S., M. Yamabe, Y. Yamaguchi, Y. Kobayashi, T. Konno & K. Tada. 1980. Establishment and characteristic of a human acute monocytic leukemia cell line (THP-1). Int. J. Cancer **26:** 171–176.
5. Maniatis, T., E. F. Fritsch & J. Sambrook. 1983. Molecular Cloning: A Laboratory Manual. Cold Spring Harbor Laboratory. Cold Spring Harbor, NY.

Dietary Protein and Cholesterol Metabolism: Effect of Soy Protein on Intestinal Apo B-48 Synthesis and Cholesterol Absorption

D. N. KIM, H.-T. HO, K. T. LEE, AND W. A. THOMAS

Department of Pathology
Albany Medical College
Albany, New York 12208

The hypocholesterolemic effect of vegetable proteins as compared to animal proteins in experimental animals is observed and is well known.[1] In humans, the hypocholesterolemic effect of vegetable proteins is observed mostly in hypercholesterolemic individuals and not generally among normocholesterolemic individuals. Similar effects are observed in swine.[1]

Studies on the mechanism of protein effects on cholesterol metabolism have been focused in several areas including: (1) intestinal, absorption and excretion of steroids,[1] (2) hepatic and intravascular metabolism of lipoproteins,[2] and (3) hormonal.[3]

In earlier studies in swine where the effects of soy protein and casein were compared using a high fat cholesterol diet and classical cholesterol balance methods, we have observed an increase in fecal steroid excretion and reduced cholesterol absorption in the soy protein group.[1]

The possibility of effects of different proteins on apolipoprotein synthesis in the enterocytes has been suggested by Tanaka, Imaizumi and Sugano[4] based on the increase in intestinal apo A-I synthesis in rats fed casein as compared to soy protein.

The current report is an extension of our study on cholesterol absorption focusing on the intestinal mechanism of soy protein actions by direct measurement of cholesterol and apolipoprotein transport in mesenteric lymph.[5]

Eight young male Yorkshire swine approximately 8 weeks old were fed a high-fat, high-cholesterol diet with either casein or soy protein as the source of protein for 5 weeks. Serum cholesterol concentrations in the casein group was 334 ± 46 mg/dl and in the soy protein group 122 ± 8 mg/dl. Thus the soy protein group exhibited significantly less hypercholesterolemic effect.

Under anesthesia, the mesenteric lymph duct was cannulated. A mixture of [^{14}C]-cholesterol and [^{3}H]-leucine was infused into the upper jejunum. The swine had been fed 1/5 of their daily ration 2 hr before. The lymph was collected hourly for 3 hr and fractionated into chylomicron, VLDL, IDL and HDL by sequential ultracentrifugation. The lymphatic transport of cholesterol was significantly higher in the casein group. The transports of triacylglycerol were similar in the two groups. The specific activities and transport of B-48 were lowered in the soy protein group. The transport of apo B-48 was positively related to the transport of cholesterol in chylomicron and VLDL fractions of mesenteric lymph.

Dietary proteins probably influence the apolipoprotein B-48 synthesis in the enterocytes and the amount of apo B-48 in turn affects cholesterol transport into the lymphatics.

REFERENCES

1. KIM, D. N., K. T. LEE, J. M. REINER & W. A. THOMAS. 1983. Effects of soy protein on cholesterol metabolism in swine. *In* Animal and Vegetable Proteins in Lipid Metabolism and Atherosclerosis. A. J. Gibney & D. Krichevsky, Eds. 101. Alan R. Liss, Inc. New York, NY.
2. SIRTORI, C. R., G. GALLI, M. R. LOVATI, P. CARRARA, E. BOSISIO & M. G. KINLE. 1984. Effects of dietary proteins on the regulation of liver lipoprotein receptors in rats. J. Nutr. **114:** 1493.
3. NOSEDA, G. & C. FRAGIACOMO. 1980. Effects of soybean protein diet on serum lipids, plasma glucagon, and insulin. *In* Diets and Drugs in Atherosclerosis. 61. G. Noseda, B. Lewis & R. Paoletti, Eds. Raven Press. New York, New York.
4. TANAKA, K., K. IMAIZUMI & M. SUGANO. 1983. Effects of dietary proteins on the intestinal synthesis and transport of cholesterol and apo A-I in rats. J. Nutr. **113:** 1388.
5. HO, H.-T., D. N. KIM & K. T. LEE. 1989. Intestinal apolipoprotein B-48 synthesis and lymphatic cholesterol transport are lower in swine fed high-fat, high-cholesterol diet with soy protein than with casein. Atherosclerosis **77:** 15.

Structure and Function of *N*-Linked Sugar Chains of Apolipoprotein B-100

TAKAHIRO TANIGUCHI, YUICHI ISHIKAWA,
MASAHIKO TSUNEMITSU, YOSHINORI ASAOKA,
KEN MATSUMOTO, AND HISASHI FUKUZAKI

First Department of Internal Medicine
Kobe University School of Medicine
7-5-1 Kusunoki-cho, Chuo-ku
Kobe 650, Japan

Apolipoprotein B-100(apo B-100) is a glycoprotein organizing the structure of lipoprotein complexes and a ligand for low density lipoprotein (LDL) receptor. Human apo B-100 has been reported to contain 16 mol of *N*-linked sugar chains.[1] To investigate the role of the carbohydrate moieties of apo B-100, we elucidated the structures of *N*-linked sugar chains of humans, Watanabe heritable hyperlipidemic (WHHL) rabbits, an animal model of human familial hypercholesterolemia, and fasting Japanese White rabbits. We also examined their relation to serum cholesterol level.

Human apo B-100 was obtained from delipidated LDL, which was isolated from normolipidemic healthy human plasma by sequential ultracentrifugation and purified by anti apo B-100 monoclonal antibody column chromatography.[2] Rabbit apo B-100 was isolated from the gels of preparative SDS-PAGE by electroelution after delipidation of LDL with isopropyl alcohol/water (1:1, v/v) and ethanol-ether (3:1, v/v). *N*-linked sugar chains of apo B-100 were liberated from the polypeptide portion by hydrazinolysis following *N*-acetylation and NaB^{3}H$_4$ reduction. Their structures were elucidated by sequential exoglycosidase digestion in combination with methylation analysis after fractionation by paper electrophoresis and Bio-Gel P-4 column chromatography.[2]

The oligosaccharide mixture liberated from each apo B-100 was separated into one neutral (N) and two acidic (A1, A2) fractions by paper electrophoresis in molar ratio of 7:8:5 in humans, 5:2:2 in one of 5 WHHL rabbits, and 4:2:5 in fasting rabbits. The neutral fraction contained high-mannose type oligosaccharides consisting of Man$_5$GlcNAc$_2$ to Man$_9$GlcNAc$_2$ as shown in FIGURE 1. The acidic fractions contained monosialylated and disialylated biantennary complex type oligosaccharides. As minor components in the monosialylated fraction, the oligosaccharides which were the absence of one terminal galactose residue and 1 mol each of the galactose and *N*-acetylglucosamine residue, and the hybrid type oligosaccharide were detected. The structures of neuraminidase-treated acidic fractions (A1N, A2N) are shown in FIGURE 1.

When we analyzed the 5 WHHL rabbits, the heterogeneity of *N*-glycosylation of apo B-100 was observed. The molar ratio of acidic oligosaccharides (A1 + A2) and the serum cholesterol level correlated inversely in the WHHL rabbits ($r = -0.973$, $p < 0.0005$) (FIG. 2). The sialic acid molar ratio (SAMR) of apo B-100 WHHL rabbits was calculated by taking the value of that of the fasting rabbits as 1.0. The inverse correlation of SAMR and the serum cholesterol level ($r = -0.997$, $p < 0.001$) was observed in the 5 WHHL rabbits. These results suggest that *N*-glycosylation of apo B-100 is involved in cholesterol metabolism in WHHL rabbits.

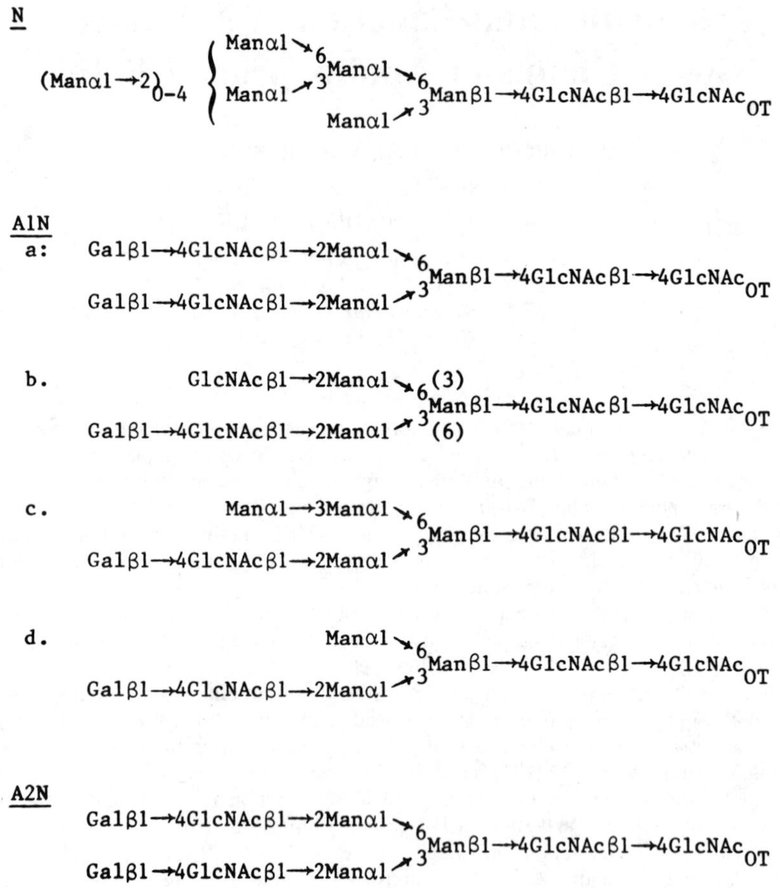

N

$$(Man\alpha1\rightarrow2)_{0-4} \begin{cases} Man\alpha1 \searrow_6 \\ Man\alpha1 \nearrow^3 Man\alpha1 \searrow_6 \\ Man\alpha1 \nearrow^3 \end{cases} Man\beta1\rightarrow4GlcNAc\beta1\rightarrow4GlcNAc_{OT}$$

A1N

a: $Gal\beta1\rightarrow4GlcNAc\beta1\rightarrow2Man\alpha1 \searrow_6$
$Gal\beta1\rightarrow4GlcNAc\beta1\rightarrow2Man\alpha1 \nearrow^3 Man\beta1\rightarrow4GlcNAc\beta1\rightarrow4GlcNAc_{OT}$

b. $GlcNAc\beta1\rightarrow2Man\alpha1 \searrow_6(3)$
$Gal\beta1\rightarrow4GlcNAc\beta1\rightarrow2Man\alpha1 \nearrow^3(6) Man\beta1\rightarrow4GlcNAc\beta1\rightarrow4GlcNAc_{OT}$

c. $Man\alpha1\rightarrow3Man\alpha1 \searrow_6$
$Gal\beta1\rightarrow4GlcNAc\beta1\rightarrow2Man\alpha1 \nearrow^3 Man\beta1\rightarrow4GlcNAc\beta1\rightarrow4GlcNAc_{OT}$

d. $Man\alpha1 \searrow_6$
$Gal\beta1\rightarrow4GlcNAc\beta1\rightarrow2Man\alpha1 \nearrow^3 Man\beta1\rightarrow4GlcNAc\beta1\rightarrow4GlcNAc_{OT}$

A2N

$Gal\beta1\rightarrow4GlcNAc\beta1\rightarrow2Man\alpha1 \searrow_6$
$Gal\beta1\rightarrow4GlcNAc\beta1\rightarrow2Man\alpha1 \nearrow^3 Man\beta1\rightarrow4GlcNAc\beta1\rightarrow4GlcNAc_{OT}$

FIGURE 1. Proposed structures of oligosaccharides in N, A1N, and A2N fractions.

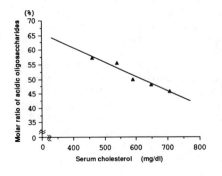

FIGURE 2. Correlation between the molar ratio of acidic oligosaccharides and serum cholesterol level in WHHL rabbits.

REFERENCES

1. YANG, C.-Y., Z.-W. GU, S.-A. WENG, T. W. KIM, S.-H. CHEN, H. J. POWNALL, P. M. SHARP, S.-W. LIU, W.-H. LI, A. M. GOTTO, JR. & L. CHAN. 1989. Structure of apolipoprotein B-100 of human low density lipoproteins. Arteriosclerosis **9:** 96–108.
2. TANIGUCHI, T., Y. ISHIKAWA, M. TSUNEMITSU & H. FUKUZAKI. 1989. The structures of the asparagine-linked sugar chains of human apolipoprotein B-100. Arch. Biochem. Biophys. **273:** 197–205.

Effect of Monocyte Colony-Stimulating Factor (M-CSF) on Lipoprotein Metabolism

SHUN ISHIBASHI, NOBUHIRO YAMADA,[a] HITOSHI SHIMANO,
HISAMORI INABA, NATSUKO MORI, AND
FUMIMARO TAKAKU

Third Department of Internal Medicine
Faculty of Medicine
University of Tokyo
7-3-1 Hongo, Bunkyo-ku
Tokyo 113, Japan

Recent investigations have indicated the involvement of many cytokines in cholesterol metabolism. Tumor necrosis factor (TNF)/cachectin elevates plasma very low density lipoproteins (VLDL) concentrations. In addition, granulocyte-monocyte colony-stimulating factor (GM-CSF) was reported to decrease plasma cholesterol levels.[1] The similar plasma cholesterol lowering activity was also demonstrated in monocyte-colony stimulating factor (M-CSF).[2] On the other hand, foam cells observed in atheromatous fatty streaks are derived from monocytes/macrophages through interaction of plasma lipoproteins. We therefore attempted to investigate the effects of M-CSF on the lipoprotein metabolism of macrophages.

M-CSF were obtained from Morinaga Milk Inc. (Tokyo, Japan).[3] Human monocytes were prepared from blood of healthy volunteers and cultured for 10 days with and without M-CSF, and used as macrophages. Thereafter, the cholesterol ester formation from [^{14}C]oleate and the cellular uptake and degradation of ^{125}I-labeled lipoproteins were measured. Since the cellular DNA contents were hardly affected by M-CSF, the values were indicated as normalized for cellular DNA. Cholesterol esterification was stimulated in the presence of LDL or acetyl-LDL. M-CSF enhanced the stimulation by both lipoproteins. The degree of the enhancement varied greatly among different preparations of macrophages. This might be due to the variation of the responsiveness of macrophages to M-CSF. On average, the cholesterol esterification stimulated by 10 μg/ml of acetyl-LDL was enhanced by 24-fold as shown in TABLE 1. This enhancement of cholesterol esterification might be mainly caused by the increased uptake of ^{125}I-acetyl-LDL, because M-CSF enhanced the uptake and degradation of ^{125}I-acetyl-LDL by 7.5-fold (TABLE 2). However, the values for the cholesterol esterification were always greater than those for the degradation. This suggests that M-CSF increase not only the uptake of the lipoproteins but also the efficiency of esterification of cholesterol derived from the lipoproteins hydrolyzed in lysosome. This direct action of M-CSF on acyl-CoA:acyltransferase needs further investigation.

As for LDL, the cholesterol esterification exceeded the degradation also (TABLES 1 and 2). This might be because M-CSF directly modulate the esterifying enzyme as well as the uptake of LDL as in the case of acetyl-LDL. However, the addition of butylated hydroxytoluene (20 μM) to the incubation medium decreased the uptake of ^{125}I-LDL.

---

[a]To whom all correspondence should be addressed.

TABLE 1. Effects of M-CSF on Cholesterol esterification in Macrophages

	LDL (N = 12)	Acetyl-LDL (N = 13)
	(n moles/μg DNA/24 h)	
M-CSF (−)	0.08 ± 0.02[a]	0.56 ± 0.16
M-CSF (+)	0.58 ± 0.29	6.83 ± 2.5

[a]The mean ± SE.

Thus, it is possible that M-CSF increased the production of oxydized-LDL, which are taken up by macrophages through the scavenger pathway, and this could be responsible for the increased uptake of LDL.

From these results, it is suggested that M-CSF stimulates the LDL-receptor activities in tissue rich in macrophages and macrophage-like cells, thereby increases the clearance of plasma LDL and reduces the plasma cholesterol level. Furthermore, M-CSF might enhance the removal of lipoproteins deposited in atheromatous lesions. All of these effects should be beneficial for preventing atherosclerosis, which appears to promise its clinical use.

TABLE 2. Effects of M-CSF on Cellular Degradation of ^{125}I-labeled Lipoproteins by Macrophages

	LDL (N = 5)	Acetyl-LDL (N = 6)
	(ng/μg DNA/24 h)	
M-CSF (−)	6.2 ± 2.5[a]	152 ± 39
M-CSF (+)	46 ± 17	886 ± 331

[a]The mean ± SE.

REFERENCES

1. NIMER, S. D., R. E. CHAMPLIN & D. W. GOLDE. 1988. J. Am. Med. Assoc. **260:** 3297–3300.
2. MOTOYOSHI, K. & F. TAKAKU. 1989. Lancet 326–327.
3. MOTOYOSHI, K., K. YOSHIDA, K. HATAKE, M. SAITO, Y. MIURA, N. YANAI, M. YAMADA, T. KAWASHIMA, G. G. WONG, P. A. TEMPLE, A. C. LEARY, J. S. WITEK-GIANNOTI, M. FUJISAWA, A. YUO, T. OKABE & F. TAKAKU. 1989. Exp. Hematol. **17:** 68–71.

Effect of Cholesterol Loading on the Translocation of Cholesterol between the Intracellular Pool and the Cell Surface Pool

MORITSUGU SHINOHARA,[a] ABU TORAB M. A. RAHIM,
AKIRA MIYAZAKI, NORIE ARAKI, MOTOAKI SHICHIRI,[a]
YOSHIMASA MORINO, AND SEIKOH HORIUCHI[b]

Department of Biochemistry
[a]Department of Metabolic Medicine
Kumamoto University Medical School
2-2-1 Honjo
Kumamoto 860, Japan

Foam cells are derived from monocytes-macrophages. Thus, an understanding of cholesterol loading and its effect on the cholesterol metabolism of macrophages is crucial to unraveling atherogenic processes. Synthesized *de novo* from acetate, cholesterol enters the "intracellular pool" which is then translocated by a vesicular transport system to the "cell surface pool." In nonloaded macrophages, amounts of cholesteryl esters are negligible (<1%) and >90% of cellular cholesterol is accounted for by the "cell surface pool." Upon cholesterol leading, cholesteryl ester accumulation occurs in the "intracellular pool" and is associated with the activation of acyl CoA:cholesterol acyl transferase (ACAT). It has been shown in nonloaded cells that cholesterol translocation occurs exclusively from the intracellular pool to the cell surface pool.[1] However, recent experiments showed that cholesterol loading with acetyl-LDL induced cholesterol translocation from the "cell surface pool" to the "intracellular pool" to be converted to cholesteryl esters.[2] This possibility was tested in the present study with rat peritoneal macrophages.

RESULTS

(i) Macrophages were converted to foam cells by 50 μg/ml acetyl-LDL. The cells were washed and incubated for 12 h with [³H]cholesterol to label the cell surface pool. The incorporation of radioactivity into cholesteryl esters was less than 3% of cellular cholesterol. (ii) In contrast, when the cell surface pool was first labeled with [³H]cholesterol and loaded with acetyl-LDL, the radioactive incorporation into cholesteryl esters was significantly increased to 9% of total cholesterol (cellular cholesterol plus cholesterol released into the medium). Under the conditions, the cholesterol-oxidase accessible pool (cholestenone) was reduced by 31%, whereas the radioactivity released into the culture medium was increased from 6% to 33%, (FIG. 1). (iii) When cells were first labeled with [³H]cholesterol and chased with 25-hydroxycholesterol, an ACAT activator, the radioactivity incorporated into cholesteryl esters was 2%.

---

[b]Corresponding author.

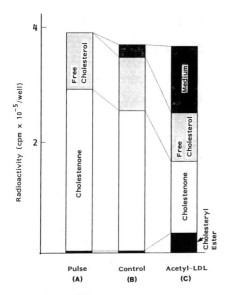

FIGURE 1. Labeling with [³H]cholesterol and subsequent loading with acetyl-LDL. Cell surface cholesterol was labeled with [³H]cholesterol. Some dishes were harvested (A) and cells in other dishes were further chased for 8 h with (C) or without (B) acetyl-LDL. Cells were then treated with cholesterol oxidase, extracted with lipid and analyzed by thin layer chromatography.

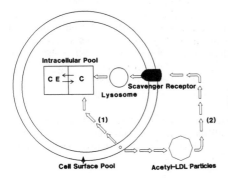

FIGURE 2. Two possible routes for incorporation of cell surface [³H]cholesterol into cholesteryl esters upon foam cell formation.

DISCUSSION

Two routes are possible for cell surface cholesterol to be incorporated into cholesteryl esters of the intracellular pool (FIG. 2). The first is a direct route from the cell surface pool to the intracellular pool, while in the second route, cell surface cholesterol is first trapped by acetyl-LDL particles by an exchange reaction and taken up then through the scaverger receptor pathway. The present results favor the second route. Therefore, an active machinery for cholesterol translocation (the 1st route in FIG. 2) is unlikely to occur to rat peritoneal macrophages, even when these cells are loaded with cholesteryl esters.

REFERENCES

1. LANGE, Y. & B. V. RAMOS. 1983. *J. Biol. Chem.* **258:** 15130–15134.
2. TABAS, I. *et al.* 1988. *J. Biol. Chem.* **263:** 1266–1272.

The Long-Chain Acyl-CoA Synthetase: Structure and Regulation

HIROYUKI SUZUKI AND TOKUO YAMAMOTO[a]

Tohoku University Gene Research Center
1-1 Tsutsumidori-Amamiya, Aoba
Sendai 981, Japan

Long-chain acyl-coenzyme A (acyl-CoA) synthetase plays a key role in both the synthesis of cellular lipids and the degradation of fatty acids via β-oxidation. In spite of the importance of the enzyme in lipid metabolism, little is known about its regulation. In rat liver, the long-chain acyl-CoA synthetase is localized in microsomes, the outer mitochondrial membrane and the peroxisomal membrane. Accumulated evidence suggests that the same long-chain acyl-CoA synthetase is localized in microsomes, mitochondria and peroxisomes. To analyze the structure and regulation of the enzyme, we isolated nearly full-length cDNAs encoding rat and human long-chain acyl-CoA synthetases.

Rat and human long-chain acyl-CoA synthetase cDNAs were isolated. Rat long-chain acyl-CoA synthetase cDNAs were identified using synthetic oligonucleotide probes derived from partial amino acid sequences of purified enzyme. Rat long-chain acyl-CoA synthetase is predicted to contain 699 amino acids. Significant sequence similarity was found between long-chain acyl-CoA synthetase and firefly luciferase. Both long-chain acyl-CoA synthetase and luciferase react with carboxyl groups of the two substrates and ATP to form adenylated intermediates in the first reactions and release AMP in the second reactions. Based on the similarity of the reactions catalyzed by the two enzymes, the amino acid sequence of the long-chain acyl-CoA synthetase, similar to the part of luciferase, may constitute a region where ATP and the carboxyl group of fatty acid interact to form acyl-AMP.

The long-chain acyl-CoA synthetase mRNA is abundant in liver, heart and epididymal adipose tissue. The long-chain acyl-CoA synthetase mRNA is increased 7- to 8-fold in rat liver by feeding a diet containing high carbohydrate or fat, consistent with the physiological significance of the enzyme in fatty acid metabolism.

[a]Corresponding author.

Alterations in Prostaglandin Metabolism in Cultured Human Umbilical Vein Endothelial Cells Affected by Atherogenic Risk Factors during Pregnancy

H.-J. BAUCH, W. ERDBRÜGGER, B. KARBOWSKI, B. KEHREL, AND W. H. HAUSS

Institut für Arterioskleroseforschung an der Universität
Domagkstrasse 3
D-4400 Münster, Federal Republic of Germany

INTRODUCTION

Many cell biological dysfunctions which are important for the development of arteriosclerotic vascular lesions are influenced by prostaglandins (PG's).[1] To study whether or not atherogenic risk factors cause alterations in PG-metabolism which might contribute to atherogenesis, we investigated PG-metabolism in cultured human umbilical vein endothelial cells (HUVEC) affected by smoking, hypertension or diabetes mellitus during pregnancy.

MATERIALS AND METHODS

Detailed information on endothelial cell culture, incubation of HUVEC with ^{3}H-arachidonic acid, isolation of prostaglandins from culture media, separation and quantitative determination of prostaglandins by thin layer chromatography and laser densitometric analysis of the autoradiograms is published elsewhere.[2]

RESULTS AND DISCUSSION

HUVEC obtained from healthy control mothers (C) mainly synthesized the prostanoids PGI_2, $PGF_{2\alpha}$ and PGE_2. HUVEC affected by the above-mentioned atherogenic risk factors during pregnancy and cells obtained from mothers suffering from placental insufficiency exhibited alterations in PG-metabolism (FIG. 1).

Compared with certain controls in all HUVEC affected by the atherogenic risk factors diabetes mellitus, smoking and hypertension during pregnancy, and in cells obtained from mothers suffering from placental insufficiency, a remarkable reduction of PGE_2 synthesis from 80% to 90% was observed. Only in these cells, but not in those obtained from healthy control mothers, the formation of an arachidonic acid metabolite, tentatively identified by thin-layer chromatography as thromboxane A_2 (TxA_2) was observed. The amount of TxA_2 found was up to 5% of total PGs (TABLE 1).

PGI_2 synthesis was reduced in HUVEC from smoking or diabetic mothers and it was

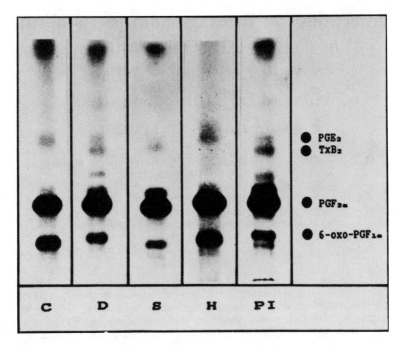

FIGURE 1. Pattern of arachidonic acid (AA)-metabolites in culture media of HUVEC from healthy controls (C) and HUVEC affected by diabetes mellitus (D), smoking (S), hypertension (H) and placental insufficiency (PI) during pregnancy.

strikingly suppressed in cells from mothers suffering from placental insufficiency. As seen from the standard deviations (SD) the formation of PGI_2 generally showed a wide inter-individual variance in all HUVEC affected by atherogenic risk factors. This was most remarkable for cells obtained from hypertensive and diabetic mothers (TABLE 1).

The synthesis of $PGF_{2\alpha}$ was quite similar to HUVEC from healthy control, hypertensive and diabetic mothers. The formation of this metabolite was reduced in cells from smoking individuals. It was elevated in HUVEC from mothers suffering from placental insufficiency (TABLE 1). Compared with cells from healthy controls the ratio of $PGI_2/PGF_{2\alpha}$ was remarkably decreased in cells obtained from mothers suffering from placental

TABLE 1. Prostanoid Synthesis (AU ± SD) in Cultured HUVEC Affected by Atherogenic Risk Factors during Pregnancy or Obtained from Mothers Suffering from Chronic Placental Insufficiency

	Metabolite			
HUVEC from:	PG I_2	PG E_2	PG $F_{2\alpha}$	Tx A_2
Healthy control mothers	3.43 ± 1.41	1.50 ± 0.42	8.76 ± 1.54	n.d.
Diabetic individuals	2.53 ± 2.32	0.18 ± 0.29	9.01 ± 2.85	0.68 ± 0.29
Smoking mothers	2.15 ± 2.15	0.44 ± 0.10	5.45 ± 0.87	0.50 ± 0.29
Hypertensive individuals	3.78 ± 2.42	0.26 ± 0.47	10.13 ± 3.28	0.71 ± 0.85
Mothers suffering from placental insufficiency	1.32 ± 0.76	0.11 ± 0.19	11.24 ± 2.87	0.61 ± 0.10

insufficiency, whereas it remained nearly unaffected in HUVEC obtained from individuals only exposed to atherogenic risk factors.

The present results show that the formation of the vasodilatory and platelet anti-aggregatory PGE$_2$ is commonly reduced in all HUVEC affected by atherogenic risk factors. Furthermore, the synthesis of the potent vasoconstrictory and platelet aggregatory TxA$_2$ seemed to be induced in these cells. The atherogenic risk factors diabetes mellitus, smoking and hypertension often cause placental insufficiency which then is already accompanied by severe arteriosclerotic changes in the fetal arteries.[3,4] The formation of both vasodilatory and platelet anti-aggregatory PGI$_2$ and PGE$_2$ generally is remarkably reduced in all HUVEC from individuals suffering from placental insufficiency. In these cells the synthesis of vasoconstrictory and platelet aggregatory PGF$_{2\alpha}$ and TxA$_2$, however, is clearly enhanced. These findings show that alterations in endothelial PG-metabolism could be observed during atherogenesis increasing with the severity of the vascular disease. The aforementioned prostanoids further control several cell biological events which play a prominent role in the development of arteriosclerosis.[5-8] Thus alterations in PG-metabolism in endothelial cells could play an important role in the formation of early arteriosclerotic vascular lesions.

REFERENCES

1. SCHRÖR, K. 1985. Basic Res. Cardio. **80:** 502–514.
2. ERDBRÜGGER, W., H.-J. BAUCH, B. KARBOWSKI, B. KEHREL & W. H. HAUSS. 1989. *In* Prostaglandins in Clinical Research. K. Schrör & H. Sinzinger, Eds. 389–394. Alan R. Liss Inc. New York, NY.
3. ASMUSSEN, I. & K. KJELDSEN. 1975. Circ. Res. **36:** 579–589.
4. NAEYE, R. L. 1977. Obstet. Gynecol. **50:** 583–588.
5. GRYGLEWSKI, R. J. 1980. CRC Crit. Rev. Biochem. **34:** 291–338.
6. NILSSON, J. & A. G. OLSSON. 1984. Atherosclerosis **53:** 77–82.
7. SMITH, W. L. 1986. Annu. Rev. Physiol. **58:** 251–262.
8. BAUCH, H.-J., B. KEHREL, P. VISCHER, M. JOHN & W. H. HAUSS. 1987. *In* Frühveränderungen bei der Atherogenese. E. Betz, Ed. 46–55. Zuckschwerdt Verlag. Munich.

Changes in Vascular Reactivity following Endothelial Denudation

J. A. MANDERSON, T. M. COCKS,[a] AND G. R. CAMPBELL

Department of Anatomy
University of Melbourne
Grattan Street
Parkville, Victoria 3052, Australia
and
[a]Baker Medical Research Institute
Commercial Road
Prahran, Victoria 3181, Australia

INTRODUCTION

Coronary artery spasm has been suggested as the mechanism underlying the development of myocardial ischemia in patients with variant angina.[1,2] Such transient episodes of vasospasm, with associated ECG changes, can be provoked in patients by the administration of ergonovine,[3] or histamine.[4] Furthermore, angiographic evidence in humans and from animal models suggests that these sites of vasospasm often correspond to areas of luminal stenosis produced by intimal lesions. We have studied the development of an experimental intimal thickening, or neointima, produced by balloon catheter injury, and have specifically examined the effects of this on the reactivity of the artery to vasoconstrictors.

METHODS

The right carotid arteries of male NZ white rabbits were denuded of endothelium using a 2F balloon catheter. The arteries were studied at 2 and 6 weeks using an *in vitro* myograph to measure isometric circumferential force. Ring segments were taken from areas of the injured artery covered by regenerated endothelium (white) and from areas lined by smooth muscle cells (blue). Prior to the construction of dose-response curves each ring was set at an internal circumference (and corresponding passive tension) equivalent to 90% of the circumference the artery would have *in situ* when relaxed and perfused with a transmural pressure of 100 mmHg.[5] Dose-response curves were then produced to either 5HT or the thromboxane A_2-mimetic U46619. When the maximum contractions were reached the ability of the arteries to relax to endothelium-dependent dilators was tested. The organ baths were then rinsed and a second set of curves constructed to KCl or to methoxamine.

RESULTS

At 2 and 6 weeks after endothelial denudation there was no difference in the average maximum contractile force (Emax) developed in response to either 5HT (FIG. 1) or U46619 (data not shown). Analysis of the EC50 values indicated the injured arteries had

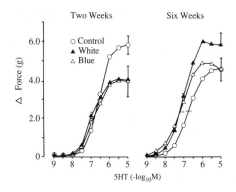

FIGURE 1. Dose-response curves for 5HT in control arteries and in white and blue areas of the ballooned arteries. The vertical and horizontal bars represent the SEM of the Emax and EC50 respectively.

an enhanced sensitivity to 5HT (2-fold) at 2 weeks which was more pronounced at 6 weeks (4-fold). Similarly there was also an increase in sensitivity (2-fold) to U46619 at both time points.

At 2 weeks the denuded arteries developed much less tension in response to methoxamine than the controls (FIG. 2). This decreased Emax was associated with a large decrease in sensitivity to methoxamine (6-fold at 2 weeks and 3-fold at 6 weeks). By 6 weeks the Emax to methoxamine had returned to a level similar to the controls. At both times the denuded arteries had a decreased Emax to KCl.

There were no differences in reactivity to any of these vasoconstrictors between the white and blue areas of the injured arteries. This suggests that endothelium-derived vasoactive substances were not involved in this model even though we have previously shown that areas lined by regenerated endothelial cells can relax in response to methacholine and substance P, whereas areas lined by smooth muscle cells were unresponsive.[6]

CONCLUSIONS

1. Following endothelial denudation and development of a neointima there are selective changes in reactivity of the carotid artery to vasoconstrictors including a

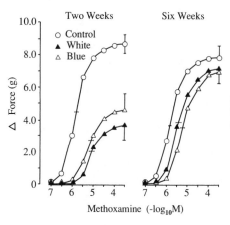

FIGURE 2. Dose-response curves for methoxamine in control and in white and blue areas of the ballooned arteries.

decreased responsiveness to KCl and to the α_1-agonist methoxamine concomitant with an increased sensitivity to 5HT and U46619.

2. The observed changes in reactivity may be related to the changes in SMC phenotype that occur in the media and neointima following endothelial denudation.

3. Our results suggest that the changes in SMC phenotype that occur in atherosclerotic plaques and adjacent areas may predispose these areas to hypercontraction in response to platelet-derived vasoconstrictors.

REFERENCES

1. BROWN, B. G. Arch. Intern. Med. 1981. **41:** 716–722.
2. GORLIN, R. Am. Heart J. 1982. **103:** 598–603.
3. SCHROEDER, J. S. *et al.* 1977. Am. J. Cardiol. **40:** 487–489.
4. GINSBURG, R. *et al.* 1981. Am. Heart J. **102:** 819–822.
5. MULVANY, M. J. & W. HALPERN. 1977. Circ. Res. **41:** 19–26.
6. COCKS, T. M. *et al.* 1987. Blood Vessels. **24:** 192–200.

Inhibition by Low Density Lipoproteins of Endothelium-Dependent Relaxation and Its Mechanism in Porcine Coronary Arteries

TAKAKO TOMITA, MASANORI EZAKI,
TOMOHIRO MITSUBORI, AND YASUHIDE INOUE

University of Shizuoka School of Pharmaceutical Sciences
395 Yada, Shizuoka-shi
Shizuoka-ken 422, Japan

Besides well-known effects of low density lipoprotein (LDL) on the cardiovascular system, several lines of investigation have suggested that LDL induce rather rapid cellular activation. We previously reported that thrombin produced a reproducible and consistent relaxation in strips of intact porcine coronary arteries and LDL dose-dependently inhibited the relaxation.[1,2] The present study has been undertaken to investigate further the inhibitory effect of LDL on endothelium-dependent (ET-dept) relaxation to hemostatic substances, and to explore the mechanism underlying the inhibition by LDL in porcine coronary arteries.

Cumulative thrombin (0.03–0.5 U/ml) induced marked concentration-dependent vasodilation in intact arteries precontracted with $PGF_{2\alpha}$, while in endothelium-denuded arteries thrombin showed a slight contractile response. Pretreatment with methylene blue (10^{-5} M) almost completely abolished the thrombin-induced vasodilation, whereas pretreatment with indomethacin (5×10^{-6} M) did not significantly affect the responses. Despite remarkable relaxation to cumulative thrombin in the absence of LDL, the presence of LDL markedly inhibited the relaxation. A further addition of sodium nitroprusside (10^{-6} M) resulted in a complete vasodilation, suggesting that the LDL inhibitory effects are mediated by the endothelium. However, reduction in the LDL concentration to a half (0.5 mg protein/ml) did not exert such inhibitory effects. Unlike the case of LDL, the presence of HDL (1 mg protein/ml) did not affect the relaxation. The inhibitory effects of LDL were completely abolished 50 min after LDL was washed out with 3 changes of normal Tyrode's buffer. ADP (10^{-6}–10^{-5} M) in the presence of theophyline (10^{-4} M), calcium ionophore A23187 (10^{-7} M), platelet activating factor (PAF, 10^{-4} M) also induced ET-dept relaxation. LDL completely abolished the relaxation and the inhibition was fully reversed by washing (TABLE 1).

As thrombin reportedly produces PAF in cultured endothelial cells, PAF relaxed the coronary artery through the endothelium, and 70% of PAF acetylhydrolase activity in human plasma was found in the LDL fraction, it was speculated that the inhibitory effects of LDL were mediated by the decomposition of PAF by PAF acetylhydrolase present in LDL. The inhibitory principles in LDL lost the activity by heating at 60°C for 10 min, and by acid treatment at pH 2 for 30 min at room temperature. But diisopropylfluorophosphate (DFP) treatment did not influence the inhibitory effect. PAF acetylhydrolase activity in LDL was completely lost by the acid and DFP treatment. Therefore, this enzyme seems not to be involved in the inhibition by LDL. An alternative hypothesis for the mechanism of LDL-inhibition is the activation of lysolecithin acyltransferase(LAT) by LDL in the endothelium. LAT activity was demonstrated in cultured bovine endothelial cells, and the inhibitors like thimerosal activate the production of endothelium-dependent relaxing factors. So, the effect of LDL on LAT activity was examined. LDL greatly enhanced LAT activity dose-dependently. Heat, acid and cyclohexanedione treatments resulted in loss of the LDL enhancing effect on LAT, but DFP treatment did not influence the effect (TABLE 2).

The effective deactivation procedures for the inhibitory principles in LDL to the ET-dept relaxation coincided well with those for the enhancing principles to LAT. Thus, it is concluded that LDL may play a new pathophysiological role in the promotion of coronary vasospasm through rapid and reversible inhibition in ET-dept relaxation to hemostatic substances. Together with this evidence, our results of the LDL modification study suggested that the profound enhancing effect of LDL on LAT activity in the endothelium was the underlying mechanism for the inhibition of ET-dept relaxation by LDL.

TABLE 1. Reversible Inhibition by Low Density Lipoprotein of Endothelium-Dependent Relaxation to Hemostatic Substances in Porcine Coronary Arteries[a]

Stimulated with	Relaxation [% of $PGF_{2\alpha}$ (10^{-5} M)]		
	Absence of LDL	Presence of 1 mg/ml LDL	After LDL Washed Out
		Mean ± SD (n)	
Thrombin (0.3U/ml)	72.4 ± 6.1 (11)	14.0 ± 4.0 (11)[b]	66.7 ± 6.4 (11)[c]
ADP (10^{-5} M)	62.6 ± 8.8 (4)	23.8 ± 3.3 (4)[b]	41.5 ± 11.0 (4)[c,d]
Ionophore A23187 (10^{-7} M)	104.0 ± 2.3 (6)	0.3 ± 0.3 (6)[b]	97.1 ± 6.0 (6)[c]
PAF (10^{-4} M)	82.9 ± 7.0 (6)	−0.2 ± 1.2 (6)[b]	85.3 ± 9.0 (6)[c]

[a]The strip of left anterior descending coronary arteries was mounted vertically under 1.5 g of resting tension in organ baths filled with normal Tyrode's solution. Endothelium-dependent relaxation to thrombin, ADP, ionophore A23187 and PAF was examined in $PGF_{2\alpha}$ (10^{-5} M)-precontracted porcine coronary arteries in the absence and the presence of LDL (1 mg protein/ml), and 50 min after LDL was washed out with three changes of Tyrode's solution. Data are expressed as percentages of relaxation as 100% of $PGF_{2\alpha}$ (10^{-5} M)-induced contraction. LDL (d = 1.006–1.063) was prepared from porcine serum by discontinuous density gradient ultracentrifugation. For the LDL experiment, normal Tyrode's solution in which strips were equilibrated was replaced with the solution containing LDL (1 mg protein/ml). After equilibrated in the LDL solution (less than 3 min), the strips were contracted with $PGF_{2\alpha}$.
[b]Significance p <0.001 vs absence.
[c]Significance p <0.001 vs. presence.
[d]Rather poor recovery due to cumulative dose.

TABLE 2. Effects of LDL and its Modification on Lysolecithin Acyltransferase Activity[a]

Additions	LAT Activity (nmol/mg Protein/h) Mean ± SD (n)	Fold Activation
Exp. 1		
+ none	3.2 ± 0.2 (3)	1.00
+ native LDL (0.5 mg/ml)	12.0 ± 0.6 (4)	3.68
+ (0.8 mg/ml)	19.4 ± 1.6 (5)	5.96
+ (1.0 mg/ml)	27.8 ± 2.5 (5)	8.55
+ (1.5 mg/ml)	26.2 ± 1.0 (4)	8.06
Exp. 2.		
+ none	3.2 ± 0.2 (3)	1.00
+ TMS (1×10^{-4} M)	4.6 ± 0.6 (4)	1.45
+ native LDL	17.5 ± 1.7 (5)	5.46
+ native LDL + TMS (1×10^{-4} M)	5.6 ± 0.8 (4)[c]	1.76
+ heat-LDL	2.7 ± 0.3 (3)[c]	0.84
+ acid-LDL	5.1 ± 0.2 (3)[b]	1.60
LDL only	0.1 ± 0.2 (3)	0.31
Exp. 3		
+ none	3.2 ± 0.2 (3)	1.00
+ native LDL (1 mg protein/ml)	27.7 ± 2.5 (5)	8.55
+ DFP (0.5 mM)-LDL	26.9 ± 2.5 (3)	8.28
+ DFP (5 mM)-LDL	25.9 ± 1.6 (4)	8.00
+ cyclohexanedione-LDL	1.6 ± 1.7 (5)[c]	0.48
LDL only	0.9 ± 0.1 (4)	0.29

[a]Enzyme solution (200 μl, 0.1–0.8 mg protein) of lysolecithin acyltransferase prepared from porcin serum (d = 1.21–1.25) was incubated for 2 hr with ^{3}H-lysolecithin (100 μl, 10^5 dpm/100 nmol) in the absence and the presence of either native LDL or modified LDL (100 μl, 0.4 mg protein) at 37°C. The formed ^{3}H-lecithin was resolved by TLC. LDL modifications were carried out as follows. Heat (60°C, 10 min), acid (pH 2, 30 min at room temperature, and then neutralized), DFP (0.5, 5 mM, 60 min at room temperature, and dialyzed), cyclohexanedione (0.1 mM, 35°C, 2 hr, pH 8.1 and dialyzed), Thimerosal (10^{-4} M, directly added to the incubation mixture).
[b]Significance $p < 0.001$ vs native LDL.
[c]Significance $p < 0.01$ vs native LDL.

REFERENCES

1. INOUE, Y. *et al.* 1988. Chem. Pharm. Bull. **34:** 4626–4629.
2. TOMITA, T. *et al.* 1990. Circ. Res. **66:** 18–27.

Clinical and Angiographic Characteristics of Coronary Artery Spasm

YOUNG BAE PARK, DAE WON SOHN, BYUNG HEE OH,
YUN SHIK CHOI, JUNG DON SEO, AND YOUNG WOO LEE

Division of Cardiology
Department of Internal Medicine
Seoul National University Hospital
28 Yongon-dong, Chongno-gu
Seoul 110-744, Korea

Coronary artery spasm, alone or superimposed on a fixed obstruction due to atherosclerosis, is an important mechanism in producing myocardial ischemia. At present, coronary artery spasm is thought to play a significant role in the conversion of stable to unstable angina and in the development of silent myocardial ischemia as well as variant angina.

Spontaneous or ergonovine-provoked spasms were demonstrated angiographically in 61 patients among 1620 coronary angiograms between April 1986 and April 1989.

Coronary artery spasm affects men more frequently than women, in a ratio of 14 to 1. Twenty-four patients were in the sixth decade, 17 patients in the seventh decade and 16 patients in the fifth decade.

Thirty-one patients complained of resting angina, and 17 patients complained of both resting and exertional angina. In 9 patients, chest pain was atypical, though notably in 31 patients, chest pain occurred during the midnight to early morning hours (FIG. 1). Chest pain developed with coronary artery spasm during the procedures in 41 patients, while in 20 patients spasms were not accompanied by chest pain, suggesting a possible role of coronary artery spasm in producing silent myocardial ischemia.

A twelve-lead ECG in 48 patients during coronary artery spasm showed an ST segment elevation on lesion-related leads in 26 patients, an ST segment depression in 6 patients, and only T wave changes or reciprocal changes in 6 patients. In 10 patients there was no ECG change.

Spasms were demonstrated on normal-looking coronary artery in 41 patients, and were superimposed on insignificant coronary artery lesion in 12 patients and on significant fixed coronary artery lesion in 10 patients. Two patients showed spasms on two sites, one on normal-looking coronary artery and the other on insignificant fixed lesion.

Spasms on the right coronary artery and left anterior descending artery were almost equally demonstrated contrary to previous reports (TABLE 1). In 2 patients, coronary artery spasms were shown on triple vessels. In provoked spasms, total doses of ergonovine were 0.05 mg in 9, 0.15 mg in 13, and 0.35 mg in 12 patients. Coronary artery spasms were demonstrated in the infarct-related arteries of 7 patients with acute myocardial infarction (6 anterior wall MI and 1 inferior MI).

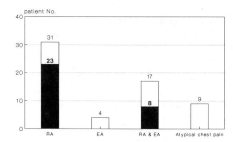

FIGURE 1. Angina in patients with coronary artery spasm. ■ patients with midnight to early morning chest pain. RA: resting angina; EA: exertional angina.

TABLE 1. Angiographic Sites of Coronary Artery Spasm[a]

	LAD	LCx	RCA	LAD + LCx	LAD + RCA	LCx + RCA	Triple	Total
Spont	14		9	1	2	1		27
EG	10		17	1	3	1	2	34
Total	24		26	2	5	2	2	61

[a]Spont: spontaneous spasm; EG: ergonovine provoked spasm; LAD: lt. anterior descending artery; LCx: lt. circumflex artery; RCA: rt. coronary artery.

Thymus Function as Initiation of Atherosclerosis

The Effect of Experimental Atherosclerosis

YOSHIHIRO FUKUO, MIKIO NAGASHIMA, YOJI KOBAYASHI,
AND AKIRO TERASHI

Second Department of Internal Medicine
Nippon Medical School
3-5-5 Iidabashi, Chiyoda-ku
Tokyo 102, Japan

INTRODUCTION

The thymus is known to be the most crucial organ in the body's immunological system. Recently, it was reported that foam cells, the hallmark of the atherosclerotic lesion, are believed to be derived from macrophages, on the basis of Fc receptor activity.[1] There is known to be a close relationship between lymphocytes and macrophages. In this study, we examined the effect of thymectomy on cholesterol metabolism and macrophage functions in experimentally induced atherosclerosis in a cholesterol-fed guinea-pig model.

MATERIALS AND METHODS

(1) Thymectomy and 1% cholesterol-feeding. Twenty-four guinea pigs were divided into two groups: Tx, n = 12, sham, n = 12. Thymectomy was performed on half the guinea pigs in each group. Following thymectomy, 1% cholesterol was fed to one group for 3 months. (2) The levels of T-cho, triglycerides, HDL-cho and phospholipid were determined. (3) The endothelia of the two groups were studied by electronmicroscopy (SEM). (4) Analysis was made of the lipid contents in various tissues. The lipid contents in liver, kidney, spleen and aorta were measured by IATRO scan. (5) E-rosette formation was examined to determine the functioning of T-lymphocytes. Furthermore, morphological changes, the capacity to reduce nitro blue tetrazolium (NBT) in alveolar macrophages, were studied.

RESULTS

(1) Changes of serum lipoprotein by thymectomy. The levels of T-cho in the 1%-fed Tx group were increased significantly compared with the control group. There was no significant difference in the TG levels. The HDL-cho levels in the cholesterol-fed Tx group were lower than in the control. (2) Electronmicroscopical examination. Although there were no typical changes on the endothelium of the sham-operated group, degeneration and thicking lesions of the endothelium were observed in the aorta of the Tx guinea pig. The attachments of platelets and leukocytes were also observed in the endothelia of the Tx groups (FIG. 1). (3) Analysis of lipid contents in aortas. The accumulation of ester-cho in the aorta of the Tx guinea pig was markedly increased, whereas in the aorta

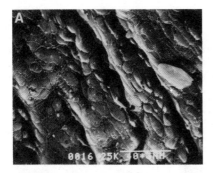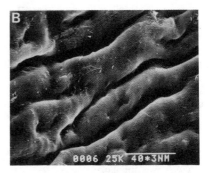

FIGURE 1. Electronmicroscopical examination of the aorta of **(A)** the Tx group and **(B)** the sham-operated group. Degeneration and thickening of lesions of the endothelium were observed in the aorta of the Tx guinea pig. The attachment of platelets and leukocytes was also observed in the endothelium of the Tx group. There is no typical change in the endothelium of sham-operated group.

of the control it was almost undetectable (FIG. 2). (4) There was no significant difference in E-rosette formation among these groups. Regarded as morphological changes of AL-Mø, pseudopod formations were detected in the Al-Mø of the Tx group. Moreover the activities of NBT reductase in the Al-Mø increased remarkably in the Tx group.

DISCUSSION AND CONCLUSION

The close functional relationship between macrophages and T lymphocytes suggested that T cells could be present in the atherosclerotic plaque.[2] It was recently shown that

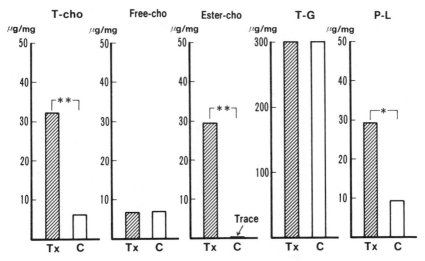

FIGURE 2. Analysis of lipids contained in the aortas of guinea pigs. The accumulation of ester-cho in the aorta of the Tx group was markedly increased, whereas in the aorta of the control it was undetectable. *Hatched columns*, Tx (n = 4); *open columns*, control (n = 4). *$p < 0.01$; **$p < 0.001$.

IFN-γ is locally released by activated T lymphocytes in the atherosclrotic plaque, and that IFN-γ inhibits endothelial excretion of PDGF and IL-1 which is a promoter for smooth muscle cells.[3] However, the net effect of thymus function during the vascular response to atherosclerosis is still unknown. This time we examined the effect of thymectomy on experimental atherosclerosis in cholesterol-fed guinea pigs. The thymectomized guinea pig showed significantly higher levels of serum cholesterol in contrast to lower levels of HDL-cho as compared with the sham-operated guinea pigs. Hislogically marked athero-sclerotic changes were observed in the aorta of the Tx group. Furthermore, pseudopod formations were detected in the Al-Mø of the Tx group. This means the differentiation of Mø in Tx were more activated than control group. The capacity in reductase NBT of the AL-Mø increased remarkably in the Tx group. This means the activities of NBT reductase in the AL-Mø were enhanced remarkably in the Tx group. These results suggest that the activity of Mø might be enhanced by thymectomy. From these studies we can propose that there is a possible role of the thymus in the pathogenesis of atherosclerosis.

REFERENCES

1. GERRITY, R. G. 1981. The role of the monocyte in atherogenesis. 1. Transition of blood-borne monocytes into foam cells in fatty lesions. Am. J. Pathol. **103:** 181–190.
2. STILL, W. J. S., P. R. MARRIOTT. 1964. Comparative morphology of the early atherosclerotic lesion in man and cholesterol atherosclerosis in the rabbit: an electron microscopic study. J. Atheroscler. Res. **4:** 373–386.
3. SUZUKI, H., K. SHIBANO, M. OKANE et al. 1989. Interferon-gamma modulates messenger RNA levels of c-sis (PDGF-B chain), PDGF-A chain, and IL-1 beta genes in human vascular endothelial cells. Am. J. Pathol. **134:** 35–43.

Evidence for the Acceleration of Atherogenesis in Dialysis Patients by Serum Factors Affecting Prostaglandin Synthesis in Endothelial Cells

H.-J. BAUCH, P. VISCHER, A. LAUEN, H. RAIDT,[a]

U. GRAEFE,[a] AND W. H. HAUSS

Institut für Arterioskleroseforschung an der Universität
[a]Institut für Nephrologie an der Universität
Domagkstrasse 3
D-4400 Münster, Federal Republic of Germany

INTRODUCTION

Many clinical investigations have shown that in dialysis patients arteriosclerosis develops often and progresses with great rapidity in these individuals.[1,2] The factors leading to this "accelerated arteriosclerosis" are still largely unknown. During atherogenesis, disorders in prostaglandin (PG) metabolism have been observed in a variety of patients.[3,4] Recent data suggest that naturally occurring circulating factors may be involved in the regulation of PG production, mainly PGI_2 formation.[5,6] To determine whether sera from dialysis patients contain factors influencing prostaglandin synthesis in the vascular endothelium and thereby contribute to genesis and acceleration of arteriosclerosis, the effects of pooled uremic sera on prostaglandin metabolism were studied in an *in vitro* model using cultured pig aortic endothelial cells (PAEC).

PATIENTS AND METHODS

Thirty-eight dialysis patients entered the study. Patients taking drugs influencing PG-metabolism were excluded. According to clinical criteria[7] dialysis patients were separated into two groups: those without arteriosclerosis (n = 19) and those with arteriosclerosis (n = 19). The latter group was divided into two subgroups: those with moderate arteriosclerosis (n = 9) and those with severe arteriosclerosis (n = 10).

PAEC were prepared and cultured according to the methods described by Vischer *et al.*[8] Cells were cultured for 24 h using those conditions. After 24 h in culture, cells were washed three times with serum-free Dulbecco's minimal essential medium (DMEM). Afterwards PAEC were kept in DMEM supplemented with 10% pooled sera from dialysis patients containing 10 µCi ^{3}H-arachidonic acid (spec. act. 210 Ci/mmol) for 24 h.

PGs were isolated from the culture media and separated by thin-layer chromatography. The amount of radioactivity incorporated into PGI_2 (measured as its stable metabolite 6-oxo-$PGF_{1\alpha}$), $PGF_{2\alpha}$ and PGE_2 was determined using autofluorography and laser densitometric analysis.

RESULTS AND DISCUSSION

Compared with pooled sera from patients with normal renal function (creatinine <1.2; n = 16) pooled sera from dialysis patients (n = 38) exhibited a strong inhibitory effect

TABLE 1. Effect of Pooled Serum from Different Groups of Patients on the Formation of Prostaglandins (AU ± SD) in Cultured PAEC

Group	Metabolite		
	PG I$_2$	PG E$_2$	PG F$_{2\alpha}$
Healthy controls (n = 16)	5.28 ± 0.64	2.40 ± 0.32	39.60 ± 1.48
Dialysis patients (HDP) (n = 38)	2.40 ± 0.01	0.76 ± 0.04	34.40 ± 1.00
HDP without AS (n = 19)	3.68 ± 0.76	1.60 ± 0.01	36.40 ± 0.76
HDP with AS (n = 19)	2.32 ± 0.60	0.52 ± 0.20	30.40 ± 1.80
HDP with moderate AS (n = 9)	4.00 ± 0.72	0.72 ± 0.08	33.60 ± 1.96
HDP with severe AS (n = 10)	1.48 ± 0.36	0.60 ± 0.28	29.20 ± 1.92
HDP without AS normotensive patients (n = 3)	2.20 ± 0.01	0.76 ± 0.06	17.6 ± 0.40
HDP without AS hypertensive patients (n = 3)	0.50 ± 0.10	0.30 ± 0.10	4.9 ± 0.70

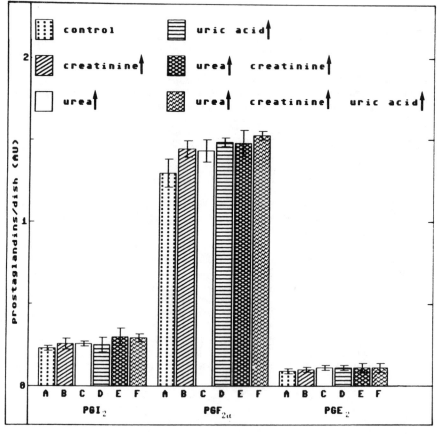

FIGURE 1. Effect of elevated concentrations of urea, uric acid and/or creatinine on PG-metabolism in cultured PAEC.

on PGI$_2$- and PGE$_2$-synthesis in cultured PAEC, whereas the formation of PGF$_{2\alpha}$ was only slightly affected. This inhibitory effect was more pronounced when PAEC were incubated with sera from dialysis patients suffering from arteriosclerosis (n = 19) compared with sera from dialysis patients free from arteriosclerotic vascular diseases (n = 19). The inhibitory effect of sera from dialysis patients on PG-synthesis in PAEC was most striking when sera from dialysis patients suffering from severe arteriosclerosis (n = 10) were examined (TABLE 1).

With respect to single atherogenic risk factors, sera from hypertensive (n = 3) and normotensive (n = 3) nonsclerotic dialysis patients were assayed. These patients were not affected by other atherogenic risk factors and showed a comparable spectrum of symptoms and routine laboratory parameters. Sera from hypertensive individuals strongly inhibited PGI$_2$-synthesis up to 77% and PGE$_2$-formation up to 65% compared with sera from normotensive subjects. Synthesis of PGF$_{2\alpha}$ was also decreased by 72% in this bioassay (TABLE 1).

The concentration of creatinine, urea and uric acid is usually increased in sera from dialysis patients. We therefore added those compounds to sera from patients with normal renal function, giving serum levels typical for dialysis patients. Investigating the effect of these spiked sera on the formation of PGs, it could be excluded, that high serum levels of creatinine, urea and/or uric acid were responsible for the inhibitory effect of uremic sera on PG-synthesis in PAEC (FIG. 1).

In summary, these data show that sera from dialysis patients either contain factors which suppress the PG-formation or lack substances which stimulate PG-synthesis. Both, inhibitory and stimulating factors, have been found in sera; yet see REFERENCES 9–11. As sera from dialysis patients contain substances which preferentially impair the formation of the cytoprotective prostaglandins PGI$_2$ and PGE$_2$, these serum factors might contribute to an accelerated atherogenesis in dialysis patients.

REFERENCES

1. WORLD HEALTH ORGANISATION. 1978. Demographic Year Book. Genf.
2. EVANS, R. W., D. L. MANNINEN, L. P. GARRISON, L. G. HART, C. R. BLAGG, R. A. GUTMAN, A. R. HULL & E. G. LOWRIE. 1985. N. Engl. J. Med. **312:** 553–559.
3. SILBERBAUER, K., G. SCHERNTHANER, H. SINZINGER, H. PIZA-KATZER & M. WINTER. 1979. N. Engl. J. Med. **300:** 366–367.
4. FITZGERALD, G. A., B. SMITH, A. K. PEDERSON & A. R. BRASH. 1984. N. Engl. J. Med. **310:** 1065–1068.
5. SEID, J. M., P. B. B. JONES & R. G. G. RUSSEL. 1983. Clin. Sci. **64:** 387–394.
6. SINZINGER, H. 1985. Wien. klin. Wschr. **97:** 71–73.
7. KANNEL, W. B., P. A. WOLF & R. J. GARRISON. 1987. *In* The Framingham Study. NIH Publication No. 87-2284.
8. VISCHER, P. & E. BUDDECKE. 1985. Exp. Cell Res. **158:** 15–28.
9. REMUZZI, G., C. ZOJA, D. MARCHESI, A. SCHIEPATI, G. MECCA, R. MISIANI, M. B. DONATI & G. DEGAETANO. 1981. Br. Med. J. **282:** 512–518.
10. DEMBÈLÈ-DUCHESNE, M. J., H. THALER-DAO, C. CHAVIS & CRASTES DE PAULET. 1981. Prostaglandins **22:** 979–985.
11. HARROWING, P. D. & K. J. WILLIAMS. 1980. Br. J. Pharmacol. **70:** 183–191.

Initiation of Atherosclerosis: Giant Endothelial Cells, Intimal Constriction, and Late Replacement of Damaged Endothelial Cells

TOSHIAKI SUNAGA AND SEI EMURA

Department of Internal Medicine
Saga Medical School
Saga 849, Japan

Endothelial cell injury and the related changes are regarded as a major factor in the initiation of atherosclerosis. Morphological developments at the initial atherosclerotic stage subsequent to endothelial injury are less well known.

MATERIALS AND METHODS

Forty male rabbits were used for the experiment: the first group of 10 were infused with adrenaline solution (0.1–10 μg/Kg/min for 15 min); the second group of 10 with noradrenaline (0.1–10 μg/Kg/min for 15 min); and a third group of 20 were fed 1% cholesterol feed for 12–18 weeks. All anesthetized animals were sacrificed by intracardiac perfusion with 110 mmHg of glutaraldehyde for 15–60 min. Sample tissues were taken from the thoracic aorta; upon removal, the tissue was cut into small pieces and promptly immersed in fixative. Electronmicroscopic observation was performed by the ordinary method.

RESULTS

Centriole-Containing Giant Endothelial Cells, Cilia under Catecholamine Infusion and Hypercholesterolemic Rabbits

The rates of large and projecting endothelial cells observed in the three groups were 15%, 5% and 10%, respectively.

In fatty streaks, elongated large endothelial cells appeared on the surface.

The sizes of large endothelial cells were approximately 50–60 μ in length and 10–20 μ in width.

A rapid increase in endothelial cell turnover seems to be induced by catecholamine administration or hyperlipidemia.

Endothelial cells characteristically take in relatively large amounts of carbon particles.

Large and elongated endothelial cells were often observed in fatty streaks. A possible explanation for this change would be that a stretching force along the long axis is at work.

These findings would account for the proliferation and the incomplete mitosis of endothelial cells.

Pathologically, the uneven surface of endothelial cells produced turbulent blood flows, thereby promoting injury to the endothelium.

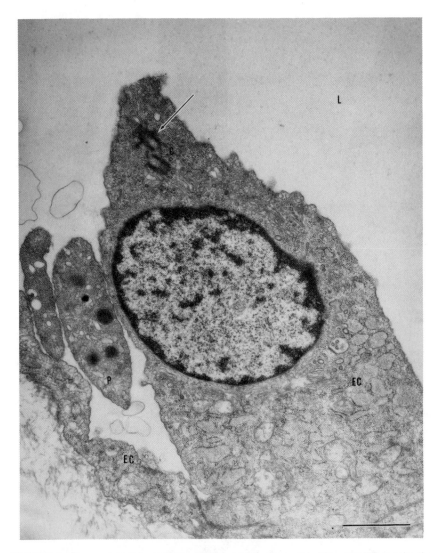

FIGURE 1. Giant endothelial cell (EC) projecting into the lumen (L). This giant EC contains the centriole (C), and in the valley between giant and normal ECs two platelets can be seen to be adhering to the normal EC.

Constrictive State of the Endothelial Lining

Constrictive changes caused stretch and shrinkage at junctions of the endothelium and the smooth muscle, and gave rise to the uneven endothelial surface with deep concaves.

At this stage, a group of neighboring endothelial cells formed a valley and squeezed themselves in the inner media through the fenestra of the internal elastic lamina. Giant ECs were often observed in those valleys.

The attachment area exhibited swollen vacuole-formation or structures resembling myelin figures.

These changes produced a marked change in blood flow, creating turbulences therein.

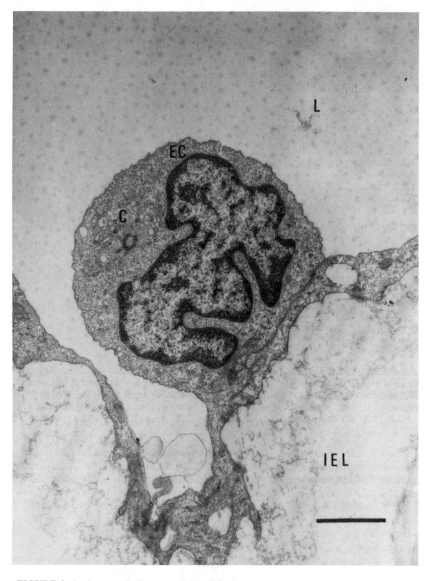

FIGURE 2. In the constrictile state, a giant EC covers the sunken area of endothelial lining.

Replacement of Damaged Endothelial Cells

Repair of damaged endothelial cells in the early stages was provided by the sprout of an intact endothelial cell or by prolongation of the marginal fold (60–80%).

Resurfacing of severely damaged endothelial cells was provided by smooth muscle cells after the initial repair (20%).

The timing of the beginning of repair seemed to be an important factor in determining whether lesion would develop at or not at the site.

We reported here the emergence of giant endothelial cells at the time of injury to the endothelium.

Appearance of these endothelial cells seems to be related to the initiation of atherosclerosis.

REFERENCES

1. SUNAGA, T. 1975. Cellular elements lying just beneath the endothelial cell: its origin and its relationship to the subendothelial thickening. I. J. Jap. Coll. Angiol. **15:** 277.
2. GERRITY, B. C., B. A. CAPLAN, M. RICHARDSON, J. F. CADE, J. HIRSH & C. J. SCHWARTZ. 1976. Endotoxin—Induced Endothelial Injury and Repair. II. Focal Injury in Enface Morphology: (H)-thymidine uptake and circulating endothelial cells in the dog. Exp. Mol. Pathol. **24:** 59.
3. REIDY, M. A. & S. M. SCHWARTZ. 1983. Endothelial injury and regeneration. IV. Endotoxin: a nondenuding injury to arotic endothelium. Lab. Invest. **25:** 25.

Collagen Metabolism in Atherogenesis

AKIRA OOSHIMA AND YASUTERU MURAGAKI

Department of Pathology
Wakayama Medical College
Kyu-bancho
Wakayama City, Wakayama 640, Japan

Migration of medial smooth muscle cells into the media after endothelial injuries is one of the main features of atherosclerosis.[1] Proliferating intimal smooth muscle cells produce a large amount of connective tissue components including collagen, leading to sclerotic lesion. Higher collagen biosynthetic activity has been reported in experimentally-induced rabbit atherosclerosis.[2] An analysis of the α-chain in aortic collagen by interrupted gel electrophoresis[3] revealed that type V collagen is proportionately increased in the sclerotic plaque of intima as compared to the adjacent media and adventitia.[4] In this report, we have attempted an immunohistochemical localization of collagen in atherosclerotic plaque utilizing monoclonal antibodies recently produced in our laboratory.

The produce monoclonal antibodies, BALB/c mice were immunized intraperitoneally with 50 μg of type I, III, IV, V and VI collagens extracted from human placenta[5] emulsified with an equal volume of complete Freund's adjuvant. The same amount of antigen without the adjuvant was injected 5 times at an interval of two weeks. Three days after the last injection, the mice were sacrificed and their spleen cells were hybridized with myeloma cell line with polyethylene glycol.[6] After HAT selection, positive hybrids were screened by an enzyme-linked immunosorbent assay (ELISA).[7] Specificity of monoclonal antibodies were determined by an immunoblot or inhibition ELISA.

Direct or indirect immunofluorescence[8] was adopted to localize collagen types. In brief, an aorta taken from a human autopsy case was immediately frozen in acetone-dry ice and cut 4μ in thickness with a cryostat. Sections were fixed in cold acetone for 5 min. To avoid nonspecific binding of the antibody, the sections were treated with 2% BSA for 30 min at room temperature. After washing with PBS, the sections were incubated with monoclonal antibodies (5μ/ml) for 30 min or 4°C overnight. The second antibody (FITC-labeled anti-mouse IgG or IgM) was then reacted with sections for 30 min at room temperature. After washing with PBS, the sections were mounted with 50% glycerine.

As shown in FIGURE 1A–E, type I, III, IV, V, and VI collagens were localized in the human aorta. Type I and III collagens were codistributed in sclerotic plaque and coincide with collagenous bundles in the interstitial connective tissue. Type III collagen tended to localize in finer bundles of connective tissue (FIG. 1A,B). Type IV collagen was localized in the basement membrane area that surrounds the intimal smooth muscle cells (FIG. 1C). Type VI collagen was localized widely in the sclerotic plaque from the vicinity of the basement membrane area to the interstitial fibrous connective tissue (FIG. 1E). In contrast with the distribution of type I, III, IV, and VI collagens, a positive immunoreaction of type V collagen was demonstrated in the cytoplasm of proliferating intimal smooth muscle cells in the sclerotic plaque (FIG. 1D). No positive immunoreaction was seen in the extracellular matrix. Compared to the medial smooth muscle cells, much higher immunoreaction was noted in the cytoplasm of intimal smooth muscle cells proliferating in atherosclerotic plaque.

An increased proportion of type V collagen has been reported in atherosclerosis,[4,9] chronic inflammation,[10] and breast cancer.[11] Stenn *et al.* reported that continual synthesis

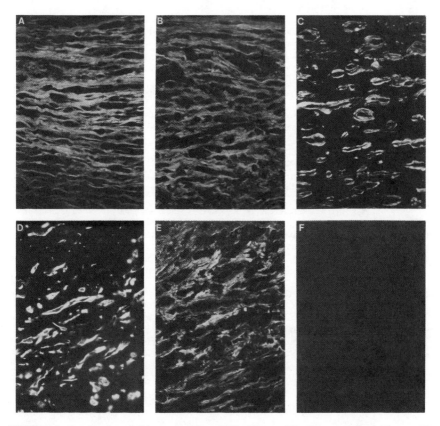

FIGURE 1. Localization of **(A)** type I, **(B)** type III, **(C)** type IV, **(D)** type V, and **(E)** type VI collagen in atherosclerotic plaque. Indirect immunofluorescence. **(F)** Control section for immuno-fluorescence. Normal mouse serum ($\times$ 40) was used in place of monoclonal antibodies.

is required for migration of epidermal squamous cells.[12] In cultured fibroblast, an addition of PDGF to the culture medium has been shown to induce a selective enhancement of synthesis of type V collagen.[13] We noticed that in cultured smooth muscle cells from rat thoratic aorta grown in MEM supplemented with 10% calf serum, type V collagen was shown in the cytoplasm as a fine, filamentous structure, suggesting that this collagen may be a family of cytoskeletal proteins and related to the migration of smooth muscle cells in atherogenesis.

In conclusion, all types of collagen (I, III, IV, V, and VI) were increased in the atherosclerotic plaque compared to the adjacent media of the aorta. Increased deposition of type V collagen was the most noticeable among the other collagen types and can be utilized for a marker for evaluation of the atherosclerotic process.

REFERENCES

1. Ross, R. & J. A. Glomset. 1976. The pathogenesis of atherosclerosis. N. Engl. J. Med. **295:** 369–377; 420–425.

2. FULLER, G. C., A. L. MATONEY, D. O. FISHER, N. FAUSTO & G. J. CARDINALE. 1976. Increased synthesis and the kinetic characteristics of prolyl hydroxylase in tissues of rabbits with experimental arteriosclerosis. Atherosclerosis **24:** 483–490.
3. SYKES, B., B. PUDDLE, M. FRANCIS & R. SMITH. 1976. The estimation of two collagens from human dermis by interrupted gel electrophoresis. Biochem. Biophys. Res. Commun. **72:** 1479–1480.
4. OOSHIMA, A. 1981. Collagen αB chain: Increased proportion in human atherosclerosis. Science **213:** 666–668.
5. MAYNE, R., J. G. ZETTERGREN, P. M. MAYNE & N. W. BEDWELL. 1980. Isolation and partial characterization of basement membrane-like collagens from bovine thoratic aorta. Artery **7:** 262–280.
6. KÖHLER, G. & C. MILSTEIN. 1975. Continuous cultures of fused cells secreting antibody of predefined specificity. Nature **256:** 495–497.
7. RENNARD, S. I., R. BERG, G. R. MARTIN, J. M. FOIDART & P. G. ROBEY. 1980. Enzyme-linked immunoassay (ELISA) for connective tissue components. Anal. Biochem. **104:** 205–214.
8. COONS, A. H., H. J. CREECH & R. N. JONES. 1941. Immunological properties of an antibody containing a fluorescent group. Proc. Soc. Exp. Biol. Med. **47:** 200.
9. MORTON, L. F. & M. J. BARNES. 1982. Collagen polymorphism in the normal and diseased blood vessel. Investigation of collagen types I, III and V. Atherosclerosis **42:** 41–51.
10. NARAYANAN, A. S., L. D. ENGEL & R. C. PAGE. 1983. The effect of chronic inflammation on the composition of collagen types in human connective tissue. Collagen Rel. Res. **3:** 323–334.
11. NARAYANAN, A. S. & R. C. PAGE. 1983. Biosynthesis and regulation of type V collagen in diploid human fibroblasts. J. Biol. Chem. **258:** 11694–11699.
12. BARSKY, S. H., C. N. RAO, G. R. GROTENDORST & L. A. LIOTTA. 1982. Increased content of type V collagen in desmoplasia of human breast cancer. Am. J. Pathol. **108:** 276–283.
13. STENN, K. S., J. A. MADRI & F. J. ROLL. 1979. Migrating epidermis produces AB_2 collagen and requires continual collagen synthesis for movement. Nature **277:** 229–232.

Closing Remarks

ROBERT W. WISSLER

ODE (OWED) TO TOWADA LAKE

As we came to blue Towada Lake
We did not merely come to bake
In brilliant sunshine nor to try to take
Some shining silvery fish which crystal waters make

We came to share the knowledge we have found
In studies we have made the world around
Where work by many yielded data sound
And offered many facts with meanings which abound

With understanding of the atheromatous disease
Which often causes heart or brain to freeze
And not to function in a way to please
The afflicted person, thus he's ill at ease

And these new findings which will help us to prevent
Or to repair the catastrophic sad event
And so this knowledge gained will make a dent
That the monograph resulting is clearly meant

To spread like ripples when a stone is tossed
Throughout the world and not be lost
And we'll go home before the snow and frost
Will not allow a traveler's return at any cost

We'll settle down, we workers young and old
Some in climates warm and some in weather cold
To use the knowledge that we've gained to help unfold
More new results which will begin to mold

A concept new of form, standing the test of time
And yielding a clearcut plan to help us climb
New peaks of promise which some will call sublime
With much more meaning than this foolish rhyme

And then we'll realize fully and retain for evermore
That which we learned here and from Saratoga Springs before
So precious, and not merely for new knowledge gained galore
It is a sparkling esprit de corps that makes our spirits soar

With new relationships which this environment lends
And from us our thanks to Japanese scientists this note sends
As we indicate that which is owed to Towada Lake my friends
Is a new kind of friendship which never ends

Robert W. Wissler
1989

Index of Contributors